Web 2.0-Based E-Learning:
Applying Social Informatics for Tertiary Teaching

Mark J.W. Lee
Charles Sturt University, Australia

Catherine McLoughlin
Australian Catholic University, Australia

Information Science REFERENCE

INFORMATION SCIENCE REFERENCE
Hershey • New York

Director of Editorial Content: Kristin Klinger
Director of Book Publications: Julia Mosemann
Acquisitions Editor: Lindsay Johnston
Development Editor: Mike Killian
Production Editor: Jamie Snavely
Cover Design: Lisa Tosheff
Printed at: Lightning Source

Published in the United States of America by
Information Science Reference (an imprint of IGI Global)
701 E. Chocolate Avenue
Hershey PA 17033
Tel: 717-533-8845
Fax: 717-533-8661
E-mail: cust@igi-global.com
Web site: http://www.igi-global.com

Library of Congress Cataloging-in-Publication Data

Web 2.0-based E-learning : applying social informatics for tertiary teaching / Mark J.W. Lee and Catherine McLoughlin, editors.
p. cm.
Includes bibliographical references and index.
Summary: "This book deals with Web 2.0 and how social informatics are impacting higher education practice, pedagogical theory and innovations"--Provided by publisher. ISBN 978-1-60566-294-7 (hardcover) -- ISBN 978-1-60566-295-4 (ebook)
1. Education, Higher--Effect of technological innovations on. 2. Web-based instruction--Social aspects. 3. Web 2.0--Social aspects. 4. Learning-- Physiological aspects. I. Lee, Mark J. W., 1981- II. McLoughlin, Catherine.
LB2395.7.W434 2010
378.1'7344678--dc22

2009054308

British Cataloguing in Publication Data
A Cataloguing in Publication record for this book is available from the British Library.

Dedicated to tertiary teachers around the world who have unselfishly contributed their invaluable wisdom, experience, and time.

List of Reviewers

Bryan Alexander, *National Institute for Technology and Liberal Education, USA*
Matthew Allen, *Curtin University of Technology, Australia*
Cameron Barnes, *University of New England, Australia*
Sue Bennett, *University of Wollongong, Australia*
Anne Bartlett-Bragg, *University of Technology, Sydney, Australia*
Curtis J. Bonk, *Indiana University, USA*
Rosemary Chang, *The University of Melbourne, Australia*
Matt Crosslin, *The University of Texas at Arlington, USA*
Nada Dabbagh, *George Mason University, USA*
Stephen Downes, *National Research Council, Canada*
Peter Duffy, *The Hong Kong Polytechnic University, Hong Kong*
Jennifer Duncan-Howell, *Queensland University of Technology, Australia*
Henk Eijkman, *University of New South Wales at the Australian Defence Force Academy, Australia*
Rebecca English, *Queensland University of Technology, Australia*
Geoff Fellows, *Charles Sturt University, Australia*
Brian Ferry, *University of Wollongong, Australia*
Mark Frydenberg, *Bentley University, USA*
Kathleen Gray, *The University of Melbourne, Australia*
Tony Herrington, *Curtin University of Technology, Australia*
Joanne Jacobs, *Queensland University of Technology, Australia*
Shelley Kinash, *Bond University, Australia*
Agnes Kukulska-Hulme, *The Open University, UK*
Mark J. W. Lee, *Charles Sturt University, Australia*
Joe Luca, *Edith Cowan University, Australia*
Florence Martin, *University of North Carolina Wilmington, USA*
Joseph P. Mazer, *Ohio University, USA*
Catherine McLoughlin, *Australian Catholic University, Australia*
Ulises Mejias, *State University of New York at Oswego, USA*
Harvey Mellar, *Institute of Education, UK*
Rich Murphy, *University of Nebraska-Lincoln, USA*
Mark Nichols, *Laidlaw College, New Zealand*

Table of Contents

Detailed Table of Contents

This chapter describes the evolution of social software and related pedagogical constructs from pre- and early Internet networked learning environments to current Web 2.0 applications, as well as examining the theoretical underpinnings of social learning environments and the pedagogical implications and affordances of social software in e-learning contexts. The authors also offer a framework to guide and inform the use of social software to facilitate customized and personalized e-learning experiences in higher education.

This chapter explores how the new range of web-based tools and services provides learners with opportunities to create their own digital artifacts, personal learning environments, and social networks, and discusses the integration of established educational principles with the application of these tools and services. The author argues that new the tools enable new design models that will better serve the cause of preparing learners for a knowledge-based society, but rejects the notion that the tools themselves will revolutionize education and make formal institutions redundant.

research skills, including but not limited to academic writing, communication, and time management, as well as the use of blogs as platforms for networking, sharing, and community building.

This chapter gives an account of an initiative involving the use of wikis to facilitate blended learning activities to support multiple cohorts of students undertaking a pre-service teacher education program. A five-stage wiki activity framework is proposed, which was used to help scaffold and structure the participants' professional learning. Data obtained from an analysis of software logs, responses to discussion board-based stimulus questions, and the results of a summative survey were used to evaluate the adopted framework and approach.

This chapter explores how a combination of Web 2.0 and mobile technologies can be used to support and enhance learning and teaching. It draws on data from interviews with six experienced tertiary practitioners to describe and analyze a number of examples that are representative of the power and potential of "Mobile 2.0" to blur the boundary between formal and informal learning, examining the benefits and challenges from both a theoretical and practical perspective.

This chapter introduces the use of wikis and written and voice web applications as supporting tools for collaborative writing in the foreign language learning domain. In particular, the authors report on a study in which advanced Spanish foreign language learners' used these tools to complete a group writing assignment. Empirical evidence collected from students' essays, wiki drafts, chat transcripts, and questionnaire responses attest to the outcomes and effectiveness of the authors' recommendations.

This chapter considers the implications of Web 2.0 for academic staff development. With the aid of fictional accounts, the authors portray the shortcomings of currently predominant institutional approaches to the training of tertiary teaching staff. They offer suggestions on how these need to change in order for the transformative potential of Web 2.0 for online learning to be realized, and for truly student-centered, constructivist learning experiences to be achieved.

This chapter contains the author's predictions of what lies ahead for the World Wide Web over the next decade, taking into consideration recent and emerging developments, and the likely impact on tertiary education. It provides coverage of "Web 3.0" concepts such as cloud computing, the Semantic Web, and the three-dimensional (3-D) Web. A possible future online learning scenario is described and analyzed as a means of helping readers visualize the educational possibilities afforded.

This chapter revisits the fundamental characteristics of Web 2.0 and attempts to place into perspective the implications for learners, teachers, and institutions, following the discussion in the preceding chapters. The author shares two approaches for understanding and leveraging the power of the new technologies. The first of these is an example of applying Web 2.0 practices to catalyze dialogue and the sharing of learning and teaching ideas, and the second advocates greater use of metaphors as a mechanism for meaning making with regard to the use of the new technologies for learning.

Foreword

It was the best of times, it was the worst of times, it was the age of wisdom, it was the age of foolishness, it was the epoch of belief, it was the epoch of incredulity, it was the season of light, it was the season of darkness, it was the spring of hope, it was the winter of despair, we had everything before us, we had nothing before us, we were all going direct to heaven, we were all going direct the other way—in short, the period was so far like the present period, that some of its noisiest authorities insisted on its being received, for good or for evil, in the superlative degree of comparison only. (Charles Dickens, A tale of two cities)

It is an exciting time, and this collection of well-thought-out responses should prove an invaluable starting point for the effective application of new social learning technologies to teaching and learning in higher education. A short time ago I was speaking at an e-learning forum in Hong Kong and was asked, "Now that we have Web 2.0, what about Web 3.0?"—an interesting question! This book also seeks to suggest possible answers by exploring the edges of current and potential future practice. Web 2.0 was a term coined by Tim O'Reilly five years ago when he was trying to identify a shift in the types of Internet applications that were becoming more available; that could possibly provide greater interactivity; and that supported more varied ways of linking like-minded users. As Tony Bates early in this volume collates the definitions from a variety of sources including the now ubiquitous Wikipedia, we are immediately led into a world that more easily supports the social construction of knowledge.

With Web 2.0 tools we are talking about the increasing possibilities of shared construction of meaning; we are also talking about the possibility of new ways of representing ideas and communicating them to others. Several years ago Gunter Kress employed the word "transduction" to refer to the technique that effective teachers employ to communicate a concept to their students. Essentially, this means being able to convert between the forms for representing an idea, such as converting numbers to graphical forms to show the trend and the rate at which something is happening. This ensures that the concept can be visually represented, hence requiring less explanation and less cognitive effort than interpreting a string of numbers. A range of options becomes available with new web-based tools that support the visualization of ideas and how they might be shared with others in select groups or even more broadly. In the early days of educational computing, the tools used to present these representations were often drawn from integrated office application packages. Increasingly, these suites of tools are now being made available through Internet-based sites (e.g., Google Docs and Spreadsheets at http://docs.google.com). Not only do they provide similar functionality, they also enable new forms of sharing and co-construction.

Not only is transduction facilitated, but the generation of new representations does not necessarily destroy the original. The advent of annotation tools that "float over" web pages or sites enables the creator to maintain his/her original content while enabling others to add to and comment on it and to link new ideas, and even other sites, to the ideas and representations. Annotation enables a social component to knowledge construction and it is not constrained to text, as it may also include aural and visual media forms. Consider the site http://www.voicethread.com/, for example, on which users begin with a short movie or animation, and can "scribble" over the top of the images or make voice comments, or even type a few thoughts, all of which are linked to the original material but none of which change its form. Other tools support annotation, co-construction of knowledge, and its representation in a series of different versions: Xtranormal (http://www.xtranormal.com/), for example, shares an animation created by one person with others, who in turn can re-edit and rescore the original and provide it back to the community for further comment and modification.

The attributes of the new Web 2.0 tools enable teachers and learners to relate and work with ideas in new ways that traditional websites and the earlier learning management systems (LMSs) do not allow. With social construction we are no longer talking about a single author, yet we can still retrieve the details of who has contributed to each element of the shared artifact. This is the case with wikis, for instance, which typically enable a log or "history" to tell the story of how the current presentation came to be constructed and displayed in the way it currently is. Group projects, for the first time, can be reviewed in terms of both the individual and cohesive group contributions. Blogs enable shared resources but also can be controlled by the creator, a function not available in current teacher-managed forums and chat rooms inside traditional LMSs. Given the rapid emergence and development of new "open" sites and tools it seems unlikely that the LMS designers will really ever catch up, and maybe we can all achieve a freedom of personal expression!

The early chapters in this book present a comprehensive introduction to the options and tools broadly represented by the term "Web 2.0." These chapters situate new options in current thinking about learning and what the technologies enable epistemologically.

The second section explores a range of innovative cases that have harnessed some of these attributes to achieve educational outcomes. In many of these cases, the authors are talking about the new geographical relationships possible between teacher and student and among students. Included among these relationships is the need to review the role of mobility and tools that support the development of students' voices. Most impressive is the distribution of geographical sites from which the cases are drawn—this illustrates the match of these tools and approaches with the authors' varied cultural contexts of learning.

The third section of the book considers current implications and muses about possible futures. In some ways, cloud computing and 3-D environments are elements that are in the current mix of tools but still being explored. All the explorations challenge us to manage a world in which learning is not constrained by representations, by where information is located, nor by how it is manipulated. Mark and Catherine have edited a collection that should challenge us to re-examine our pedagogies, our notions of who is in control, our notions of where and how learning occurs, and most importantly, our notions of fun, play, and creativity in the endeavor.

Professor John G. Hedberg
Millennium Innovations Chair of ICT and Education
Head, Department of Education
Macquarie University

***John G. Hedberg**, Ph.D., is Professor, Millennium Chair of ICT and Education, and Head of the Department of Education at Macquarie University. Over the years, he has worked on several research projects about the use of ICTs in learning, and is an internationally recognized expert and authority in this area. Past/recent projects include: the use of mobile phones as social software tools in orienteering tasks in geography; designing learning objects for small screen display; using cognitive tools to develop mathematics problem-solving repertoire; Internet literacy; and the production of multimodal artifacts in history and science. John has designed training needs assessments and evaluation systems, and conducted workshops on the instructional design and evaluation of e-learning environments. He has been keynote speaker at numerous conferences throughout Australia and in Canada, the United States, Singapore, Malaysia, China, and Europe.*

Preface

Social software tools, most notably those that have emerged as a result of the Web 2.0 movement, have spread widely and permeated all sections of society, modes of communication, and the worlds of business and work as well as that of education over the last few years. O'Reilly (2005a, 2005b) demonstrated and described how Web 2.0 differs from "Web 1.0" in terms of the syndication and authoring capabilities of the new social computing applications and the modus operandi of the individuals, groups, and communities that use them to connect, create and share ideas, and communicate. Although there are multiple interpretations of the term "Web 2.0" (see for example, Atkinson, 2006), for the purposes of this book we define it broadly as a second generation or more personalized, communicative form of the World Wide Web that emphasizes active participation, connectivity, collaboration, and sharing of knowledge and ideas among users. Web 2.0 has also been referred to as the "read/write Web" (Price, 2006; Richardson, 2006), as it goes beyond the provision of viewable/downloadable content to enabling users to actively contribute and shape the content.

More recently, O'Reilly and Battelle (2009) have revisited the concept of Web 2.0, in an attempt to elaborate on how the networked applications that are growing daily at an exponential rate are systems for harnessing collective experience. They comment that "The Web is no longer a collection of static pages of HTML that describe something in the world. Increasingly, the Web is the world—everything and everyone in the world casts an 'information shadow,' an aura of data which, when captured and processed intelligently, offers extraordinary opportunity and mind-bending implications" (p. 2, emphasis added).

Over the past decade or so, the term "social informatics" (Kling, 1999; Kling, Rosenbaum, & Sawyer, 2005) has also emerged to reflect the centrality of recognizing that the design, adoption, and use of information and communication technologies (ICTs) are profoundly and intricately linked to people's actions and the environmental and social contexts in which those actions occur. Social informatics and its applications, powered by Web 2.0 technologies including but not limited to web logs (blogs), wikis, Twitter, Really Simple Syndication (RSS), podcasting, social networking sites, tag-based folksonomies, grassroots video, and peer-to-peer (P2P) media sharing utilities (and the list goes on), are now being embraced and embedded across all fields of endeavor. These applications are claimed by many to have a transformative effect on teaching and learning in tertiary and higher education (Allen, 2004; Alexander, 2006).

Web 2.0-based social informatics, with its associated raft of social software tools, is seen to hold considerable potential for addressing the needs of today's diverse students, meeting their demands for flexible, ubiquitous, media-rich learning experiences through customization, personalization, and opportunities for networking and collaboration. Vast and continually growing numbers of people are frequenting social media sites on the Internet, which are proving fertile spaces for informal and incidental learning. With the ease of use of Web 2.0 tools, user-generated content is now proliferating as digital-age students are developing and demonstrating the skills needed to be authors, creators, and co-producers of content. In higher education, course materials and learning content have traditionally come from experts such as teachers and textbook authors. However, such "supplied" content is but one of many resources available to assist students in developing knowledge and skills, and has severe limitations, particularly if used in isolation and in a fashion that pre-empts learner exploration and discovery. As a result of the simplicity and speed with which social software can be used to create, share, tag, and upload media, student-produced content can be used to augment the pool of learning resources now available. In what has been dubbed a "rip, mix, and burn" culture, students can become creators, media producers, and critics (Hughes & Lang, 2006; Lamb, 2007). The new tools can be used in creative ways to give today's learners a greater sense of agency and a more active role in learning, and teachers are often challenged as adopters of new forms of communication and networking.

At the same time, however, there continues to be much debate over Web 2.0-based pedagogical applications and associated theoretical implications, although there is correspondingly little published research in the area of higher education pedagogy and how universities, teachers, and learners have responded to the recent and impending changes. In soliciting and planning the contributions to this book, the editors consciously sought contributions from all over the world that would address central concerns and challenges faced by tertiary education institutions in adopting emerging ICTs, and in engaging staff and students in productive ways of exploiting these new instruments, services, and facilities for learning, teaching, communication, and assessment.

THE IMPLICATIONS OF WEB 2.0 FOR TERTIARY EDUCATION

As Web 2.0 enables more user-centered behavior and the passing of the locus of control from teachers to students, paradigms of teaching and learning are shifting. Historically, e-learning experiences delivered by tertiary education providers have tended to emphasize individual learning, where students have some freedom but are limited by institutionally-controlled systems and platforms like learning management systems (LMSs) and lack the opportunity to tailor or personalize the learning process as a whole. Hilton (2006) describes the impact of Web 2.0 as a combination of both negative and positive energies (i.e., "sunrise" versus "perfect storm") and as a disruptive and subversive force that is bound to change the face of higher education. With greater availability of information and steady moves toward universal accessibility, the traditional gateways to information provided by the conventional university lecture and library are becoming redundant as such information is available online and to a mass audience. Universities therefore need to re-evaluate their focus and mission in order to support knowledge creation by capitalizing on the new tools and applications to foster interaction, collaborative dialogue, and critical discussion among its clients in ways that are consistent with the philosophy and ethos of Web 2.0, rather than simply remaining as custodians of inert knowledge.

Productive, student-centered pedagogies call for collaborative learning and participation in communities of learning and practice, as well as for a large element of self-managed learning to be fostered, all of which can be supported by Web 2.0 tools if implemented and used in conjunction with pedagogically sound models and learning designs. In academia, this may mean moving beyond the confines of LMSs and tapping into a wider pool of expertise to include community-generated ideas and learning resources. In turn, such a change may result in the empowerment of learners with greater agency, control, and autonomy not only in how they learn, but also in the resources and services they choose to draw upon to support them.

The Learner Experience

Evidence is mounting that teaching and learning contexts need to become more complex and diversified to reflect the reality of the knowledge economy and networked society, and as students increasingly participate in online social networking activities outside the formal boundaries of school and university. There have been several recent reports that detail the growth and uptake of Web 2.0 tools among university students (see for example Committee of Inquiry into the Changing Learner Experience, 2009; Minocha, 2009; Fitzgerald & Steele, 2008), signaling that social software is being used by many to forge new interpersonal ties, to consolidate existing ties, as well as to engage in various forms of social discourse encompassing the sharing of audio, photo, and video files. The increased engagement of individuals in these types of activities is having an impact on higher education, as university entrants often have familiarity with and competence in the use of social computing tools, and they have expectations in terms of accessibility to ICT, of staff competence in enriching teaching with technology, and of being provided with flexible, personalized learning experiences that suit their individual needs, interests, and preferences.

Nevertheless, in a study of the learner experience conducted in the UK by the Committee of Inquiry into the Changing Learner Experience (CLEX, 2009), it was reported that students who have experienced social media as tools for social connectivity may not associate these with teaching and learning, and therefore they may require a reorientation to the educational applications of such tools. Kennedy et al. (2008) also caution against making assumptions or overgeneralizations about students' use of Web 2.0 technologies outside the classroom and how this might carry over into formal education settings. They present evidence from a large cross-institutional Australian study suggesting that levels of uptake and day-to-day use of collaborative and self-publishing technologies like blogs that have often been associated with the so-called "digital native" generation (Prensky, 2001a, 2001b; see also Chapter 16 in this book) may in fact be much lower than commentators have speculated. Students may also possess high levels of technical ICT skills, but may need to develop critical digital literacy skills to assist them to learn effectively using these tools. Many students lack proficiency in searching for, retrieving, and evaluating information, and it cannot be assumed that all students enter university with these competencies (Lorenzo & Dziuban, 2006; Katz & Macklin, 2007). While many, if not most, may have used the technology for social and personal (e.g., entertainment) purposes, the use of such tools to support learning and study may be unfamiliar, or seem irrelevant or pointless. Teaching and learning with these tools therefore requires academic staff to demonstrate their relevance and to adopt innovative approaches that take advantage of the unique capabilities and affordances of these tools, as opposed to using them simply for the sake of novelty.

Imperatives for Tertiary Educators and Institutions

It must be recognized that the adoption of Web 2.0 in higher education is not achievable without challenge and change, and that change is almost invariably met by resistance. These issues are tackled by many authors in the book, especially in the section on emerging paradigms in teaching and learning (Section 1) and also in Section 2, which is dedicated to illustrative case studies of effective practice. The chapters and case studies elucidate the many challenges that higher education institutions face in keeping up with developments in technology-mediated learning. For example, one of the challenges facing providers of e-learning in higher education is to focus on the opportunities for promoting personalization and individuality within the learning experience. One approach to this end is to augment learning landscapes by incorporating personal learning preferences, interests, and resources created by students with pedagogically sound institutional platforms and frameworks that use Web 2.0 tools and applications. However, there is a lack of consensus on which paradigms of learning are best used to underpin the pedagogical changes that are currently happening. Additionally, it is arguable that although many LMSs are purported to enable "Web 2.0"-based learning because they include tools such as blogs, wikis, and podcasts, it is arguable that most do not embody the Web 2.0 philosophy; indeed, confining students and teachers to a "walled garden" within which online teaching takes place is at odds with the very essence of Web 2.0, irrespective of the tools supported and used. (See Chapters 5 and 14 for insightful discussions and alternative perspectives on this issue.)

Although Web 2.0, user-generated content, and the open content movement significantly increase the volume of information available to students and expose them to a vast array of ideas and representations, as mentioned earlier, many students currently do not have the competencies necessary to navigate and use the overabundance of information available—they lack, for instance, the skills required to locate and recognize valid, reliable, and current sources (see Windham, 2005; Katz & Macklin, 2007). In a recently published EDUCAUSE Learning Initiative (ELI) white paper, it is recommended that tertiary students be assisted and encouraged to develop sound information literacy skills in effectively finding, evaluating, and creating information. Additionally, beyond search and retrieval, information is contextualized, analyzed, visualized, and synthesized, all of which involve complex critical-thinking skills (Lorenzo & Dziuban, 2006; Jenkins, Purushotma, Clinton, Weigel, & Robison, 2006). While encouraging the production and use of learner-generated content in teaching contexts, there is still a need for students to observe the canons of academic integrity in their own work. Students must be made aware of the expectations regarding citation of sources when engaging in emerging forms of collaborative scholarship and self-expression using social computing tools. In this regard, concerns about copyright, ownership, and intellectual property must be carefully and systematically dealt with by educators and institutions. Fortunately, there are signs of optimism that institutions of higher learning globally have commenced the development of the various competencies in their curricula, as can be seen through some of the many examples in this book (see, in particular, Chapter 6).

A further challenge, and one that is addressed in several of the chapters in this book, entails fostering learner self-direction and self-regulation through the use of social software. The design of appropriate learner-centered interventions and tasks in ways that are congruent with Web 2.0 ethos is not the same as endorsing a "sink or swim" philosophy whereby students are left to their own devices and expected to use social computing tools to learn without the help of suitable instructional support and task scaffolding. In fact, such "open-ended" approaches that neglect to acknowledge the importance of teacher guidance have been heavily criticized by a number of educational researchers (e.g., Mayer, 2004). Tertiary educators, therefore, are confronted with the challenge of negotiating balance in the way of promoting learner control, knowledge creation, autonomy, and agency by offering flexible options and choice, while simultaneously providing learners with the needed guidance and structure and adding value to the learning process (McLoughlin & Lee, 2010). Worldwide, there are a growing number of designs for tasks and learning environments that seek to achieve the aforementioned balance, while integrating Web 2.0 tools as well as the creation, sharing, and use of student-generated content. Once again, many examples of such designs are showcased in this book (see Section 2, in particular).

Staff confidence and competence in using and applying the new tools to support learning constitute yet another critical issue. Effective use of technology to enhance learning demands that teaching staff be armed with both operational and pedagogical competence to maximize benefits for students. Therefore, professional learning in the area of innovative pedagogies is necessary. Instructors and educators need to possess full awareness of the potential and range of social software tools, and be equipped with procedural knowledge of how Web 2.0 applications can support teaching and assessment in meaningful and authentic ways. In this digital age, teachers who adopt social software tools should not do so merely to appear conversant with the tools, but also need to demonstrate the capacity to integrate the tools into effective pedagogical strategies and designs to add value to existing courses and foster authentic exchange and dialogue with and among students. (Refer to Chapter 19 for further discussion on the implications of Web 2.0 for academic staff/faculty development.)

Theoretical and Practical Challenges Addressed by the Book

There continues to be much ongoing debate and deliberation about pedagogical innovation fuelled by Web 2.0 and social informatics, along with questions relating to the theoretical, practical, policy, and other implications associated with the use of the new tools in tertiary learning settings. In this regard, there has been a paucity of evaluative research that provides conclusive evidence about the effectiveness or otherwise of particular approaches and tools; perhaps owing in part to the attention and hype that has surrounded the area, many published reports on Web 2.0-based e-learning have been merely "show-and-tell," rhetorical in nature, and bereft of sound theoretical underpinnings. Existing research is highly contextualized, disconnected, and primarily focused on specific, isolated cases, with few studies generalizable to a variety of courses, institutions, disciplines, countries, cultures, and/or student audiences. The diverse chapters in this book address this gap in the research literature.

While the requirement for more unified, transdisciplinary, and systemic empirical investigation is of supreme import, academics worldwide must also not downplay or overlook the value and significance of continuing scholarly dialogue and discussion about what works and why, and which combinations of pedagogic strategies and Web 2.0 tools best target particular desired outcomes. A concerted effort is needed at all levels of tertiary/higher education, from individual to department or discipline through to institutional and sectoral levels, to actively participate in and contribute to the discussion, as well as to work collaboratively to leverage and extend the products and ideas arising from the discussion in ways that promote evidence-based practice. This can be achieved through the development and validation of pedagogical and theoretical models and frameworks that guide and inform practice. It is equally important to ensure that there is feedback from practice to theory, and that both help shape and drive the future research agenda in the field.

All in all, this book provides an informed and well-researched starting point for those seeking answers to some of the many questions surrounding research and practice—and the intersection of research and practice—in the field of pedagogical and institutional change in the Web 2.0 era, and in the effective integration of Web 2.0 tools into tertiary teaching and learning. Questions such as the following are addressed throughout the chapters of this book:

- Does Web 2.0 represent a major conceptual or paradigmatic shift in how we conceive and make use of the Internet as a means of delivering teaching and learning?
- Do the new technologies have anything fundamentally new or different to offer us in the way of improving our pedagogy? What can we do to avoid falling victim to the novelty and hype, and to "technology-driven pedagogy" (Salaberry, 2001)?

- Is Web 2.0 changing the culture of, and/or redefining the competencies needed by, teachers and learners?
- What examples of "best practice" and "good principles" are available, and how can we learn from them?

OVERALL AIMS AND ORGANIZATION OF THE BOOK

The book is structured into three parts or sections, each comprising several chapters that consider current issues, topics, and challenges in adopting Web 2.0 tools in higher education. Each of the 21 chapters deals with an aspect of how Web 2.0 and social informatics are impacting on higher education practice, pedagogical theory and innovation, and/or the roles of teachers, learners, and institutions. Many of the chapters also contain a discussion of scenarios for future learning uses and spaces. The chapters are built on evidence-based practice, and there are case studies of exemplary and innovative applications involving the use of social software in face-to-face, online, and blended learning contexts globally. The content of each of the chapters is outlined below.

Section 1: Emerging Paradigms and Innovative Theories in Web-Based Tertiary Teaching and Learning

Chapter 1 is the first of five opening chapters whose function is to lay the groundwork and "set the scene" for the book. It presents an overview of the history of social software and shows how the changes in each phase have been incremental and developmental, such that new tools that have emerged in the Web 2.0 age are premised on the continuation of a tradition of computer-mediated communication (CMC) and collaboration tools, rather than a radical transformation of social interaction capabilities. The authors maintain that tools for networked social interaction have naturally evolved through a number of phases such as "augmenting human thinking," "computer-mediated communication," "group collaboration," and "collective intelligence," which can be perceived as the result of current Web 2.0-enabled information aggregation and social networking capabilities. Nevertheless, according to them, Web 2.0 has changed the nature of social interaction and brought about a new "pedagogical ecology" that has implications for higher education in general and e-learning in particular.

In Chapter 2, the author's focus is on integrating established educational principles of virtual learning with the application of emerging Web 2.0 tools and technologies. He considers the implications of the technological and social changes for the design of learning materials, workplace training, and assessment/accreditation of learners. While rejecting the notion that the new tools of themselves will revolutionize education and make formal institutions redundant, he argues that there are rich opportunities for the creation of new design models for education and training that will better prepare citizens and workers for a knowledge-based society.

The book then continues with Chapter 3, which echoes many of the concerns of Chapters 1 and 2, and further explores the themes of how the new suite of Web 2.0 tools and practices is challenging and redefining scholarship and pedagogy, along with the accompanying need for higher education institutions to adopt innovative approaches to teaching and learning that capitalize on social media. A pedagogical framework, "Pedagogy 2.0," is proposed that addresses the themes of participation in networked communities, personalization of the learning experience, and learner productivity in the form of knowledge creation and innovation.

Next, Chapter 4 presents the concept of Learner-Generated Contexts (LGCs) as a potential framework for encouraging and engendering the more effective use of technology to support learner-driven learning, and to promote high levels of personal meaning, relevance, and authenticity in such learning. Building on their previous work, the authors concentrate upon the theoretical grounding for the consideration of LGCs as a model to guide, inform, and organize learning design, in addition to illuminating institutional practices and factors that contribute to the success or otherwise of such efforts.

Chapter 5 stresses the importance of taking into account the student perspective, or more specifically, students' perceptions and expectations of the learning environment, in the design of technology-based or technology-enhanced educational programs, courses, and interventions. It examines the notions of personal learning environments (PLEs) and distributed learning environments (DLEs) as examples of approaches that place students at the center of the learning process, drawing upon and developing their ability to organize and configure their own learning environment(s). It gives an account of a study in which an experimental course design heavily supported by Web 2.0 tools was evaluated by applying an ecological approach of affordances. In the course, students were granted freedom and autonomy to select social media applications and services, and were tasked with assembling and customizing their own PLEs and DLEs, within which they used the chosen tools in self-determined ways according to the affordances they perceived. They were then asked to represent their conceptual understanding of their environments and the activities they performed in visual form, which the authors analyzed to reveal a number of findings. The chapter concludes with a summary of the salient issues and aspects of the authors' findings as relevant to educators and instructional designers.

Section 2: Towards Best Practice: Case Studies and Exemplars of Web 2.0-Based Tertiary Teaching and Learning

Upon entering the second section of the book we move from a focus on theoretical and pedagogical models and theories to a focus on practice, beginning with Chapter 6, which discusses the importance of assisting learners in acquiring and refining personal knowledge management (PKM) skills to enable them to perform successfully in the Web 2.0 environment within tertiary education and as lifelong learners. The authors present a practical, reusable model consisting of two types or classes of PKM skills, namely basic PKM competencies associated with creating, organizing, and sharing information, and higher-order PKM skills that relate to the advanced management of an individual's personal knowledge structures and artifacts. A learning design framework with specific, practical examples is included to provide guidance for those seeking to plan learning activities aimed at developing students' PKM skills.

Chapter 7 reports on the application of a connectivist (Siemens, 2005) approach to create authentic learning spaces for teaching Web 2.0 concepts in a freshman (first-year) college-level information technology course. Drawing on his experience teaching students both about and using Web 2.0, the author makes a number of valuable suggestions in relation to good practices for fostering learning by using Web 2.0 tools to create connections between people, ideas, and technology. The chapter shows how, by integrating collaborative and social media applications in authentic learning environments and creating opportunities for students to become both consumers and producers of classroom materials, students can experience and become immersed in the "culture of participation" that lies at the heart of Web 2.0.

Chapter 8 illustrates how the blog can be a useful repository of information and resources, in addition to serving as a platform for the synthesis and presentation of ideas to a public audience. Blogs in higher education can also facilitate the creation of an online community where academic events are flagged, resources and shared research are advertised, and ideas and comments are exchanged. The authors report on an empirical investigation into the self-motivated course-related blogging activities of undergraduate and Master's students, and research-related blogging activities of doctoral students. The chapter demonstrates how blogging may be used to assist students in developing and honing study and research skills, as well as how writing in the public domain can encourage networking, commitment to goals, and articulation of research ideas, thus cultivating confident writers capable of critical and reflective thinking.

Chapter 9 tells of how wikis were used to support the development of professional practice in an initial teacher training program at a British university. Student teachers undertook blended learning activities and used a course wiki to augment and support face-to-face sessions, employing it both as a repository to store and retrieve their work as well as a discussion space to engage in dialogue with peers and tutors outside the classroom. This illustrates both the personal and social dimensions of learning with Web 2.0 tools, and is an excellent example of how collaborative content creation, review, and editing that are hallmarks of Web 2.0 can be integrated with pedagogical approaches to provide useful scaffolding and support in professional learning. The author also shares with readers the five-stage framework that was used to structure the student teachers' wiki-based activities.

The authors of Chapter 10 introduce the concept of "Mobile 2.0," which entails the convergence of Web 2.0 and mobile technology—for example, social networking via an Internet-capable cellular telephone or "smartphone," or photo sharing on a mobile blog—and suggest strategies to integrate such informal activities into formal learning and teaching. The chapter begins with an analysis of the practical challenges and barriers that educators and institutions face in the adoption of mobile tools and resources for tertiary education purposes. Drawing on data from interviews with six experienced tertiary teaching practitioners, the authors describe and analyze a number of examples that point to the particular power of mobile learning (m-learning) to blur the lines between study and other aspects of learners' lives, which can have both positive and negative consequences. The chapter encourages educators to look beyond the hype around technological advances in mobile devices and connectivity to focus on the opportunities that exist to use the distinctive affordances of Mobile 2.0 in productive ways to meet the needs of learners.

Chapter 11 examines the use of wikis in conjunction with other text and voice-based web applications to support collaborative writing. The authors studied the writing processes of Spanish foreign language learners who were working collaboratively using wikis to complete an essay assignment. It was observed that students maintained an interest in accuracy as well as a focus on global rather than local aspects of their writing outputs. In addition, the combination of wikis and synchronous chats gave students a platform on which to state a clear thesis, provide supporting evidence, and work on the organization of the essay in a manner often missing in individual work. The chapter provides advice in terms of pedagogical strategies, supported by social software tools, which can be used to help students become better writers in their second language.

An exploration of how podcasting can be used to support and enhance the student experience forms the topic of Chapter 12, with an emphasis on tertiary-level distance education contexts. The chapter critically examines the unique features and attributes of podcasting that distinguish it from older audio-based educational technologies. By surveying the literature to identify innovative practices of educators across the globe in the use of both student- and instructor-generated podcasts, four thematic areas representing the benefits of podcasting for distance e-learning and blended learning are exemplified: increasing learner motivation and engagement, facilitating and enhancing learning outcomes, supporting mobility and lifestyle learning, and fostering a sense of community.

Chapter 13 provides an overview of the nexus between student learning and student engagement outside the classroom, and explores how Web 2.0 tools can be used in creative ways to support non-teaching areas (such as libraries, guilds, student services, and other bodies) in a university. It highlights the role of non-teaching units in contributing to student satisfaction, and shows how this can be supported through the establishment and maintenance of online communities using social software. The chapter uses a case study of a specially designed project to demonstrate issues and challenges, and offers recommendations for staff, including advice on establishing a successful Web 2.0-based online community within a university.

Chapter 14 addresses the question of whether or not, and if so how, the use of LMSs can be reconciled with the Web 2.0 ethos. Drawing on examples and anecdotes from the authors' institution, an Australian university that operates primarily as a provider of distance education, the chapter explores options for integrating Web 2.0-based e-learning tools, technologies, and strategies with LMS-based pedagogy. The authors reason that the goals and ideals of Web 2.0 and Pedagogy 2.0 (see Chapter 3) can be realized, or at least stimulated, within an institutional LMS environment, provided concrete steps are actually taken to align the environment with the desired goals and ideals.

In Chapter 15, the author looks at the emergence of social networking systems and applications and their impact on tertiary education, through an analysis and exploration of one such application, namely the popular website Facebook. He highlights the educational possibilities, problems, and pitfalls of incorporating Web 2.0 social network structures in teaching approaches, as well as putting forward suggestions for the effective exploitation of these emergent social networks to enhance student learning.

The authors of Chapter 16 report on a project in which Web 2.0 technologies were introduced to students purportedly belonging to the so-called "digital native" generation. They present the results and findings of studies critical of the generational metaphor, and argue against stereotyping and taking as given unsubstantiated claims or assertions about particular groups of students. Instead, the authors posit that young people may need to develop skills often associated with the digital natives to prepare them for work and life in our increasingly connected and networked world. They observe that often, students need and desire more support and structure than what is assumed within an academic context. The chapter ends with a recommendation that educational uses of social software technologies be more strongly and explicitly connected to curricular activities, which calls for a more concerted pedagogical effort and a higher degree of institutionalization.

Chapter 17 examines the role and importance of assessment in the Web 2.0-based e-learning era, explaining how Web 2.0 tools can be used to promote learner-centered assessment and "assessment for learning." It presents a number of cases of peer, self, and other online or e-assessments that display a range of characteristics for the next generation of assessment tasks and strategies. The author concludes that in order for assessment activities and tools to become more effective in the digital age, they need to be embedded within solid pedagogical frameworks (a number of which are reviewed from the literature), which in turn require a supportive infrastructure that takes into account the key elements of tool development, staff training, rethinking of assessment tasks, and learning from assessment tasks.

Section 3: Web 2.0 and Beyond: Current Implications and Future Directions for Web-Based Tertiary Teaching and Learning

The authors of the four chapters in the final section of the book were specifically asked to adopt a forward-looking viewpoint so as to illuminate and project current implications and possible future directions for web-based tertiary teaching and learning. Chapter 18 addresses a theoretical gap in the literature by scrutinizing the educational implications of the epistemological shifts associated with and/or brought about by the Web 2.0 movement. It returns to and builds on the idea, alluded to in Chapter 2, that in order for Web 2.0-based e-learning to be successful, there needs to be a degree of consistency between our own epistemic assumptions and those embedded in Web 2.0. The author argues that the new understanding of the nature of knowledge and learning as social rather than individual phenomena, which transcends Web 2.0 and will outlive any given set or suite of tools and technologies, has very different consequences for learning, teaching, and research, and for the ways in which tertiary teachers and their students approach the creation, dissemination, and validation of knowledge. The chapter concludes with strategies for critical engagement with the new epistemic learning space, and with questions to guide future research and practice.

Chapter 19 argues that while the current wave of Web 2.0 technologies has the potential to transform e-learning for the better, in order to realize this potential universities must rethink how they develop academics' online teaching skills. The predominant emphasis on training academics to teach online using centralized LMSs has yielded mixed results; too much of the focus has been on "top-down" models of change, in contrast with the way in which Web 2.0 itself favors "bottom-up" approaches emanating from the grassroots, that is, approaches that leverage the power, ease of use, and flexibility of social software technologies. Such bottom-up approaches have a better chance of yielding the constructivist, student-centered pedagogy that is espoused by many but rarely implemented or enacted in online learning environments. Fictional accounts are used in an effort to capture and depict the issues involved and their implications for capacity and capability building of academic staff.

In Chapter 20, the author contemplates how the World Wide Web could change over the next 10 years into a situation increasingly referred to as "Web 3.0," and how these changes might affect education. The term "Web 3.0" implies that Web 2.0 may not necessarily represent a revolution, but rather marks one step or phase in a continuous evolution of the Web and of social informatics at large (see also Murugesan, 2009). The chapter looks at how Web 3.0 concepts such as cloud computing, the Semantic Web, and the three-dimensional (3-D) Web are currently being explored and realized. A possible future online learning scenario is also described and analyzed to help envisage the possibilities for tertiary education.

Finally, the book's concluding chapter, Chapter 21, revisits the fundamental characteristics of Web 2.0, and in light of the preceding chapters, attempts to place into perspective the implications for learners, teachers, and institutions. The author's contention is that the impact of Web 2.0 on teaching and learning practice can be both positive and negative, and that consequently, educational institutions need to develop new, reactive and proactive policies and strategies. The chapter finishes with two approaches to making sense of and harnessing the power of the new technologies: the first involves applying Web 2.0 practices to facilitate greater dialogue and sharing of learning and teaching ideas; the second advocates greater use of metaphors as a mechanism for understanding Web 2.0 technologies in an educational context.

REFERENCES

Alexander, B. (2006). Web 2.0: A new wave of innovation for teaching and learning? *EDUCAUSE Review, 41*(2), 32–44. Retrieved January 20, 2007, from http://www.educause.edu/ir/library/pdf/erm0621.pdf

Allen, C. (2004, October 13). *Tracing the evolution of social software.* Life With Alacrity. Retrieved June 4, 2007, from http://www.lifewithalacrity.com/2004/10/tracing_the_evo.html

Atkinson, R. (2006). Web 2.0: Next-g, a sequel, or more of the same? *HERDSA News, 29*(2), 20–22.

Committee of Inquiry into the Changing Learner Experience. (2009). *Higher education in a Web 2.0 world.* Bristol, UK: CLEX. Retrieved August 20, 2009, from http://clex.org.uk/CLEX_Report_v1-final.pdf

Fitzgerald, R., & Steele, J. (2008). *Digital Learning Communities (DLC): Investigating the application of social software to support networked learning.* Sydney: Australian Learning and Teaching Council. Retrieved October 17, 2009, from http://www.altc.edu.au/system/files/resources/grants_cg_report_dlc_uc_feb09.pdf

Hilton, J. (2006). The future for higher education: Sunrise or perfect storm? *EDUCAUSE Review, 41*(2), 58–71. Retrieved January 19, 2008, from http://net.educause.edu/ir/library/pdf/erm0623.pdf

Hughes, J., & Lang, K. (2006). Transmutability: Digital decontextualization, manipulation, and recontextualization as a new source of value in the production and consumption of culture products. In *Proceedings of the 39th Annual Hawaii International Conference on System Sciences* (p. 165a). Los Alamitos, CA: IEEE Computer Society.

Jenkins, H., Purushotma, R., Clinton, K., Weigel, M., & Robison, A. J. (2006). *Confronting the challenges of participatory culture: Media education for the 21st century.* Chicago: MacArthur Foundation. Retrieved October 17, 2009, from http://digitallearning.macfound.org/atf/cf/%7B7E45C7E0-A3E0-4B89-AC9C-E807E1B0AE4E%7D/JENKINS_WHITE_PAPER.PDF

Katz, I. R., & Macklin, A. S. (2007). Information and communication technology (ICT) literacy: Integration and assessment in higher education. Systemics, *Cybernetics and Informatics, 5*(4), 50–55. Retrieved November 17, 2007, from http://www.iiisci.org/Journal/CV$/sci/pdfs/P890541.pdf

Kennedy, G. E., Dalgarno, B., Gray, K., Judd, T., Waycott, J., Bennett, S., … Churchward, A. (2007). The Net Generation are not big users of Web 2.0 technologies: Preliminary findings. In R. Atkinson & C. McBeath (Eds.), *ICT: Providing choices for learners and learning.* Proceedings of the 24th Australasian Society for Computers in Learning in Tertiary Education (ASCILITE) Conference (pp. 517–525). Singapore: Nanyang Technological University. Retrieved January 12, 2008, from http://www.ascilite.org.au/conferences/singapore07/procs/kennedy.pdf

Kling, R., Rosenbaum, H., & Sawyer, S. (2005). *Understanding and communicating social informatics: A framework for studying and teaching the human contexts of information and communication technologies.* Medford, NJ: Information Today.

Kling, R. (1999). What is social informatics and why does it matter? *D-Lib Magazine, 5*(1). Retrieved June 1, 2009, from http://www.dlib.org/dlib/january99/kling/01kling.html

Lamb, B. (2007). Dr. Mashup; or, why educators should learn to stop worrying and love the remix. *EDUCAUSE Review, 42*(4), 12–25. Retrieved January 19, 2008, from http://net.educause.edu/ir/library/pdf/erm0740.pdf

Lorenzo, G., & Dziuban, C. (2006). *Ensuring the Net Generation is net savvy.* Boulder, CO: EDUCUASE. Retrieved July 18, 2009, from http://www.educause.edu/ir/library/pdf/ELI3006.pdf

Mayer, R. E. (2004). Should there be a three-strikes rule against pure discovery learning? The case for guided methods of instruction. *American Psychologist, 59*(1), 14–19. doi:10.1037/0003-066X.59.1.14

McLoughlin, C., & Lee, M. J. W. (2010). Personalised and self-regulated learning in the Web 2.0 era: International exemplars of innovative pedagogy using social software. *Australasian Journal of Educational Technology, 26*(1), 28–43. Retrieved February 23, 2010, from http://www.ascilite.org.au/ajet/ajet26/mcloughlin.pdf

Minocha, S. (2009). *A study on the effective use of social software by further and higher education in the UK to support student learning and engagement.* Bristol, UK: Joint Information Systems Committee. Retrieved August 14, 2009, from http://www.jisc.ac.uk/media/documents/projects/effective-use-of-social-software-in-education-finalreport.pdf

Murugesan, S. (Ed.). (2009). *Handbook of research on Web 2.0, 3.0, and X.0: Technologies, business, and social applications.* Hershey, PA: Information Science Reference.

O'Reilly, T. (2005a, October 10). *Web 2.0: Compact definition?* [Web log post]. O'Reilly Radar. Retrieved November 28, 2006, from http://radar.oreilly.com/archives/2005/10/web_20_compact_definition.html

O'Reilly, T. (2005b). *What is Web 2.0: Design patterns and business models for the next generation of software.* Retrieved December 15, 2006, from http://www.oreillynet.com/pub/a/oreilly/tim/news/2005/09/30/what-is-web-20.html

O'Reilly, T., & Battelle, J. (2009). *Web squared: Web 2.0 five years on.* Sebastopol, CA: O'Reilly Media. Retrieved November 1, 2009, from http://assets.en.oreilly.com/1/event/28/web2009_websquared-whitepaper.pdf

Prensky, M. (2001a). Digital natives, digital immigrants. *On the Horizon, 9*(5), 1–6. doi:10.1108/10748120110424816

Prensky, M. (2001b). Digital natives, digital immigrants, Part II: Do they really think differently? *On the Horizon, 9*(6), 1–6. doi:10.1108/10748120110424843

Price, K. (2006, October 2–4). *Web 2.0 and education: What it means for us all.* Paper presented at the 2006 Australian Computers in Education Conference, Cairns, Australia.

Richardson, W. (2006). *Blogs, wikis, podcasts, and other powerful tools for classrooms.* Thousand Oaks, CA: Sage.

Salaberry, M. R. (2001). The use of technology for second language learning and teaching: A retrospective. *The Modern Language Journal, 85*(1), 39–56. doi:10.1111/0026-7902.00096

Siemens, G. (2005). Connectivism: A learning theory for the digital age. *International Journal of Instructional Technology and Distance Learning, 2*(1), 3–10. Retrieved May 2, 2007, from http://www.itdl.org/Journal/Jan_05/article01.htm

Windham, C. (2005). The student's perspective. In D. G. Oblinger & J. L. Oblinger (Eds.), *Educating the Net Generation* (pp. 5.1–5.16). Boulder, CO: EDUCAUSE.

Acknowledgment

The editors wish to recognize the assistance and support of all those who were involved in the collation and review process of this book, including but not limited to our international panel of reviewers, without which the finished product would not have been possible. We also acknowledge the support of our respective institutions, Charles Sturt University and the Australian Catholic University.

Special thanks also go to the publishing team at IGI Global, in particular to Heather Probst, Julia Mosemann, Mike Killian, Kristin Klinger, Jan Travers, and Jamie Snavely, whose contributions, strategic guidance, and administrative support throughout the whole process from inception of the initial idea to final publication have been invaluable.

In closing, we would especially like to thank all of the authors for their extremely valuable insights and excellent contributions to this book.

Mark J. W. Lee and Catherine McLoughlin
October 2009

Section 1
Emerging Paradigms and Innovative Theories in Web-Based Tertiary Teaching and Learning

Chapter 1
Back to the Future:
Tracing the Roots and Learning Affordances of Social Software

Nada Dabbagh
George Mason University, USA

Rick Reo
George Mason University, USA

ABSTRACT

This chapter provides a developmental perspective on Web 2.0 and social software by tracing the historical, theoretical, and technological events of the last century that led to the emergence—or re-emergence, rather—of these powerful and transformative tools in a big way. The specific goals of the chapter are firstly, to describe the evolution of social software and related pedagogical constructs from pre- and early Internet networked learning environments to current Web 2.0 applications, and secondly, to discuss the theoretical underpinnings of social learning environments and the pedagogical implications and affordances of social software in e-learning contexts. The chapter ends with a social software use framework that can be used to facilitate the application of customized and personalized e-learning experiences in higher education.

INTRODUCTION

Is social software merely a continuation of a broad class of older computer-mediated communication (CMC) and collaboration tools, or does it represent a significant transformation of social interaction capabilities? In this chapter, we trace the evolution of social software tools, beginning with their use to augment computational and communication capabilities and foster collaboration and social interaction, and progressing to their Web 2.0-enabled information aggregation capabilities. Throughout this chronological depiction, we emphasize the socio-pedagogic affordances and implications of social software. We conclude the chapter with a social software use continuum to guide the design of e-learning experiences in academic contexts.

DOI: 10.4018/978-1-60566-294-7.ch001

BACKGROUND

Before the name or construct of Web 2.0 became popular, the terms "social software" and "social computing" were being used interchangeably to describe the advent of a new wave of tools that support social interaction and collaboration in education. Therefore, we perceive social software as a subset of Web 2.0 and a continuation of older CMC and collaboration tools such as instant messaging (IM), newsgroups, groupware, and virtual communities (Kesim & Agaoglu, 2007; Alexander, 2006; Rheingold, 2003). Subsequently, we consider Web 2.0 as a more current and encompassing term that includes a broad range of web technologies, services, and tools, and refers to a renewed pattern of web technology adoption and innovation in the business sector (O'Reilly, 2007). Despite the chronological delineation between Web 2.0 and social software, the latter term has become more commonplace in academia and is the one preferred by EDUCAUSE (http://www.educause.edu/). Figure 1 illustrates our view of the relationship between Web 2.0, social software, and CMC.

The proliferation of the Web 2.0 "pattern" of technology-enabled social collaboration involves both new tools and new social behaviors and practices (Alexander, 2006; Cormier, 2008; Carroll, 2008). However, the roles of technology and sociology in the development of these online tools are often confused, and the actual novelty of Web 2.0 may be less than some proclaim. It is helpful, therefore, to distinguish between the social and technical sides of Web 2.0.

Figure 1. Web 2.0, social software, and CMC

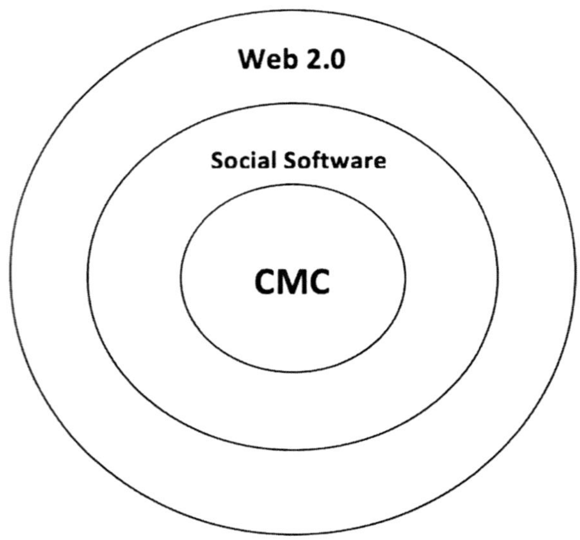

Social Side of Web 2.0

Web 2.0 was defined in an April 20, 2007 Burton Group report as "an ambiguous concept—a conglomeration of folksonomies and syndication, wikis and mashups, social networks and reputation, ubiquitous content, and perhaps even kitchen sinks" (Lindstrom, 2007, p. 6). The Burton Group report also suggests that "The value of Web 2.0 can be summarized in 2 words—participative and collaborative—served with a supersized helping of ubiquitous content" (p. 6). In a more recent (February 2008) Project 10X report, Davis (2008) characterizes Web 2.0 as the "Social Web" and describes it as the second stage of Internet growth that is all about "connecting people" and "putting the 'i' in user interface, and the 'we' into Webs of social participation" (p. 3). These definitions and attributes emphasize the social side of Web 2.0, as does O'Reilly's (2005) depiction of the four key attributes of Web 2.0 applications: collective intelligence, data on an epic scale, architecture of participation, and user-generated content.

The social side of Web 2.0 was also emphasized in the 2007 *Horizon report* (New Media Consortium, 2007), which highlighted the concepts of *user-created content* and *social networking* as new trends that will have a significant impact on college and university campus learning environments. Educational researchers and practitioners have further delineated some of the social affordances of Web 2.0 applications as: establishing group identity and personal reputations, building social contexts of knowledge, enabling personalization, and erecting recommendation and folk knowledge systems (Butterfield, 2003; Sessums, 2006).

Technical Side of Web 2.0

It is widely agreed that dramatic improvements in our information technology (IT) infrastructure have led to the emergence of Web 2.0 (see Jones, 2008). The exponential increases in personal computer power, high-speed broadband connectivity, and cheap, efficient, small-sized electronics, combined with the convergence of voice, data, and video into a single system, are enabling expansive computing environments that can synchronize online social interaction more effectively with offline activity. This cascade of IT developments and other business factors have led analysts to proclaim the advent of a new platform or generation of the Web (i.e., Web 2.0). IT researchers emphasize key technical factors or mechanisms of Web 2.0 that harvest, mine, scrape, filter, or aggregate user content and other information, and may include broader patterns of technology such as rich Internet applications, AJAX (asynchronous JavaScript and XML), Flash, Web services, and mashups.

Although the technical developments have certainly paved the way for or enabled the social side of Web 2.0, we believe that it is more meaningful as educators to take a Darwinian approach to the pedagogical affordances of technology, in order to better understand the linkage between the technical and social sides of Web 2.0 and to establish that this linkage has been continuous, gradual, and developmental in nature. As Madden and Fox (2006) conclude in their report for the Pew Internet and American Life Project, the heart of the Internet has always been its facility for social connectivity (see also Berners-Lee, 2000), and the actions or affordances that Web 2.0 technologies make possible to this end are in fact "nothing new" (p. 5) when compared to the social sites of the 1990s. In the next section, we engage in a "back to the future" analysis by tracing the roots and evolution of social software from pre-Internet to post-Web 1.0, revealing the technological and pedagogical trajectory that led to the emergence of current Web 2.0 and social software tools, systems, and applications.

EVOLUTION OF SOCIAL SOFTWARE

To answer the question of whether social software is simply a continuation of older CMC and collaboration tools as opposed to representing a significant transformation of our social interaction capabilities, we trace the technological and pedagogical evolution of social software across the history of the Internet, which we break into four periods: (1) pre-Internet (before 1969), (2) Internet (1969 to 1992), (3) Web 1.0 (1992 to 2000), and (4) Web 2.0 (after 2000). Within each period, we provide examples of social software tools, technologies, and networked learning environments that preceded and anticipated the social side of Web 2.0 (see Table 1). While other authors (e.g., Allen, 2004) have examined the evolution of social software with a focus on technical terminology, our goal is to underscore the influence of social constructivist principles as a developmental blueprint leading to current social software learning environments (SSLEs).

Pre-Internet Period: Before 1969

The history of social computing started with a declarative act of what Campbell (2007) calls the "digital imagination" and is portrayed by Press (1993) as "an information processing machine was needed to augment intellect" (p. 1). Long before the arrival of digital computers and the Internet, Paul Otlet, whom Wright referred to as the "forgotten forefather," envisioned in 1934 a "mechanical database stored on millions of 3x5 index cards" in the form of "a moving desk shaped like a wheel, powered by a network of hinged spokes

Table 1. Social software evolution timeline

Period	Social computing context	Examples
Pre-Internet (pre-1969)	Thinking machines Integrated domain Proto-learning networks Hypertext Computer-based conferencing	• Memex • oNLineSystem (NLS) • Galactic Network • Xanadu
Internet (1969 to 1992)	Computer-mediated communication Networked supported collaboration Personal computing environments Groupware	• ARPANET • Usenet • Virtual Communities (The WELL) • MUDs/MOOs • EIES • CSCW
Web 1.0 (1992 to 2000)	World Wide Web Groupware-based social interaction Open source movement Communities of practice	• CSILE • CSCL • Knowledge webs
Web 2.0 (post-2000)	Social software platforms Collective intelligence Network effect User-generated content Architecture of participation	• Wikipedia • Virtual worlds (Second Life) • Experience and resource-sharing tools • Folksonomies • Social bookmarking • RSS/XML

beneath a series of moving surfaces" (Wright, 2003, "The Web that wasn't," para. 1) that would allow scholars to search, read, write, and annotate documents. Next, Vannevar Bush envisioned the creation of "thinking machines" that mimic brain function and could be put to use to augment human cognition. Bush's (1945) article, "As we may think," contains his vision of The Memex, which he conceived as a mechanical information browser with the ability to capture trails or trains of thought that simulate brain associations and retrace them via machine. The Memex stands as one of the earliest conceptions of a hypertext system. Ted Nelson brought the concept of a hypertext system to fruition in 1963 in his Xanadu project, which anticipated the architecture of a deep hypertext document system that eventually resulted in the World Wide Web (WWW).

Throughout the 1960s and 70s, Engelbart, working at Xerox PARC, expanded on the visionary work of Bush and others and demonstrated his concept of an "integrated domain;" that is, how a networked computer system incorporating videoconferencing and other communication tools called the oNLineSystem (NLS) could augment collaborative capabilities and not just individual mental functions. In the 1960s, Licklider envisioned a networked computing system called "Galactic Network" to connect people and augment their knowledge and learning ability (Alexander, 2006). What stands out in the pre-Internet period is a vision of how computing machines, hypertext systems, and computer networks could augment human intelligence and group collaboration. These researchers perceived the pedagogical affordances of technology and their visions became a precursor to the Internet period where network-enabled social interactions began in earnest.

Internet Period: 1969 to 1992

At the dawn of the Internet, the technological infrastructure and standards for interoperability to support computer-to-computer communication were still being developed. The original purpose of the U.S. Department of Defense's ARPANET

(Advanced Research Projects Agency Network), the first major implementation of the Internet, was to interconnect geographically dispersed and technically disparate computers at university research centers (Press, 1993). Throughout the 1970s the network expanded through small government-funded projects such as Usenet (a contraction for "User Network") and NSFNET (National Science Foundation Network), as well as through various bifurcations and mergers, to create the complex interconnection of computers that is now the Internet, which today hosts approximately 600 million nodes. The 1980s ushered in the personal computing revolution, the commercial Internet, and by the end of the decade, networked-supported CMC became the dominant trend for collaboration within educational research centers. The fundamental ideas and technologies that underlie the modern personal computing environment were, however, essentially developed by the mid-1970s (Press, 1993).

Additionally, during this period the sparking of the "digital imagination" occurred in the educational community, and it was expressed in various networked learning applications. As early as 1971, Ivan Illich, in his book, *Deschooling society*, advocated for network-styled "learning webs" (Illich, 1971, p. 76) that use database-driven systems to interconnect learners, experts, and educational content, anticipating the knowledge webs of the 1990s and the social networking applications of the 21st century. The 1970s saw the emergence of influential educational projects that explored the constructivist pedagogical affordances of networked learning systems. These included Computer-Supported Intentional Learning Environments (CSILE) and other multiuser applications such as multi-user dungeons (MUDs), MUDs, object-oriented (MOOs), and multi-user virtual environments (MUVEs). CSILE, developed in the 1980s by Scardamelia and Bereiter (see Scardamalia, Bereiter, McLean, Swallow, & Woodruff, 1989; Scardamalia, Bereiter, & Lamon, 1994), grew out of CSCL (computer-supported collaborative learning) and was designed to support collaboration and knowledge management in K–12 educational settings. CSILE had a significant impact on current, Web 2.0 social software applications because it was considered to be the first networked system for knowledge-building communities.

One digital imaginer in particular, Turoff, advanced the state of networked learning ideas in this period. Turoff coined the term "computer-mediated communication" (CMC) and in 1973 developed the Delphi method, a way to generate consensus on decisions by cycles of voting (see Turoff, 2002). Turoff also played an important role in the development of many early government projects that were premised on CMC and the use of social computing for knowledge management and collaborative learning. But Turoff's major contribution to the history of social computing was the NSF-funded Electronic Information Exchange System (EIES), which featured a computerized conferencing system for research communities and functioned as a means for human groups to exercise "collective intelligence" (Rheingold, 1993, pp. 113–14). Turoff was also involved in several research projects based on social constructivist principles such as group decision support, computer-supported collaborative work (CSCW), groupware, and others, which used CMC tools and processes to enable social interaction and user participation activities like voting, rating, and ranking that can be viewed as precursors to current reputation systems and tagging functionality now present in modern Web 2.0-based social software applications. Turoff and his associates conducted numerous related research activities in CMC from 1976 to 1991 at the New Jersey Institute of Technology's Computerized Conferencing and Communications Center, (see history in Turoff & Hiltz, 1995). Computerized conferencing systems like the EIES and various groupware and CMC systems in the Internet period were natural outgrowths of Englebart's vision of an "integrated domain" and the NLS from the pre-Internet period. Meanwhile, a telecommunications industry convergence was underway and people were beginning to imagine the possibilities of a fully digital domain so well connected to computerized devices that it could serve as a worldwide information platform.

Web 1.0 Period: 1992 to 2000

The personal computing context preceding the arrival of the WWW had essentially all the functional features we have today, although access to the Internet lacked an intuitive interface and speed to accelerate connectivity. But the Internet was about to get a facelift and a speed boost that would, without question, change the world forever. In 1989, at CERN, the European Organization for Nuclear Research, Tim Berners-Lee circulated a new hypertext document system to aid collaborative work; by 1992 the system was released to the public as the WWW. In 1993, the Mosaic web browser interface was developed by the National Center for Supercomputing Applications (NCSA) at the University of Illinois at Urbana-Champaign, and it provided a convenient desktop graphical user interface that facilitated global communication and information exchange. Popular Internet systems like email, discussion boards, search engines (e.g., Archie), Gopher, as well as various university and commercial services, migrated their tools to this more user-friendly web space while new services like eBay and Amazon were created to take commercial advantage of the new medium. As CMC tools began to connect people around the globe, one can easily understand how Internet technologies became more social (Alexander, 2006). Rheingold (1993) was one of the first to tell the story of how people were flocking to the Internet for all kinds of social activities. He noted the irony of how what started as a military project had evolved into a "citizen's thinking tool," and predicted that many of the social learning experiments underway at the time would influence and shape future generations of CMC tools on the Internet.

Stahl (2007) describes eight CSCL project prototypes tested in the 1990s that progressively aimed to demonstrate how groupware-based social interaction could improve knowledge building. For example, WebGuide, a web-based prototype program for a K-12 audience, was used to investigate methods for capturing and identifying the overlapping ideas or "perspectives" from individuals and their groups. Stahl (2000) elaborated on the term "perspectives" as follows: "The idea of perspectives traces its lineage to hypertext ideas like 'trail blazing' (Bush, 1945), 'transclusion' (Nelson, 1981), and 'virtual copies' (Mittal et al., 1986)—techniques for defining and sharing alternative views on large hypermedia spaces" (p. 85). These terms and concepts correspond to current Web 2.0 ideas and functions like social bookmarking, social tagging, and folksonomies, and are rooted in social constructivist principles.

Another source of influence on the development of the Web comes from the open source software (OSS) movement. This movement, which generates free software code through communities of developers, has provided key alternatives to proprietary computer software programs beginning with Apache for web servers in the early 1970s. The OSS movement produced the Linux operating system in 1991, the Mozilla web browser in the late 1990s, as well as a range of other essential software whose development continues on to the present day. The open source community promulgated a culture of participation by putting the power to develop "disruptive technologies" in the hands of communities of interest with strong egalitarian ethos. Indeed, the success of the OSS movement is often attributed to its self-organizing community of practice (CoP) that harnesses the "collective intelligence" of software user-developers—a characteristic that makes it a prime example of social constructivist learning in action.

The bursting of the dot-com bubble (1996–2001) marks the end of this Web 1.0 period and a time of irrational exuberance of investment in technology ventures. When the bubble burst and was overshadowed by the events of September 11, 2001, many came to the realization that the Web was not a "super platform" on which any kind of innovative business technology approaches would automatically succeed. However, a global super platform was being built out of the convergence of increasingly more powerful technological infrastructures, improved systems interoperability, the social connection incentives of businesses and interest groups, and a new generation of digital imaginers personified by the innovative web applications of young software developers.

Web 2.0 Period: 2000 to Present

No single technology can be said to mark the commencement of the Web 2.0 period; rather, Web 2.0 is better thought of as a meme or idea describing patterns of emerging technology. O'Reilly (2005) and his associates first observed a few of these patterns forming among the flood of new tools and services appearing on the Web. These tools and services seemed to be changing the rules for how people interact with and through technology, resulting in new constructs and perspectives such as wisdom of crowds, data on an epic scale, architecture of participation, and user-generated content, as described earlier in this chapter.

The new Web as a user-centric and socially connective technology platform has caused a proliferation of "must-have" Web applications that have quickly amassed large numbers of members and subsequently become acquired by large companies like Google and Yahoo!. Wikipedia, the community-written encyclopedia, was formally launched on January 15, 2001 (Wikipedia, 2007). In the same year, the iTunes digital media player application was introduced by Apple. iPods entered the market in 2003, demonstrating that the fall of Napster was not the death knell for high-tech companies, in fact, just the opposite was true. iCohere (http://www.icohere.com/) was established as a software and consulting firm focused on creating collaborative communities.

Additionally in this period, a core set of social networking tools and services have emerged such as Friendster founded in 2002; MySpace, launched in 1999; LinkedIn, launched in 2003; and Facebook, which started as a college network, also in 2003. These social networking tools have collectively changed the rules of social interaction because of their inherent flexibility, user friendliness, and wide availability. Another core set of social software tools that has emerged in this period is one that enables resource sharing and tagging, examples of which are the social bookmarking site delicious (formerly del.icio.us, launched 2003), the photo sharing site Flickr (2004 public release), and the video sharing site YouTube (launched 2005). This toolset, which also includes web logs (blogs) and wikis, has led to the emergence of new constructs such as "social bookmarking," "social tagging," and "folksonomies," underscoring the theory of affordances discussed later in this chapter. We briefly define these constructs below and their implications for e-learning.

Folksonomies are user-generated or "grassroots" taxonomies and hence are dynamic and socially or collaboratively constructed, in contrast to established, hierarchical taxonomies that are typically created by experts in a discipline or domain of study. For example, the food pyramid is a well-established taxonomy created by the U.S. Food and Drug Administration (FDA). Even though the food pyramid has been revised several times, this is done by experts in the field of health and nutrition and based on empirical research. Folksonomies, on the other hand, are subjective and classifications of "things" or artifacts (e.g., photos, documents, URLs) are relative to each user (Peterson, 2006), emerging as a result of "personal free tagging" (Vander Wal, 2005) or "social tagging" (Seldow, 2007).

Specifically, *tagging* involves the ability for any user of a resource-sharing technology to label an object by entering one or more descriptors (tags) for that object in addition to its name, title, or other identifier. Other users can then label their objects using the same tags, or search for objects using these tags, creating a global collection of "things" that are linked or indexed by common metadata. This tagging process or phenomenon "uses the language of a community to form connections" and has been identified by Professor Chris Dede of Harvard's School of Education as "socio-semantic networking" (Seldow, 2007, p. 5). Folksonomic classification or "social tagging" can be a powerful teaching tool, especially if an instructor's pedagogical approach is more constructivist (e.g., implementing a CoP) than objectivist (i.e., primarily lecturing and testing).

Last but not least, we have begun to see explicit social constructivist learning tools released during the Web 2.0 period. Moodle, an open source course management system, was intentionally designed based on social constructivist principles and developed with the open source LAMP (Linux, Apache, MySQL, PHP) tool suite in 2001 by Dougiamas, an Australian programmer who still directs the growing Moodle community. Fle3 (Future Learning Environment 3) is another example of web application software based on CSCL pedagogy that was prototyped in Scandinavia in 1998–99 but was not released until 2002. MUVEs such as massively multiplayer online role-playing games (MMORPGs), Second Life, and OpenCroquet have emerged in this period as well; Dede (1996) predicted the effectiveness of MUVEs in supporting meaningful and distributed learning well before the Web 2.0 period.

Summary

This overview of social software history reveals how the technological changes in each period are developmental in nature, such that new tools that emerged in the Web 2.0 period are premised on the continuation of a tradition of CMC and collaboration tools rather than a radical transformation of social interaction capabilities as some are proclaiming. Tools for networked social interaction have naturally evolved through the periods described, beginning with a focus on "augmenting human thinking" and progressing to "computer-mediated communication," "group collaboration," and eventually, "collective intelligence," which can be perceived as the result of current Web 2.0-enabled information aggregation and social networking capabilities. Despite this evolutionary trend, Web 2.0 tools have changed the nature of social interaction resulting in a new pedagogical ecology that has implications for higher education and e-learning. We examine this pedagogical ecology next.

THEORETICAL AND PEDAGOGICAL UNDERPINNINGS OF SOCIAL SOFTWARE

Few would argue against the idea that social constructivism and distributed cognition offer a solid theoretical framework within which to ground the pedagogical affordances of social software. In fact, Web 2.0 and social software tools are enabling an unprecedented opportunity to enact the fundamental principles of social constructivism and distributed cognition, which entail *learning as a social process* (Duffy & Cunningham, 1996; Brown, Collins, & Duguid, 1989). Learning as a social process is based on the idea that "knowledge is always under construction (fluid, dynamic)" and acquired "through enculturation [into a CoP]" (Dabbagh & Bannan-Ritland, 2005, p. 9).

Cormier (2008) describes "knowledge … [as] a moving target" (p. 1) and proposes a "rhizomatic model of education" (p. 3) powered by the Internet in which "the community is the curriculum" (p. 3) and "not the path to understanding or accessing the curriculum" (p. 3). McLoughlin and Lee (2008) posit that while "the directive for the teacher to be a 'guide on the side' as opposed to a 'sage on the stage' has been with us for many years, Web

2.0 equips us with new ways in which to realize this goal while continuing to recognize the role of the teacher as an expert" (p. 5). We agree with these claims and believe that *learning as a social process* and telecommunications technology (the genesis of social software) are inextricably linked, and that overall, the linkage or interaction between learning theory and technology is systematically redefining and transforming our learning spaces, perspectives, and interactions. So how did this compatible bonding of pedagogy and technology come about, and what are its implications for learning in general and e-learning in particular?

Pedagogical Ecology

Jaffee (2003) uses the construct "pedagogical ecology" to characterize the linkage between pedagogy and technology, positing that pedagogical ecology emphasizes the non-neutrality of the learning space, and subsequently, the consideration of the expectations and potentials that each learning medium brings forth to the teaching and learning process. Supporters of this view (e.g., Kozma, 1994; Frielick, 2004) argue that each learning medium, setting, or context, has a unique set of characteristics, and that understanding the pedagogical affordances of these characteristics is essential to understanding their ecological influence on teaching and learning. For example, Frielick (2004) suggests that "the teaching/learning setting (the classroom, the lecture theatre, the e-learning environment, the department, and even the institution itself) can be viewed as a system that is characterized by mental events" (p. 330). Frielick adds that this system can be described as an ecosystemic process that transforms, influences, and shapes the quality of learning outcomes. We concur with Frielick and argue that Gibson's theory of affordances provides a viable thesis with which to view the reciprocal and transformative interaction between pedagogy and technology (Dabbagh, 2004).

Gibson (1979) espoused an ecological (environmental/contextual) approach to psychology and argued that learning is based on action and perception (information pickup) rather than memory and retrieval (information processing). Gibson proposes that objects and artifacts (e.g., technologies) have certain affordances (possibilities for action) that lead organisms (e.g., people) to act based on their perceptions of these affordances. Later in this book, the authors of Chapter 5 argue that Gibson's theory of affordances has been misconstrued in educational technology settings or interpreted to take into consideration *only* the objective properties of the tools or the functionalities supplied by the tools' developers. However, we believe that instructional designers and faculty need to be aware of the concrete or intended affordances of these tools in order to harness their pedagogical potential and design appropriate learning activities. So the question for faculty and instructional designers becomes, "What is it about this technology that makes users [students] want to interact with it in this way?" and "What perceiving abilities does it provide or enable?" and "How can we leverage or harness this technology in educational contexts?"

Patterns of technology use across the decades have shaped our teaching and learning experiences, and consequently, our learning theories and models. This is where "the relativistic nature" of the ecological view (see Chapter 5) comes into play. For example, broadcast technologies that focus primarily on transmitting information, which were the norm in traditional distance learning environments, resulted in pedagogical models and constructs that can be characterized as primarily behaviorist or prescriptive in nature, Examples of such models and constructs include programmed instruction (PI), computer-assisted instruction (CAI), stimulus–response–reinforcement (SRR), and Gagne's events of instruction (Saettler, 1990; Dabbagh, 2002; Dabbagh & Bannan-Ritland, 2005), among others. Figure 2 illustrates the pedagogical ecology of traditional distance learning environments.

As telecommunications and network technology evolved following the birth of the Internet and the WWW, new affordances for use emerged leading to new pedagogical trends in distance learning. For example, learning spaces and interactions became unbounded and distributed so that learning could happen anytime, anywhere, using a variety of media; the "physical" distance between the learner and the instructor or the learner and other learners became blurred or relatively unimportant; learning resources proliferated, prompting a reconsideration of what constitutes an acceptable academic source; and the concept of learning in groups, or collaborative learning, flourished. As a result, new pedagogical models began emerging such as distributed learning, open/flexible learning, learning communities and CoPs (Dabbagh & Bannan-Ritland, 2005). Figure 3 illustrates the pedagogical ecology of distributed or networked learning environments.

Internet and web-based technologies premised new learning interactions (affordances) that were not thought possible before, such as the coupling of experts from all around the world with novices, the accessibility of global resources, the ability to publish instantly to an international audience, the opportunity to take virtual field trips, the opportunity to communicate with a wider range of people, and the ability to share and compare information, negotiate meaning, and co-construct knowledge. These activities emphasize learning as a function of interactions with others and with the shared tools of the community, supporting and epitomizing the principle of *learning as a social process* described earlier (Brown et al., 1989; Brown & Adler, 2008).

A Three-Component Model

Figure 2 and Figure 3 suggest a recursive and transformative interaction between three components of a learning environment that work collectively to shape our learning spaces, perspectives and interactions. These components are: (1) learning technologies; (2) instructional strategies or learning activities; and (3) pedagogical models or constructs (Dabbagh & Bannan-Ritland, 2005). Figure 4 illustrates the recursive and transformative interaction between these three components, which is ecosystemic (Frielick, 2004). The arrows in Figure 4 depict a cyclical and iterative relationship between the three components of the model, in which patterns of technology use shape our learning interactions (enacted through

Figure 2. Pedagogical ecology of traditional distance learning environments

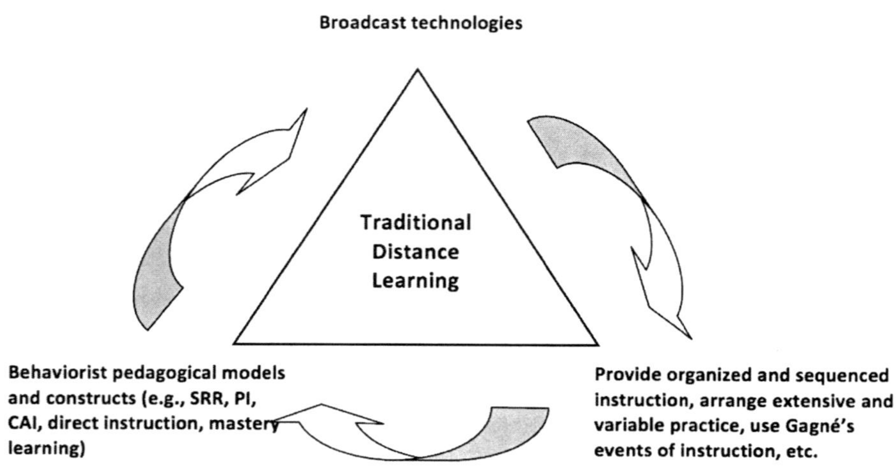

Figure 3. Pedagogical ecology of networked distance learning environments

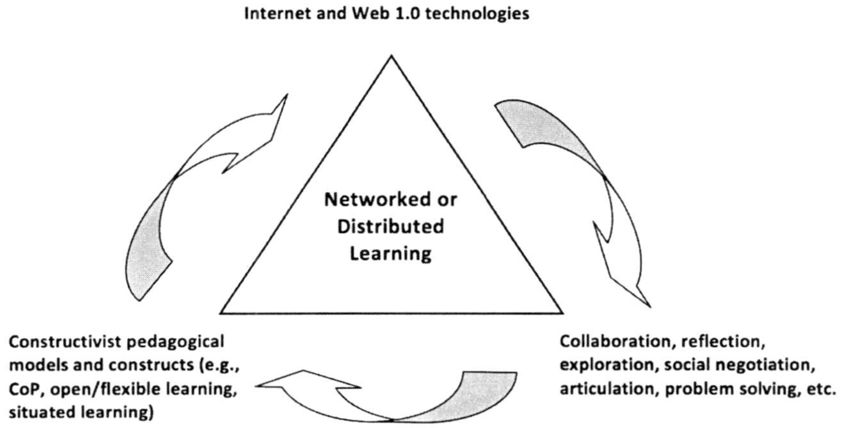

instructional strategies and learning activities) and our sociocultural practices, which in turn shape our pedagogical models and constructs leading to the emergence or re-emergence of new learning technologies. The three-component model embodies the non-neutrality of the learning space and emphasizes the pedagogical affordances of learning technologies, or pedagogical ecology, as discussed earlier.

More specifically, the three-component model suggests that as new technologies continue to emerge, bringing forth new learning affordances, pedagogical practices and social structures are transformed. So what are the perceived affordances of Web 2.0-enabled social software? How is social software transforming our learning spaces and interactions? Figure 5 implies that SSLEs best capture the pedagogical ecology of social software tools. SSLEs are affording new learning activities such as blogging, podcasting, social bookmarking, and socio-semantic networking, enabling pedagogical models that are globalizing education (e.g., open education, borderless education, transnational education) (Dabbagh & Benson, 2007)

Figure 4. Pedagogical ecology of technology-mediated learning environments in general

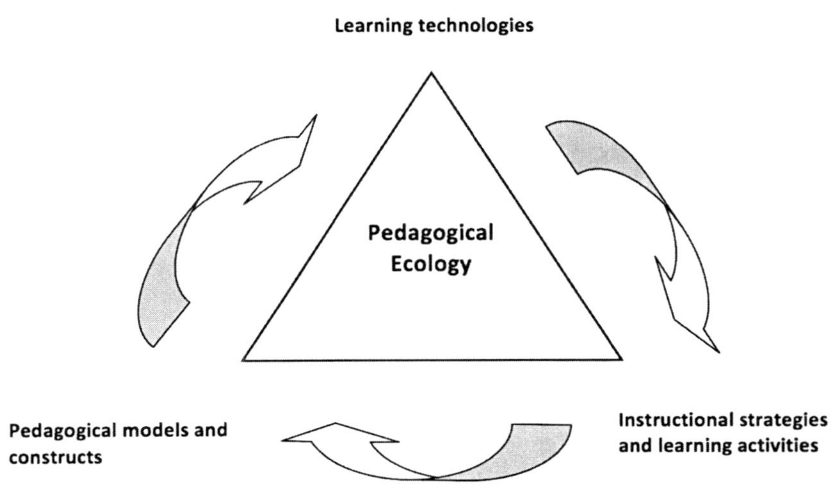

in addition to personalizing, contextualizing, and socializing education (e.g., personal learning environments [PLEs—see Chapter 5], immersive learning, informal learning, rhizomatic education) (Sclater, 2008; Cormier, 2008; Frielick, 2004).

IMPLICATIONS FOR SOCIAL SOFTWARE USE IN E-LEARNING

While the three-component model provides a theoretical and conceptual grounding within which to situate SSLEs, higher education faculty would benefit from a more applied representation or classification of social software use to help them integrate social software tools into their e-learning practice. However, attempting the development of such a classification is often difficult due to the multifunctional and emergent nature of the tools. For example, a wiki can be used in multiple ways, including but not limited to collaborative editing, group discussion, content repository, and even course delivery, making it a very flexible e-learning tool (Watson & Harper, 2008; EDUCAUSE Learning Initiative, 2005). Additionally, Skype has evolved from a tool for placing free, online VoIP calls, to a full-featured computer conferencing application; Facebook now has widgets for adding course spaces and interfacing with traditional learning management systems (LMSs) such as Blackboard. Despite the emergent nature of social software, there have been several attempts at classifying both Web 2.0-based and pre-Web 2.0 social software tools to aid their use in educational and non-educational contexts.

We begin with Laurillard (1993), who classified educational media based on a principled teaching strategy defining the learning process as a dialogue between teacher and student that embodies the following characteristics: discursive, adaptive, interactive, and reflective. Gunawardena, Lowe, and Anderson (1997) developed a model for examining the social construction of knowledge in computer conferencing environments. The model has five developmental stages beginning with the sharing and comparing of information (Stage 1), progressing to the co-construction of knowledge through social negotiation (Stage 3), and leading to the agreement and application of newly constructed meaning (Stage 5). Gunawardena et al. argue that this model is necessary for the generation of new knowledge in collaborative learning contexts. Salmon (2004) also developed a five-stage model that depicts how CMC tools can be

Figure 5. Pedagogical ecology of social software learning environments (SSLEs)

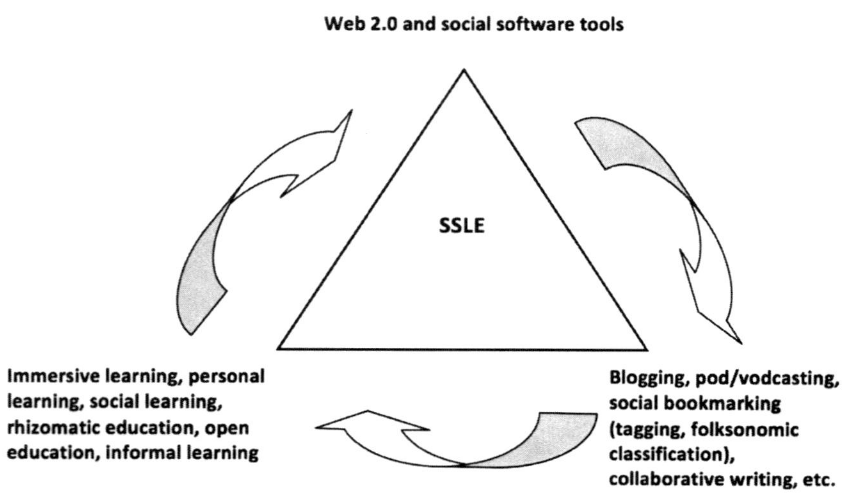

used to generate varying levels of interactivity to support social interaction and knowledge creation. The stages include: (1) access and motivation; (2) online socialization; (3) information exchange; (4) knowledge construction; and (5) development. Salmon's model enables participants to gain both technical and e-moderating skills. Web 2.0 classifications include Obasanjo's (2004) five broad classes of social software that enable groups to communicate, share experiences, discover friends, manage relationships, and play games, as well as O'Reilly's (2007) four-level hierarchy of Web 2.0 applications that captures how these tools increasingly leverage user contributions to embrace and empower the broader network.

The classification that we developed is similar to the above models in that it is based on the learning affordances of the tools however it differs in that it is specifically grounded in the pedagogical ecology of SSLEs as depicted in Figure 5. Hence it is fluid, dynamic, and transformative (i.e., less static). Moreover, it is more applied in that it is user and use oriented and thus based on a continuum (rather than hierarchy) of social software use in which the user can activate the features of the tool to enable the degree of interaction and sharing desired and/or required for learning.

We perceive social software tools as providing three levels of social software use in e-learning contexts, which are described in turn below.

Level 1: Personal Information Management

At the lowest level of social interactivity are people who use social software tools to manage personal information only (both online or offline). They do not activate any of the social sharing or networking features the tools provide, and do not have an observable presence on the "grid," so to speak. Users may "pull in" other people's content, but the goal is to create a private learning environment rather than sharing self-generated content with others. Usage at this level involves passive use of systems preferences and features. The focus is on managing private information for personal productivity or e-learning tasks such as online bookmarks, to-do lists, multimedia libraries or archives, and personal journals/writing.

Level 2: Basic Interaction or Sharing

This level embraces users' capacity for communication, social interaction, and collaboration via social software. Most social software tools provide a public and globally-accessible interface and a variety of built-in features that enable social interaction through various strategies such as expressing individual identity, gaining awareness of the presence of others, engaging in conversations, establishing relationships, forming groups and reputations, and sharing experiences and resources publicly (Butterfield, 2003; Sessums, 2006). At this level, customization prevails and users manually configure the look, feel, and function of their tools. Collectively, this behavior helps foster a nascent culture of knowledge sharing and can spawn relatively small common interest networks and groups.

This level is also about using social software to foster learning by increasing or improving users' capabilities for aggregating and incorporating various types of digital resources into the e-learning experience. Examples of such resources include open educational content, traditional learning objects, micro-content like tags, short message service (SMS) messages, or collaboration objects from various online learning systems and social activities. Folksonomic activity is a prime example for this level. Folksonomies or grassroots taxonomies, described earlier in this chapter, are an emergent property that results from the aggregation of social (public) tagging activity. Another example of Level-2 activity involves RSS-based syndication services. RSS (Really Simple Syndication) can open up the collaboration space to wider public audiences by notifying subscribers what others are doing and by redistributing content from individual or group collections. RSS expands the functionality and broadens the user base of learning object repositories such as Multimedia Educational Resource for Learning and Online Teaching (MERLOT at http://www.merlot.org/). The RSS redistribution capability makes it easier to bring learning objects or open educational resources into (and out of) course tools via RSS feeds. Moreover, third-party web meta-information aggregation services like Technorati, Digg, and Rollyo provide differing strategies to enhance the overall process of redistributing, re-publishing, and remixing educational content and social information. User-friendly customization capabilities thatprovide the impetus for individual members to engage in social interaction also drive the aggregative activities that can lead to the formation of novel systemic behavior as the scale of interaction intensifies (Wiley & Edwards, 2002).

Level 3: Social Networking

The social networking level represents the highest degree of social interaction. We see this level as somewhat resembling O'Reilly's (2007) concept of "Web 2.0-ness," which stems from the application or tool being usable solely online on the global Internet, where it can leverage the power of network dynamics. The mechanism that directs this process is known as the network effect: when enough people begin using a particular social software tool, or interacting (sharing and aggregating) in an online community, the value of the network increases for everyone involved, and a multiplier dynamic can set in that escalates the benefits of the service for all (Weinberger, 2002; O'Reilly, 2007). Social software mediates the learning process at this level by filtering it through the collective intellect, which in turn reshapes meaning for social software tool users.

While the three levels apply to all types of social software tools, Table 2 illustrates how this continuum of usage applies to a core set of educational social software tools such as blogs, wikis, media sharing applications (e.g., Flickr, YouTube), RSS readers, and social bookmarking utilities (e.g., delicious). We end the chapter with a simple example of how the social software use continuum can be applied in an e-learning context involving wikis.

LEVELS OF SOCIAL SOFTWARE USE APPLIED TO WIKIS

Wikis epitomize the social constructivist idea that knowledge derives from social interactions, since it is a social software tool that makes it easy for multiple users to create and edit web pages collaboratively. A wiki provides a shared interactional space or platform for fostering collaborative knowledge construction. This collaborative space mediates the online interaction of users through what Perkins (1992) calls a "rich" (as opposed to "minimalist") learning environment (p. 48)—with tools for offloading memory demands, managing tasks, accessing information, and building modular content structures. Wikis allow their owners to manage public access. Additionally, the interface is designed to permit the public or registered users to easily edit content. In this way, wikis are inherently designed to support all the levels of the social software use continuum.

For example, at Level 1, a wiki could be used as a private or personal online workspace in a manner similar to how one works offline with word processing software. In an e-learning scenario, an instructor can recommend that students who do not have a word processor, or who are busy travelers and need to access all their learning content online (mobile learners), use one of the free, commercially hosted wiki tools such as Wikispaces (http://www.wikispaces.com/). This way, students can self-manage their documents online, and they do not necessarily have to share their work. Level 2 usage takes advantage of wiki features that activate the possibilities for creating a collaborative workspace. Such features include

Table 2. Continuum of social software use

Tools	Level 1: Private Information Management →	Level 2: Basic Interaction or Sharing →	Level 3: Social Networking
Common tool features for each level	• Setup for private use/personalization • Disable search engine indexing	• Enable public view • Setup personal profile • Configure tool for resource sharing	• Configure to pull in other people's knowledge or content via comments, RSS feeds, etc. • Enable information "push" via subscription, follow, watchlist, notifications, etc. • Build tool-based communities/ groups/ collections • Employ promotional activities • Setup multimodal, two-way communication pathways
Blog	• Use as private online journal	• Create multimedia blog posts • Enable blogroll	• Dynamic access to related/recommended content (e.g., TrackBack) • Enable comments, TrackBack, RSS feeds • Add blog to RSS aggregation services (e.g., Technorati)
Wiki	• Use as private content management space	• Password protected collaborative editing and commenting	• Public collaborative editing and commenting • Enable users view history/recent changes
RSS reader (Bloglines)	• Private news/media feed archive	• Enable personal archive sharing	• Access social filtering features to network with like-minded tool users or discover content via recommendations
Social bookmarking (delicious)	• Private bookmark archive	• Personal and collective tagging	• Create/join user networks to access other people's links • Use group tags; subscribe to tags
Social media (Flickr, YouTube)	• Set up private media archive or channel (consume only)	• Create/add media content and apply Creative Commons licenses	• Create/join public user groups or channels
Start pages (iGoogle, PageFlakes)	• Private multimedia information management web pages built on widgets	• Enable subscriptions	• Invite/enable group or open editing of content
Social networking sites (MySpace, Facebook)	• Privacy controls available but public access the default	• Add contacts, friends, etc.	• Enable a range of conversation/ chat, comment, discussion management services (e.g., wall graffiti)

inviting new members, adding comments, and enabling RSS feeds for each content page. Instructors of e-learning courses can encourage students to form independent groups using wikis to work on collaborative projects. Students can compile project content in a public area, edit documents collaboratively, and invite the instructor, experts, and/or peers to comment on or annotate their content. Instructors can also manage multiple group projects via RSS at this level, making it easy to provide feedback and monitor learner progress. Also, at Level 2, the collaborative space established naturally progresses to a higher level of experience sharing and content aggregation due to the accumulation of users' digital resources and use of wiki features such as RSS feeds and widgets. An e-learning instructor can use a central wiki for several classes, enabling a learning community that builds reusable knowledge on an area of study. With their familiar web page structure, wikis are one of the most versatile social software tools for assembling and maintaining content of various types.

Finally, at Level 3, wiki use would involve large numbers of learners who contribute content, provide feedback on existing content, or act as site "gardeners" to weed out and correct inaccurate content, although there are some who may participate solely as consumers—thereby contributing to the popularity of the site and the network effect. Wikipedia is the prime example of the power of Level 3 social networking use that e-learning could aspire to accomplish. Of course, this is not easy to achieve, and the size of the network, in addition to institutional restrictions, poses limits for academic class applications.

CONCLUSION

Social software is the realization on a *web-based platform* of the fundamental principles of social constructivism. As we have argued in this chapter, the pedagogical ecology of social software harnesses the principles of social constructivism in an unprecedented fashion. Social software tools are enabling the design of SSLEs that are stretching the scope and deepening the interconnectedness of learning activities leading to the "globalization" of e-learning and the "flattening" of our world as Thomas Friedman (2007) purports. Knowledge in SSLEs is perceived as belonging to, and distributed in, communities of practice or "environments of participation" in which the learner practices the patterns of inquiry and learning, and the use of shared resources is part of the preparation for membership in a particular community (Firdyiwek, 1999). This is an exciting time for e-learning. Instructors and faculty in higher education contexts can leverage social software use to design SSLEs that truly foster or instantiate communities of learners. Higher education institutions should seriously consider the impact of SSLEs and adapt to the fact that Web 2.0 levels the playing field between the wisdom of the crowds and traditional authority.

REFERENCES

Alexander, B. (2006). Web 2.0: A new wave of innovation for teaching and learning? *EDUCAUSE Review, 4*(2), 32 –44. Retrieved June 13, 2006, from http://www.educause.edu/ir/library/pdf/ERM0621.pdf

Allen, C. (2004, October 13). Tracing the evolution of social software [Web log post]. *Life With Alacrity*. Retrieved February 12, 2006, from http://www.lifewithalacrity.com/2004/10/tracing_the_evo.html

Berners-Lee, T. (2000). *Weaving the Web*. New York: HarperCollins.

Brown, J. S., & Adler, R. P. (2008). Open education, the long tail, and Learning 2.0. *EDUCAUSE Review*, *43*(1), 18–32.

Brown, J. S., Collins, A., & Duguid, P. (1989). Situated cognition and the culture of learning. *Educational Researcher*, *18*(1), 32–42.

Bush, V. (1945). As we may think. *Atlantic Monthly*, *176*(1), 101–108.

Butterfield, S. (2003, March 24). An article complaining about 'social software' and a rebuttal from Ross Mayfield [Web log post]. *Syllogue*. Retrieved February 10, 2006, from http://www.sylloge.com/personal/2003_03_01_s.html#91273866

Campbell, G. (2007). *Jon Udell's interviews with innovators*. Retrieved December 20, 2007, from http://itc.conversationsnetwork.org/shows/detail3451.html

Carroll, D. (2008). Dorion Carroll: Technorati. In Jones, B. L. (Ed.), *Web 2.0 heroes: Interviews with 20 Web 2.0 influencers* (pp. 55–78). Indianapolis, IN: Wiley.

Cormier, D. (2008). Rhizomatic education: Community as curriculum. *Innovate: Journal of Online Education, 4*(5). Retrieved July 2, 2008, from http://www.innovateonline.info/index.php?view=article&id=550

Dabbagh, N. (2002). Evolution of authoring tools. *Educational Technology*, *42*(4), 24–32.

Dabbagh, N. (2004). Distance learning: Emerging pedagogical issues and learning designs. *Quarterly Review of Distance Education*, *5*(1), 37–49.

Dabbagh, N., & Bannan-Ritland, B. (2005). *Online learning: Concepts, strategies, and application*. Upper Saddle River, NJ: Prentice Hall.

Dabbagh, N., & Benson, A. (2007). Technology, globalization, and distance education: Pedagogical models and constructs. In Levy, J., Thompson, J., & Hayden, M. (Eds.), *Handbook of Research in International Education* (pp. 188–198). Thousand Oaks, CA: Sage.

Davis, M. (2008). *Semantic wave 2008 report: Industry roadmap to Web 3.0 & multibillion dollar market opportunities. Executive Summary.* Washington, DC: Project 10X.

Dede, C. (1996). Emerging technologies and distributed learning. *American Journal of Distance Education*, *10*(2), 4–36. doi:10.1080/08923649609526919

Duffy, T., & Cunningham, D. (1996). Constructivism: Implications for the design and delivery of instruction. In Jonassen, D. H. (Ed.), *Handbook of Research for Educational Communications and Technology*. New York: Simon & Schuster Macmillan.

EDUCAUSE Learning Initiative. (2005). *7 things you should know about wikis*. Retrieved October 28, 2009, from http://www.educause.edu/ir/library/pdf/ELI7004.pdf

Firdyiwek, Y. (1999). Web-based courseware tools: Where is the pedagogy? *Educational Technology*, *39*(1), 29–34.

Friedman, T. L. (2007). *The world is flat: A brief history of the twenty-first century* (3rd ed.). New York: Picador.

Frielick, S. (2004). Beyond constructivism: An ecological approach to e-learning. In R. Atkinson, C. McBeath, D. Jonas-Dwyer, & R. Phillips (Eds.), *Beyond the comfort zone: Proceedings of the 21st Australasian Society for Computers in Learning in Tertiary Education (ASCILITE) Conference* (pp. 328–332). Perth, Australia: The University of Western Australia. Retrieved from http://www.ascilite.org.au/conferences/perth04/procs/pdf/frielick.pdf

Gibson, J. J. (1979). *The ecological approach to visual perception*. Boston: Houghton Mifflin.

Gunawardena, C., Lowe, C., & Anderson, T. (1997). Analysis of a global online debate and the development of an interaction analysis model for examining social building of knowledge in computer conferencing. *Journal of Educational Computing Research*, *17*(4), 397–431.

Illich, I. (1971). *Deschooling society*. New York: Harper & Row.

Jaffee, D. (2003). Virtual transformation: Web-based technology and pedagogical change. *Teaching Sociology*, *31*(2), 227–236. doi:10.2307/3211312

Jones, B. L. (Ed.). (2008). *Web 2.0 heroes: Interviews with 20 Web 2.0 influencers*. Indianapolis, IN: Wiley.

Kesim, E., & Agaoglu, E. (2007). A paradigm shift in distance education: Web 2.0 and social software. *Turkish Online Journal of Distance Education, 8*(3), 66–75. Retrieved June 16, 2008, from http://tojde.anadolu.edu.tr/tojde27/pdf/article_4.pdf

Kozma, R. B. (1994). A reply: Media and methods. *Educational Technology Research and Development, 42*(3), 11–14. doi:10.1007/BF02298091

Laurillard, D. (1993). *Rethinking university teaching: A framework for the effective use of educational technology*. New York: Routledge.

Lindstrom, P. (2007). *Securing "Web 2.0" Technologies*. Boulder, CO: EDUCAUSE Center for Applied Research.

Madden, M., & Fox, S. (2006, October 5). *Riding the waves of "Web 2.0": More than a buzzword, but still not easily defined.* Retrieved January 10, 2008, from http://pewresearch.org/pubs/71/riding-the-waves-of-web-20

McLoughlin, C., & Lee, M. J. W. (2008). Future learning landscapes: Transforming pedagogy through social software. *Innovate: Journal of Online Education, 4*(5). Retrieved July 2, 2008, from http://www.innovateonline.info/index.php?view=article&id=539

New Media Consortium. (2007). *The Horizon Report: 2007 edition.* Austin, TX: NMC. Retrieved July 2, 2008, from http://www.nmc.org/pdf/2007_Horizon_Report.pdf

O'Reilly, T. (2005, October 10). Web 2.0: Compact definition? [Web log post]. *O'Reilly Radar*. Retrieved July 23, 2006, from http://radar.oreilly.com/archives/2005/10/web_20_compact_definition.html

O'Reilly, T. (2007, July 17). Levels of the game: The hierarchy of Web 2.0 applications [Web log post]. *O'Reilly Radar*. Retrieved January 23, 2008, from http://radar.oreilly.com/archives/2006/07/levels_of_the_game.html

Obasanjo, D. (2004, October 5). Social software is the platform of the future [Web log post]. *Dare Obasanjo aka Carnage4Life*. Retrieved October 10, 2004, from http://www.25hoursaday.com/weblog/PermaLink.aspx?guid=06ff2206-27a3-4d55-81d8-bbee37073d6d

Perkins, D. N. (1992). Technology meets constructivism: Do they make a marriage. In Duffy, T. M., & Jonassen, D. H. (Eds.), *Constructivism and the technology of instruction: A conversation* (pp. 45–55). Hillsdale, NJ: Lawrence Erlbaum.

Peterson, E. (2006). Beneath the metadata: Some philosophical problems with folksonomy. *D-Lib Magazine, 12*(11). Retrieved March 16, 2007, from http://www.dlib.org/dlib/november06/peterson/11peterson.html

Press, L. (1993). Before the Altair—the history of personal computing. *Communications of the ACM, 36*(9), 27–33. doi:10.1145/162685.162697

Rheingold, H. (1993). *The virtual community*. Reading, MA: Addison-Wesley.

Rheingold, H. (2003, May 8). *Re: My working definition of social software ...* [Web log comment]. *Plasticbag.org*. Retrieved June 10, 2005, from http://www.plasticbag.org/archives/2003/05/my_working_definition_of_social_software.shtml

Ryder, M. (1995, February 8–12). *USENET: A constructivist learning environment.* Paper presented at the Association for Educational Communications and Technology (AECT) National Convention, Anaheim, CA.

Saettler, P. (1990). Cognitive science and educational technology: 1950–1980. In Saettler, P. (Ed.), *The evolution of American educational technology* (pp. 318–342). Englewood, CO: Libraries Unlimited.

Salmon, G. (2004). *E-moderating: The key to teaching and learning online* (2nd ed.). London: Routledge Falmer.

Scardamalia, M., Bereiter, C., & Lamon, M. (1994). The CSILE project: Trying to bring the classroom into world 3. In K. McGilly (Ed.), *Classroom lessons: Integrating cognitive theory and classroom practice*. (pp. 201–228). MA: MIT Press.

Scardamalia, M., Bereiter, C., McLean, R. S., Swallow, J., & Woodruff, E. (1989). Computer supported intentional learning environments. *Journal of Educational Computing Research*, *5*(1), 51–68.

Sclater, N. (2008). *Web 2.0, personal learning environments, and the future of learning management systems*. Boulder, CO: EDUCAUSE Center for Applied Research. Retrieved October 28, 2009, from http://www.educause.edu/ir/library/pdf/ERB0813.pdf

Seldow, A. (2007, June 5–7). *Social tagging in education and the workplace*. Paper presented at the 3rd Annual Innovations in e-Learning Symposium, Fairfax, VA. Retrieved October 28, 2009, from http://innovationsinelearning.gmu.edu/2007/presentations/Seldow%20-%20Social%20Tagging%20in%20Education%20and%20the%20Workplace.pdf

Sessums, C. D. (2006, January 21). Notes on the significance of the emergence of blogs and wikis [Web log post]. *Christopher D. Sessums: Blog*. Retrieved October 12, 2006, from http://elgg.net/csessums/weblog/6172.html

Stahl, G. (2000). Collaborative information environments to support knowledge construction by communities. *AI & Society*, *14*(1), 71–97. doi:10.1007/BF01206129

Stahl, G. (2006). *Group cognition: Computer support for building collaborative knowledge*. Cambridge, MA: MIT Press.

Turoff, M. (2002). *Murray Turoff's homepage*. Retrieved December 23, 2007, from http://is.njit.edu/turoff

Turoff, M., & Hiltz, S. R. (1995). *An overview of research activities in computer mediated communications from 1976 to 1991 conducted by the Computerized Conferencing and Communications Center at NJIT*. Retrieved December 23, 2007, from http://web.njit.edu/~turoff/Administrative/ccc.htm

Usenet. (2007, December 17). In *Wikipedia. The free encyclopedia*. Retrieved December 23, 2007, from http://en.wikipedia.org/wiki/Usenet

Vander Wal, T. (2005). Folksonomy definition and Wikipedia [Web log post]. *Off the Top: vanderwal.net*. Retrieved March 14, 2007, from http://www.vanderwal.net/random/entrysel.php?blog=1750

Watson, K., & Harper, C. (2008). Supporting knowledge creation: Using wikis for group collaboration. EDUCAUSE Center for Applied Research. Retrieved October 28, 2009, from http://www.educause.edu/ir/library/pdf/ERB0803.pdf

Weinberger, D. (2002). *Small pieces loosely joined: A unified theory of the Web*. New York: Perseus.

Wikipedia. (2007, December 23). In *Wikipedia, the free encyclopedia*. Retrieved December 23, 2007, from http://en.wikipedia.org/wiki/Wikipedia

Wiley, D., & Edwards, E. K. (2002). *Online self-organizing social systems: The decentralized future of online learning*. Retrieved July 7, 2008, from http://opencontent.org/docs/ososs.pdf

Wright, A. (2003). *Forgotten forefather: Paul Otlet*. Retrieved July 7, 2008, from http://www.boxesandarrows.com/view/forgotten_forefather_paul_otlet

KEY TERMS AND DEFINITIONS

Affordances: Grounded in Gibson's (1979) theory of affordances. Implies possibilities or potentials for action and alerts us to how an object can be interacted with, or how an object can be specifically designed to enable a particular action.

Distributed Learning: A pedagogical model or construct that refers to learning anytime, anywhere, using a variety of media.

Folksonomies: Subjective classifications of "things" or "artifacts" (e.g., photos, documents, URLs) that emerge as a result of users entering descriptors of such artifacts. Often used interchangeably with "tagging," "social tagging," and "socio-semantic tagging."

Networked Learning: Formal or informal learning that is made possible by computing devices that are connected to one another over computer networks.

Pedagogical Ecology: Characterizes the linkage between pedagogy and technology and emphasizes the non-neutrality of the learning space and the expectations and potentials that each learning medium brings forth to the teaching and learning process.

Social Constructivism: Refers to a set of epistemological principles that privilege sociocultural factors over individual psychological ones in the construction of reality and the learning process.

Social Networking: Refers to a type of online tool used to establish and maintain connection with friends and acquaintances (e.g., Facebook, LinkedIn, MySpace). This term is also used in the chapter to refer to a general process of online social interaction, and more specifically, to the third level of social software use that leverages the power of large-scale network dynamics.

Social Software: Describes the advent of a new wave of tools that support social interaction and collaboration in education. The term appears to be more commonplace than "Web 2.0" in educational discourse and literature. It is described in the chapter as a as a subset of Web 2.0 and a continuation of older computer-mediated communication (CMC) and collaboration tools.

SSLE: Social Software Learning Environment. Describes the pedagogical ecology of social software tools that instantiate learning activities and social interactions such as blogging, podcasting, social bookmarking, and socio-semantic networking. SSLEs produce new pedagogical affordances and models and their use on a large scale can transform pedagogical practices and social structures.

Web 2.0: A popular term used to describe a broad range of web technologies, services, and tools. Also used to define a renewed pattern of web technology adoption and innovation in the business sector.

Chapter 2
Understanding Web 2.0 and its Implications for E-Learning

Tony Bates
Tony Bates Associates, Canada

ABSTRACT

A whole new range of web-based tools and services now provides learners with the opportunity to create their own digital learning materials, personal learning environments, and social networks. What are the implications for the design of learning materials, workplace training, and accreditation of learners? This chapter focuses on integrating educational principles of virtual learning with the application of these new technologies. The argument is made that these tools provide an opportunity for new design models for education and training that will better prepare citizens and workers for a knowledge-based society. It rejects, though, the notion that these tools of themselves will revolutionize education and make formal institutions redundant.

INTRODUCTION

A whole new range of web-based tools and services, including but not limited to blogs, e-portfolios, virtual worlds, massively multiplayer online games (MMOGs), Really Simple Syndication (RSS), podcasting, and synchronous tools such as Skype and Elluminate, now provides learners with the opportunity to create their own digital learning materials, personal learning environments, and social networks. Some, such as Stephen Downes (2006), have argued that with these new tools,

Learning is centered around the interests of the learner ... Learning is immersive—learning by doing—and takes place not in a school but in an appropriate environment (such as a living arts centre). (Slide 27)

Downes argues that so far, the mainstream education system has either tried to ban these tools outright, or has tried to do what traditional educators have always done with technology,

DOI: 10.4018/978-1-60566-294-7.ch002

namely incorporate them into a classroom-based environment.

Although agreeing in many ways with Downes' position and arguments, this chapter recognizes the diversity of approaches to teaching and learning, and therefore offers an approach to the use of Web 2.0 tools that focuses on choice for both teachers and learners. The argument is made that these tools could facilitate new models of design for education and training that will better prepare citizens and workers for a knowledge-based society. The chapter rejects, however, the notion that the tools of themselves will revolutionize education and make formal institutions redundant, because many learners require structure and guidance. Furthermore, whatever organizational arrangements are made (or not made) to support learning, these new technologies need to be integrated with a variety of educational approaches if all learners are to be accommodated.

The term "Web 2.0" was coined by Tim O'Reilly in 2004. Wikipedia defines Web 2.0 as follows:

the changing trends in the use of World Wide Web technology and web design that aim to enhance creativity, communications, secure information sharing, collaboration and functionality of the web. Web 2.0 concepts have led to the development and evolution of web culture communities and hosted services, such as social-networking sites, video sharing sites, wikis, blogs, and folksonomies. ("Web 2.0," 2008, para. 1)

Web 2.0 is a neat term, reflecting a new version of the Web in the language of computer science. However, although the term describes new technologies that have emerged over the last few years, "Web 2.0" reflects as much a social as a technological development. At the same time, Web 2.0 has been given an educational twist, through the parallel term "E-learning 2.0" (Downes, 2005), which involves e-learning based on Web 2.0 tools. Therefore in this chapter, while addressing some of the social philosophy implicit in many discussions of Web 2.0, the focus is primarily on the educational functionality and implications of these new tools, and an attempt is made to situate them not only in a socio-philosophical context, but also in the context of economic development, and educational theory and practice.

While the terms "Web 2.0" and "E-learning 2.0" suggest a clean break from earlier applications of the Web, in education the differences, although significant, are due more to a gradual development and evolution of tools and teaching practice than a sudden "big bang." Indeed, there is cause for concern that the term "Web 2.0" has been hijacked to describe one particular application of second-generation web tools, while excluding other new web tools equally of value to education. Thus some understanding of the history of the application of information and communications technologies (ICTs) in education is important in order to provide the necessary context for understanding Web 2.0 in education.

E-LEARNING 1.01–1.02 (1978–2005)

One of the first recorded uses of the Internet for teaching is the use of computer-mediated communication systems (CMCS) at the New Jersey Institute of Technology in the 1970s (Hiltz & Turoff, 1978; Hiltz, 1986). This was a "blended" learning model, combining classroom teaching with online discussion between students and teacher. A variety of software programs to support computer-mediated communication (CMC) were developed in the 1980s. One of the most used at this time was CoSy, developed by the University of Guelph in Canada. An important feature of CoSy was that it enabled threaded discussion, that is, postings were linked directly to a specific previous posting to which the student or teacher was replying, rather than just being listed by the timing of the posting. In 1988, the author of the present chapter used CoSy as an instructor on *DT200: An Introduction to Information Technology*, a second-year distance education course developed by The Open University in the UK, with 1,500 students a year (see Mason, 1989). This again was a blended model, but delivered wholly at a distance, with content provided mainly through specially designed printed material, audiocassettes, and broadcast television programs. CoSy was used to provide students with the opportunity to discuss issues raised in the other medium. Thus the use of computers for collaborative learning through discussion forums is not new. This could be described as "E-learning 1.01."

Up until 1990, educational applications of the Internet were limited mainly to email and discussion forums such as CoSy. It was difficult to store or send large amounts of content over the Internet, because of the narrow bandwidth available at the time to most users (56 Kbps using dialup modems), and the difficulty and cost of creating and transmitting large amounts of textual material. This limitation was removed by the development of the World Wide Web, the Wikipedia entry for which states:

Using concepts from earlier hypertext systems, the World Wide Web was begun in 1989 by English scientist Tim Berners-Lee, working at the European Organization for Nuclear Research (CERN) in Geneva, Switzerland. In 1990, he proposed building a "web of nodes" storing "hypertext pages" viewed by "browsers" on a network, and released that web in 1992. Connected by the existing Internet, other websites were created, around the world, adding international standards for domain names & the HTML language. ("World Wide Web," 2008, para. 1)

Initially, the importance of the Web was that it allowed large amounts of content (in particular, text and graphics) to be created, stored, searched for, and transmitted cheaply over the Internet, by breaking down the information into tiny packets and reassembling them again at the destination computer.

It took post-secondary education about three years to understand how the Web could be used for teaching and learning. Initially professors created their own web pages or online courses using hypertext markup language (HTML), then very quickly commercial products became established, providing teachers with "off-the-shelf" online learning environments that included "pages" for online course materials, tests and assignments, discussion forums, and access to other web-based resources. These are now called learning management systems (LMSs). WebCT was designed originally by Murray Goldberg at the University of British Columbia (UBC), and was one of the first LMSs. Subsequently, UBC sold WebCT to an American venture capital conglomerate, and in 2005 WebCT was bought over by its leading competitor, Blackboard. Over 90% of two- and four-year colleges in the USA had an LMS system in 2007 (Lokken & Womer, 2007).

At the same time, and partly in response to Blackboard's near monopoly now of commercial LMSs, there has been a move, particularly by large research universities and some government agencies, towards the development and implementation/use of open source LMSs, such as Moodle and Sakai. Gartner Research, based on the results of their 2007 Higher Education E-Learning Survey, estimated that open source LMSs constituted 26% of the market and that this was likely to grow to 35% by the end of 2008 (Lowendahl, Zastrocky, & Harris, 2008). Open source LMSs have the advantage of being free, in that, unlike commercial LMSs, there are no user license fees. However, by the nature of open source software, there are so far undetermined but nevertheless, according the 2007 Gartner survey, very real costs in installation, adaptation, and maintenance of open source LMSs, which have not yet been clearly identified.

Just as important as the use of LMSs has been the way the Web has been used to deliver teaching. In the *classroom aids* model, the teacher decides on the use of the computer, and uses it mainly to add to the classroom experience, for instance, by

Figure 1. Different forms of e-learning (from OECD, 2005; Bates & Poole, 2003)

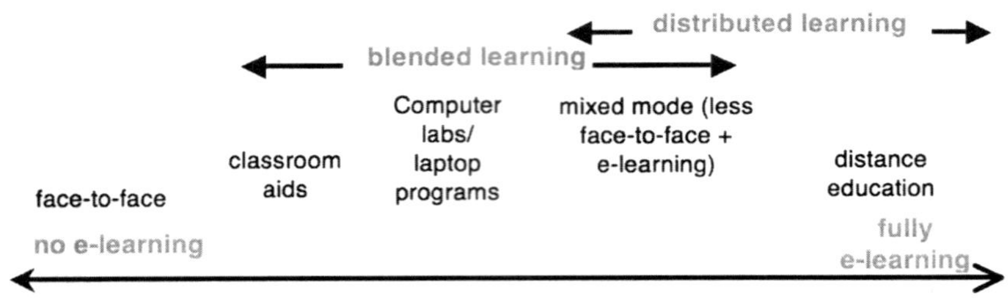

providing a list of readings, lecture PowerPoints, assignment questions, and URLs to additional online resources.

With *laptop programs* (where the students bring their own or a leased computer to class), or programs using computer labs, where the institution provides the computers, the students and the teachers are active users of the computer, but still in a fixed-time-and-place classroom.

In the *mixed-mode (or hybrid) model*, students still spend some time in class, but class time is reduced to give students more time for online study. There are several versions of mixed-mode teaching, from dropping from three class sessions a week to one, with the rest done online, to the Royal Roads University (http://www.royalroads.ca/) model, where students study online before and after a semester spent on campus.

Lastly, there are courses where the student studies entirely online, which of course is one form of distance education. Figure 1, then, shows e-learning as a continuum. Note that blended learning can be any one of the three "middle" modes (Bates & Poole, 2003).

By far the greatest use of computer and communications technologies is to support—rather than replace—classroom teaching (80% of e-learning applications, according to Allen & Seaman, 2008). However, what is important here is the trend. More and more universities and colleges are now adding fully online courses. A study conducted for the American Association of Community Colleges found that 24% of all students were taking at least one fully online course in 2007. Some colleges were making it compulsory for a student to take at least one of their courses online before graduating (Lokken & Womer, 2007). Across the North American post-secondary system, fully online programs have been increasing by an average of 20% per annum since 2002 (Allen & Seaman, 2008).

Thus by and large we have two main forms of e-learning in post-secondary education, both based on the use of LMSs: blended learning—using a mix of classroom and face-to-face teaching (although the proportion may vary substantially)—and fully online learning. However, whether the Web is used as a classroom aid, or for blended learning, or for fully online courses, nearly all these applications are based on the use of an LMS. An LMS these days, whether commercial or open source, is a "heavy" piece of software, with a million lines of code or more. It is institutionally driven, linking teaching with administration. The teaching through an LMS is controlled by the instructor, who chooses content and activities, including the organization of the asynchronous online discussion forums. This is what Stephen Downes (2005) is referring to when he talks about "E-learning 1.0."

THE TOOLS OF WEB 2.0 (2005–)

Around 2005, a new range of web tools began to find their way into general use, and increasingly into educational use. These can be loosely described as Web 2.0 tools, as they reflect a different culture of web use from the former "centre-to-

Table 1. Examples of Web 2.0 tools

Type of tool	Example(s)	Application
Blogs	• Stephen's Web (http://www.downes.ca/)	Allows an individual to make regular postings to the Web, e.g., a personal diary or an analysis of current events
Wikis	• Wikipedia (http://en.wikipedia.org/)	An "open" collective publication, allowing people to contribute or create a body of information
Social networking	• Facebook (http://www.facebook.com/) • MySpace (http://www.myspace.com/)	A social utility that connects people with friends and others who work, study, and live around them
Multimedia archives	• Podcasts • YouTube (http://www.youtube.com/) • Flickr (http://www.flickr.com/) • iTunes • e-portfolios	Allows end-users to access, store, download, and share audio recordings, photographs, and videos
Synchronous communication tools	• Skype • Elluminate • Adobe Connect	Allows free "real-time" audio and visual communication over the Web
3-D virtual worlds	• Second Life (http://secondlife.com/)	Real-time semi-random connection/communication with virtual sites and people
Multiplayer games	• Lord of the Rings Online (http://www.lotro.com/)	Enables players to compete against or collaborate with each other or a third party/parties represented by the computer, usually in real time
Mobile learning	• Mobile phones • Ubiquitous computing devices and applications	Enables users to access multiple information formats (voice, text, video, etc.) at any time, any place
Open content	• MIT OpenCourseWare (http://ocw.mit.edu/)	Digital learning materials available free over the Internet, for use either by instructors or learners

periphery" push of institutional websites. Table 1 shows some of the tools and their uses (this is, of course, by no means an exhaustive list—there are many more possible examples).

The main feature of Web 2.0 tools is that they empower the end-user to access, create, disseminate, and share information easily in a user-friendly, open environment. Usually the only cost is the time of the end-user. There are often few controls over content, other than those normally imposed by a state or government (such as libel or pornography), or where there are controls, they are imposed by the users themselves. Some have called Web 2.0 the "democratization" of the Web.

In general, Web 2.0 tools are based on very simple software in that they have relatively few lines of code. As a result, new tools are constantly emerging, and their use is either free or very low cost. However, not all the new tools developed since 2005 are social software tools, and not all are free or low cost (e.g., many commercial games).

Web 2.0 tools have proved increasingly popular in both social and business applications. One feature of such tools is to empower the end-user—the learner or customer—to self-access and manage data (e.g., online banking) and to form personal networks (e.g., through Facebook).

EDUCATIONAL APPLICATIONS: E-LEARNING 2.0?

Web 2.0 tools are so relatively new to education that educators have yet to find new designs for teaching and learning that fully exploit such tools. Most uses to date have been within the framework of a teacher-controlled model of instruction. For instance, teachers may add their own blog to an online course, or encourage students to chat or work offline then post their work back in the "teaching" area. They may use Elluminate to deliver a live lecture with slides, or a podcast to catch an update from a visiting expert, or to transmit a recorded classroom lecture. Note that Web 2.0 tools can be used quite independently of an LMS (although they can also be made available within or in parallel to an LMS). Nevertheless, there are now an increasing number of examples of teaching and learning using Web 2.0 tools that exploit the learner's capacity to access, create, and publish materials.

Social and Collaborative Networking

The first Internet educational tool, well preceding the invention of the Web, was discussion software that allowed multiple users to discuss asynchronously online in a common, if virtual, area (CMC—see Hiltz, 1986). This technology has gradually evolved through discussion forums into community-based collaborative networks. Social software, such as discussion forums, allows students to test, question, and construct their own, personalized knowledge.

In the personal networking areas, there are several tools that "are fostering collaboration webs that span almost every discipline … [Collaborative workspaces] are easy to create, and they allow people to jointly collaborate on complex projects using low-cost, simple tools" (New Media Consortium, 2008, p. 14). These collaborative workspaces serve as hubs where groups of people with common interests can gather and share resources—such as relevant references or publications—related to their interests.

Multimedia Archives

Multimedia archives such as YouTube, Flickr, and Google Video, and the increasing access to cheap digital video cameras or integrated video and audio recording in mobile phones, now enable learners to create their own digital e-portfolios of work, incorporating text, graphics, audio, and video. These tools again are relatively simple to use. YouTube, for example, provides a video toolbox (see http://www.youtube.com/video_toolbox/) that includes a set of guidelines for producing good-quality video material. Posting video to sites such as YouTube is free, quick, and easy.

This means that learners can now go out and do local fieldwork, and create digital multimedia web-based portfolios of their work, either individually or collaboratively (see Lorenzo & Ittelson, 2005). This raises questions regarding online assessment as well as the design of teaching and learning experiences (see Joint Information Systems Committee [JISC], 2007; see also Chapter 17). Learners can demonstrate what they are able to do and what they have learned, record their experiences, and allow others—such as potential employers—to access their work.

Synchronous Technologies

The case could be made that tools such as Elluminate that allow synchronous two-way communication (mainly audio, supplemented with graphics such as PowerPoint) and Skype are not "authentic" Web 2.0 tools. This is because they are most commonly used to reflect the "old" paradigm of an instructor giving a lecture, and are also more expensive to use than social software such as blogs, wikis, or social networking sites (e.g., Facebook). However, synchronous communication tools take advantage of improved compression technology and wider bandwidth capacity, and can also be organized and managed by end-users or learners for communication. Certainly for certain educational tasks such as learning a language, these tools provide much more flexibility than the previous generation of web tools.

Virtual Worlds

Virtual worlds (or Massively Multiplayer Virtual Worlds—MMVWs) are complex digital environments that allow participants to project a non-physical presence of themselves—an *avatar*—into a generated three-dimensional (3-D) reality, and within that reality to interact with other participants. Users can build and modify this world to a large degree. Second Life (SL) is the best-known virtual world with the largest number of users. Senges, Praus, and Bihr (2007) reported six million accounts in SL in 2006. By June 2008, this had grown to 14 million accounts (Parsons, 2008), although active accounts are much fewer.

Senges et al. (2007) identified a number of educational applications of SL (see Kay & FitzGerald, 2008 for a detailed list of educational applications of SL). The National Oceanic and Atmospheric Administration has built immersive environments where participants can virtually experience tsunamis and simulated weather fronts, combined with explanations about the causes and strategies to reduce harm (see Earth System Research Laboratory, 2008). Hydro Hijinks, developed by students at Montgomery College, USA, is a diplomacy adventure game set in a scenario where farmers are suffering a water shortage, and players have to discover the cause of the water shortage (see morebrainsmedia, 2006).

More recently, Cigna Healthcare has created a virtual environment in SL to educate people on how to improve their health. Like many insurance companies, Cigna offers healthcare advice to those it insures as an attempt to keep its long-term costs lower and its insurance rates more affordable. The Cigna Virtual Healthcare Community is an "island" in SL where users can walk through 3-D interactive displays with their avatars, play educational games, listen to seminars on nutrition and health, and receive virtual health consultations (Takahashi, 2008). There are several projects in SL in the language learning domain, involving the creation of environments where learners can practice languages and meet other foreign language speakers. Several architectural projects have used SL for collaborative design (see, for instance, Studio Wikitecture at http://studiowikitecture.wordpress.com/). Robert C. Amme, a research professor of physics, and his colleagues at the University of Denver received a $200,000 grant from the U.S. Nuclear Regulatory Commission to build a simulated nuclear reactor to train the next generation of environmental assessment specialists (Guess, 2007).

The relative novelty of SL means that there are as yet no well-established educational designs for exploiting the uniqueness of the virtual world. Some merely replicate traditional classroom practice. It is also not yet possible to build a business model that will set costs against benefits. It is thus still very much an experimental environment for learning (Senges et al., 2007). Nevertheless, especially with such a large potential number of participants, a learner in SL is presented with a wide array of learning opportunities, enabling knowledge to be constructed through a combination of social interaction, collaboration, exploration, and experimentation, in real time.

Digital Games

There have been major advances in games technology over recent years. A few games have been designed or adapted for educational purposes ("serious gaming environments"), mainly for the K-12 sector (Prensky, 2006). However, educational games to date have had limited application and utility, mainly because of the high cost of development and lack of appropriate and sound instructional design (Burgos, Tattersall, & Koper, 2007).

Nevertheless, there is strong potential for taking some of the building blocks of games technology, such as "off-the-shelf" software for scenery animation, hand–eye coordination, and crowd behavior, and adapting them to educational purposes, thereby cutting down the cost of building all software from scratch.

Mobile Learning

Worldwide, more people have mobile phones than personal computers. Green (2007) reports that more than two-thirds of all classes in North American colleges now have wireless access. The rapid expansion of wireless technology has stimulated interest in mobile learning—delivery of education and training to people on the move.

Mobile learning has been developed in a number of ways. The simplest is the use of RSS feeds to alert students to course news and information, such as the imminent deadline for the next assignment. However, as mobile technology has become more sophisticated, with larger, clearer screens, touch-controlled keyboards, and motion-controlled navigation, the potential for educational applications has also increased.

One major application is to use mobile phones for student data collection, in the form of real-time polling and interviews, photographs, and video for project work, etc. that students can then organize and post on a class website (Alexander, 2004; JISC, 2005). (See also Chapter 10 in this book, on "Mobile 2.0.")

Open Content

Another major development has been the move to digital open content. Institutions such as the Massachusetts Institute of Technology (see the MIT OpenCourseWare initiative at http://ocw.mit.edu/) and The Open University in the UK (see the OpenLearn website at http://openlearn.open.ac.uk/) have been making available their educational content free of charge for educational purposes. Intellectual property management, and recognition of instructors' contribution to content creation, has been managed through cooperative copyright management sites such as Creative Commons (http://www.creativecommons.org/), which allows instructors to make available content with some protection against improper or commercial use.

The move to more open content has several implications. Teachers and learners now have an increasing range of quality-assured learning materials that they can access, free of charge, for educational purposes. Teachers no longer need to create all their own material online; learners are no longer restricted to the content and curriculum provided by the university or college at which they are enrolled. Thus one can imagine an "open content" approach to a subject, where the instructor is a guide, providing goals and criteria for assessment, but where the students track down, assess, and organize appropriate learning materials.

Educational Implications of the New Web 2.0 Tools

Learners now have powerful tools for creating their own learning materials or for demonstrating their knowledge and skills. Courses can be structured around individual students' interests, allowing them to seek appropriate content and resources to support the development of negotiated competencies or learning outcomes. Content is now open; learners can go and seek, use, and apply information beyond the bounds of what a professor or teacher may dictate. Increasingly, quality educational content will become free, open, and abundant. Students can create and customize their own online personal learning environments (see also Chapter 5 in this book).

This represents a major power shift from teachers to learners. Some commentators (e.g., Downes, 2006) have argued that traditional institutions such as schools and universities are now no longer needed for learning purposes, as the tools of Web 2.0 allow learners to control what and how they learn. The idea of abolishing schools of course is not a new idea—Ivan Illich (1973) wrote about deschooling and learning webs long ago—but the Internet multiplies infinitely the number of connections an individual may now make to the point where it becomes much easier for those who wish to learn this way to do so. Supercool School (http://www.supercoolschool.com/) now uses Facebook to network learners with a common interest who teach themselves: no curriculum, no formally appointed teachers, and no examinations.

However, although the technology continually changes, some things do not. Many of the services that educational institutions currently provide—such as guidance, learner support, and accreditation—will still be needed. Many students are not, at least initially, independent learners (see Candy, 1991), and many deliberately seek guidance and help from teachers and institutions. One reason we have educational institutions that are supported by the public is because, to quote former U.S. Secretary of Defense Donald Rumsfeld (2002), "there are known unknowns; that is to say we know there are some things we do not know." This is one reason why students choose to go to university, or why parents send children to school. Many students come to a learning task without the necessary skills or confidence to study independently from scratch (Moore & Thompson, 1990). They need structured support, structured and selected content, and recognized accreditation. The advent of new tools that at last give students more control over their learning will not change their need for a structured educational experience. However, learners can be taught the skills needed to become independent learners (Moore, 1973; Marshall & Rowland, 1993). The new tools will make this learning of how to learn much more effective, but still only, in most cases, within an initially structured environment.

At the same time, research by the Sloan Consortium, which found that over 80% of online teaching in the USA was performed to support traditional classroom teaching (Allen & Seaman, 2006), suggests that most teachers working online are not changing their teaching method sufficiently to make full use of the new Web 2.0 tools. One reason is that institutions are locked into supporting LMSs such as Blackboard or Moodle. Even more importantly, most instructors are locked into a classroom-based, 9:00–4:00, five-days-a-week, 13-weeks-a-year semester system—essential for classroom teaching, but meaningless in a fully online environment. For many students, this structured education is necessary, even when they begin to move online, and such tools as LMSs also have administrative advantages like linking student records to teaching activities. Nevertheless, this mode of teaching does not empower learners in the way that some of the newer Web 2.0 tools can. Downes (2006) argues that these new tools allow for *immersive* learning—learning everywhere and at any time, within all aspects of life, without the need for formal, time-and-place-dependent institutions.

The use of Web 2.0 tools raises the inevitable issue of quality. How can learners differentiate between reliable, accurate, authoritative information and inaccurate, biased, or unsubstantiated information, if they are encouraged to roam free? What are the implications for expertise and specialist knowledge, when everyone has a view on everything? As Andrew Keen (2007) has commented, "we are replacing the tyranny of experts with the tyranny of idiots." Not all information is equal, nor are all opinions. Unless we are to descend into subjective, quarreling beasts (the tyranny of idiots, as expressed by Keen), expertise remains critical for progress. Many students look for structure and guidance, and it is the responsibility of teachers to provide it. A middle ground is therefore needed between the total authority and control of the teacher, and complete anarchy as seen in the children roaming free on the desert island in the novel *Lord of the flies* (Golding, 1954). The new Web 2.0 tools allow for such a middle ground, but only if teachers have a clear pedagogy or educational philosophy to guide their choices and use of the technology.

The point here is that the choice of technology and the design of the learning experience is an academic decision that will vary depending on the type of students being taught and the nature of the subject. However, perhaps the most important factor determining choice of the actual tools to be used in online learning will be the educational theory or approach (the pedagogy, for want of a better term) most favored by those responsible for the teaching or learning.

DIFFERENT PEDAGOGICAL APPROACHES TO WEB-BASED LEARNING

There are many different theories of learning, and most of these theories reflect underlying but different philosophical beliefs about the nature of knowledge (epistemologies). This is a large and complex topic and can be dealt with only briefly in this chapter. For a good discussion of the overall epistemological issues raised by ICTs, see Lyotard (1979/1984) and Lankshear, Peters, and Knobel (2000).

It is necessary here to make a distinction between epistemologies and theories of learning. An epistemology basically describes the basis on which we know or believe something to be true. This can be illustrated by the famous debate between Thomas Huxley and Bishop Wilberforce in 1860 on the origin of man. Huxley argued that man was descended from the apes, based on Darwin's work on the origin of species. Huxley's argument was in the form of a scientific theory grounded in empirical evidence. Wilberforce argued that man was created by God, based on evidence from the Bible. The basis for their beliefs were by and large irreconcilable, because they started from fundamentally different views of what constitutes "evidence" for their belief. There are many different epistemologies, including rationalism (based on logic), objectivism (empirically tested knowledge), scholasticism (authorized interpretation of historical sources such as the Bible or Qur'an), and constructivism.

A theory of teaching or learning will be strongly influenced by one or more epistemological positions. However, an epistemology does not in itself address issues of teaching or learning. Learning or teaching theories are applications of a more general set of epistemological positions or beliefs about the nature of knowledge. Thus behaviorism is an approach to teaching and learning reflecting an objectivist epistemology, but then so are some forms of cognitive psychology or artificial intelligence.

Three epistemologies will be dealt with here—objectivism, constructivism, and connectivism—that are relevant to the application of Web 2.0 tools. It should be noted, however, that there are other epistemologies that could be applied. The point here is that it is important for teachers to be aware of different epistemologies and to be sure that their use of Web 2.0 tools is consistent with their own preferred epistemological positions.

Objectivism

An objectivist view of knowledge is that truth exists outside the human mind. In particular, there are undeniable facts, concepts, and principles that are constant, reflecting an unchanging reality, and independent of personal beliefs (Popper, 1972). Scientific laws are examples of an objectivist approach to knowledge. Whatever one may happen to believe, there is a law of gravity. The apple will fall downwards, at a certain speed that is predictable with enough known "facts."

For teachers who hold an objectivist position, there is a body of knowledge to be learned and defined by experts. This is organized into subject disciplines or content areas. The job of the teacher is to transmit that body of knowledge. Teaching is about moving knowledge from those that know to those that do not know. The learner's task is to understand, memorize, reproduce accurately what has been learned, and perhaps apply that knowledge to specific, well-defined contexts. Good teaching is authoritative, correct, well organized, clear, and not to be questioned. Learning is assessed by the production of correct answers and efficient reasoning based on the facts and concepts taught in the course. Objectivist teaching can be found in all subject areas, but for obvious reasons it is particularly strong in the natural sciences, computer sciences, engineering, and law. Objectivist instructional design is based strongly on behavioral approaches, systems thinking, and quantitatively measured outputs (see, for instance, Dick & Carey, 1996).

Constructivism

Constructivists believe that all knowledge is a human construct (Gould & Brown, 2003). Even the laws of science are what scientists believe at a particular time, and are open to change as a result of not just new facts, but also new ideas, and agreement is reached through discussion. Particularly important to constructivists is that all knowledge is relative, personal, and dynamic. For instance, the concept of heat is understood early in life through sensation. A baby learns about heat by touching something hot, like a stove. As the child grows older, he or she realizes that heat is relative, and can be quantified. For a child in Vancouver, a daily temperature of 30 degrees Celsius is hot, and a temperature of minus 30 is cold. However, this is not true for a child in Riyadh or one in Iqualuit, where the concepts of a hot or cold day are quite different. As the child gets older, he or she may learn that heat is the transfer of energy between two objects due to temperature differences. Thus the concept of heat is dynamic, relative, and personal. One person's understanding of heat will be different from that of another, because their experiences are different. There may be enough shared understanding of heat for them to agree on what it is, but their understandings of it will not be quite the same.

For constructivists, teaching is about observation, comparison, questioning, reflection, discussion, and above all, the assimilation and accommodation of new experiences with previous forms of understanding. This is done through reflection (internal contemplation) and discussion. Discussion, in particular, is important, because this is how we test and challenge new ideas or unfamiliar concepts. Thus learning is both a personal and a social activity.

The teacher's job is to create an environment in which questions are raised, problems are presented for solution by the learners, and discussion and argument can take place. In this environment, learners are more equal in that they are encouraged to challenge not only other learners but also the teacher. Assessment is based on the quality of argument or reasoning, not the reproduction of facts or concepts. Constructivist approaches to teaching and learning are also found in all subject areas, but are more common in the humanities, social sciences, and education. (See Jonassen, Davidson, Collins, Campbell, & Bannan Haag, 1995 for a discussion of how constructivism can be applied to online learning.)

Connectivism

Connectivism is a theory advanced by George Siemens (2005). A connectivist view of knowledge is that the nature of knowledge is radically transformed by the technology of the Internet. Lyotard (1979/1984), for example, has argued that the nature of knowledge derived from the use of information technologies is radically different from the knowledge derived through scientific thinking. According to Lyotard, knowledge derived from science and rationalism has an intrinsic value, whereas knowledge in the information society has a commercial or utilitarian value. Siemens argues that knowledge is advanced and transformed by the contributions of those connected to particular networks, which are in turn connected to other networks (collective intelligence). The interconnectedness of people through the Internet allows for the learning that occurs overall to be greater than the learning of each individual connected (the "wisdom of crowds"—Surowiecki, 2004). For Siemens, it is more important to be connected to the "right" nodes to "catch" new knowledge than to be outside the network with "old" knowledge, or connected to networks that are less "useful". According to him, "Nodes that successfully acquire greater profile will be more successful at acquiring additional connections" (p. 6); "The pipe is more important than the content within the pipe" (p. 8). Thus knowledge is constantly shifting and changing. Recognizing patterns within the chaos of shifting knowledge is a core skill to be learned, as is recognizing the networks of connections that matter.

Although he describes it as a theory of learning, and his ideas certainly have profound implications for teaching and learning, Siemens' position is more of an epistemology—a view of the nature of knowledge—than a theory of teaching and learning. Thus there are hints of possible actions to be taken, but at this stage of development, there are no clear guidelines for teachers and learners. However, Web 2.0 tools and practices will likely be critical elements of any teaching or learning that is consciously built around the concept of connectivism.

Choosing Epistemological Positions

Teachers are always making choices about how to teach based on their views of what constitutes knowledge, and the best means to help learners acquire that knowledge. Frequently teachers will use a variety of approaches, depending on the nature of the subject matter and the needs of individual learners. For instance, an objectivist, didactic approach—delivering information in a well-structured and organized way—may be necessary to get learners quickly to a position where they can start asking questions or solving problems in a more constructivist manner. Nevertheless, the design of teaching will be influenced by the dominant epistemological position of teachers, and this will need to "match," to some extent, the needs of learners. It is important, then, to ensure that learners are developing the skills and competencies they will need in the "outside world," which brings the discussion to the teaching and learning needs of a knowledge-based society. In particular, this will provide some guidance on the appropriate choice and use of Web 2.0 tools.

LEARNING IN A KNOWLEDGE-BASED SOCIETY

In any country, there are at least three somewhat different economies operating at the same time (Porter, 1990):

- *Resource-based economies:* These are primarily land- and sea-based economies: agriculture, mining, fishing. Increasingly over time, they have become more knowledge-based, but the majority of workers in these industries have learned their skills in traditional ways, either from relatives or on the job. The numbers working in these industries in economically advanced countries has rapidly declined, even though in countries such as Canada and Australia resource-based economies still are major contributors to gross national product (Smith, 2007). Nonetheless, they employ relatively few workers, because the number of workers in relation to economic output is very low, due to innovation, mechanization, and the high value of the goods produced per worker.
- *Industrial-based economies:* These are based primarily on manufacturing, that is, converting the raw materials of the resource-based industries into goods through factories. Such economies are mainly urban. Labor is a major cost, and economies

of scale—manufacturing the same product many times—is essential, because of the high fixed cost of equipment. The organization of labor is mainly hierarchical, with owners, managers, supervisors, skilled workers, and unskilled workers. Skilled workers are relatively narrowly trained within a specific occupation; only the owners and managers require advanced levels of education, although as manufacturing becomes more automated, labor costs are reduced and knowledge and skill levels for some workers increase. In spite of the above, even industrial-based companies now are relying more and more on knowledge-based products and services. For instance, Volkwagen estimates that 70% of the value of a modern car is knowledge-based, mainly in the form of its electronic systems and the costs of research and design. In the past, manufacturing provided large numbers of workers with steady work and relatively high wages.

- *Knowledge-based economies:* These are primarily based on the production, transmission, management, and organization of information, mostly digital information (Drucker, 1969). Typical knowledge-based industries are telecommunications, financial services (banking, insurance), health services, entertainment (movies, games), biotechnology, information technology companies (computing, etc.), and education. These economies are "virtual," that is, they are not dependent on a particular, single location (although companies operating in them may have headquarters), they are global, and they require workers with a high level of education and multiple skills. Often, knowledge-based companies are small, with between two and 100 employees. They are networked to other organizations, highly flexible, and emerge, combine, and disappear very quickly, although in some areas there are dominant industry players (e.g., Microsoft, Google).

Over time, there has been a significant shift in economies (Porter, 1990). Because labor is a major cost in industrial organizations, manufacturing has been moving from high-cost labor markets to lower-cost labor markets. To retain their global competitiveness, economically advanced countries have been switching from industrial-based to knowledge-based economies. Their advantage is that knowledge-based industries require workers with high levels of education and knowledge, which countries such as Canada and the USA, with over 50% of an age group going on to some form of post-secondary education, have in abundance. It should be noted though that the skills of knowledge-based workers are markedly different from those of industrially based workers, except at the senior management level. Thus the shift to a knowledge-based economy is dependent on large numbers of highly educated workers with different skills from those of industrially based workers (Conference Board of Canada, 1991).

The shift in economies has been quite dramatic. Figure 2 and Figure 3 show this effect on employment in Canada. Figure 2 shows the division of the workforce between the three economies from the middle of the 19th century to the present day. Before 1850, nearly 80% of jobs in Canada were based on working the land and sea. As the Industrial Revolution impacted on Canada, many people left the countryside and migrated to jobs in factories. Between the 1930s to around 1985, nearly 75% of employed Canadians worked in manufacturing (Marcus, 1952).

Figure 3 shows a dramatic change in Canadian employment from 1985 onwards. Manufacturing jobs in Canada have dropped from nearly 75% in 1985 to under 15% by 2007. They have almost entirely been replaced by jobs in the service sector. The service sector hides, though, the important dif-

Figure 2. Shifting jobs: Canada

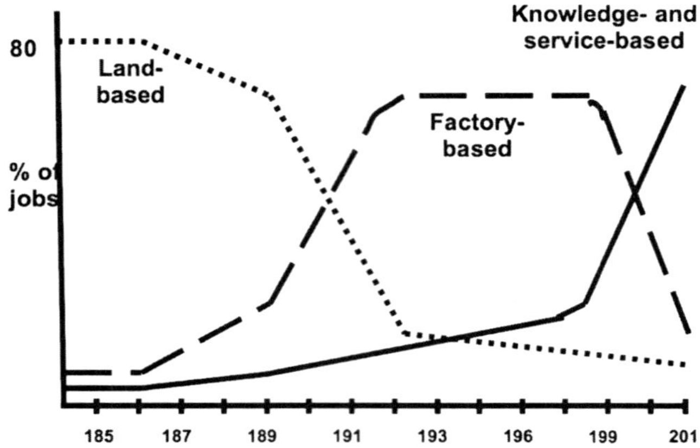

Figure 3. Percentage share of Canadian industrial employment (Source: The Globe and Mail, April 27, 2006, B9)

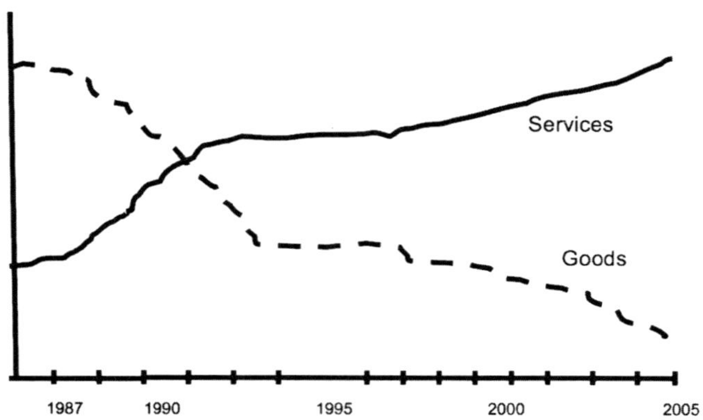

ferences between high-paying knowledge-based jobs and low-paying, unskilled or semi-skilled service jobs (e.g., shop assistants). Nevertheless, despite this huge drop in manufacturing jobs, Canada's unemployment rate is at an all-time low, and its economy has been booming (Note that the figures reflect the proportion of jobs in each sector, *not* the proportion of gross domestic product [GDP]. The resource sector—mining and oil in particular, which are land-based—is a major contributor to Canada's GDP, but employs relatively few people.)

Although the timing and magnitude of the change may vary, similar patterns will be found in many other economically advanced countries (according to the *Financial Times* in the UK, for example, the British economy reached the "cross-over" point between employment in goods and services in 2008 [Laitner, 2008]). The reason is that manufacturing jobs have migrated to countries with low labor costs. However, much of the value of goods produced in low-labor economies is created (and retained) in economically advanced countries. For instance, the Conference Board of Canada (2008, p. 2) states that

Every US$300 Apple iPod adds $150 to the official U.S. imports from China, but only $3 of its

value is actually created in China. About $147 is created in the rest of Asia, and another $149 in the United States.

The point here is that economically advanced countries are increasingly depending on knowledge-based workers to maintain and increase their standard of living. In an industrial society, less than 15% of those in the workforce (mainly owners, managers, and those working in financial services) needed post-secondary education. In knowledge-based economies, more than 50% need post-secondary education (the Alberta Provincial Government, 2008 has put this figure at 62.7% of all jobs by 2011).

Education therefore needs to be focused particularly on the knowledge and skills required in knowledge-based companies. What are those skills? The Conference Board of Canada (1991) surveyed employers in knowledge-based companies and identified the following:

- good communication skills (reading/writing/speaking/listening);
- ability to learn independently;
- social skills: ethics, positive attitudes, responsibility;
- teamwork;
- ability to adapt to changing circumstances;
- thinking skills: problem solving; critical/logical/numerical;
- knowledge navigation: where to get/how to process information;
- entrepreneurial skills: taking initiative to seize an opportunity;
- IT and computing skills.

It might be argued that these are not very different from the kinds of skills one would expect from any traditional liberal arts program. The catch, though, is that these skills are required *in addition to* specialist qualifications in engineering, management, health sciences, business, etc. It will still be essential to build the foundations of knowledge in these areas, such as mathematics, accountancy, anatomy, etc. Furthermore, skills such as problem solving are not generic: problem solving in medicine is different from problem solving in business. The skill needs to be embedded within the content area. This means teaching content and designing learning activities in such a way as to develop these skills.

A second feature of knowledge-based work is that knowledge workers must continue to go on learning (Senge, 1990). The knowledge bases of medicine, IT, and biotechnology, for example, are constantly changing. To stay competitive, knowledge-based companies and their employees must continually change and adapt through a process of lifelong learning. Thus universities and colleges face two challenges: with regard to those entering from high schools, how to develop the thinking skills identified as needed within a knowledge-based society within a traditional undergraduate program; and equally as important, how to provide ongoing opportunities for learning for those who have already graduated and are in the workforce.

This is where the epistemological basis for teaching and learning becomes critical. Constructivism, with its emphasis on learner-centered teaching, discussion, and communication between learners, and connectivism, with its emphasis on Internet-mediated knowledge construction and digital literacy, seem to provide a better basis for developing the skills needed in knowledge-based economies than what is possible with a predominantly objectivist approach. Noteworthy, however, is Lyotard's (1979/1984) observation about the changing nature of knowledge as having commercial rather than intrinsic value in a knowledge-based society.

CHANGING STUDENTS

In discussing the topic of changing students, it may be useful to begin with a warning from a study commissioned by the British Library and JISC, the UK universities' computer network organization. The study used log file analysis of actual search behavior of a wide range of users of different ages (Centre for Information Behaviour and the Evaluation of Research [CIBER], 2008):

There are very, very few controlled studies that account for age and information seeking behavior systematically: as a result there is much misinformation and much speculation about how young people supposedly behave in cyberspace. (p. 14)

Nevertheless, Marc Prensky (2001) claims:

Our students have changed radically. Today's students are no longer the people our educational system was designed to teach ... today's students think and process information fundamentally differently from their predecessors. (p. 1)

He argues that students now entering university have grown up all their lives with technology—mobile phones, computers, video games, and so on—and therefore are "digital natives." As a result of this exposure to technology, digital natives access and process information more quickly, multitask more easily, prefer graphics to text and random to sequential access, thrive on instant gratification and rewards, and prefer games to serious work. This makes them different from "digital immigrants," that is, people who did not grow up with this technology, but have learned to adapt to it later in life. As a result, according to Prensky, educational institutions need to change their approach to accommodate the needs of such learners, but it is difficult for most teachers to do this, since they are digital immigrants, not natives.

It is certainly true that many digital natives are early and heavy adopters of Web 2.0 tools such as MySpace, Facebook, YouTube, and Twitter. These mesh well with their prior experience and needs. However, there is little research or systematically collected empirical evidence at this stage that the skills digital natives have developed in their personal and social lives carry over into academic work. Laurillard (2002, p. 218) points out, for instance, that

academic knowledge is distinct from experiential knowledge. It is a reflection on experience, rather than being synonymous with experience per se. It also includes knowledge of how that knowledge came to be known.

The British Library/JISC study (CIBER, 2008) looked at the "Google generation," defined as those born after 1993, and asked the following question (among others) in relation to this generation: "[Are they] searching for and researching content in new ways and ... [is this] likely to shape their future behaviour as mature researchers?" (p. 5). This study reported that

young people scan online pages very rapidly (boys especially) and click extensively on hyperlinks—rather than reading sequentially. Users make very little use of advanced search facilities, assuming that search engines "understand" their queries. They tend to move rapidly from page to page, spending little time reading or digesting information and they have difficulty making relevance judgments about the pages they retrieve. (p. 14)

Although this somewhat supports Prensky's position, the CIBER study goes on to challenge a number of apparent myths about "digital natives," with varying degrees of confidence. However, one point they do make clearly is that

the evidence indicates that more people across all age groups are using the Internet and Web 2.0 technologies widely and for a variety of purposes. The young... may have been the earliest adopters but now older users are fast catching up... the so-called Silver Surfers. In many ways the Google generation label is increasingly unhelpful. (p. 21)

The study concludes:

much writing on the topic of this report overestimates the impact of ICTs on the young and underestimates its effect on older generations. A much greater sense of balance is needed. (p. 21)

This empirical study reinforces a few—and challenges many—of the assumptions made by Prensky (see also Chapter 16 in this book for a further, critical examination of the "digital natives" concept). The CIBER study identifies that young people's use of Google is relatively superficial, and does not lead to deep processing of information. Thus, although young people may enter post-secondary education with familiarity of new technologies, they may not necessarily know how best to use it for academic purposes. From this perspective there is still an important role for teachers. On the other hand, bearing in mind Siemens' (2005) aforementioned view that the pipe is more important than the content, young people's fast and voluminous searching behavior may nevertheless be important in its own right in a networked world.

The issues, then, are (1) to what extent new technology requires a re-examination of the fundamental principles and beliefs that underpin academic study, so as to accommodate to the exigencies of a networked society; and (2) to what extent the non-academic technology behavior of young people can be harnessed for more traditional academic study. Because different teachers will come to different conclusions about these issues, it is necessary to provide some way of analyzing the potential educational use of Web 2.0 tools, and this needs to be done by linking it to different epistemological positions that teachers may adhere to.

ANALYZING WEB 2.0 TOOLS FROM AN EDUCATIONAL PERSPECTIVE

Figure 4 presents a diagrammatic analysis of various e-learning tools. This represents the author's personal interpretation of the tools, and other teachers may well rearrange the diagram differently, depending on their particular applications of these tools. The position of any particular tool in the diagram will depend on its actual use. LMSs can be used in a constructivist way, and blogs can be very much teacher controlled if the teacher is the only one permitted to use a blog on a course, for example. However, the aim here is not to provide a cast-iron categorization of e-learning tools, but simply to offer a framework to assist teachers in deciding which tools are most likely to suit a particular teaching approach. Indeed, other teachers may prefer a different set of pedagogical values as a framework for analysis of the different tools.

However, to give an example from Figure 4, a teacher may use an LMS to organize a set of resources, guidelines, procedures, and deadlines for students, who then may use several of the Web 2.0 tools, such as YouTube, to collect data. The teacher provides a space and structure within the LMS for students' learning materials in the form of an e-portfolio, into which students can upload their work. Students in small groups can use the discussion features in Facebook to work on projects together. Note that this figure also permits traditional teaching modes, such as lectures and seminars, to be included and compared.

It can be seen that Web 2.0 tools now enable teachers to set online group work, based on cases or projects, and students can collect data in the field, without any need for direct face-to-face contact with either the teacher or other students. Learners can access learning materials through open content, and also access other experts on a topic through their websites, social network profiles, and blogs. Learners can post media-rich assignments either individually or as a group; these assignments, after being assessed, can be loaded

Figure 4. Analysis of Web 2.0 tools from an educational perspective

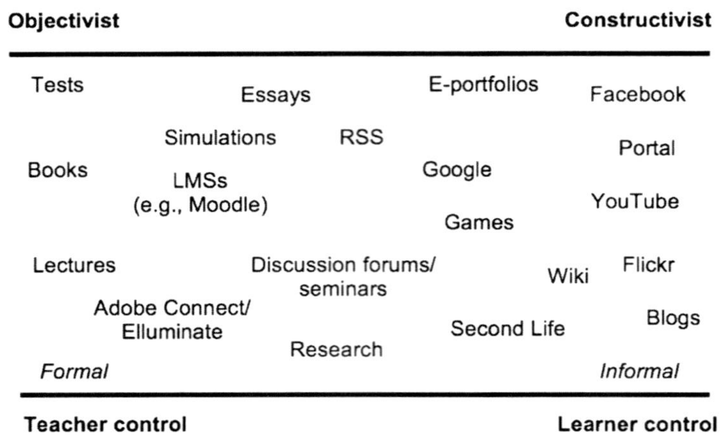

by learners into their own personal learning environments for later use when seeking employment or transfer to graduate school.

The above example from Figure 4 assumes the context of a course being studied for academic credit, but the framework would also fit the non-institutional or informal approach to the use of Web 2.0 for learning, with a focus on tools such as Facebook, blogs, and YouTube. These applications would be much more learner driven, with the learner having complete choice and control over the tools and their uses.

WHO DECIDES?

In an institutional setting, who should decide on the form of e-learning (blended or fully online/distance), on the overall teaching approach (teacher or learner centered), and on the choice of technologies (an LMS and/or Web 2.0 tools)? Traditionally, and particularly in post-secondary education, it has been the individual instructor. However, increasingly, there are strong reasons to adopt a whole-program approach to decision making in this area.

This would mean all the teachers in a program, such as a Bachelor of Arts or a Master's in Business Administration, coming together to discuss not only the content of the program, but also how it should be delivered. The program team would develop an overall plan for the program, which would try to answer the following questions:

- What kind(s) of students (full-time, part-time, off-campus) are we trying to reach with this program?
- What is their experience in using technology for learning?
- How well will this program prepare our learners for knowledge-based work? What skills are we trying to develop in this program? What will distinguish an "A" student from the rest in this program?
- What kind of content do we want learners to access? Where is it? Do we have to create it from scratch, or does it already exist on the Web? Can learners find their own material? If so, what guidelines or criteria should we provide?
- What is our overall philosophy of teaching going to be in this program? How will our teaching approach support the skills we have identified as being important? Do the early courses have to start didactically, with a lot of supplied information? Do we have to de-

liberately help students become independent learners? How relevant are the learners' own life experiences likely to be for this program? How can we best draw on these?

- How can technology help us achieve our goals in this program? How will the use of technology change during the program? Which tools should we be using, and why?
- What support will we need in the use of technology, both for those teaching and for those learning? What prior training is required?

In making these decisions, it will help if the following points are borne in mind:

- E-learning is well suited for developing the skills needed in a knowledge-based society, in particular how to find, evaluate, organize, and apply information relevant to specific work areas. Using technology for learning prepares learners for knowledge-based work.
- E-learning is particularly suited for lifelong learners, those already in the workforce, who may already have at least a first degree, who have jobs and families, and/or who do not want to come on campus on a regular basis.
- Web 2.0 tools provide learners with powerful means to create their own learning materials and personal learning environments.
- Web 2.0 tools of themselves do not teach or result in effective or meaningful learning—there must be a particular purpose or rationale for their use, and teacher support and guidance in most cases are still likely to be essential. However, they may be provided in different ways from conventional teaching.
- There is tremendous scope for innovative uses of Web 2.0 tools, but this requires an institutional environment that encourages and rewards exploration and risk taking.
- Decisions about the use of e-learning are best taken in a whole-program context, rather than by individual teachers working in isolation.

CONCLUSION

ICTs, and in particular the new Web 2.0 tools, present a major challenge to all educational and training organizations. Web 2.0 represents not just a new generation of tools, but a significant shift in approaches to teaching and learning that challenge the very existence of formal educational institutions. At the same time, many of these new tools can be integrated within a more structured context, and provide significant educational benefits through empowering students to create and manage their own digital learning materials.

There is no sign that the pace of change in ICTs is slowing. If anything, the context is even more complex and challenging now than ever before. In such a volatile context, it is critical that educational organizations have processes in place that encourage dynamic change, innovative uses of technology, and monitoring and evaluation of what works and what does not. Above all, it is important not only to recognize the new opportunities that these tools offer, but also to make sure that they are used in educationally meaningful ways. Despite these cautions, used wisely, Web 2.0 tools can help bridge the gap between the requirements of academic rigor and the lifestyles of modern learners.

REFERENCES

Alberta Provincial Government. (2008). *Alberta access planning framework*. Edmonton, AB: Alberta Advanced Education and Technology.

Alexander, B. (2004). Going nomadic: Mobile learning in higher education. *EDUCAUSE Review, 39*(5), 28–35. Retrieved December 6, 2008, from http://www.educause.edu/ir/library/pdf/ERM0451.pdf

Allen, E. I., & Seaman, J. (2006). *Making the grade: Online education in the United States, 2006*. Needham, MA: Sloan Consortium.

Allen, E. I., & Seaman, J. (2008). *Staying the course: Online education in the United States, 2008*. Needham, MA: Sloan Consortium.

Bates, A. W., & Poole, G. (2003). *Effective teaching with technology in higher education: Foundations for success*. San Francisco: Jossey-Bass.

Burgos, D., Tattersall, C., & Koper, R. (2007). Re-purposing existing generic games and simulations for e-learning. *Computers in Human Behavior, 23*(6), 2656–2667. doi:10.1016/j.chb.2006.08.002

Candy, P. (1991). *Self-direction for lifelong learning*. San Francisco: Jossey-Bass.

Centre for Information Behaviour and the Evaluation of Research. (2008). *Information behaviour of the researcher of the future.* London: CIBER, University College London. Retrieved December 6, 2008, from http://www.bl.uk/news/pdf/googlegen.pdf

Conference Board of Canada. (1991). *Employability skill profile: The critical skills required of the Canadian workforce.* Ottawa, ON: Conference Board of Canada.

Conference Board of Canada. (2008). *Canada's "missing" trade with Asia.* Ottawa, ON: Conference Board of Canada.

Dick, W., & Carey, L. (1996). *The systematic design of instruction* (4th ed.). New York: HarperCollins.

Downes, S. (2005, October). E-learning 2.0. *eLearn Magazine*. Retrieved December 6, 2008, from http://www.elearnmag.org/subpage.cfm?section=articles&article=29-1

Downes, S. (2006). *Understanding learning networks*. Keynote presentation delivered at the Fourth EDEN Research Workshop, Castelldelfels, Spain. Retrieved December 6, 2008, from http://www.downes.ca/files/spain.ppt

Drucker, P. (1969). *The age of discontinuity: Guidelines to our changing society*. New York: Harper & Row.

Earth System Research Laboratory. (2008). *Outreach at ERSL*. Retrieved December 20, 2008, from http://www.esrl.noaa.gov/outreach/index.html

Golding, W. (1954). *The lord of the flies*. London: Faber & Faber.

Gould, C., & Brown, D. (2003). *Constructivism and practice*. Lanham, MD: Rowman & Littlefield.

Green, K. C. (2007). *The 2007 National Survey of Information Technology in U.S. Higher Education*. Encino, CA: The Campus Computing Project. Retrieved December 6, 2008, from http://www.campuscomputing.net/sites/www.campuscomputing.net/files/2007-CCP_0.pdf

Guess, A. (2007, August 20). In Second Life, there's no fallout. *Inside Higher Ed*. Retrieved from http://insidehighered.com/news/2007/08/20/secondlife

Hiltz, S. R. (1986). The virtual classroom: Using computer-mediated communication for university teaching. *The Journal of Communication, 36*(2), 95–104. doi:10.1111/j.1460-2466.1986.tb01427.x

Hiltz, S. R., & Turoff, M. (1978). *The network nation: Human communication via computer*. Reading, MA: Addison-Wesley.

Illich, I. (1973). *Deschooling society*. Harmondsworth, UK: Penguin.

Joint Information Systems Committee. (2005). *Innovative practice with e-learning: A good practice guide to embedding mobile and wireless technologies into everyday practice*. Bristol, UK: JISC. Retrieved December 6, 2008, from http://www.jisc.ac.uk/media/documents/publications/innovativepe.pdf

Joint Information Systems Committee. (2007). *Effective practice with e-assessment: An overview of technologies, policies and practice in further and higher education*. Bristol, UK: JISC. Retrieved December 6, 2008, from http://www.jisc.ac.uk/media/documents/themes/elearning/effpraceassess.pdf

Jonassen, D. H., Davidson, M., Collins, M., Campbell, J., & Bannan Haag, B. (1995). Constructivism and computer-mediated communication in distance education. *American Journal of Distance Education*, *9*(2), 7–26. doi:10.1080/08923649509526885

Kay, J., & FitzGerald, S. (2008). *Educational uses of Second Life*. Retrieved December 6, 2008, from http://sleducation.wikispaces.com/educationaluses

Keen, A. (2007). *The cult of the amateur: How today's Internet is killing our culture*. New York: Doubleday.

Laitner, A. (2008, June 10). EU in working week discussions. *Financial Times*.

Lankshear, C., Peters, M., & Knobel, M. (2000). Information, knowledge and learning: Some issues facing epistemology and education in a digital age. *Journal of Philosophy of Education*, *34*(1), 17–40. doi:10.1111/1467-9752.00153

Laurillard, D. (2002). *Rethinking university teaching: A conversational framework for the effective use of learning technologies* (2nd ed.). London: RoutledgeFalmer. doi:10.4324/9780203304846

Lokken, F., & Womer, L. (2007). *Trends in e-learning: Tracking the impact of e-learning in higher education. 2006 distance education survey results*. Washington, DC: Instructional Technology Council. Retrieved December 6, 2008, from http://www.itcnetwork.org/file.php?file=/1/ITCAnnualSurveyFeb2007.pdf

Lorenzo, G., & Ittelson, J. C. (2005). *An overview of portfolios*. Boulder, CO: EDUCAUSE. Retrieved December 6, 2008, from http://www.educause.edu/ir/library/pdf/ELI3001.pdf

Lowendahl, J.-M., Zastrocky, M., & Harris, M. (2008). *Gartner Higher Education E-Learning Survey 2007: Clear movements in the market*. Stamford, CT: Gartner.

Lyotard, J.-F. (1984). *The postmodern condition: A report on knowledge*. (G. Bennington & B. Massumi, Trans.). Minneapolis, MN: University of Minnesota Press. (1979).

Marcus, E. (1952). The cyclical adjustment pattern of an "open economy": Canada, 1927–1939. *The Economic Journal*, *62*(246), 305–317. doi:10.2307/2227006

Marshall, L., & Rowland, F. (1993). *A guide to learning independently*. Buckingham, UK: Open University Press.

Mason, R. (1989). An evaluation of CoSy on an Open University course. In Mason, R., & Kaye, A. (Eds.), *Mindweave: Communication, computers, and distance education* (pp. 221–226). New York: Pergamon.

Moore, M. G. (1973). Towards a theory of independent learning and teaching. *The Journal of Higher Education*, *44*(9), 661–679. doi:10.2307/1980599

Moore, M. G., & Thompson, M. (1990). *The effects of distance education: A summary of the literature*. University Park, PA: American Center for Distance Education, Pennsylvania State University. morebrainsmedia. (2006, March 26). *Hydro Hijinks Version 2* [Video file]. Retrieved December 6, 2008, from http://www.youtube.com/watch?v=JS2JT9IV3CM

New Media Consortium. (2008). *The Horizon Report: 2008 edition*. Austin, TX: NMC. Retrieved December 6, 2008, from http://www.nmc.org/pdf/2008-Horizon-Report.pdf

OECD. (2005). *E-learning in tertiary education: Where do we stand?* Paris: OECD.

Parsons, C. (2008, July 13). Second Life offers healing, therapeutic options for users. *San Francisco Chronicle*. Retrieved December 6, 2008, from http://www.sfgate.com/cgi-bin/article.cgi?f=/c/a/2008/07/11/LVL211GP5C.DTL

Popper, K. (1972). *Objective knowledge: An evolutionary approach*. London: Oxford University Press.

Porter, M. E. (1990). *The competitive advantage of nations*. New York: Free Press.

Prensky, M. (2001). Digital natives, digital immigrants. *Horizon*, *9*(5), 1–6. doi:10.1108/10748120110424816

Prensky, M. (2006). *Don't bother me Mom—I'm learning: How computer and video games are preparing your kids for 21st century success and how you can help!* St. Paul, MN: Paragon.

Rumsfeld, D. H. (2002, February 12). *DoD news briefing—Secretary Rumsfeld and Gen. Myers* [News transcript]. Retrieved December 6, 2008, from http://www.defense.gov/transcripts/transcript.aspx?transcriptid=2636

Senge, P. M. (1990). *The fifth discipline: The art and practice of the learning organization*. New York: Doubleday.

Senges, M., Praus, T., & Bihr, P. (2007). *Virtual worlds: A Second Life beginner's guide*. Barcelona: Open University of Catalonia. Retrieved December 6, 2008, from http://www.thewavingcat.com/wp-content/uploads/2007/07/uoc_virtual_worlds_a_second_life_beginners_guide.pdf

Siemens, G. (2005). Connectivism: A learning theory for the digital age. *International Journal of Instructional Technology and Distance Learning*, *2*(1), 3–10. Retrieved October 2, 2007, from http://www.itdl.org/Journal/Jan_05/Jan_05.pdf

Smith, K. H. (2007). *Innovation and growth in resource-based economies*. Melbourne, Australia: Committee for Economic Development of Australia.

Surowiecki, J. (2004). *The wisdom of crowds: Why the many are smarter than the few and how collective wisdom shapes business, economies, societies, and nations*. New York: Doubleday.

Takahashi, D. (2008, July 1). Cigna deploys a Second Life island for health education. *VentureBeat*. Retrieved December 6, 2008, from http://venturebeat.com/2008/07/01/cigna-deploys-a-second-life-island-for-health-education/

Web 2.0. (2008). In *Wikipedia, the free encyclopedia*. Retrieved December 3, 2008, from http://en.wikipedia.org/wiki/Web_2.0

World Wide Web. (2008, December 3). In *Wikipedia, the free encyclopedia*. Retrieved December 3, 2008, from http://en.wikipedia.org/wiki/World_Wide_Web

Chapter 3
Pedagogy 2.0:
Critical Challenges and Responses to Web 2.0 and Social Software in Tertiary Teaching

Catherine McLoughlin
Australian Catholic University, Australia

Mark J. W. Lee
Charles Sturt University, Australia

ABSTRACT

Worldwide, tertiary educators and institutions are discovering that new models of teaching and learning are required to meet the needs of today's students, and their demands for autonomy, connectivity, and socio-experiential learning. The educational applications of the new wave of Web 2.0-based social software tools compel us to consider how the affordances and potential for generativity and connectivity offered by these tools, as well as the broader societal changes that the Web 2.0 movement forms part of, impact on pedagogy and teaching, and open up the debate on how we conceptualize the dynamics of student learning. This chapter explores the ways in which scholarship and pedagogy are being challenged and redefined in the Web 2.0 era, and the accompanying need for students to develop new skills and competencies to prepare them for work and lifelong learning in a dynamic, networked society and knowledge economy. In response to these challenges the authors propose a pedagogical framework, "Pedagogy 2.0," which addresses the themes of participation in networked communities of learning, personalization of the learning experience, and learner productivity in the form of active knowledge creation and innovation, and discuss how emerging social practices, ethos, and modes of communication influence the roles of teachers and learners.

INTRODUCTION

In contrast to earlier e-learning efforts that simply replicated traditional models of learning and teaching in online environments, social software, together with other components of the Web 2.0 movement, offers rich opportunities to move away from the highly centralized industrial model of learning of the past decade, toward achieving individual empowerment of learners through designs

DOI: 10.4018/978-1-60566-294-7.ch003

that focus on collaborative, networked communication and interaction (cf. Rogers, Liddle, Chan, Doxey, & Isom, 2007; Sims, 2006). Hilton (2006) discusses how a number of "disruptive forces" are shaping the future of higher education. These include the unbundling of content, the shift from "provider push" to "demand pull," the arrival of ubiquitous access to information and services, and the rise of the "pure property" view of ideas that is not consistent with the Web 2.0 philosophy and spirit of collaboration and sharing.

For the purposes of the current discussion, the focus is on social software that enables participation, collaboration, self-direction, creativity, and generativity, as these are arguably the cornerstones of what it means to be educated in a networked age (Bryant, 2006; Oblinger, 2008). Social software tools are a defining characteristic of Web 2.0, and many are already being widely used to support learning. For example, one of the most basic social software tools, the web log (blog), has been used for diverse purposes, including teaching composition, as a reflective writing tool, as a platform for housing e-portfolios, and to facilitate shared and guided exploration; it has proven a resounding success in many schools and universities (Ganley, 2004; Richardson, 2006a). With the rich and varied functionality of social computing in mind, together with its "always-on" culture and participatory attributes, it is useful to consider the potential value adding of these emerging tools and technologies for learners in the new millennium.

HOW WEB 2.0 AND SOCIAL SOFTWARE TOOLS IMPACT ON EDUCATION, LEARNING, AND WAYS OF KNOWING

The Affordances of Web 2.0-Based Social Software Tools

Web 2.0 does not involve radical changes in the technical specifications of the Web, but most proponents of the concept describe it in terms of new possibilities and applications. O'Reilly (2005), who first coined the term, believes that these new applications have emerged due to a morphing sociocultural context, giving rise to the perception of revolutionary new uses for the same technologies. What, then, are the implications of Web 2.0 for education? Social software tools such as blogs, wikis, social networking sites, media sharing applications, and social bookmarking utilities are also pedagogical tools that stem from their *affordances* of sharing, communication, and information discovery. An affordance is an action that an individual can potentially perform in his or her environment by using a particular tool (Gibson, 1977, 1979; Norman, 1988). In other words, an affordance is a "can do" statement that does not have to be predefined by a particular functionality, and refers to any application that enables a user to undertake tasks, whether these capabilities are known or unknown to him or her. For example, blogging entails typing and editing posts, which are not affordances, but which make possible the affordances of idea sharing and interaction. Kirschner (2002) states that educational affordances can be defined as the relationships between the properties of an educational intervention and the characteristics of the learner that enable certain kinds of learning to take place. In considering the educational applications of information and communication technologies (ICTs), it is imperative to acknowledge the technologies are related to many other elements of the learning context (e.g., task design) that can shape the possibilities they offer to learners, how learners perceive those possibilities, and the extent to which learning outcomes can be attained.

According to Anderson (2004), "The greatest affordance of the Web for educational use is the profound and multifaceted increase in communication and interaction capability" (p. 42), which is even more evident in Web 2.0 when compared to the set of hyperlinked but largely static information sources that characterized "Web 1.0." The affordances of Web 2.0 are now making learner-centered education a reality, with tools that enable collaborative writing (wikis, Google Docs & Spreadsheets), media sharing applications (Flickr, YouTube, TeacherTube), and social networking sites (MySpace, Facebook, Friendster, Bebo, Ning) capable of supporting multiple communities of learning. These tools foster and encourage informal conversation, dialogue, collaborative content generation, and the sharing of information, supplying learners with access to a wide raft of ideas and representations of knowledge.

The attributes and affordances of social software tools also make possible an expanded repertoire of online behavior, distributed collaboration, and social interaction. Mejias (2005, p. 1) observes that "social software can positively impact pedagogy by inculcating a desire to reconnect to the world as whole, not just the social part that exists online," which stands in contrast to the isolating and decontextualized experience of much text-based traditional education. Many current social software applications straddle real and virtual social worlds, as they entail both online and offline interactions and visual/verbal connectivity. For example, Flickr and YouTube facilitate the sharing of photos and videos respectively with both "real world" and "virtual" friends. Social networking sites allow users to build an online identity by customizing their personal profiles with a range of multimedia elements, as well as communicating asynchronously with existing contacts and establishing new relationships, with some such sites additionally allowing users to interact in real time using their web cameras and microphones. These practices are being harnessed for knowledge sharing, creative production, and the development of ideas, while allowing for personal sense making and reflection (National School Boards Association, 2007; Bryant, 2007; Downes, 2007).

There are also associated changes in what and how people learn, and the ways in which they access information. Knowledge is no longer controlled and stable, but open to interpretation, review, and modification by anyone, anywhere. The traditional macrostructures of the disciplines are being replaced by dynamic microstructures created by networked individuals working collaboratively. These networks are able to link people and summon the "wisdom of crowds" (Surowiecki, 2004), so that the collective intelligence of groups can be harnessed to generate ideas that are fresher, richer, and more sophisticated than the contributions of individual users. Lindner (2006) quotes Parkin (2005, p. 31), who observes: "it's not content or even context, but process that gets us going," indicating that participating, doing, and experiencing rather than knowing what or where, and creating knowledge rather than consuming it, is the new mindset and *modus operandi* of learners, online communities, and the knowledge economy at large. All in all, we have an environment in which digital technology and information are paramount, and in which "learning to learn" is now far more important than memorizing or rote learning explicit knowledge and facts.

Implications for the Design of Learning Environments

The expansion and growth in popularity of Web 2.0 services and tools, as well as the accompanying increase in prevalence of user-generated content, have implications for learning environments in tertiary education, and are already influencing pedagogical choices and approaches (Williams & Jacobs, 2004). There is a shift away from the production of online content by traditional, "authoritative" sources, toward content generated by web users themselves. In academia, these users are students, who now have the tools, spaces, and skills to contribute ideas and publish their views, research, and interpretations online. It is important to remember that these tools can also be used in combination and engage people through communication, co-production, and sharing. Through these activities, social and cognitive benefits accrue to both individuals and the community of users who support and take part in them (Boyd, 2007; Barsky & Purdon, 2006).

For example, course content and learning resources can come from many sources, as a result of the ease with which social software can be used to create, share, augment, tag, and upload content. In what has been described as a "rip, mix, and burn culture" and a "digital democracy," all participants can become creators of content (Goodman & Moed, 2006; Hughes & Lang, 2006; Lamb, 2007). In academia, this means moving beyond the confines of learning management systems (LMSs) and tapping into a wider pool of expertise to include community-generated resources for learning (Eisenstadt, 2007; Lamb, 2007).

The participatory media genres and tools are cheap, easy to use, and versatile, and enable sharing, reproduction, and recreating of ideas and content in dynamic virtual communities. One commentator remarks: "The potential payoff for using open and discoverable resources … and remixable formats is huge: more reuse means that more dynamic content is being produced more economically, even if the reuse happens only within an organization. And when remixing happens in a social context on the open Web, people learn from each other's process" (Lamb, 2007, p. 18). These changes are having a profound and immediate effect on the learning landscape, and on the nature of literacies and skills required of learners, as many authors and researchers have recently noted (Eisenstadt, 2007; Berg, Berquam, & Christoph, 2007; Lankshear & Knobel, 2007). As students engage with social technologies and begin to generate and remix content, share it with a global audience, and connect to wide range of communities, their expectations for "always-on" services and relevant, participatory, interactive, flexible learning experiences expand and become drivers of change in tertiary education (Milne, 2007).

Nevertheless, challenges remain for tertiary education institutions in terms of how they will manage change, and set up physical infrastructures and spaces for learners to maximize networking and knowledge exchange (Bleed, 2001; Joint Information Systems Committee, 2006; Carrick Institute for Learning and Teaching in Higher Education, 2007). In the UK in particular, research on the applications of social software is informing innovative approaches to education in all sectors, and is driving a strong agenda for personalization of curricula and the foregrounding of lifelong learning skills, innovation, and creativity as essential learning outcomes (Owen, Grant, Sayers, & Facer, 2006).

RETHINKING PARADIGMS OF LEARNING AND KNOWLEDGE

The rise of Web 2.0 and social software sits against the backdrop of much broader changes in the educational landscape and in society at large, changes that are impacting profoundly upon paradigms of learning and knowledge. Before investigating the transformative effects of social software tools on existing tertiary teaching practice and pedagogy, an overview of the emerging paradigms, grounded in explanatory theoretical frameworks, will serve as a useful signpost of the directions in which tertiary education is headed. A number of terms and metaphors signal the move from traditional pedagogies to more active forms of teaching and learning engagement, where learners have greater levels of agency, autonomy, and social connectedness.

Applying a New Metaphor: Students as Knowledge Producers

The manner in which we conceptualize learning evokes a number of possible scenarios or metaphors. Sfard (1998), for example, distinguishes between two metaphors of learning, the acquisition metaphor and the participation metaphor. The former represents a view of learning that is mainly a process of acquiring chunks of information, usually delivered by a teacher. An alternative model, according to Sfard, is the participation metaphor, which sees learning as a process of participating in various cultural practices and shared learning activities. However, in order to keep pace with knowledge-building processes that are emerging in the Web 2.0 era, it appears to be necessary to go beyond the acquisition and participation dichotomy. The knowledge creation metaphor of learning (Paavola & Hakkarainen, 2005) mirrors the societal shift toward a networked knowledge age, in which creativity, originality, and the capacity to gain knowledge from networks are highly valued. It builds on common elements of Bereiter's (2002) theory of knowledge building, Nonaka and Takeuchi's (1995) model of knowledge creation, and Engeström's (1987, 1999) theory of expansive learning. The "trialogic" nature of the knowledge creation metaphor reminds us that learning is an intensely social activity, where ideas are generated in conjunction with others in the community through mutual exchange, contribution, and sharing of ideas.

Learning as knowledge creation is mediated by a range of digital tools and affordances that support networking, socialization and communication, and engagement with communities of learning (Lee, McLoughlin, & Chan, 2008). Students, enabled by social software tools, are capable of being both producers and consumers ("prosumers") of knowledge, ideas, and artifacts. As novices or newcomers to a community of practice, they not only engage in "legitimate peripheral participation" (Lave & Wenger, 1991) to develop their own mastery of knowledge and skills through interaction with experts such as their instructors, but also have a responsibility to play a part in the ongoing advancement of the community's existing body of knowledge, as they move toward full participation in the sociocultural practices of the community (Lee, Eustace, Hay, & Fellows, 2005). In a knowledge-building community, all members work together to make responsible decisions, intent not only on imparting and preserving the community's existing knowledge but also on generating novel and innovative contributions to benefit the community and ensure its continued progress and growth.

"Knowledge creation" and "knowledge building" are now terms that are used internationally in management, corporate organizations, and institutions of higher learning that value innovation and creativity (Leadbeater, 2006; Nonaka & Toyama, 2003). This paradigm can be appropriately applied to learning environments where digital tools and affordances enable engagement in self-directed activities, and learners have freedom and choice to move beyond mere participation in groups and communities to become active creators of ideas, resources, and knowledge artifacts. In today's knowledge-based society, characterized by rapid change, dynamic communication, and continual knowledge advancement, core competencies needed include self-direction, problem solving, critical inquiry, creativity, teamwork, and communication skills, all of which can be fostered through pedagogies that leverage digital tools, content, and services in appropriate ways (Bryant, 2006).

Learning as Navigating the Knowledge Seas

Given the rapid expansion of available information, particularly on the World Wide Web, and the great diversity in the backgrounds, needs, and interests of individual students in tertiary education courses worldwide, it is neither realistic nor feasible for an instructor or course to be expected to provide students with all the information and resources they need or desire throughout their professional and personal lives. Moreover, in the knowledge age, information in many fields is quickly surpassed or rendered out of date. Teachers are, however, expected to educate students in digital and information literacy skills and assist them in developing the ability to access, evaluate, and apply relevant information and concepts from reliable sources using constructivist pedagogies (Eshet-Alkalai, 2004; Heeren, 2007; Ward, 2008). With the ubiquity of information and communications technologies (ICTs) in universities today, navigationism (Brown, 2005, 2006) has emerged as a broader and more inclusive concept than constructivism, and one whose focus is on the importance of "'navigating' the ocean of available knowledge" (Brown, 2005, p. 7).

Navigationism recognizes that successful learning occurs as a result of learners being able to solve contextual, real-world problems through collaboratively exploring, evaluating, manipulating, and integrating available information from an array of sources, as opposed to passively acquiring information from texts selected by the teacher. To this end, it advocates the development of information navigation skills that "will have more to do with being able to be your own private, personal reference librarian, one that knows how to navigate through the incredible, confusing, complex information spaces and feel comfortable and located in doing that" (Brown, 1999, p. 6, cited in Brown, 2005).

Learning Through and Within Communities and Networks of Knowledge

In the present era, new and dynamic forms of community are emerging that are self-directed and open to a global audience. These offer new forms of social and intellectual engagement to students, often based on sharing objects and artifacts, in what has been described as "object-centered sociality" (Engeström, 2005a, 2005b). Flickr allows the posting and sharing of photos and descriptors; social bookmarking utilities (Furl, delicious) allow people to connect through shared metadata and user-created tagging; social writing platforms enable collaborative text composition, synchronous and/or asynchronous editing, and the addition of personal commentary. Social networking practices also enable the creation of virtual communities based on shared motives and/or common interests, leading to relationship building. These social, informal experiences are very often the foundation of learning (Gee, 2003). Individuals are motivated to link personal interests to broader social networks, thereby situating responses and contributions within a dynamic community that provides feedback and reciprocity (Owen et al., 2006).

Contemporary and future learning environments must therefore take into account the social and networked nature of knowledge as well as the opportunities afforded by participation in knowledge generation in technology-rich communities and environments (van Weert, 2006; Brown & Duguid, 2000). Connectivism is gaining popularity as a theory that seeks to describe the social, interconnected, and community-based characteristics of learning in contemporary times. In the words of its originator, Siemens (2005):

> *Personal knowledge is comprised of a network, which feeds into organizations and institutions, which in turn feed back into the network, and then continue to provide learning to individual. This cycle of knowledge development (personal to network to organization) allows learners to remain current in their field through the connections they have formed. (p. 8)*

Connectivism strives to overcome the limitations of behaviorism, cognitivism, and constructivism, by synthesizing the salient features and elements of several educational, social, and technological theories and concepts to create a new and dynamic theoretical construct for learning in the digital age. It employs a network with nodes and connections as a central metaphor for learning. In this metaphor, a node may be any entity, whether tangible or intangible, that can be connected to other nodes, including but not limited to information, data, feelings, and images. In connectivism, learning is the process of creating connections between nodes to form a network, a view that accurately mirrors the ways in which people engage in socialization and interaction in the Web 2.0 world through social networking sites and the "blogosphere." As in the knowledge creation metaphor, connectivism acknowledges the centrality of learning through the generation of ideas, supported by social activity, enabled by personal networks, interactivity, and engagement in experiential tasks.

NEW CONCEPTUALIZATIONS OF PEDAGOGY

Overall, emerging paradigms of learning and teaching emphasize the significance of individuals being able not only to find, identify, manipulate, and evaluate information and knowledge, but also to share in the knowledge production process. These paradigms view learners as active co-producers of knowledge rather than passive consumers of content, and learning is seen as a participatory, social, and networked process supporting personal life goals and needs. In assessing the value and impact of learning networks for learning and knowledge creation, researchers suggest that pedagogical innovation is needed,

and requires the development of learning episodes ... that have dialogue and communication as core features. From this perspective, there is a far greater emphasis on networked rather than linear models of learning and on providing culturally relevant experiential and purposeful learning episodes than the consumption of abstract knowledge (Rudd, Sutch, & Facer, 2006, p. 5).

The importance of integrating digital resources and social software tools stems from the fact that such resources are part of the knowledge society and economy, and are now woven into how we communicate, think, and generate knowledge and ideas in everyday life. While technology itself should not be the sole driving force for pedagogical change, changes in society are interconnected and intertwined with technology (Collis & Moonen, 2008). Thus, in the digital age and Web 2.0 world, fuelled by high connectivity and ubiquitous, demand-driven learning, we are beginning to see the growth of approaches and conceptualizations that enable us to expand our vision of pedagogy. Table 1 depicts a number of conceptualizations of pedagogy that resonate with or are representative of the new paradigms discussed in the previous section, and that are inspired and enabled by Web 2.0 and social software, along with their associated values and principles.

These terms signal changes in pedagogy from teacher-controlled, prescriptive, and didactic modes to learner-driven, social, collaborative, and participatory approaches to task design and learner engagement. However, rather than harnessing the technologies that are already integrated into learners' daily lives, educational institutions often take on a fortress mentality, "battening down the hatches" and excluding mobile technologies and social software tools that are considered disruptive or distracting. Being highly outcomes driven and assessment focused, many colleges and universities see learners not as active, critical participants in their own learning, but as passive consumers of information within LMSs where content is predetermined and learning pathways are limited.

If we consider and compare the conceptualizations of pedagogy depicted in Table 1 to the narrow, transmissive approaches that are often adopted in education, a number of discontinuities become apparent. The big change is happening in e-learning paradigms where new tools and software enable students to create, share, and showcase their own ideas and content. The learner is conceived of as mobile, active, and engaging with peers in collaborative knowledge generation. Downes (2005) notes that social software tools allow learning content to be created and distributed in ways that move beyond pre-packaged course content consumed by students, promoting the view that learning and the content associated with it

Table 1. Terms indicating innovative conceptualizations of pedagogy

Term	Source(s)	Description
Networked learning	Polsani, 2003	A "form of education whose site of production is the network," i.e., that enables lifelong and life-wide learning processes through connections and access to networks where there are multiple layers of information and knowledge.
E-learning 2.0	Downes, 2005	A new conceptualization of e-learning inspired and enabled by Web 2.0 technologies and practices. Conventional e-learning or "e-learning 1.0" systems and applications focused on the composition, organization, packaging, and delivery of instructional content. In contrast, in e-learning 2.0 content is syndicated for aggregation by students using their own personal tools and applications, from where it is remixed and repurposed with the students' own individual needs in mind. E-learning 2.0 also places increased emphasis on recognizing that learning is becoming a social and creative activity, and advocates the use of platforms for supporting learners' individual needs and choices as opposed to the imposition of particular applications chosen by teachers and administrators.
Social learning 2.0	Anderson, 2007b	Learning is essentially social and dialogic, and is no longer restricted to didactic modes of instruction. Social learning 2.0 emphasizes the benefits of learner engagement with social tools and reinforces the importance of community for learning in the modern age, conceptualizing it in terms of "groups," "networks," and "collectives" (see also Anderson, 2007a; Dron & Anderson, 2007).
Microlearning	Hug, Lindner, & Bruck, 2006; Lindner, 2006	Learning through relatively small learning units and short-term activities. Microlearning processes often derive from interaction with micro-content, which involves small chunks of learning content and flexible technologies that can enable learners to access them easily, anywhere, on demand and on the move. In a wider sense, it describes the way in which informal and incidental learning and knowledge acquisition are increasingly occurring through micro-content, micro-media, or multitasking environments, especially those that are based on Web 2.0 and mobile technologies.
Nanolearning	Masie, 2005, 2006	An analogue of nanotechnology. Similar to microlearning, in emphasizing the trend toward the atomization of learning beyond the learning object (Menell, 2005) to comprise personalized smaller units of information that can be learned and recombined. This ensures greater relevance for learners as well as enabling just-in-time learning to serve personal and work needs.
University 2.0	Barnes & Tynan, 2007	A new generation of universities using social computing technologies in an attempt to be more responsive to the needs and demands of millennial learners. These universities are reframing their focus so that they are no longer simply custodians of a fixed body of knowledge, but rather service providers through which students are connected to wider social, academic, and professional networks that are not confined to the institution, and in which both formal and informal learning occur.
Curriculum 2.0	Edson, 2007	Curriculum is negotiated, driven by learner needs, personalized, and based on assisting learners in developing skills in managing and accessing knowledge, as well as being in control of their own learning pathways and choices.

involve creative processes. Arguing along similar lines, Boettcher (2006) suggests that there is a need to carefully re-evaluate the role of content in courses, particularly given a tertiary education climate in which the value of textbooks and prescribed content is being questioned (Moore, 2003; Fink, 2005), and in which the open source and open content movements (Beshears, 2005; Massachusetts Institute of Technology, 2009; Multimedia Educational Resource for Learning and Online Teaching, 2009) are gaining momentum. Today's younger students perceive little value in the absorption or rote learning of factual information, given the accessibility and ease of use of search engines and web-based reference sites such as Google and Wikipedia (Berg et al., 2007; Oblinger, 2008). Instead, true educational value arguably lies in the enablement of personalized learning experiences that empower students to take charge of their learning journeys, collaborating with peers and experts and drawing on multiple sources both within and outside of the formal learning environment to produce their own ideas, content, and resources.

PEDAGOGY 2.0: A FRAMEWORK FOR INNOVATION

Evidence suggests that the boundaries of current pedagogies are being stretched and challenged by the potential offered by Web 2.0-based social software applications for dynamic, user-generated content, as well as by the ability of pervasive computing and wireless networking tools to ensure constant connectivity and participation in communities of learning and practice. With social software, there is a recognizable shift to include both formal and informal spaces for learning. As the tools afford greater learner autonomy and flexibility, the learning experience becomes more personalized and responsive, not only with respect to learners' goals, but also to their future needs in a knowledge-based society.

Earlier in this chapter, the importance of access to and use of social software tools and services was emphasized as these are integral to communicating and generating digital content in the knowledge society, while also enabling global collaboration and networking. The need for pedagogical innovation is urgent and immediate. As Richardson (2006b) remarks:

In an environment where it's easy to publish to the globe, it feels more and more hollow to ask students to "hand in" their homework to an audience of one. When we're faced with a flattening world where collaboration is becoming the norm, forcing students to work alone seems to miss the point. And when many of our students are already building networks far beyond our classroom walls, forming communities around their passions and their talents, it's not hard to understand why rows of desks and time-constrained schedules and standardized tests are feeling more and more limiting and ineffective. (para. 10)

We therefore propose a framework for innovative teaching and learning practices, *Pedagogy 2.0*, which capitalizes on the core energies and affordances of Web 2.0, while facilitating personal choice, participation and collaboration, and creative production. These overlapping elements are depicted in Figure 1.

Pedagogy 2.0 is envisioned as an overarching concept for an emerging cluster of practices that favor learner choice and self-direction, and engagement in flexible, relevant learning tasks and strategies. Though it is intended neither as a prescriptive framework nor a technology-driven mandate for change, it distills a number of guidelines characterizing effective learning environments, such as choice of resources, tasks, learning supports, and communication modalities. Each of the core elements, that is, the three Ps of personalization, participation, and productivity, can be applied to teacher and student roles and enable transformation and extension of current practices.

Participation as an Element of Pedagogy 2.0

More engaging, socially based models for teaching and learning are needed to replace the traditional, "closed classroom" models, which place emphasis on the institution and instructor. A defining feature of Pedagogy 2.0 is that alongside the increased socialization of learning and teaching, there is a focus on a less prescriptive curriculum and a shift toward student–teacher partnerships, with teachers as co-learners or associates in the learning process (Eustace, 2003; Lee, 2005). As such, this element of Pedagogy 2.0 is reflective of the "participation" as opposed to the "acquisition" model of learning (Sfard, 1998). In the words of Lee (2005):

we have already managed to overcome the confines of the physical classroom, but ... still remain unknowing prisoners of the instructor-centred online classroom. To move further ahead, we will need to demolish these virtual walls so as to create social learning spaces, in which learners and ... [instructors] ... become associates in a

Figure 1. Key elements of Pedagogy 2.0

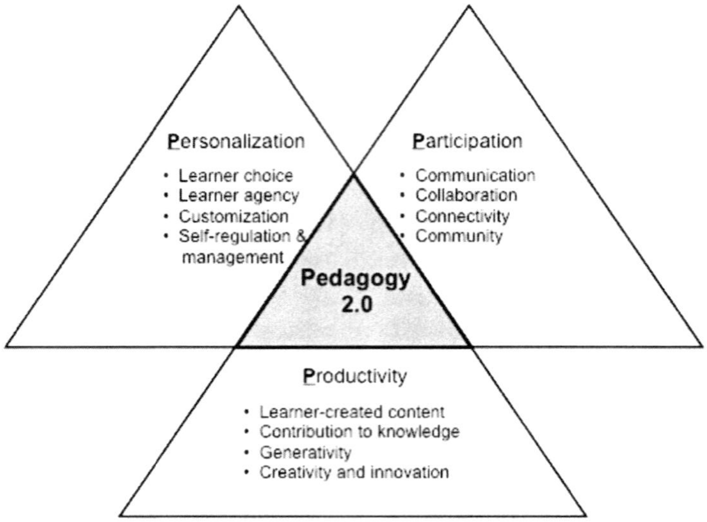

community of practice, participating in networks of interaction that transcend the old-fashioned constructs of institutions and organisations. (p. 17)

While the use of popular social software technology in itself is of value in motivating learners, the tools also allow learners to engage deeply with their peers, instructors, other subject-matter experts, and the community at large. The additional connectivity achieved by linking people, tools, and data is part of an emerging global network or "architecture of participation" (O'Reilly, 2005; Barsky & Purdon, 2006). Pedagogy 2.0 therefore adds a further dimension to participative learning by increasing the level of socialization and collaboration with peer groups, experts, and community, and by fostering connections that go beyond the walls of the classroom or institution.

Personalization as an Element of Pedagogy 2.0

Pedagogy 2.0 challenges university and college teachers to harness the many resources that exist outside the formal spaces of the institution to foster authentic learning that is personally meaningful and relevant to learners, and to capitalize on the interests and digital literacy skills that learners already possess. It is widely accepted that learning effectiveness can be improved by giving the learner control over, and responsibility for, his or her own learning; this is the foundation for such approaches as problem-based and inquiry-based learning (Desharnais & Limson, 2007). Indeed, the notion of personalized learning is fundamentally not new to educators and is often linked to the term "learner-centered" education, a desirable state in which learners know how to choose and make decisions relating to their personal learning needs. Even so, there continue to be significant gaps and differences in the espoused and enacted constructivist pedagogies of teachers (Lim & Chai, 2007).

By harnessing digital technologies and social software tools, three key areas pivotal to the development of personalization through teaching are summarized by Green, Facer, Rudd, Dillon, and Humphreys (2005). According to them, pedagogy must:

- ensure that learners are capable of making informed educational decisions;
- diversify and recognize different forms of skills and knowledge;
- include learner-focused forms of feedback and assessment.

The ability to study online already affords students a degree of personalization, as they can access resources aligned to their own needs and interests, at times and in places of their choosing. Furthermore, Web 2.0 and social software tools enable even greater levels of choice and allow learners to make decisions about which tools best suit their goals and needs for connection and social interaction. Apart from choosing which resources and sites to subscribe and contribute to, which tools to use, and how and where to use them, we are witnessing a shift in the modalities of expression that are now available. Text alone is not always the preferred mode of communication, as web-based multimedia production and distribution tools incorporating rich audio (podcasting, Skype), photo (Flickr), and video (vodcasting, YouTube) capabilities are growing. There is much scope to cater to the preferences, abilities, and learning styles of students through these different modalities. The ultimate challenge for educators is to enable learner autonomy, agency, and control through the provision of flexible options and choice, while still ensuring that students have access to timely and appropriate forms of support and scaffolding (Dron, 2007; McLoughlin & Lee, 2010).

A promising area of development in e-learning that has been the subject of much ongoing discussion and investigation is centered around the notion of the personal learning environment (PLE—see for example Liber & Johnson, 2008; Barrett & Garrett, 2009; Syed-Khuzzan, Goulding, & Underwood, 2008). According to Siemens (2007), a PLE is "a collection of tools, brought together under the conceptual notion of openness, interoperability, and learner control" (para. 2). The PLE concept represents the latest step toward an alternative approach to e-learning. Unlike LMSs, which take a course-centric view and result in online learning environments set firmly in frameworks and decisions made by teachers and administrators, PLEs are learner centric (Attwell, 2007). The idea is to give learners greater control over their own learning experiences, and to support a wider variety of learning practices, tools, and resources than is currently employed. To this end, PLEs allow learners to shape and mold their own "personal learning landscapes" (Tosh & Werdmuller, 2005) by acting as platform for them to select and customize their own learning toolsets according to their individual needs, priorities, circumstances, and contexts (Downes, 2005). In a PLE, it is the learner, not the teacher, educational technologist, or institution, who has primary control over the tools available and the ways in which they can be used. (Chapter 5 of this book includes further coverage of PLEs, their design, and the implications for learner personalization and choice.)

Productivity as an Element of Pedagogy 2.0

The knowledge creation metaphor of learning (Paavola & Hakkarainen, 2005), discussed earlier, acknowledges that in addition to acquiring knowledge and participating in learning activities, students are also capable of creating and generating new and original ideas, concepts, and knowledge. In the Web 2.0 era, the importance of enabling and encouraging this form of creativity and productivity is of prime significance. Educators are beginning to realize that teacher-supplied content has limitations, particularly if it preempts learner discovery, research, and active student involvement in the knowledge creation process.

In the past, content created by students in formal tertiary education contexts has generally been restricted to essays, papers, and reports used to demonstrate their absorption and/or understanding of content selected and developed by teachers, instructional designers, and textbook authors (Sener,

2007a). Even since the advent of e-learning, such student work products have typically been presented only to an audience of one (the teacher); this is clearly incongruent with the open culture of personal publishing (Downes, 2004) and does not take advantage of the outpouring of digital user-generated content between peers, groups, and networks now occurring on the Web. Learners can now engage in creative authorship by being able to produce and manipulate digital images and video clips, tag them with chosen keywords, and make both the media content and metadata available to their friends and peers worldwide through Flickr and YouTube. Many individuals create and maintain Facebook or MySpace profiles, while others write blogs and build wiki spaces where like-minded people comment on, improve, and augment the contributions of peers and fellow community members, all of which are examples of the new genre of dynamic, self-published content.

The importance and value of promoting innovative forms of knowledge creation and productivity enabled by Web 2.0 and social software tools are thus becoming increasingly apparent in tertiary education. In addition to completed project/assignment work or deliverables, student-generated content may also incorporate evidence of the process of learning that is representative of the complexity and "messiness" of problem-based learning, such as successive attempts at a task or drafts of solutions, descriptions of mistakes made, and/or difficulties encountered. Such "interactive, spontaneous 'performance' content" (Boettcher, 2006, "How much content do we need?," para. 4) in multiple media forms can now be easily captured *in situ* within the real-world or authentic contexts where knowledge construction naturally occurs, to be shared with others both internal and external to the formal education environment, thanks to the power and ubiquity of social software tools. Moreover, with "Mobile Web 2.0" or "Mobile 2.0," the wireless connectivity and data gathering capabilities of modern wireless mobile devices (e.g., photo blogging, video recording, voice recording, text input) can be used by learners to further simplify, accelerate, and enhance peer-to-peer content creation and distribution processes (Cochrane, 2008; see also Chapter 10 of this book for more on Mobile 2.0).

In addition to the above examples, student-generated content may include chat and instant messaging logs, reflective writing in the form of diaries or blog posts, as well as syntheses, summaries, and reviews, created by students working individually or cooperatively in teams. Finally, it may encompass "found" content, such as the results of students' own wide reading and exploration of web sites, journals, magazines, blogs, video clips, and podcasts that they bring to and share with one another in the learning environment.

All in all, Web 2.0 empowers "the people formerly known as the audience" to contribute ideas and content (Rosen, 2006, para. 1), which has both important implications and promising potential for tertiary teaching and learning. However, it is noteworthy that while the end *products* of student content generation are likely to be of value to the learner, peers, and future student cohorts, not to mention a wider Internet community, it is debatably the creative and generative *processes* involved and the knowledge construction that occurs that are of chief import in terms of preparing students for work and life in the Web 2.0 era (Boettcher, 2006).

IMPLEMENTING AND REALIZING PEDAGOGY 2.0

Current Examples of Pedagogy 2.0

The three Ps of Pedagogy 2.0 may be used not only as a conceptual framework for designing learning experiences and interventions, but also as a means of examining and evaluating the innovative practices of tertiary teachers across the globe who are making use of Web 2.0 and social software tools in innovative, learner-centered ways. Three brief examples are presented in this subsection to demonstrate how this can be done. Indeed, the three Ps are exhibited by many of the examples showcased in Section 2 of this book, in a multitude of different ways—It is hoped that the model will serve as a useful lens through which to view and analyze the examples appearing in the present publication, as well as those observed or encountered by readers in their day-to-day experiences and practice.

The first example of the three Ps of Pedagogy 2.0 in action involves second-year undergraduate information technology students at Charles Sturt University, Australia, who produce short, three-to-five-minute talkback radio-style podcasts for pre-class listening by first-year students enrolled in a subject that the second-year students successfully completed in an earlier semester (Lee, Chan, & McLoughlin, 2006; Chan & Lee, 2005). This is an innovative form of peer teaching, whereby the brainstorming of script ideas as well as design, editing, and recording of the podcasts is driven by student producers (productivity), with minimal teacher intervention in the process. By engaging in active dialogue and exchange and participating in collaborative peer review/critique of podcast scripts (participation), the student producers extend and adapt content for distribution to an audience of peers. Both the student producers and student listeners are afforded a high degree of choice, with the former group being able to determine the topics for the podcasts based on their previous experience studying the subject, and the latter group being able to decide how to use the content to support their study, as well as consuming the content at times and places of their choosing, using a range of devices including mobile/portable devices with MP3 playback capabilities (personalization).

In another example in which the three Ps are manifested, Dr. Kenneth Mentor of the University of North Carolina at Pembroke (UNCP), USA makes use of a wiki-based encyclopedia in his courses, with the goal being for students to create and maintain encyclopedia entries on a variety of subjects related to law, criminal justice, sociology, and criminology (Mentor, 2005; Sener, 2007c). In previous courses, Mentor's students authored web pages as class assignments; the *Online Encyclopedia of Criminal Justice* (2009) project extends those efforts in two notably powerful ways: firstly, using a wiki allows content created by students to be readily shared in virtual "public spaces" and to a broader audience beyond the classroom walls, and secondly, the wiki's ease of use enables the creation of substantial amounts of content within a short timeframe (productivity). In addition to generating and entering initial content, students also perform the roles of editing, revising, and organizing the content, which becomes part of the shared pools of resources accessible to all learners. Learners have a great deal of autonomy and choice in determining when, where, and how to contribute to the collection of information on the wiki, as well as deciding which topics or entries to create, read, add to, and/or modify (personalization). Although UNCP students initially wrote all content, the site is now available for educators to use for class assignments, and users outside the university are allowed to register and contribute. In this way, Mentor's students are active participants not only in the context of the course they are studying, but also in a wider, academic and professional community that transcends the boundaries of the classroom and institution in which they are based (participation).

The third and final example of Pedagogy 2.0 hails from the health sciences domain, where students at Mt. San Jacinto College, also in the USA, use the social networking site Ning to facilitate a project related to drug use and abuse (Helms, 2007a, 2007b; D. Helms, personal communication). Operating in groups, they each take on one of four roles: Web Designer, Multimedia Designer, Researcher, and Copyrighter, and work collaboratively to research a specific drug with the goal of creating Web 2.0-based web pages to teach others about the dangers associated with that drug (productivity). Ning allows the students to integrate various forms of multimedia in personalized ways (personalization) by drawing on the vast resources already published on the Web, for example in image libraries and on media sharing sites such as YouTube, without the need to learn complex web authoring and programming techniques. The students also use the blogging and threaded discussion features of Ning to engage in constructive and reflective discourse (participation) about the content they have produced.

Potential Problems and Pitfalls

While there are many signs of optimism and promise, it is vital to appreciate that the implementation of a Pedagogy 2.0 approach is not without its issues and challenges. Research has shown that many tertiary education students currently lack the competencies necessary to navigate and select relevant sources from the overabundance of information available (Katz & Macklin, 2007). In the age of personal publishing and user-generated content, essential digital literacy and information fluency skills are required to locate quality sources and assess them for objectivity and currency. Students need to develop expertise and confidence in finding, evaluating, creating, and sharing ideas, which often calls for complex critical thinking (Brown, 2005; Lorenzo & Dziuban, 2006). Fortunately, evidence is mounting that in combination with appropriate instructional strategies, the use of social software can lead to opportunities for higher-order thinking and metacognitive development (e.g., Miller, 2006; Sener, 2007b; Lee et al., 2006; McLoughlin, Lee, & Chan, 2006). Moreover, in fostering learning processes that encourage student-generated content there is still a need for gatekeepers and quality assurance mechanisms to maximize the validity and reliability of such content, however moving beyond teacher-centered models of evaluation and assessment, the review, editing, and quality assurance of the content can be done collaboratively and in partnership with learners, while simultaneously drawing on input from the wider community (i.e., evaluation based on the "wisdom of crowds").

Other issues and challenges lie in the area of assessment (see also Chapter 17), where educators and institutions must take steps to ensure that academic integrity and rigor are maintained, while promoting learner engagement and the development of activities, tools, and processes that are effective and efficient for both students and academics. In participating in emerging forms of collaborative authorship and self-expression for academic purposes, students must be made aware of the expectations in terms of originality and acknowledgment/attribution of ideas, including citation of sources of scholarship (Oblinger, 2007). A dilemma here is that established practices such as the major referencing standards and styles, as well as the associated marking and feedback practices adopted by tertiary teachers, are scarcely applicable and in some cases inapplicable to the dynamic capabilities and features of Web 2.0 (Gray, Thompson, Clerehan, Sheard, & Hamilton, 2008). Both students and staff require assistance and guidance in moving forward, and further progress to this end is contingent on appropriate policies and procedures being devised and implemented at the institutional and sectoral levels, albeit with input from stakeholders at all levels. Universities and colleges still appear to be battling to find solutions to Internet plagiarism and other problems of academic misconduct belonging to earlier era (Darbyshire & Burgess, 2006). For example, in the U.S., recently-enacted legislation mandates that any tertiary distance or correspondence education provider must "have processes through which the institution establishes that the student … is the same student who participates in and completes the program and receives the academic credit" (Higher Education Opportunity Act, 2008, §495); this is being interpreted by many to necessitate the introduction of costly, complex, and potentially invasive technological mechanisms for student authentication. Meanwhile, tertiary education is being surpassed by Web 2.0 innovations and is missing out on opportunities to leverage the new tools and technologies to provide meaningful and relevant learning and assessment experiences for students. There is a need to reframe the discussion to focus on pedagogical strategies, instructional design, and curricular approaches to avoiding academic dishonesty (Journal of Online Learning and Teaching, 2009; Pilati & Perry, 2009).

A related issue is that in the Web 2.0 age and in attempting to achieve the goals of Pedagogy 2.0, there is much onus on tertiary education institutions, government agencies, and accrediting bodies to formulate policies and strategies to deal with questions that arise in relation to copyright and ownership. The issues of identification and preservation of student work in the online environment (or more specifically, on the wider Internet) must also be carefully and systematically tackled. Overall, university leaders must act swiftly to address the four important yet potentially conflicting areas of institutional quality identified by Collis and Moonen (2008): major accreditation frameworks, external stakeholders' expectations, endorsement of learning resources and activities, and concerns in regard to intellectual property.

Further extant challenges have to do with fairness and equity considerations. It cannot simply be assumed or taken as given that all students have access to Web 2.0 technologies and pedagogies; while a key rationale behind the use of these technologies and pedagogies in an academic setting is the building of community and promotion of inclusivity, there may in fact be adverse effects in this regard if certain individuals or groups of students do not have the necessary technical tools and infrastructure at their disposal, or if they lack the requisite skills to operate the technology. There exists a real risk of creating new digital divides and deepening existing ones if measures are not implemented to ensure that these students are not unfairly disadvantaged, or their interests marginalized in any way.

Last but not least, tertiary educators may not be fully aware of the potential and range of social software tools, and may need opportunities for professional development to reveal how Web 2.0 applications can support teaching and assessment in meaningful and authentic ways. They must avoid basing curricular and instructional design decisions on broad generalizations and extrapolations of anecdotal observations of their students' preferences, attitudes, and behaviors (Kennedy et al., 2008; Lee & Chan, 2007), or worse still, on short-term or fleeting trends and technological innovations (Salaberry, 2001; Joyes 2005/2006). Tertiary educators must be wary of potential safety, security, and privacy issues involved in the use of Web 2.0 tools, while also being cognizant that they may feel unwelcome in their students' online social networks and communities. While the educators endeavor to exploit technologies students use in their day-to-day lives with the hope of enhancing their formal learning experiences, such attempts may be perceived by the students as intrusions into "their space" (Green & Hannon, 2007). In other words, students may exhibit unanticipated, polarized, or less than favorable reactions when educational uses of social networking are formalized and assessed (Ipsos MORI, 2008).

CONCLUSION: FUTURE LEARNING LANDSCAPES INFORMED BY THE PRINCIPLES OF PEDAGOGY 2.0

Current educational and social research is making an increasingly strong case for a conceptualization of learning as networked, collaborative, and social activity, supported by a range of ICT affordances, including those provided by Web 2.0-based social software tools. While the adoption of these social software tools may provide opportunities to meet the increasingly diverse needs of institutions and learners, they may also be used to support both local communities and wider professional contexts, facilitating lifelong and life-wide learning. These next-generation practices provide an opportunity for tertiary education institutions to look at wider implementation issues around technical infrastructure, but they must also address pedagogical challenges such as the integration of informal learning experiences, the limitations of existing physical and virtual learning environments, and the personalization of learning experiences. There may be a culture shock and/or skills crisis when "old world" educators are confronted with the expectation of working in unfamiliar environments and scenarios, using tools with which they lack expertise and confidence. For these reasons, there is a need to make time for talking, awareness raising, and discussion of what pedagogic approaches and tools work best for achieving the desired learning outcomes.

In summary, Web 2.0 and social software tools can be used to promote learner autonomy and increased levels of socialization and interactivity, while enabling user-controlled, peer-to-peer knowledge creation and network-based inquiry. The authors envision that the affordances of these technologies, coupled with a paradigm of learning focused on knowledge creation and networking, offer the potential for transformational shifts in teaching and learning practices, whereby learners can access peers, experts, the wider community, and digital media in ways that enable reflective, self-directed learning. Nonetheless, it must be recognized that technology is not of itself the sole driver of pedagogical change. Furthermore, Web 2.0 is part of a constellation of broader environmental factors that includes but is not limited to changing student expectations and demographics and institutional pressures for improved, innovative, and cost-efficient modes of teaching. There are promising signs that existing Pedagogy 2.0 practices, by capitalizing on the three Ps of personalization, participation, and productivity, will result in a learning landscape and a diverse range of educational experiences that are socially contextualized, engaging, and community based.

However, obstacles and barriers remain. Web 2.0, Pedagogy 2.0, and the new views of learning they encapsulate and espouse are likely to be met by resistance and inertia. Can tertiary teachers and administrators, whose traditional frame of reference is formality, comprehend the value of informal, non-formal, and incidental learning that takes place through social networking and beyond the formal spaces of lecture halls, libraries, and laboratories? Can they extend these formal spaces to link with dynamic and open communities that are constantly sharing, revising, and creating new ideas? Can academia, with its established legacy of transmissive pedagogy, rise to the challenge and effect the kind of teaching revolution and changes that are both necessary and inevitable in the new age? The goal is to facilitate learning, be less prescriptive, and be open to new media, tools, and strategies, while nurturing innovation and creativity, independent inquiry, and the development and refinement of new literacy skills. This can be achieved by employing the tools, resources, and opportunities that can leverage what our students do naturally and spontaneously—socialize, network, and collaborate. Overall, for the principles of Pedagogy 2.0 to come to fruition, institutional change is needed to dissolve educational silos and equip educators with the desire, skills, and facilities to enable them to be responsive to learner needs, while encouraging learners themselves to become active associates or partners in co-creating pathways that will give them the skills and competencies needed to be successful in the networked age.

In describing the wave of social and technological changes affecting higher education, Hilton (2006) uses two competing metaphors to depict the challenges of the Web 2.0 era: "a perfect storm, born from the convergence of numerous disruptive forces … [and] the dawn of a new day, a sunrise rife with opportunities arising from these same disruptive forces" (p. 59). Taking a positive view, we believe that change is imminent and unavoidable; student-driven demand, coupled with a new approach to pedagogy that leverages the flexibilities and creative options of Web 2.0 and social software tools, can and is already beginning to make the teaching and learning process much more dynamic, creative, and generative. As evidenced in the examples throughout this book, there is a great deal of innovation and experimentation with social software on an international scale, and many educators are transforming their pedagogy to create learning experiences that are participatory, personalized, and geared to the production of digital knowledge artifacts by learners that can be shared in social contexts that might otherwise be minimal in traditional teacher-centered classrooms or within the confines of the "walled garden" of an institutionally-controlled LMS.

Pedagogy 2.0 therefore enables new pathways to learning with peers and connections to the wider community to flourish, and makes active, self-directed, self-managed learning a reality. Success in the knowledge economy demands that we exploit the educational value of Web 2.0 and social software to promote student-generated content and foster the cultivation of digital competencies in ways that allow learners to develop their critical thinking, knowledge-building, and creative skills.

REFERENCES

Anderson, T. (2004). Toward a theory of online learning. In Anderson, T., & Elloumi, F. (Eds.), *Theory and practice of online learning* (pp. 33–60). Athabasca, AB: Athabasca University.

Anderson, T. (2007a, April 30). On groups, networks and collectives [Web log post]. *Virtual Canuck*. Retrieved July 2, 2007, from http://terrya.edublogs.org/2007/04/30/on-groups-networks-and-collectives/

Anderson, T. (2007b, June 25–29). *Social Learning 2.0*. Keynote paper presented at World Conference on Educational Multimedia, Hypermedia, and Telecommunications 2007, Vancouver, BC. Retrieved June 27, 2007, from http://www.slideshare.net/terrya/educational-social-software-edmedia-2007/

Attwell, G. (2007). Personal learning environments: The future of e-learning? *eLearning Papers, 2*(1). Retrieved December 11, 2007, from www.elearningeuropa.info/files/media/media11561.pdf

Barnes, C., & Tynan, B. (2007). The adventures of Miranda in the brave new world: Learning in a Web 2.0 millennium. *ALT-J Research in Learning Technology*, *15*(3), 189–200.

Barrett, H. C., & Garrett, N. (2009). Online personal learning environments: Structuring electronic portfolios for lifelong and life-wide learning. *Horizon*, *17*(2), 142–152. doi:10.1108/10748120910965511

Barsky, E., & Purdon, M. (2006). Introducing Web 2.0: Social networking and social bookmarking for health librarians. *Journal of the Canadian Health Libraries Association, 27*(3), 65–67. Retrieved March 29, 2008, from http://article.pubs.nrc-cnrc.gc.ca/RPAS/RPViewDoc?_handler_=HandleInitialGet&calyLang=eng&journal=jchla&volume=27&articleFile=c06-024.pdf

Bereiter, C. (2002). *Education and mind in the knowledge age*. Mahwah, NJ: Lawrence Erlbaum.

Berg, J., Berquam, L., & Christoph, K. (2007). Social networking technologies: A "poke" for campus services. *EDUCAUSE Review, 42*(2), 32–44. Retrieved February 3, 2008, from http://educause.edu/ir/library/pdf/erm0721.pdf

Beshears, F. M. (2005, October 4). Viewpoint: The economic case for creative commons textbooks. *Campus Technology*. Retrieved March 10, 2007, from http://campustechnology.com/articles/40535/

Bleed, R. (2001). A hybrid campus for the new millennium. *EDUCAUSE Review, 36*(1), 17–24. Retrieved January 20, 2008, from http://net.educause.edu/ir/library/pdf/erm0110.pdf

Boettcher, J. V. (2006, February 28). The rise of student performance content. *Campus Technology*. Retrieved November 10, 2009, from http://campustechnology.com/Articles/2006/02/The-Rise-of-Student-Performance-Content.aspx?p=1

Boyd, D. (2007). The significance of social software. In Burg, T. N., & Schmidt, J. (Eds.), *BlogTalks reloaded: Social software research & cases* (pp. 15–30). Norderstedt, Germany: Books on Demand.

Brown, J. S., & Duguid, P. (2000). *The social life of information*. Boston: Harvard Business School Press.

Brown, T. H. (2005). Beyond constructivism: Exploring future learning paradigms. *Education Today, 2005*(2). Retrieved January 11, 2006, from http://www.bucks.edu/IDlab/Beyond_constructivism.pdf

Brown, T. H. (2006). Beyond constructivism: Exploring future learning paradigms. *Horizon, 14*(3), 108–120. doi:10.1108/10748120610690681

Bryant, L. (2007). Emerging trends in social software for education. In *Emerging technologies for learning* (Vol. 2, pp. 9–18). Coventry, UK: Becta. Retrieved October 28, 2008, from http://partners.becta.org.uk/upload-dir/downloads/page_documents/research/emerging_technologies07_chapter1.pdf

Bryant, T. (2006). Social software in academia. *EDUCAUSE Quarterly, 29*(2), 61–64. Retrieved March 14, 2008, from http://net.educause.edu/ir/library/pdf/eqm0627.pdf

Carrick Institute for Learning and Teaching in Higher Education. (2007). *Places & spaces for learning seminars*. (Draft report). Retrieved November 13, 2009, from http://www.altc.edu.au/system/files/resources/Consolidated%20Report%20P%20%20S%20Seminars%20without%20slides%20ref%20v%200%205%20_5_.pdf

Chan, A., & Lee, M. J. W. (2005). An MP3 a day keeps the worries away: Exploring the use of podcasting to address preconceptions and alleviate pre-class anxiety amongst undergraduate information technology students. In D. H. R. Spennemann & L. Burr (Eds.), *Good practice in practice: Proceedings of the Student Experience Conference* (pp. 58–70). Wagga Wagga, Australia: Charles Sturt University. Retrieved November 30, 2005, from http://www.csu.edu.au/division/studserv/sec/papers/chan.pdf

Cochrane, T. (2008). Mobile Web 2.0: The new frontier. In R. Atkinson & C. McBeath (Eds.), *Hello! Where are you in the landscape of educational technology? Proceedings of the 25th Australasian Society for Computers in Learning in Tertiary Education (ASCILITE) Conference* (pp. 177–186). Melbourne, Australia: Deakin University. Retrieved December 3, 2008, from http://www.ascilite.org.au/conferences/melbourne08/procs/cochrane.pdf

Collis, B., & Moonen, J. (2008). Web 2.0 tools and processes in higher education: Quality perspectives. *Educational Media International, 45*(2), 93–106. doi:10.1080/09523980802107179

Conole, G., & Dyke, M. (2004). What are the affordances of information and communication technologies? *ALT-J Research in Learning Technology, 12*(2), 113–124.

Darbyshire, P., & Burgess, S. (2006). Strategies for dealing with plagiarism and the Web in higher education. *Journal of Business Systems, Governance and Ethics, 1*(4), 27–39. Retrieved April 2, 2007, from http://www.jbsge.vu.edu.au/issues/vol01no4/Darbyshire-Burgess.pdf

Desharnais, R. A., & Limson, M. (2007). Designing and implementing virtual courseware to promote inquiry-based learning. *Journal of Online Learning and Teaching, 3*(1), 30–39. Retrieved October 11, 2007, from http://jolt.merlot.org/vol3no1/desharnais.pdf

Downes, S. (2004). Educational blogging. *EDUCAUSE Review, 39*(5), 14–26. Retrieved January 21, 2007, from http://net.educause.edu/ir/library/pdf/ERM0450.pdf

Downes, S. (2005, October). E-learning 2.0. *eLearn Magazine*. Retrieved January 11, 2006, from http://www.elearnmag.org/subpage.cfm?section=articles&article=29-1

Downes, S. (2007). Learning networks in practice. In *Emerging technologies for learning* (Vol. 2, pp. 19–27). Coventry, UK: Becta. Retrieved October 28, 2008, from http://partners.becta.org.uk/upload-dir/downloads/page_documents/research/emerging_technologies07_chapter2.pdf

Dron, J. (2007). *Control and constraint in e-learning: Choosing when to choose*. Hershey, PA: Information Science Publishing.

Dron, J., & Anderson, T. (2007). Collectives, networks and groups in social software for e-learning. In T. Bastiaens & S. Carliner (Eds.), *Proceedings of World Conference on E-Learning in Corporate, Government, Healthcare, and Higher Education 2007* (pp. 2460–2467). Chesapeake, VA: Association for the Advancement of Computers in Education.

Edson, J. (2007, June 25). Curriculum 2.0: User-driven education. *The Huffington Post*. Retrieved December 10, 2007, from http://www.huffingtonpost.com/jonathan-edson/curriculum-20-userdri_b_53690.html

Eisenstadt, M. (2007). Does Elearning have to be so awful? (Time to mashup or shutup). In J. M. Spector, D. G. Sampson, T. Okamoto, Kinshuk, S. A. Cerri, M. Ueno, & A. Kashihara (Eds.), *Proceedings of the Seventh International Conference on Advanced Learning Technologies* (pp. 6–10). Los Alamitos, CA: IEEE Computer Society.

Engeström, J. (2005a, June 10–11). *Object-centered sociality*. Paper presented at Reboot 7, Copenhagen. Retrieved July 23, 2008, from http://aula.org/people/jyri/presentations/reboot7-jyri.pdf

Engeström, J. (2005b, April 13). Why some social network services work and others don't—Or: the case for object-centered sociality [Web log post]. *Zengestrom.com*. Retrieved July 23, 2008, from http://www.zengestrom.com/blog/2005/04/why_some_social.html

Engeström, Y. (1987). *Learning by expanding*. Helsinki: Orienta-Konsultit Oy.

Engeström, Y. (1999). Innovative learning in work teams: Analyzing cycles of knowledge creation in practice. In Engeström, Y., Miettinen, R., & Punamäki, R.-L. (Eds.), *Perspectives on Activity Theory* (pp. 377–404). Cambridge, UK: Cambridge University Press.

Eshet-Alkalai, Y. (2004). Digital literacy: A conceptual framework for survival skills in the digital era. *Journal of Educational Multimedia and Hypermedia, 13*(1), 93–106.

Eustace, K. (2003). Educational value of e-learning in conventional and complementary computing education. In S. Mann & A. Williamson (Eds.), *Proceedings of the 16th Annual Conference of the National Advisory Committee on Computing Qualifications* (pp. 53–62). Hamilton, New Zealand: NACCQ.

Fink, L. (2005, September 16). Making textbooks worthwhile. *Chronicle of Higher Education*. Retrieved March 10, 2007, from http://chronicle.com/weekly/v52/i04/04b01201.htm

Ganley, B. (2004, October 11). Images, words and students finding their way [Web log post]. *Bgblogging*. Retrieved November 19, 2009, from http://bgblogging.com/2004/10/11/images-words-and-students-finding-their-way/

Gee, J. P. (2003). *What video games have to teach us about learning and literacy*. New York: Palmgrave.

Gibson, J. J. (1977). The theory of affordances. In Shaw, R., & Bransford, J. (Eds.), *Perceiving, acting, and knowing: Toward an ecological psychology* (pp. 67–82). Hillsdale, NJ: Lawrence Erlbaum.

Gibson, J. J. (1979). *The ecological approach to visual perception*. Boston: Houghton Mifflin.

Goodman, E., & Moed, A. (2006, November 4–8). *Community in mashups: The case of personal geodata*. Paper presented at the 20th ACM Conference on Computer Supported Cooperative Work, Banff, AB. Retrieved March 19, 2008, from http://mashworks.net/images/5/59/Goodman_Moed_2006.pdf

Gray, K., Thompson, C., Clerehan, R., Sheard, J., & Hamilton, M. (2008). Web 2.0 authorship: Issues of referencing and citation for academic integrity. *The Internet and Higher Education, 11*(2), 112–118. doi:10.1016/j.iheduc.2008.03.001

Green, H., Facer, K., Rudd, T., Dillon, P., & Humphreys, P. (2005). *Personalisation and digital technologies*. Bristol, UK: Futurelab. Retrieved October 23, 2007, from http://www.futurelab.org.uk/resources/documents/opening_education/Personalisation_report.pdf

Green, H., & Hannon, C. (2007). *Their space: Education for a digital generation*. London: Demos. Retrieved December 2, 2007, from http://www.demos.co.uk/files/Their%20space%20-%20web.pdf

Heeren, E. S. (2007*). Exploring the new literacies: Instruction and assessment practices of middle school master teachers of Internet literacy*. Unpublished Ed.D. dissertation, The University of Memphis, Memphis, TN.

Helms, D. (2007a). *Drug use and abuse*. Retrieved November 2, 2007, from http://druguseandabuse.ning.com/

Helms, D. (2007b). *Group project*. Retrieved November 2, 2007, from http://www.msjc.edu/hs/hs123_group_project.html

Higher Education Opportunity Act of 2008, Pub. L. No. 110-315, 122 Stat. 3078 (2008).

Hilton, J. (2006). The future for higher education: Sunrise or perfect storm? *EDUCAUSE Review, 41*(2), 58–71. Retrieved January 19, 2008, from http://net.educause.edu/ir/library/pdf/erm0623.pdf

Hug, T., Lindner, M., & Bruck, P. A. (Eds.). (2006). *Microlearning: Emerging concepts, practices and technologies after e-Learning. Proceedings of Microlearning 2005: Learning & working in new media*. Innsbruck, Austria: Innsbruck University Press. Retrieved October 15, 2007, from http://www.microlearning.org/micropapers/microlearning2005_proceedings_digitalversion.pdf

Hughes, J., & Lang, K. (2006). Transmutability: Digital decontextualization, manipulation, and recontextualization as a new source of value in the production and consumption of culture products. In *Proceedings of the 39th Annual Hawaii International Conference on System Sciences* (p. 165a). Los Alamitos, CA: IEEE Computer Society.

Ipsos, M. O. R. I. (2007). *Student expectations study: Key findings from online research and discussion evenings held in June 2007 for the Joint Information Systems Committee*. London: JISC. Retrieved November 9, 2009, from http://www.jisc.ac.uk/media/documents/publications/studentexpectations.pdf

Joint Information Systems Committee. (2006). *Designing spaces for effective learning: A guide to 21st century learning space design*. Bristol, UK: JISC. Retrieved July 2, 2007, from http://www.jisc.ac.uk/media/documents/publications/learningspaces.pdf

Journal of Online Learning and Teaching. (2009). *Call for papers—Special issue: Integrity and identity authentication in online education*. Retrieved March 20, 2009, from http://jolt.merlot.org/special09.htm

Joyes, G. (2005/2006). When pedagogy leads technology. *The International Journal of Technology. Knowledge & Society, 1*(5), 107–113.

Katz, I. R., & Macklin, A. S. (2007). Information and communication technology (ICT) literacy: Integration and assessment in higher education. *Systemics, Cybernetics and Informatics, 5*(4), 50–55. Retrieved November 17, 2007, from http://www.iiisci.org/Journal/CV$/sci/pdfs/P890541.pdf

Kennedy, G., Dalgarno, B., Gray, K., Judd, T., Waycott, J., & Bennett, S. … Churchward, A. (2007). The Net Generation are not big users of Web 2.0 technologies: Preliminary findings. In R. Atkinson & C. McBeath (Eds.), *ICT: Providing choices for learners and learning. Proceedings of the 24th Australasian Society for Computers in Learning in Tertiary Education (ASCILITE) Conference* (pp. 517–525). Singapore: Nanyang Technological University. Retrieved January 12, 2008, from http://www.ascilite.org.au/conferences/singapore07/procs/kennedy.pdf

Kirschner, P. A. (2002). Can we support CSCL? Educational, social and technological affordances for learning. In Kirschner, P. A. (Ed.), *Three worlds of CSCL: Can we support CSCL?* (pp. 7–47). Heerlen, The Netherlands: Open University of the Netherlands.

Lamb, B. (2007). Dr Mashup; or, why educators should learn to stop worrying and love the remix. *EDUCAUSE Review, 42*(4), 12–25. Retrieved January 19, 2008, from http://net.educause.edu/ir/library/pdf/erm0740.pdf

Lankshear, C., & Knobel, M. (2007). Researching new literacies: Web 2.0 practices and insider perspectives. *E-learning, 4*(3), 224–240. doi:10.2304/elea.2007.4.3.224

Lave, J., & Wenger, E. (1991). *Situated learning: Legitimate peripheral participation*. Cambridge, UK: Cambridge University Press.

Leadbeater, C. (2006). *The ten habits of mass innovation*. London: National Endowment for Science, Technology and the Arts. Retrieved November 3, 2007, from http://www.nesta.org.uk/assets/pdf/ten_habits_of_mass_innovation_provocation_NESTA.pdf

Lee, M. J. W. (2005). New tools for online collaboration: Blogs, wikis, RSS and podcasting. *Training and Development in Australia, 32*(5), 17–20.

Lee, M. J. W., & Chan, A. (2007). Pervasive, lifestyle-integrated mobile learning for distance learners: An analysis and unexpected results from a podcasting study. *Open Learning, 22*(3), 201–218.

Lee, M. J. W., Chan, A., & McLoughlin, C. (2006). Students as producers: Second year students' experiences as podcasters of content for first year undergraduates. In *Proceedings of the Seventh Conference on Information Technology Based Higher Education and Training* (pp. 832–841). Broadway, Australia: University of Technology, Sydney.

Lee, M. J. W., Eustace, K., Hay, L., & Fellows, G. (2005). Learning to collaborate, collaboratively: An online community building and knowledge construction approach to teaching computer supported collaborative work at an Australian university. In M. R. Simonson & M. Crawford (Eds.), *Proceedings of the 2005 Association for Educational Communications and Technology International Convention* (pp. 286–306). North Miami Beach, FL: Nova Southeastern University.

Lee, M. J. W., McLoughlin, C., & Chan, A. (2008). Talk the talk: Learner-generated podcasts as catalysts for knowledge creation. *British Journal of Educational Technology*, *39*(3), 501–521. doi:10.1111/j.1467-8535.2007.00746.x

Liber, O., & Johnson, M. (2008). Personal learning environments [Special issue]. *Interactive Learning Environments*, *16*(1). doi:10.1080/10494820701772645

Lim, C. P., & Chai, C. S. (2007). Teachers' pedagogical beliefs and their planning and conduct of computer-mediated classroom lessons. *British Journal of Educational Technology*, *39*(5), 807–828. doi:10.1111/j.1467-8535.2007.00774.x

Lindner, M. (2006). Use these tools, your mind will follow. Learning in immersive micromedia and microknowledge environments. In D. Whitelock & S. Wheeler (Eds.), *The next generation: Research proceedings of the 13th Association for Learning Technology Conference* (pp. 41–49). Oxford, UK: ALT.

Lorenzo, G., & Dziuban, C. (2006). *Ensuring the Net Generation is net savvy*. Boulder, CO: EDUCAUSE. Retrieved July 10, 2007, from http://www.educause.edu/ir/library/pdf/ELI3006.pdf

Masie, E. (2005). *Nano-learning* [Podcast transcript]. Retrieved July 2, 2006, from http://www.masieweb.com/component/option,com_alphacontent/Itemid,122/section,9/cat,29/task,view/id,1321/

Masie, E. (2006). Nano-learning: Miniaturization of design. *Chief Learning Officer*, *5*(1), 17. Retrieved August 29, 2007, from http://www.clomedia.com/content/templates/clo_article.asp?articleid=1221

Massachusetts Institute of Technology. (2009). *About OCW*. Retrieved April 8, 2009, from http://ocw.mit.edu/OcwWeb/web/about/about/index.htm

McLoughlin, C., & Lee, M. J. W. (2010). Personalised and self-regulated learning in the Web 2.0 era: International exemplars of innovative pedagogy using social software. *Australasian Journal of Educational Technology, 26*(1), 28–43. Retrieved February 23, 2010, from http://www.ascilite.org.au/ajet/ajet26/mcloughlin.pdf

McLoughlin, C., Lee, M. J. W., & Chan, A. (2006). Using student-generated podcasts to foster reflection and metacognition. *Australian Educational Computing*, *21*(2), 34–40.

Mejias, U. (2005). A nomad's guide to learning and social software. *The Knowledge Tree: An e-Journal of Learning Innovation, 7*. Retrieved November 10, 2006, from http://knowledgetree.flexiblelearning.net.au/edition07/download/la_mejias.pdf

Menell, B. (2005, November). Atomization of learning (Beyond the learning object) [Web log post]. *Learning 2.0*. Retrieved January 8, 2006, from http://learning20.blogspot.com/2005/11/atomization-of-learning-beyond.html

Mentor, K. (2005, November 15–19). *The Online Encyclopedia of Criminal Justice*. Paper presented at the Annual Meeting of the American Society of Criminology, Toronto, ON.

Miller, D. B. (2006, October 18). Podcasting at the University of Connecticut: Enhancing the educational experience. *Campus Technology*. Retrieved April 10, 2007, from http://campustechnology.com/news_article.asp?id=19424&typeid=156

Milne, A. J. (2007). Entering the interaction age: Implementing a future vision for campus learning spaces. *EDUCAUSE Review, 42*(1), 12–31. Retrieved August 30, 2008, from *http://*net.educause.edu/ir/library/pdf/ERM0710.pdf

Moore, J. W. (2003). Are textbooks dispensable? *Journal of Chemical Education*, *80*(4), 359. doi:10.1021/ed080p359

Multimedia Educational Resource for Learning and Online Teaching. (2009). *About us*. Retrieved April 8, 2009, from http://taste.merlot.org/index.html

National School Boards Association. (2007). *Creating and connecting: Research and guidelines on online social—and educational—networking*. Alexandria, VA: National School Boards Association. Retrieved June 2, 2008, from http://www.nsba.org/site/docs/41400/41340.pdf

Nonaka, I., & Takeuchi, H. (1995). *The knowledge-creating company: How Japanese companies create the dynamics of innovation*. New York: Oxford University Press.

Nonaka, I., & Toyama, R. (2003). The knowledge-creating theory revisited: Knowledge creation as a synthesizing process. *Knowledge Management Research and Practice, 1*(1), 2–10. doi:10.1057/palgrave.kmrp.8500001

Norman, D. A. (1988). *The psychology of everyday things*. New York: Basic.

Norman, D. A. (1999). Affordance, conventions, and design. *Interaction, 6*(3), 38–43. doi:10.1145/301153.301168

O'Reilly, T. (2005). *What is Web 2.0: Design patterns and business models for the next generation of software*. Retrieved December 15, 2006, from http://www.oreillynet.com/pub/a/oreilly/tim/news/2005/09/30/what-is-web-20.html

Oblinger, D. G. (2007). Becoming net savvy. *EDUCAUSE Quarterly, 30*(3), 11–13. Retrieved November 14, 2008, from http://www.educause.edu/ir/library/pdf/eqm0731.pdf

Oblinger, D. G. (2008). Growing up with Google: What it means to education. In *Emerging technologies for learning* (Vol. 3, pp. 11–29). Coventry, UK: Becta. Retrieved November 2, 2009, from http://partners.becta.org.uk/upload-dir/downloads/page_documents/research/emerging_technologies08_chapter1.pdf

Online Encyclopedia of Criminal Justice. (2009). Retrieved November 19, 2009, from http://cjencyclopedia.com

Owen, M., Grant, L., Sayers, S., & Facer, K. (2006). *Social software and learning*. Bristol, UK: Futurelab. Retrieved April 11, 2007, from http://www.futurelab.org.uk/resources/documents/opening_education/Social_Software_report.pdf

Paavola, S., & Hakkarainen, K. (2005). The knowledge creation metaphor—An emergent epistemological approach to learning. *Science and Education, 14*(6), 535–557. doi:10.1007/s11191-004-5157-0

Pilati, M., & Perry, E. (Eds.). (2009). Integrity and identity authentication in online education [Special issue]. *Journal of Online Learning and Teaching, 5*(2). Retrieved November 8, 2009, from http://jolt.merlot.org/Vol5_No2.htm

Polsani, P. R. (2003). Network learning. In Nyíri, K. (Ed.), *Mobile learning: Essays on philosophy, psychology and education*. Vienna: Pasagen Verlag.

Richardson, W. (2006a). *Blogs, wikis, podcasts, and other powerful tools for classrooms*. Thousand Oaks, CA: Sage.

Richardson, W. (2006b). *The Internet breaks school walls down*. Retrieved November 3, 2007, from http://www.edutopia.org/new-face-learning

Rogers, P. C., Liddle, S. W., Chan, P., Doxey, A., & Isom, B. (2007). Web 2.0 learning platform: Harnessing collective intelligence. *Turkish Online Journal of Distance Education, 8*(3), 16–33. Retrieved December 20, 2007, from http://tojde.anadolu.edu.tr/tojde27/pdf/article_1.pdf

Rosen, J. (2006, June 27). The people formerly known as the audience [Web log post]. *PressThink*. Retrieved October 2, 2007, from http://journalism.nyu.edu/pubzone/weblogs/pressthink/2006/06/27/ppl_frmr.html

Rudd, T., Sutch, D., & Facer, K. (2006). *Towards new learning networks*. Bristol, UK: Futurelab. Retrieved July 5, 2007, from http://www.futurelab.org.uk/resources/documents/opening_education/Learning_Networks_report.pdf

Salaberry, M. R. (2001). The use of technology for second language learning and teaching: A retrospective. *Modern Language Journal*, *85*(1), 39–56. doi:10.1111/0026-7902.00096

Sener, J. (2007a). In search of student-generated content in online education. *e-mentor, 21*. Retrieved December 20, 2007, from http://www.e-mentor.edu.pl/_xml/wydania/21/467.pdf

Sener, J. (2007b). *University of Connecticut—Beyond lecturecasting: Using podcasts for discussion and student content creation*. Retrieved March 10, 2007, from http://www.sloan-c-wiki.org/wiki/index.php?title=University_of_Connecticut_--_Beyond_Lecturecasting:_Using_Podcasts_for_Discussion_and_Student_Content_Creation

Sener, J. (2007c). *University of North Carolina at Pembroke—cjencyclopedia.com: Online Encyclopedia of Criminal Justice*. Retrieved March 10, 2007, from http://www.sloan-c-wiki.org/wiki/index.php?title=University_of_North_Carolina_at_Pembroke_--_cjencyclopedia.com:_Online_Encyclopedia_of_Criminal_Justice

Sfard, A. (1998). On two metaphors for learning and the dangers of choosing just one. *Educational Researcher*, *27*(2), 4–13.

Siemens, G. (2005). Connectivism: A learning theory for the digital age. *International Journal of Instructional Technology and Distance Learning, 2*(1), 3–10. Retrieved October 2, 2007, from http://www.itdl.org/Journal/Jan_05/Jan_05.pdf

Siemens, G. (2007, April 15). PLEs—I acronym, therefore I exist [Web log post]. *elearnspace: learning, networks, knowledge, technology, community*. Retrieved November 1, 2007, from http://www.elearnspace.org/blog/archives/002884.html

Sims, R. (Ed.). (2006). Online distance education: New ways of learning; new modes of teaching? [Special issue]. *Distance Education*, *27*(2).

Surowiecki, J. (2004). *The wisdom of crowds: Why the many are smarter than the few and how collective wisdom shapes business, economies, societies, and nations*. New York: Doubleday.

Syed-Khuzzan, S. M., Goulding, J. S., & Underwood, J. (2009). Personalised learning environments—Part 1: Core development issues for construction. *Industrial and Commercial Training*, *40*(6), 310–319. doi:10.1108/00197850810900075

Tosh, D., & Werdmuller, B. (2004). *Creation of a learning landscape: Weblogging and social networking in the context of e-portfolios*. Retrieved October 30, 2009, from http://eduspaces.net/bwerdmuller/files/61/179/Learning_landscape.pdf

van Weert, T. J. (2006). Education of the twenty-first century: New professionalism in lifelong learning, knowledge development and knowledge sharing. *Education and Information Technologies, 11*(3/4), 217–237.

Ward, C. B. (2008). Information fluency: A literary review. *Journal for Computing Teachers, 1*(1). Retrieved May 9, 2009, from http://www.iste.org/Content/NavigationMenu/Membership/SIGs/SIGCS_Computer_Science_/JCTJournalforComputingTeachers/PastIssues/2008/Fall/Ward.pdf

Williams, J. B., & Jacobs, J. (2004). Exploring the use of blogs as learning spaces in the higher education sector. *Australasian Journal of Educational Technology, 20*(2), 232–247. Retrieved May 1, 2007, from http://www.ascilite.org.au/ajet/ajet20/williams.html

KEY TERMS AND DEFINITIONS

Affordance: A term coined by Gibson (1979) to refer to the functional properties that determine the possible utility of an object or environment. Norman (1988) argued that until an affordance is perceived it is of no utility to the potential user, and in his later work drew a distinction between "perceived affordances" and "real affordances" (Norman, 1999). The term is now increasingly used in educational contexts to describe the relationships between the properties of an educational intervention and the characteristics of the learner that enable certain kinds of learning to occur (Kirschner, 2002; see also Conole & Dyke, 2004).

Architecture of Participation: A term that describes the nature of innovation in the open source movement, whereby individuals can share, create, and amend software, thereby participating in the creation of improved forms of software. This can help turn a good idea or piece of software into a best-quality product as many users and developers can adapt, change, and improve it.

Blogosphere: A term used to describe the cultural and social milieu surrounding blogging and its users, conceived by observers who liken blogging communities to a large, intricate ecological network or biosphere. The blogosphere is an example of a web-based social network. See also social networking.

Collective Intelligence: A form of intelligence that results from the cooperation, collaboration, and/or competition of a large number of individuals.

Connectivism: An emerging theory of learning, based on the integration of principles explored by chaos, network, complexity, and self-organization theories. Developed by George Siemens with input from Stephen Downes, it defines learning as a process of forming connections between specialized nodes or information sources. Connectivism views the understanding of where to find knowledge when it is needed ("know where") as being equally important as declarative or propositional knowledge ("know what") and procedural knowledge ("know how"). It also emphasizes the centrality of meta-learning, that is, learning how to learn. See also navigationism.

Digital Literacy: Encompasses the knowledge and skills required to locate, understand, evaluate, organize, and create information in various forms using digital tools. While it implies a working knowledge of current technology, it transcends the technical aspects to incorporate the ability to select and use digital information and information sources to achieve particular goals or outcomes. In the information age and knowledge economy, digitally literate people are better placed to communicate and work efficiently, and to participate in society at large.

Knowledge Creation Metaphor of Learning: Unlike theories that emphasize learning as knowledge acquisition (the acquisition metaphor) and as participation in a social community (the participation metaphor) (Sfard, 1998), a third metaphor views learning as a process of knowledge creation (the knowledge creation metaphor) (Paavola & Hakkarainen, 2005). This view focuses on mediated processes of knowledge creation that have become especially important in a knowledge society.

LMS: Learning Management System. An integrated suite of software tools designed to manage learning interventions. Commercial examples are Blackboard and WebCT, although many open-source alternatives, such as Moodle and Sakai, exist. In addition to the provision of online learning content and activities and the facilitation of online assessment, LMSs typically support a range of administrative functions including learner enrollment, workflow, records management (e.g., reporting of assessment results/outcomes), and resource management (e.g., facilities, equipment).

Mashup: Content or material that is collected from several web-based sources, then modified, remixed, and/or recombined to create a new formulation of the material. A mashup is typically a digital media file including one or more the following: text, graphics, audio, video, and animation. Mashups are commonly seen in Web 2.0 services and social software tools such as blogs, wikis, RSS and podcast feeds, media sharing applications (e.g., YouTube), and social networking sites (e.g., MySpace, Facebook). See also micro-content.

Micro-Content: Very small, basic units of digital content or media that can be consumed in unbundled micro-chunks and aggregated and reconstructed in various ways. See also mashup.

Navigationism: An emergent learning theory, developed by Tom Brown, that views learning as "'navigating' the ocean of available knowledge" (Brown, 2005, p. 7). From a navigationist perspective, successful learning occurs as a result of learners being able to solve contextual, real-world problems by jointly exploring, evaluating, manipulating, and integrating available information from a range of sources. See also connectivism.

Pedagogy 2.0: Digital tools and affordances call for a new conceptualization of teaching that is focused on participation in communities and networks for learning, personalization of learning tasks, and production of ideas and knowledge. Pedagogy 2.0 is a response to this call. It represents a set of approaches and strategies that differs from teaching as a didactic practice of passing on information; instead, it advocates a model of learning in which students are empowered to participate, communicate, and create knowledge, exercising a high level of agency and control over the learning process.

Personal Publishing: A process in which an individual actively produces his or her own content and information and publishes it on the World Wide Web. For example, the maintenance of a personal blog as an online diary is an instance of personal publishing. See also user-generated content.

PLE: Personal Learning Environment. A system, application, or suite of applications that assists learners in taking control of and managing their own learning. It represents an alternative approach to the LMS, which by contrast adopts an institution-centric, content-centric, or course-centric view of learning. Key PLE concepts include the blending of formal and informal learning, participation in social networks that transcend institutional boundaries, as well as the use of a range of networking protocols (RSS, peer-to-peer [P2P], Web services) to connect systems, resources, and users within a personally-managed space. See also LMS.

Prosumer: A portmanteau formed by contracting word "producer" with the word "consumer," signifying the blurring of the distinction between the two roles with respect to content and ideas in today's knowledge economy.

Social Networking: A social network is a social structure comprising various nodes, which generally represent individuals or organizations, that are tied together by one or more specific types of interdependency, for example, common values, shared visions, exchange of ideas, mutual financial benefit, trade, friendship/kinship, or even dislike and conflict. In the context of the Web 2.0 movement, the term is commonly used to refer to web sites like MySpace, Facebook, Ning, Friendster, and LinkedIn, which attract and support networks of people and facilitate connections between them for social and professional purposes. The "blogosphere" may also be viewed as an example of an online social network. See also blogosphere.

Student-Generated Content: Content that is produced by students, often for sharing with peers or a wider audience on the Internet, as distinct from instructor-supplied content such as course notes and textbooks. It is arguable that the main benefits to be gained from student-generated content lie in engagement in the processes of content creation and knowledge construction, as opposed to the tangible end products themselves. Also called "learner-generated content." See also user-generated content.

User-Generated Content: A term that refers to web-based content created by ordinary people or users, for example, pictures posted on Flickr or encyclopedia entries written in Wikipedia. Such "read-and-write" applications are characteristic of the Web 2.0 movement, which encourages the publishing of one's own content and commenting on or augmenting other people's. It differs from the "read-only" model of Web 1.0, in which websites were created and maintained by an elite few.

Wisdom of Crowds: A concept that relates to the aggregation of information in groups and communities of individuals. It recognizes that the innovation, problem-solving, and decision-making capabilities of the group are often superior to that of any single member of the group. The term was used as the title of a book written by James Surowiecki, published in 2004. See also collective intelligence.

Chapter 4
Learner-Generated Contexts:
A Framework to Support the Effective Use of Technology for Learning

Rosemary Luckin
Institute of Education, UK

Wilma Clark
Institute of Education, UK

Fred Garnett
Institute of Education, UK

Andrew Whitworth
University of Manchester, UK

Jon Akass
Media Citizens Ltd, UK

John Cook
London Metropolitan University, UK

Peter Day
University of Brighton, UK

Nigel Ecclesfield
Becta, UK

Tom Hamilton
University of Sussex, UK

Judy Robertson
Heriot-Watt University, UK

ABSTRACT

In this chapter the authors present the concept of Learner-Generated Contexts as a potential framework through which the more effective use of technology to support learning might be supported and engendered. In particular, they concentrate on the theoretical grounding for consideration of Learner-Generated Contexts as a context-based model and organizing principle for designing learning and as a means of elucidating what institutional practices might support or retard their development. In so doing, the authors offer a model for the learning–teaching process based upon the Russian concept of "obuchenie" and a reconsideration of pedagogic design based upon a combinatory model termed the "PAH continuum."

DOI: 10.4018/978-1-60566-294-7.ch004

INTRODUCTION

The rapid development of technologies has made it possible for people to access data and resources in their environment, to share information in multimedia formats, to collaborate, publish and track their lives beyond the constraints of physical space or temporal constraint. Developed in this chapter is the concept of a *Learner-Generated Context (LGC)*: a way to describe learning–teaching processes that takes account of these advances. It is based around the democratic principle that:

ordinary people are intrinsic participants in technical processes. They can transform technology through enlarging the margin of manoeuvre they already enjoy in the technical networks in which they are enrolled. (Feenberg, 2002, p. 174)

The agenda is not about technology use *per se*. Nonetheless the issues highlighted here have been prompted by thinking about the affordances and potentials of a range of technologies and practice; Web 2.0, mobile learning (m-learning), participative media, learning design, and learning space design. They have also been prompted by the convergence of parallel developments and observations including:

- *Technology developments.* A brief history of the last 15 years reveals a number of transformations in how people communicate and interact. The Internet and the World Wide Web have opened up our ability to publish and taken us from hypertext to multimedia, brought us networking and enabled us to communicate in more places: to socialize, collaborate, co-author, and co-publish. Increased availability of digital devices such as cameras and sensors enable us to digitally capture and store more about our environment. Mobile, ubiquitous, and pervasive technologies offer multiple choices about how we keep in touch. One of the consequences of these digital developments is to enable users to generate content; user outputs can be seen on blogs, wikis, and social networks such as YouTube, Facebook, MySpace, and Flickr. End-users are now active content producers across online and offline environments.
- *Concerns about the current education system and in particular the role of technology.* There is mixed evidence about the effectiveness of current educational technology use (e.g., du Boulay, Coultas, & Luckin, 2007; Selwyn, 2007), recognition that learners often dumb down their expectations with respect to technology when they enter formal educational establishments (Puttnam, 2007) and growing recognition of the need for policy reform.
- *A blurring of the boundaries between designers and users.* From the introduction of the first examples of technologies that were designed to support learning some have built systems without considering users but some have focused on user needs. This has supported an increasing trend towards participatory design methods. The convergence of these parallel developments results in a situation where more people have the technological means to engage in system reform. There is the potential for both a participatory democracy and for technological and design reforms to enrich learners' educational experiences, making them more effective learners and participants in a reform agenda. However, there is a particular tension within the current system around the extent to which formal educational institutions can cope with the more informal communicative approaches to digital interactions that new generations of learners possess (Luckin, Logan, Clark, Graber, Oliver, & Mee, 2008; Clark, Logan, Luckin, Mee, & Oliver, 2009).

LGC is about trying to find a *framework* that might support the more effective use of technology to support learning. It is about opening up the process through which knowledge is constructed and understanding is gained. The enterprise of the LGC group (members of which authored this chapter) is precipitated by a recognition that a combination of factors have brought educators to a particular point in the evolution of learning with technology that requires reflection on how things might work better. The group's work is inherently interdisciplinary and its (admittedly ambitious) desire is to appeal to and encompass a huge sphere of activity that includes a great deal of education.

The current working definition of a Learner-Generated Context is as follows:

a context created by people interacting together with a common, self-defined learning goal. The key aspect of Learner-Generated Contexts is that they are generated through the enterprise of those who would previously have been consumers in a context created for them.

The LGC group members share common concerns to ensure that learning is a participatory experience that is about participative technology, participative education, and participative democracy. The current popularity among learners for the creation and publication of their own material, combined with the open content and open source initiatives offer the tools for increased educational democracy. These tools support the potential for the boundaries to be redrawn between learners and teachers, formal and informal education, and the producers and consumers of knowledge. However, learners still need support to scaffold their skills and understanding (Wood, Bruner, & Ross, 1976) as part of a Learner-Generated Context process.

The chapter presents the latest iteration of the authors' specification for Learner-Generated Contexts. In particular, it concentrates upon their theoretical grounding, considering how to best facilitate the development of context-based models as the organizing principle for designing learning and what institutional practices might support or retard their development. A model for the teaching–learning process is offered, based upon the Russian concept of "obuchenie."

WHAT IS A LEARNER-GENERATED CONTEXT?

The Learner Generated Context concept is based upon the description of an educational context as a learner-centric Ecology of Resources (Luckin, 2008, 2010). These resources may be organized to meet the needs of a learner or group of learners by various individuals including teachers, parents, the government, and learners themselves. The resources within a learner's ecology include:

- the *subject* they are learning, the way in which it is recognized and validated as a skill or *knowledge*, and the epistemic community built around the subject in formal and informal ways;
- the social and physical *environments* with which the learner interacts and the way in which these are organized;
- the *resources*, both human—such as peers, teachers, and parents—and inanimate—such as the communications technologies (books, handouts, the WWW, etc.) that allow the learner access to the knowledge of others, and those that allow access to information about the world such as microscopes and telescopes.

These context elements are situated within the prior cognitive structures that exist both in the learner's subjective consciousness and the objective world, embedded into technologies, organizations, and other "persistent structures" (Nardi, 1996, p. 83) such as norms and legal procedures. (For a detailed exploration of the consequences of this environment- and resource-based approach to the design of learning, see Whitworth, 2009.)

This definition of context moves away from the idea that a context is a physical location, toward the idea that the context is the combination of interactions the learner experiences across multiple physical spaces and times. It is personal to the learner. The proposition made by Learner-Generated Contexts is that through a constant series of adjustments to this dynamic environment, learners can now take greater agency in the creation of their learning contexts. The implications of this for policy and pedagogy are considerable. (See Luckin, 2010; Luckin et al., 2005; Luckin, Shurville, & Browne, 2007 for more detail on the learner-centric Ecology of Resources framework and for more detailed examples.)

THE CASE FOR A CONTEXT-BASED MODEL OF EDUCATION/LEARNING

In this section what is meant by context is considered, along with what a context-based model for education and learning might look like. As part of the discussion other models and what makes them inadequate are covered, including a consideration of formal and informal learning. What a context-based model could offer is questioned, and why it might be better, before the section concludes with a consideration of how the development of context-based models such as Learner-Generated Contexts might be facilitated.

What Do We Mean by Context and What Might a Context-Based Model Look Like?

The suggestion that we should explore the educational context in which learning takes place is not new. There are examples within studies of contemporary educational practice that contribute descriptions of *classrooms as Social Learning Contexts* (Mercer, 1992) in which the organization of the learning resources, including the computer, influences the manner in which these resources are used and the nature of the context itself. We know that each individual class will have its own unique culture and brand of learning environment (Smagorinsky & Fly, 1993). Previous research has also indicated that the impact of technology on learning is heavily dependent upon the specifics of the educational context into which the technology is introduced (Wood, Underwood, & Avis, 1999). This work is useful in confirming the importance of looking at the wider environment within which educational interactions occur, but it is only part of the story for LGC. These research examples tend to look at environmental locations with fixed physical or temporal boundaries rather than the personal, learner-centric, and learner-generated contexts that can encompass multiple locations, which are at the heart of this article.

In the introduction context was described as something that was not tied to a physical location, nor any specific virtual location, but rather as something that belongs to an individual and is created through their interactions in the world. Every person's context is individual to them and is the ultimate form of personalization of the world and of the elements of the world that can contribute to learning. This view of context is not inconsistent with ideas from computer scientists such as Dey (2001), who consider a context to be defined by the information that characterizes a particular situation with respect to an entity—which in educational settings is a learner or a group of learners. Dourish (2004) highlights the importance of human activity and Chalmers (2004) adds an individual's experience and history to the mix. Following this approach, a context can be described as a situation defined through the relationships and interactions between the elements within that situation over time. For a learner, a context is a situation defined through interactions in and with the world that are themselves historically situated and culturally idiosyncratic. In the case of the learner, social interactions are of particular importance (Vygotsky, 1978, 1986).

This approach is also related to views proposed from an activity theory perspective by writers such as Nardi (1996) who see context as "not an outer container or shell inside of which people behave in certain ways. People consciously and deliberately generate contexts (activities) in part through their own objects" (p. 76). Context is a constant, dynamic interaction between internal and external forces. To an extent contexts are consciously and deliberately generated, but because prior practices and decisions are embedded in the infrastructural resources on which they must draw, actors do not have complete freedom to generate a context. The level of control they *do* have over their context—particularly its technostructural parameters (see below)—is exactly what the LGC model seeks to increase; to move learners out of a subordinate relationship to their context and into one of greater control.

The Ecology of Resources model of context offers a definition of context as a set of interrelated resource elements, including people and objects, the interactions between which define a particular context. It offers a description of the categories of elements that need to be taken into account when trying to explore the interactions that constitute a particular context. These categories include those noted in the introduction (skills, resources, prior cognitive schema, and so on); this idea is an essentially dynamic one. However, the nature of the interactions that our learner has with these different types of contextual element is filtered in some way. For example, knowledge and skills are filtered, organized, and validated through concepts such as "curriculum" and "qualifications." These are socially constructed concepts that have become reified through having been *designed into* the way education is organized. By doing so they become removed from public scrutiny and intervention, despite the fact that "public intervention may actually improve technology by addressing problems ignored by vested interests entrenched in the design process" (Feenberg, 1998, p. 89). Such filters impose a certain structure and fixity on the dynamic context.

What Other Models Are There? Why Are They Inadequate?

Educational ideas often have both a static, objective, and quantifiable expression as well as a more dynamic, (inter)subjective, and qualitative form (cf. Carr & Kemmis, 1986). As an illustration, consider the zone of proximal development (ZPD). This could be described quantitatively as "The discrepancy between a child's actual mental age and the level he reaches in solving problems with assistance" (Vygotsky, 1986, p. 187). However, a more dynamic, qualitative definition would define the ZPD as something that must be created through instructional interactions that "awaken" the internal developmental processes that can only operate when the child is interacting with other people in the environment (Vygotsky, 1978). This split reflects schisms often discussed in social theory literature between a technical or instrumental rationality and a more humanist or communicative perspective.

The Ecology of Resources model could be viewed statically, as merely a set of elements that could be "optimized" by design and organizational practice. Most formally constituted organizations have within them a *technostructure* (Mintzberg, 1989). Technostructures are where technology and organization meet; they are organizational artifacts that operationalize the procedures, systems, and technologies that control the work of the other wings of the organization, particularly the professional core and the support staff. In universities, historically, technostructures have been weak (Mintzberg, 1989), but the increased use of information and communication technology (ICT) to not just teach but administer the university does represent an organizational transformation; it also represents a move towards a more static and less flexible approach to the support of learning. Centralization and consolidation occur through the "closure" of technological options (Feenberg, 1998). As a result, there can be a lack of freedom to experiment with new technological possibilities, due to a strengthening of the filters around the available resources. There is, of course, a role for standardization in design (Norman, 1990)—but as a protection against arbitrariness, not as something that "closes" the possibility of further adaptation and innovation.

Models that currently underpin the education system are not communicative and learner-centric, but instrumental and organization-centric.

The organizational problems posed to higher education by the rise of ICT have been recognized even by relatively organization-centric writers. Bates (2000), for instance, advocated addressing staff development of technology at an organizational level by supplying resources for "Lone Rangers"—self-motivated, self-empowered teaching faculty, engaging in experimentation in their local context. But Bates later withdrew this support, claiming that the more mature organizational approach to technology was to centralize (for a critique of this view see Whitworth & Benson, 2007).

Diana Laurillard's (2002) conversational model of educational technology is based on pedagogical principles, though this is not quite the same as being "learner-centric." This model considers how students and teachers describe and redescribe their conception of the world, through technologies. Laurillard then takes this pedagogical idea and examines its impact upon organizational infrastructures. She specifically states that the infrastructure must *learn*, be reflexive: "An organisational infrastructure for educational technology … must enable the system to learn about itself. The decision-making hierarchy must be in a position to receive feedback on the effects of its decisions at each level in exactly the same way that the student needs feedback on their interactions with the world in order to learn" (Laurillard, 2002, p. 237). Garnett and Ecclesfield (2008) call this "developing the organisational architecture of participation" (p. 468).

Feedback mechanisms are, however, identifiable as filters, rather than as communicative exchanges that help dynamically develop the ecology of resources. In order to really be effective feedback has the potential to *transform practice*, not just provide information about that practice to "objective" actors concerned to assess the performance of an existing technostructural configuration. The dynamic nature of context, and the way it transcends easy physical and temporal definition, means that an external, "objective" researcher or observer can only ever hope to identify a snapshot of a particular context at a particular moment in time. To the individual or group at the center of a context, however, it is lived experience; but that does not mean that the dynamic development of context is a process that takes place in the forefront of conscious awareness. The consequences of this view will be explored below, but first formal and informal learning issues will be looked at.

How We Might Facilitate the Development of Context-Based Models like Learner-Generated Contexts

If a context-based model is deemed to be worthy of consideration then there is a need to explore how such models might be developed and implemented. Here, attention in turned, in particular, to the question of design.

Design "choices" are not free but in fact are greatly constrained by the "persistent structures" (Nardi, 1996, p. 83) in which they are made. Organizations embed values, procedures, systematized ways of working and even thinking, not only into the "objective" technostructure, but into their intersubjective communications networks (the use of *language* can restrict choice) and the subjective consciousnesses of their members. Organizations *push* certain "cognitive schema" at their members (Blaug, 2007) and this is why many activities within organizations take place beneath the level of conscious awareness. On the one hand, this is necessary, for no organization could function if its members were continually questioning the premises of even the most basic activity. On the other hand, this can retard "double-loop learning" (Argyris, 1999, p. 67) and thus the organization's ability to learn and adapt.

The problem with "design" as an industrial process is that it is specifically oriented towards the reduction of choice. Designed systems are built around assumptions as to what activities will take place within them, what mental models will govern these activities, and what information best fits these mental models. For any such system, processing is eased when incoming data are schema-consistent, and data that are inconsistent with this schema can be filtered out and ignored (see Blaug, 2007; via Augoustinos & Walker, 1996). Ultimately, Blaug (2007) claims that we cede portions of our cognition to the organization and the technologies that make it up: we allow these designed techno-structures to do a lot of our thinking for us. All the context-based methodologies Nardi describes recognize that there is a delegation of cognition to the system (distributed cognition) and, to an extent, activity theory allows for this explicitly: even situated action (the most individualized and spontaneous of these approaches) allows for the presence of "routines" that govern action at an unconscious level. Yet this is a "deeply passive" (Blaug, 2007, p. 38) relationship on behalf of the individual; the individual *and his or her context* become subordinate to the technostructure, rather than active within it, and able to transform it if necessary (Feenberg, 1998).

Learner-generated contexts stem not from organizational imperatives but more from the tradition of autonomous action (more redolent of non-formal learning traditions). They challenge those validity claims—claims to technological pre-eminence, the control over meaning and personal context—which are then not validated by the organizational environment within which social actors function (see Feenberg, 2002; via de Certeau, 1980/1984). They are "outbreaks of democracy" (Blaug, 2000, p. 145); whether they take place outside the formally constituted educational sphere, as people develop their own, network-based applications of technology (see Rheingold, 2002), or perhaps within it, as sub-ordinate groups in an organization "subvert" its dominant technostructural systems (see Wenger, 1998; Benson & Whitworth, 2007). Through these actions, learners increase their *awareness* of the possibilities—lifting up operations, unconscious ways of working in a technostructural context, and creatively playing with them—but also critically transforming them.

The principle of LGC begins with an apprecia-tion of the tension that is building in the current system in which learners are using technology more creatively and effectively outside of the education system than within it (Puttnam, 2007). Teachers often do not have as high a level of technical skills as their students and in which it is hard for many of them to find a way to make that the basis for a positive learning experience for students and for themselves. But this suggests that technology is a "problem type" in which even younger learners can potentially validate the claims of teachers—and vice versa (Young, 1990).

This calls into question the role of "design" in the development of an ecology of resources. Learn-ers are usually considered either the "customers" or "products" of educational organizations. When pedagogical processes are discussed they have the learner in mind, but the relationship is rarely discussed as one in which learners *generate* peda-gogical processes. The idea of learner-generated *content* (Lee & McLoughlin, 2007; Sener, 2007) is broadly used, particularly in constructivist pedagogy. But this content is being produced in a context that learners act within, consume, but do not generate or transform. LGC is what happens because a design-based approach *stems from* the cognitive separation between learners and the organization; it cannot relieve it.

The idea of learner-generated *contexts* forces reassessment of the validity of the "filter" that is the sharp boundaries around the roles of teacher and learner. Hence the authors' liking for the term *obuchenie*, which means both teaching and learning. It recognizes that critical pedagogy and the internal critique of self-reflexive staff development are related (Young, 1990; Carr & Kemmis, 1986). More significantly, this relationship is what supports LGC against criticisms that it stands in a fundamental opposition to the authority of the teacher. This idea will now be developed further, starting with a discussion of the various "ogys"—broadly based conceptions of teaching strategy at different stages of cognitive development.

THE LEARNER-GENERATED CONTEXT PROCESS

In the previous section a case was presented for the development of context-based models of learning, and it was suggested that the Ecology of Resources model might be a good starting point for thinking about the nature of the elements that might be active in the construction of learning contexts. This section considers what types of interactions between these context elements might support the construction of effective learning contexts. In particular, the interactions between teachers and learners and the issue of pedagogy are examined.

In commencing the discussion, the need to integrate the roles of learners as consumers and producers in the learning process should first be considered. As highlighted in the introduction to this chapter, we are seeing the rapid increase in the variety and availability of resources and tools that enable people to easily create and publish their own materials and to access those created by others. This extends the capacity for learning context creation beyond teachers, academics, designers, and policy makers. However, this gives rise to the following question: How can we integrate the roles of learners as consumers and producers in the learning process? In the authors' view of LGC, there are role shifts for both the learner and teacher or instructor. These role shifts can have a positive and empowering impact; however, they can also cause disruption in formal education systems, and such change may consequently be resisted. Various issues are emerging, one of which is the focus here: the need to consider what pedagogical practices or non-formal learning patterns might work in a context-based learning model.

The Ogy Model

Educators have previously adopted a hierarchical view on moves away from the term *pedagogy* towards a learner-directed style of learning, such as that described by Knowles (1984) as *andragogy*, and the more self-determined learning paradigm subsequently proposed by Hase and Kenyon (2000), referred to as *heutagogy*. This reflects the Greek origins of the words (child-leading, adult-leading, and self-leading respectively).

The increased use and development of social, collaborative, and distributed learning environments and the blurring of the boundaries between formal and non-formal learning requires that we move on from these traditional, developmental, and temporally situated understandings of what it means to learn and what it means to be a learner. We are entering a space where teachers are learners and students are teachers, where physical boundaries are being replaced or supported by virtual ones and the teacher is no longer the sole expert.

There is merit in developing the idea of a learning continuum from pedagogy through andragogy to heutagogy as part of a process in education where the "teacher" is developing learning skills in the learner. In *The e-mature learner*, Anderson (2006) characterized this as follows:

in pedagogy, what is to be learnt, and how, is both determined and directed by the teacher;

in andragogy, it is determined by the teacher and directed by the learner; in heutagogy, both determination and direction shift to the learner. Normally, concepts of pedagogy, andragogy and heutagogy are associated with age, sector or the formal stage of learner development—for example, pedagogy with schools, andragogy with adult education and heutagogy with doctoral research (p. 5, emphasis in original).

O'Beirne (quoted in *Developing the pedagogy andragogy heutagogy continuum*, "OGY & Context," para. 1) comments in response to Anderson that he is concerned about:

the lack of "social" context. What I mean is that a learner situated in the Heutagogy is not necessarily determining her learning, i.e. not self-determining and self-directing but is involved in a more socio-constructivist type learning where, as a heutagogical learner she avails of, is influenced by, develops, contributes to, criticizes and ultimately reflects on, a social networking scenario. So I think that with Heutagogy, yes, there is a shift to the learner but not the learner alone in isolation.

He questions whether talking of a continuum implies that they are mutually exclusive when we are thinking of the relationship as being "cumulative."

It can be argued that the value in a pedagogic approach is in developing the learner's understanding of a subject. The value in an andragogic approach is in developing an understanding of how to negotiate a way through the learning process. The value in a heutagogic approach is in developing the understanding that one is empowered to *look at the learning context afresh* and take decisions in that context. Thus this developmental view implies that learners need to understand how subjects are constructed, what is canonical and, in the sense of learner-generated contexts, that learning is a social process of discussion, negotiation, and partnership, where learning enables you to go out into the world equipped not only to solve problems, but also to identify new areas worthy of your attention. Heutagogy must now also reflect the embedding of certain educational values into systems of control: critical reflection on the technologies that one is presented with to construct a context and the transformation of these technologies. It is further arguable that learners have to be equipped to manage their own learning and that they need to be educated in those skills through an understanding of this (cumulative) "PAH continuum." Another way of describing this development process could be that of developing cognition, metacognition, and epistemic cognition in the learner (see Table 1).

The Obuchenie Context Model

In addition to consideration of this "PAH continuum," a closer investigation of the socio-cultural roots of the Ecology of Resources model (see Luckin, 2008 for a fuller description) offers an additional construct that contributes a desirable "fuzziness" to the debate—that of "obuchenie." Ambiguities around the Russian word *obuchenie* and the search for an apt translation of this

Table 1. The PAH continuum

	Pedagogy	Andragogy	Heutagogy
Locus of control	teacher	learner	learner
Educational sector	schools	adult education	doctoral research
Cognition level	cognitive	metacognitive	epistemic
Knowledge production context	subject understanding	process negotiation	context shaping

Vygotskian term have been the subject of much debate over the years (Davydov, 1995; Daniels, 2001; Clarke, 2003; LeBlanc & Bearison, 2004). It has been variably described as "instruction" (van der Veer & Valsiner, 1994), "teaching/learning" (Clarke, 2003), "teaching-and-learning" (Wells & Claxton, 2003, p. 152), "teaching–learning" (Davydov, 1995), and "learning" (Wertsch & Sohmer, 1995, p. 332). LeBlanc and Bearison (2004), considering *obuchenie* in formal educational contexts, suggest that it characterizes interactions in the ZPD that are "conceptualized less as displays of unidirectional guidance or support on the part of teachers to learners and more as bi-directional displays of knowledge transformed through the course of dyadic interaction" (p. 501), suggesting that the relationship between teacher and a learner is "characterized by a gradual exchange of knowledge that results in mutual cognitive growth" (p. 513). Sutton (1980) points to *obuchenie* as "a phenomenon made up of mutually interpenetrating opposites" (pp. 169–170), an argument supported by Moll (2000), who, addressing the concept of *obuchenie* in informal contexts, for example among peers or in out-of-school contexts, suggests that interactions framed as *obuchenie* have the potential to mutually enhance the cognitive approach of both teacher and learner as marked by the coordination of self-regulatory behaviors in a process of collaboration.

In this chapter, however, it is proposed that it is the very fuzziness of the word *obuchenie* that makes it a suitable construct for understanding the potentiality of learner-generated contexts and, in particular, the permeable nature of the "implicit" boundaries between teaching and learning by looking at the principles of PAH and combining these with the notion of *obuchenie*.

In contrast to traditional perceptions of PAH, the Obuchenie Context Model integrates PAH with the Ecology of Resources model and views it not as a developmental hierarchy of dyadic or bi-directional interactions between teachers and learners, but rather as a complex, "heterarchical" continuum characterized by multiple points of intersection and an evolving reciprocity of relations and interactions that fall along an "other-regulated—self-regulated" continuum.

The traditional perception of a multi-leveled, bi-directional continuum of teaching/learning in which "teacher" influence is seen to decrease as "learner" independence increases is reshaped (see Figure 1).

In turn, the combination of the Ecology of Resources and the acceptance of a fuzzy-field concept of *obuchenie* together generate the potential for understanding the systemic interaction of teacher/learner in which the elements of PAH are shaped by the interactions of the teacher/learner within the available ecology of resources, such that their individual interests/motivations lead to "agile configurations" in the process of knowledge construction so that at any one moment, teacher may be learner, learner may be teacher, and both may become mutually conditioned co-learners. This is referred to here as the Obuchenie Context Model (see Figure 2).

In this way, the Obuchenie Context Model empowers actors within the learner-generated context, in a mutually beneficial process, to gener-

Figure 1. Teacher influence

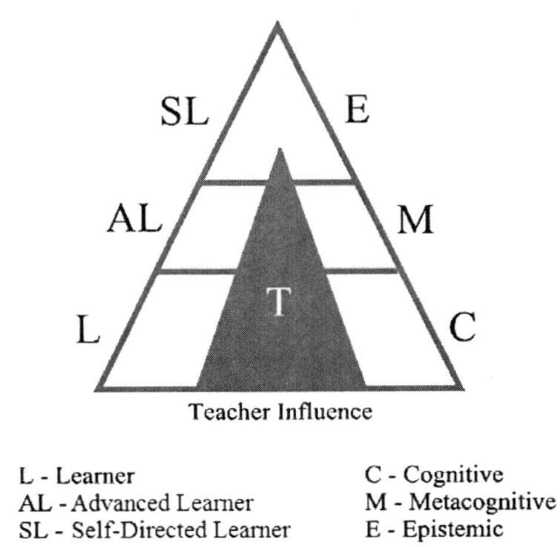

Figure 2. The Obuchenie context model

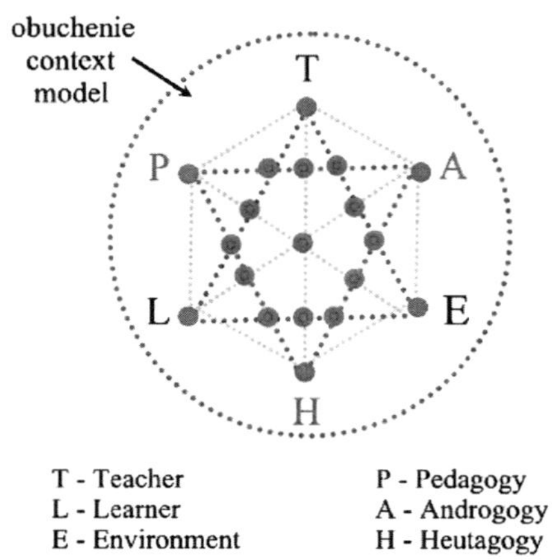

ate new knowledge models in the obuchenie-led fragmentation of traditional discourses in the life world of the organization. This, in turn, opens up networks of communication within the system, enabling both teacher and learner to reap the mutual benefit of a certain parity of voice reflected in the facilitation of self-motivated, self-reflexive enquiry between and among participants, which in turn serves to generate a form of democratic, socially-constructed, community-based defense against the traditional levers of control or colonization by the organization.

In these discussions of the processes that need to occur in order to support the creation of a Learner-Generated Context, the chapter has presented the PAH continuum and the Obuchenie Context Model as new ways of looking at old ideas. An attempt has been made to move consideration of the individual concepts of pedagogy, andragogy, heutagogy, and obuchenie into "context" mode where the boundaries of meaning around the terms are made more flexible and permeable.

The Open Context Model and Web 2.0

Web 2.0 is based on a number of elements—the Web as a platform, architecture of participation, small pieces loosely joined (now "everything is miscellaneous")—which are aimed at providing tools for users to pull together resources in ways that make sense to them. It describes a new set of user-centered experiences that are participative and interactive, which Web 2.0 tools enable and support. The authors think that learner-generated contexts are about providing the tools to enable learner-centered experiences, and the Open Context Model discusses the set of pedagogical issues that need to be addressed if the affordances of Web 2.0 are to be used to enable and support learner-centered learning. The Open Context Model provides a new pedagogic framework to enable thinking about which Web 2.0 resources are to be used for learning and why.

However, the authors do not think that new pedagogies are sufficient in themselves; a more adaptive and collaborative education system is also needed—this is discussed in more detail in Garnett and Ecclesfield (2008). The authors believe that the future of education will emerge from the changed pedagogic practice described in this chapter, allowing greater co-creation (obuchenie), enabled and supported by appropriate Web 2.0 tools in a transformed educational architecture of participation with "adaptive institutions working across collaborative networks" (Garnett & Ecclesfield, p. 472). The LGC group will continue to review and publish on all these factors, including Web 2.0, as they develop and change.

CONCLUSION

In this chapter the authors have argued for a context-based model of learning and education and have proposed that Learner-Generated Contexts can provide a framework for open, creative, and participatory learning experiences. An LGC is a contributory context that generates a culture of production that is characterized by replenishment and renewal drawing on existing resources that are expanded and enhanced. The chapter has discussed what is meant by context and offered a personalized perspective of a learner's context as *a situation defined through social interactions that are themselves historically situated and culturally idiosyncratic.* The authors have proposed a learner-centric *Ecology of Resources model consisting of a set of interrelated resource elements, including people and objects, the interactions between which provide a particular context.* In addition to this constitutional approach, in this chapter the authors have also explored the processes that need to occur in order to support the creation of a Learner-Generated Context. To this end the PAH continuum and the Obuchenie Context Model were presented. An effort was made to try to move consideration of the individual concepts of pedagogy, andragogy, heutagogy, and obuchenie into "context" mode where the boundaries of meaning around the terms are made more flexible and permeable. In this way, *the Obuchenie Context Model empowers actors within the learner-generated context,* in a mutually beneficial process, to generate new knowledge models in the obuchenie-led fragmentation of traditional discourses in the life world of the organization.

ACKNOWLEDGMENT

The authors would like to thank all those who have shown an interest in the LGC initiative, though their contributions to the LGC wiki, their attendance at events, and their willingness to engage in the debate. Thanks also go to the UK Engineering and Physical Sciences Research Council (EPSRC), which funds the work of Prof. Luckin through an Advanced Research Fellowship.

REFERENCES

Anderson, J. (2006). *The e-mature learner.* Retrieved November 29, 2008, from http://tre.ngfl.gov.uk/uploads/materials/24875/The_emature_learner_John_Anderson.doc

Argyris, C. (1999). *On organizational learning* (2nd ed.). Oxford, UK: Blackwell.

Augoustinos, M., & Walker, I. (1996). *Social cognition.* London: Sage.

Bates, A. W. (2000). *Managing technological change: Strategies for college and university leaders.* San Francisco: Jossey-Bass.

Benson, A. D., & Whitworth, A. (2007). Technology at the planning table: Activity theory, negotiation and course management systems. *Journal of Organisational Transformation and Social Change, 4*(1), 75–92. doi:10.1386/jots.4.1.75_1

Blaug, R. (2000). Outbreaks of democracy. In L. Panitch & C. Leys (Eds.), *Socialist Register 2000: Necessary and unnecessary utopias* (pp. 145–160). Pontypool, UK: Merlin. Retrieved November 29, 2008, from http://socialistregister.com/index.php/srv/article/view/5739/2634

Blaug, R. (2007). Cognition in a hierarchy. *Contemporary Political Theory, 6*(1), 24–44. doi:10.1057/palgrave.cpt.9300276

Carr, W., & Kemmis, S. (1986). *Becoming critical: Knowing through action research.* Geelong, Australia: Deakin University Press.

Chalmers, M. (2004). A historical view of context. *Computer Supported Cooperative Work, 13*(3/4), 223–247. doi:10.1007/s10606-004-2802-8

Clark, W., Logan, K., Luckin, R., Mee, A., & Oliver, M. (2009). Beyond Web 2.0: Mapping the technology landscapes of young learners. *Journal of Computer Assisted Learning, 25*(1), 56–69. doi:10.1111/j.1365-2729.2008.00305.x

Clarke, D. (2003, April 21–25). *Practice, role and position: Whole class patterns of participation*. Paper presented at the Annual Meeting of the American Educational Research Association, Chicago.

Daniels, H. (2001). *Vygotsky and pedagogy*. London: RoutledgeFalmer.

Davydov, V. (1995). The influence of L. S. Vygotsky on education theory, research, and practice. (S. T. Kerr, Trans.). *Educational Researcher*, *24*(3), 12–21.

de Certeau, M. (1984). The practice of everyday life. (S. Rendall, Trans.) Berkeley, CA: University of California Press. (1980)

Developing the pedagogy andragogy heutagogy continuum. (2008). Retrieved November 29, 2008, from http://learnergeneratedcontexts.pbworks.com/PAH

Dey, A. K. (2001). Understanding and using context. *Personal and Ubiquitous Computing*, *5*(1), 4–7. doi:10.1007/s007790170019

Dourish, P. (2004). What we talk about when we talk about context. *Personal and Ubiquitous Computing*, *8*(1), 19–30. doi:10.1007/s00779-003-0253-8

du Boulay, B., Coultas, J., & Luckin, R. (2007). *How compelling is the evidence for the effectiveness of e-Learning in the post-16 sector? A review of the literature in higher education, the health sector and work-based learning and a post-review stakeholder consultation*. Bath, UK: Eduserv. Retrieved November 29, 2008, from http://www.reveel.sussex.ac.uk/files/Version4.2.pdf

Feenberg, A. (1998). *Questioning technology*. London: Routledge.

Feenberg, A. (2002). *Transforming technology: A critical theory revisited* (2nd ed.). Oxford, UK: Oxford University Press.

Garnett, F., & Ecclesfield, N. (2008). Colloquium; Developing an organisational architecture of participation. *British Journal of Educational Technology*, *39*(3), 468–474. doi:10.1111/j.1467-8535.2008.00839.x

Hase, S., & Kenyon, C. (2000). From andragogy to heutagogy. *ultiBASE, 5*(3). Retrieved November 29, 2008, from http://ultibase.rmit.edu.au/Articles/dec00/hase1.pdf

Knowles, M. S. (1984). *Andragogy in action: Applying modern principles in adult learning*. San Francisco: Jossey-Bass.

Laurillard, D. (2002). *Rethinking university teaching: A conversational framework for the effective use of learning technologies* (2nd ed.). London: RoutledgeFalmer. doi:10.4324/9780203304846

LeBlanc, G., & Bearison, D. J. (2004). Teaching and learning as a bi-directional activity: Investigating dyadic interactions between child teachers and child learners. *Cognitive Development*, *19*(4), 499–515. doi:10.1016/j.cogdev.2004.09.004

Lee, M. J. W., & McLoughlin, C. (2007). Teaching and learning in the Web 2.0 era: Empowering students through learner-generated content. *International Journal of Instructional Technology and Distance Learning, 4*(10), 21–34. Retrieved November 29, 2008, from http://www.itdl.org/Journal/Oct_07/Oct_07.pdf

Luckin, R. (2008). The learner centric ecology of resources: A framework for using technology to scaffold learning. *Computers & Education*, *50*(2), 449–462. doi:10.1016/j.compedu.2007.09.018

Luckin, R. (2010). *Re-designing learning contexts: Technology-rich, learner-centred ecologies*. Abingdon, UK: Routledge.

Luckin, R., du Boulay, B., Smith, H., Underwood, J., Fitzpatrick, G., & Holmberg, J. … Pearce, D. (2005). Using mobile technology to create flexible learning contexts. *Journal of Interactive Media in Education*. Retrieved November 29, 2008, from http://jime.open.ac.uk/2005/22/luckin-2005-22.pdf

Luckin, R., Logan, K., Clark, W., Graber, R., Oliver, M., & Mee, A. (2008). *Learners' use of Web 2.0 technologies in and out of school in Key Stages 3 and 4*. Coventry, UK: Becta. Retrieved November 29, 2008, from http://research.becta.org.uk/upload-dir/downloads/page_documents/research/web2_technologies_ks3_4.pdf

Luckin, R., Shurville, S., & Browne, T. (2007). Initiating e-learning by stealth, participation and consultation in a late majority institution. *Organisational Transformation and Social Change*, *4*(1), 317–332. doi:10.1386/jots.3.3.317_1

Mercer, N. (1992). Culture, context and the construction of knowledge in the classroom. In Light, P., & Butterworth, G. (Eds.), *Context and cognition: Ways of learning and knowing* (pp. 28–46). London: Harvester Wheatsheaf.

Mintzberg, H. (1989). *Mintzberg on management: Inside our strange world of organizations*. London: Macmillan.

Moll, L. C. (2000). Inspired by Vygotsky: Ethnographic experiments in education. In Lee, C. D., & Smagorinsky, P. (Eds.), *Vygotskian perspectives on literary research: Constructing meaning through collaborative inquiry* (pp. 256–268). New York: Cambridge University Press.

Nardi, B. A. (1996). *Context and consciousness: Activity theory and human–computer interaction*. Cambridge, MA: MIT Press.

Norman, D. A. (1990). *The design of everyday things*. London: Doubleday.

Puttnam, D. (2007, May 8). "In class, I have to power down". *The Guardian*. Retrieved January 14, 2008, from http://education.guardian.co.uk/egweekly/story/0,2074182,00.html

Rheingold, H. (2002). *Smart mobs: The next social revolution*. New York: Perseus.

Selwyn, N. (2007). Curriculum online? Exploring the political and commercial construction of the UK digital learning marketplace. *British Journal of Sociology of Education*, *28*(2), 223–240. doi:10.1080/01425690701192729

Sener, J. (2007). In search of student-generated content in online education. *e-mentor, 21*. Retrieved November 29, 2008, from http://www.e-mentor.edu.pl/_xml/wydania/21/467.pdf

Smagorinsky, P., & Fly, P. K. (1993). The social environment of the classroom: A Vygotskian perspective on small group process. *Communication Education*, *42*(2), 159–171. doi:10.1080/03634529309378922

Sutton, A. (1980). Backward children in the USSR: An unfamiliar approach to a familiar problem. In Brine, J., Perrie, M., & Sutton, A. (Eds.), *Home, school and leisure in the Soviet Union* (pp. 160–191). London: Allen & Unwin.

van der Veer, R., & Valsiner, J. (Eds.). (1994). *The Vygotsky reader*. Oxford, UK: Blackwell.

Vygotsky, L. S. (1978). *Mind in society: The development of higher psychological processes*. Cambridge, MA: Harvard University Press.

Vygotsky, L. S. (1986). *Thought and language*. Cambridge, MA: MIT Press.

Wells, G., & Claxton, G. (Eds.). (2003). *Learning for life in the 21st century*. Oxford, UK: Blackwell.

Wenger, E. (1998). *Communities of practice: Learning, meaning, and identity*. Cambridge, UK: Cambridge University Press.

Wertsch, J. V., & Sohmer, R. (1995). Vygotsky on learning and development. *Human Development*, *38*(6), 332–337. doi:10.1159/000278339

Whitworth, A. (2009). *Information obesity*. Oxford, UK: Chandos.

Whitworth, A., & Benson, A. D. (2007, January 8–10). *Taming the Lone Ranger: The creative development of e-learning technologies within UK and US higher education institutions.* Paper presented at Creativity or conformity? Building cultures of creativity in higher education, Cardiff, UK.

Wood, D., Underwood, J., & Avis, P. (1999). Integrated learning systems in the classroom. *Computers & Education*, *33*(2/3), 91–108. doi:10.1016/S0360-1315(99)00027-5

Wood, D. J., Bruner, J. S., & Ross, G. (1976). The role of tutoring in problem solving. *Journal of Child Psychology and Psychiatry, and Allied Disciplines*, *17*(2), 89–100. doi:10.1111/j.1469-7610.1976.tb00381.x

Young, R. E. (1990). *A critical theory of education: Habermas and our children's future*. New York: Teachers College Press.

KEY TERMS AND DEFINITIONS

Context Elements: Socially constructed concepts within the Ecology of Resources model that have been reified in some way.

Ecology of Resources: A way of characterizing a learner, and the interactions that form that learner's context. Based upon Vygotsky's work on the zone of proximal development (ZPD), it provides an abstract representation of the situations, resources, and relations that can be used to explore the potential benefits of available technologies in a range of learning contexts.

Filters: Feedback mechanisms constructed around available resources within the Ecology of Resources model.

Learner-Generated Context (LGC): A context created by people interacting together with a common, self-defined learning goal. The key aspect of LGCs is that they are generated through the enterprise of those who would previously have been consumers in a context created for them.

Obuchenie: Teaching–learning process, from the Russian—a concept derived by the Russian theorist, Lev Vygotsky.

Open Context Model: A new pedagogic framework that describes a new set of user-centered experiences that are participative and interactive, and discusses the set of pedagogical issues that need to be addressed if we are to use the affordances of Web 2.0 to enable and support learner-centered learning.

PAH Continuum: The idea of a cumulative learning continuum from pedagogy through andragogy to heutagogy as part of a process in education where the "teacher" is developing learning skills in the learner.

Participation: Involvement in the collaborative, co-created, participatory architecture of the Web 2.0 environment.

Chapter 5
Considering Students' Perspectives on Personal and Distributed Learning Environments in Course Design

Terje Väljataga
Tampere University of Technology, Finland & Tallinn University, Estonia

Kai Pata
Tallinn University, Estonia

Kairit Tammets
Tallinn University, Estonia

ABSTRACT

This chapter presents the findings from an experimental postgraduate student-centered course using social media tools and services to support learning. The main aim of this research was to evaluate a course design that was heavily supported by social media. The main aspects of this course design were that students were granted the freedom to select social media tools and services and use them in a personalized way, construct personal and distributed learning spaces, and visualize their conceptual understanding of these environments and their activities. Students' perceptions of the social media they used was used to evaluate the overall course design. Their perception of the affordances of social media are presented by noting conceptual changes in how they represented the structure of their personal and distributed environments, and by how they rated their learning experience with social media. This chapter concludes with the most important aspects of course design that need to be taken into account in higher education learning environments seeking to integrate Web 2.0 tools.

DOI: 10.4018/978-1-60566-294-7.ch005

INTRODUCTION

The ongoing evolution of the Web has had a great influence on every part of our society, from leisure time and educational life to business and work. In 2004, people began to use the term "Web 2.0" to refer to the new perspective and understanding of the ways software developers and end-users use the Web (O'Reilly, 2005). Though there is considerable discussion about the appropriateness of the term Web 2.0 and its definition, the main idea is that the Web and its applications are increasingly used for creativity enhancement, information sharing, collaboration among users, and social networking. In other words, Web 2.0 attempts to capture the economic value of social interaction (Barnwal, 2007). The term "social media" (sometimes called "Web 2.0 applications") refers to applications that support customized information retrieval, personalized aggregation and monitoring, and joint publication, sharing, and interaction (Owen, Grant, Sayers & Facer, 2006). Social media generally provide open and free access to web content, connection-building, and networking opportunities for people with common interests (MacManus & Porter, 2005). Social media tools and services are providing and shaping the cultural tools that serve as "carriers" of socio-cultural patterns and knowledge (Wertsch, 1994). Thus, this new trend in the use of web technology makes it even harder to escape the implications of social networking tools for learning (Candy, 2002).

Without doubt, many of our activities have moved to the Web, which offers a medium for a number of tasks we deal with every day in the home, community, office, library, etc. There is a constant flow of new web-based tools and services, applications, and terminology (Candy, 2002). The landscape of web tools and services is continuously complemented with a new generation of open source and open access *social media* tools, services, and enhancements (e.g., delicious as an example of social bookmarking tools; LinkedIn and Facebook for community-building environments; wiki applications for collaborative work; photo-, music-, and video-sharing tools such as Flickr, YouTube). Today, people are regularly confronted with the challenge of finding the most appropriate solutions with available resources and tools. Understanding how and where to get adequate information and resources, how to filter, interpret and use information effectively, and how to produce, exchange, and transmit information has become an important set of skills in today's society (Candy, 2002). Increasingly, learners must also be able to support these activities with web-based technologies and make informed choices about various online tools and services. Thus, we increasingly rely on applications and development of Web technology that can mediate our activities (Fiedler & Pata, 2009).

This chapter examines an innovative course design in higher education with the aim of investigating students' experiences with regard to the use of social media tools and services for supporting their study activities. The chapter gives an overview of the course design and students' perceptions of the affordances of their learning environments. Based on data collected on these perceptions, conclusions are drawn regarding the overall course design.

USING WEB 2.0 TOOLS IN EDUCATION

From an educational point of view, emerging web technologies present new challenges and requirements for both educators and students. Although most new technologies are not designed specifically for educational purposes, educators must be aware (and raise their students' awareness) of current web-based tools, services, and resources.

New technologies are causing many educators to rethink pedagogy and current learning and teaching models. Some, drawing from the term Web 2.0, have labeled new educational innovations "e-learning 2.0" (Downes, 2005). Zimmerman (2000) suggests that e-learning with social media tools and services can be seen as a promising approach to establishing an innovative learning and teaching culture that helps students cope with the changing knowledge environment and learning requirements. Thus, higher education institutions are facing the situation where the use of new technologies simultaneously creates conditions for introducing new teaching practices on the one hand, and on the other hand, revising current pedagogical approaches.

Since much of our work and communication activities have moved to the Web, selection and maintenance of a set of networked tools and services to enrich learning environments is becoming an educational imperative. Facilitators need to be prepared to select and combine appropriate software tools and services to support individual and collaborative tasks, and to establish shared procedures and knowledge. Taking initiative and responsibility for one's own learning trajectory, including tools and resources (i.e., the learning environment), requires new skills that enable the student to create an environment that best suits his or her learning style and expectations. Students have the opportunity to create authentic situations, where they are not only responsible for completing tasks, but also for managing the tools and services required to mediate those tasks. The use of new social media tools and services in education can be considered a student-driven, bottom-up approach, where students have more choice than facilitators over which tools and resources to employ (Pata & Väljataga, 2007; Underwood & Banyard, 2008). This means they take control of their activities and the environment in which the activities are carried out. Developing these skills meets the needs of the post-industrial society, where each individual needs to support the fulfillment of his or her life-long learning objectives with digital tools.

Thus, in higher education, there is a need to go beyond traditional approaches in which learning environments and tools are selected and mandated by the facilitator or institution. Students need opportunities to practice and acquire expertise in selecting and integrating a meaningful combination of diverse networked tools and services so that they become independent learners. Personally composed and (at least partial) personal control over the environment that mediates and supports work and study activities is an increasingly important consideration in higher education (Väljataga & Fielder, 2008).

DRAWBACKS OF CURRENT LEARNING ENVIRONMENTS

Available research indicates that in many higher education institutions, students have had few opportunities to decide which types of tools and services to use to mediate their activities (Väljataga, Pata, Laanpere, & Kaipainen, 2007). Currently, many universities still provide proprietary, homogeneous, and centrally-administered learning management systems (LMSs—e.g., Blackboard, WebCT, Moodle) to support and enhance teaching and study activities. These systems require students to learn how to use them and adapt their activities to fit the requirements of the environment (Gonella & Pantò, 2008). Institutionalized learning environments are structured mainly around content and driven by the needs of the institution rather than individual students. Furthermore, they represent a typical, application-centered approach that only allows for the performance of a particular, pre-defined set of activities within closed and rather static systems (Arenas, 2008). Students have to act within the system under the constraints and limitations dictated by the particular application (Fiedler & Kieslinger, 2006). Such environments are centrally-controlled and managed by the facilitator, who defines the learning objectives, tasks, media, and expected outcomes. The facilitator has limited possibilities to adapt to student preferences for tools that support their personal study aims. Thus, individual differences between students in terms of prior knowledge and experiences but also their expectations are left aside. We cannot disregard students' expectations towards the learning situation and environment as these will determine their perception of what the environment enables them to do, and will consequently influence their study activities within this environment (Könings, Brand-Gruwel, van Merriënboer, & Broers, 2006; Entwistle & Tait, 1990).

Furthermore, as these LMSs are usually only accessible to students of a particular course, the possibility to engage and interact with the outside world is rather limited. In general, students do not have a chance to choose and to go beyond the barriers imposed by the institution. They can only adjust to the provided LMS application and its artificially-created boundaries. It is hard to imagine that under these circumstances acquisition of requisite digital literacy and generic skills can be successfully built up and later easily transferred to authentic settings outside of formal education. However, applying the concepts of personal and distributed learning environments offers an alternative to the closed educational environments imposed by LMSs.

PERSONAL LEARNING ENVIRONMENTS

Rapid development of the Web and the necessity to rethink pedagogy and education has guided the discourse around the notion of the personal learning environment (PLE). One can find a diversity of interpretations of what a PLE is and what it should constitute (see, for example, Johnson, Hollins, Wilson, & Liber, 2006; van Harmelen, 2008; Attwell, 2007; Dron & Bhattacharya, 2007; Kolas & Staupe, 2007; Wilson, Liber, Johnson, Beauvoir, Sharples, & Milligan, 2007; Wilson, 2008; Johnson & Liber, 2008; Severance, Hardin, & Whyte, 2008).

In general, the discourse on PLE may tend to be technology-centric, stressing the importance of the development and implementation of social media and communication tools as monolithic, all-embracing applications, or as a combination of all the different tools and services used on one platform by an individual, even if the platform is institutional (van Harmelen, 2008; Severance et al., 2008). Thus, the PLE is seen by some as the conceptual "glue" embracing all networked and interoperable tools and services (Väljataga & Fiedler, 2008). For example, Türker and Zingel (2008) consider the PLE as a software application (desktop or web-based) that allows students to organize learning resources and publish individual outcomes. van Harmelen (2006) takes a highly technological perspective claiming the PLE to be: (1) as a desktop- or laptop-based client, (2) PLE as a browser and web server; (3) social media based PLE; and (4) m-PLE referring to the personal and community learning activities. From Schaffert and Hilzensauer's (2008) point of view, LMSs and PLEs are both technological concepts that allow several pedagogical methods or personal learning strategies.

There is also a non-technological view of the PLE that is more pedagogical/philosophical (Attwell, 2007; Downes, 2006). Treating a PLE more as subjective, pedagogical approach offers a broader, more naturalistic view of what comprises a personal environment in which learning occurs (Väljataga & Fiedler, 2008). In this view, a PLE is a knowledge network (Shepherd, 2007) or a cognitive space (Underwood & Banyard, 2008) that is in a constant state of flux (Norman, 2008). It has some physical characteristics (technical facilities) and cognitive characteristics such as students' investment in studies, their sense of efficacy, motivation, etc. (Underwood & Banyard, 2008). This perspective does not focus on exact technologies that are in use at any particular point in time; rather, more attention is paid to how people and resources are connected through technology (Norman, 2008). Downes (2006) refers to the PLE as one's community, where a student is at the centre and his facilitators—if there are any—are his peers. The PLE presents a different concept of learning, where the student's attitude is critical, and he or she can use the variety of tools available to begin structuring that experience. Martin (2007) defines a PLE as an approach to learning that is more self-directed and focused on students continually seeking meaningful resources, pulling together information and applying it to their own learning. Thus, the PLE is a promising means for organizing under one umbrella all the formal and informal learning of one individual (Attwell, 2007).

For the purposes of the study presented in this chapter, the PLE is defined from a psychological/pedagogical point of view. The PLE entails all the instruments, materials, and human resources that a student is aware of and has access to in the context of an educational project at a given point in time (Fiedler & Pata, 2009, Henri, Charlier, & Limpens, 2008; Jones, 2008). A PLE is entirely "controlled" or constructed by a student and is adapted according to the student's needs and current activities (Väljataga & Fiedler, 2008). A student can alter or extend his or her PLE by replacing the components of an environment or by complementing them with additional ones. Some components can also be eliminated or temporarily excluded if they do not further serve the desired educational objectives. Accordingly, every PLE is different, depending on the student's preferences and expectations, his or her process of personal development and mental processing (Väljataga & Fiedler, 2008), and current study activities. Students can construct their environments so that the components provide the learning experience they desire.

DISTRIBUTED LEARNING ENVIRONMENTS

The term "distributed learning environment" (DLE) has as many varied definitions as "Web 2.0" and "personal learning environment" (see, for example, Converso, Schaffer, & Guerra, 1999). The notion of distributed learning came with the development of high-performance computing and communications, as well as new media such as the Web and virtual reality (Dede, 1996). These new media enable interpersonal interactions across networks and countries and the evolution of synchronous, group, and presentation-centered forms of distance education. Early technologies replicated traditional "teaching by telling" across barriers of distance and time, but then morphed into an alternative instructional paradigm: distributed learning (Dede, 1996). Distributed learning refers to the potential to create shared "learning-through-doing" environments that are available anywhere, anytime, and on demand (Dede, 1996). Furthermore, depending on the collaborative setting and its context students need/tend to ascribe various roles for themselves. Thus, students with their personal environments may form a temporary *distributed environment* for collaboration, where parts of each collaborator's personal environments partially overlap. Our understanding of DLE does not refer merely to an attempt to bring together geographically and temporarily distributed students and facilitators. Rather, it signifies a repertoire of tools and services, human and material resources managed by collaborators. Therefore, a distributed environment emerges when individuals engage in collaborative activities, and is maintained for the duration of the collaboration (Fiedler & Pata, 2009). DLEs are also dynamic in terms of their components, structure, and extension. They are adjusted and defined according to student needs, preferences, and abilities.

Distributed environments enable conversations on subject matter (terminology, concepts), processes (distribution of work, roles, media), and execution (Fiedler & Pata, 2009). However, all types of actions are highly intertwined and students can switch rapidly from one to another. In loosely coupled, networked settings, these actions may need to be mediated by an appropriate selection of tools and services. While the choice of technological components in a PLE only requires internal reflection, collaborative settings require explanation, negotiation, and mutual acceptance of selected technologies in order to form a functional distributed learning environment (Väljataga & Fiedler, 2008).

PLE AND DLE IMPLEMENTATION IN HIGHER EDUCATION

In recent years, personal and distributed learning environments have been considered as a revolutionary concept for learning engagements of individuals throughout life (Muldoon, 2008). Since lifelong learning is recognized as being crucial in a knowledge society, personal and distributed environments can be easily created for the purposes of one's study activities and combined with work and leisure pursuits. In this context PLEs should be considered as permanent, adaptable, and evolving, enabling different types of learning in different context and at different times in life (Henri et al., 2008).

The adoption and use of PLEs and DLEs in formal educational contexts embodies a paradigm shift that moves away from current institutional practices of learning and teaching (Jones, 2008) as well as learning and course management systems provided by institutions. The implementation of PLEs and DLEs should be seen as a complex intervention into an already complex educational context (Snowden & Boone, 2007), where, apart from ethical issues of intellectual property, issues like curriculum development, content delivery, and assessment also require some rethinking (Arenas, 2008).

As the PLE and DLE are not a single piece of software, but instead a collection of tools and services used by a student or a group of students to meet their needs as part of their personal learning and work endeavors, the characteristics of the PLE and DLE design may be achieved using a combination of existing devices (laptops, mobile phones, portable media devices), desktop applications (RSS news readers, instant messaging clients, browsers, calendars), and web-based services (social bookmark services, web logs [blogs], wikis) (Wilson, 2008).

The role of facilitators is to participate peripherally as experts or mentors assisting students to construct their meaning through sustained communication. Such dialogue, often established and initiated in face-to-face interaction, can continue virtually in environments supported by technology (Garrison & Kanuka, 2004).

LEARNING LANDSCAPES SUPPORTED BY WEB 2.0 TOOLS

This chapter focuses on research mainly on the technological part of PLEs and DLEs, that is, the landscape of social media tools and services that students use. The authors view learning as the process of continual change, requiring students to adapt to new situations. Current social media make possible a new level of openness, flexibility, and customization. Combining various tools and services offers quite powerful ways of managing, repurposing, and remixing information in order to support various regulative, coordinative, and executive processes in knowledge building. Planning the landscape of tools and services in personal or distributed environments requires an understanding of information flows between the different tools and services.

For instance, one can imagine a scenario in which a student makes use of blog for presenting thoughts and essays (e.g., submitting assignments). In order to be able to keep track of the other students' postings one may want to add all the blog addresses of other students to his or her blog's "blogroll" area. Feedback on assigments can be given by peers and facilitators via the comments feature of the blog. Furthermore, to keep track of the course materials and other resources one may want to create an account on delicious and "pull" the tag cloud into his or her blog. This can be considered as a minimal set of tools and services for participating in an online as well as face-to-face course. Naturally, giving the freedom to select and combine appropriate tools and services to support and manage learning activities challenges students not only to deal with the content or the problem but also the context around it. The personal choice of tools and services can be interpreted as an aspect of the learning process itself (Dalsgaard, 2006) and the creation of a personal environment for learning can be considered as one of the learning outcomes (Wild, Mödritscher, & Sigurdarson, 2008).

Many students will have had little experience in selecting and planning tools for collaborative learning activities. To be effective lifelong learners, however, students require training in how to cope with dynamic personal and collaborative learning environments. Mapping the learning environment and its different tools and services in the context of personal activities presumes that students are aware of the positive and negative aspects of the tools and services as well as having the capacity to make use of the perceived affordances.

AFFORDANCES

To analyze how students perceive the components of their personal and distributed learning environments, it may be useful and appropriate to apply the concept of affordances. The term "affordances" was coined by Gibson (1979) as part of his ecological framework of perception and action. This framework considers perception more as a direct process of translating environmental action potentialities into action. Gibson originally defined the affordances provided by an environment as opportunities for action. According to him, mutuality between an actor and the environment constitutes the basis for the actor's perception and action. However, alternative definitions of and approaches to affordances exist. For example, Greeno (1994) sees affordances as an opportunity to describe the properties of the environment that permit certain activities. Albrechtsen, Andersen, Bødker, & Pejtersen (2001) extended the affordance definition as follows: affordances are "cues for action relevance, displayed in the context of a virtual ecology of work" (p. 32). Chemero (2003) understands affordances as features of whole situations.

In this chapter the elaborated ecological notion to affordances is followed, which takes into account: (1) students with certain objectives and the task objectives; (2) students' continuous interaction with each other and the facilitator; and (3) multiple objects, tools, and services in the learning environment (Fiedler & Pata, 2009). The affordances as potentials for actions are evoked and changed dynamically. This happens in the interplay of students' and facilitators', task objectives, learning culture, the activation of previously experienced emotions and performed learning activities, human and material resources in the learning environment (see, for example, Fiedler & Pata, 2009; Barab & Roth, 2006). The affordances of the environment for a certain person are dependent on the co-participants and their different perceptions of the affordances (Gaver, 1996; Kreijns, Kirschner, & Jochems, 2002). For example, the affordances related to social bookmarking tools would be fully actualized only if other people use the same tool. The affordances of social filtering and mashing information with tags and feeds is dependent on collective writing and tagging the information. Thus perceived affordances as action potentialities determine which activities and social media tools and services would mediate the most.

To reflect upon affordances in personal or distributed learning environments, students can write them down according to a set of rules. Each affordance may consist of an action and perceptual dimensions (visual, aural, temporal). In addition to actions, the affordance description may also consist of the human and material resources such as a subject (e.g., student, community, group), artifact or tool (e.g., web page, document, image, model) and their properties (e.g., shared, interactive, etc.). Examples of affordances may be the synchronous audio chat of students, shared media artifacts, recordings of community chat, or RSS feeds from peers.

Awareness of the affordances of social media tools and services associated with PLEs and DLEs, coupled with adequate preparation while engaged in formal education, may hold the key for lifelong learners across the lifespan (Muldoon, 2008). How students perceive the affordances of social media tools and services for supporting the formation of their own landscape of tools and services is described in the sections that follow.

RESEARCH DESIGN

An experimental course was designed with the concepts of personal and distributed learning environments and affordances. This experimental course was conducted as an action research study at Tallinn University, Estonia. In this study, action research was employed by the facilitators who developed and implemented the course. Creswell (2002) explains that action research is typically undertaken in a school setting among educators—in line with Creswell's recommendations, reflection, data collection, and experimentation were all parts of this action research. The purpose of the study was to critically examine the authors' practices and to investigate the positive and negative aspects of an educational technology course in which students were encouraged to create and make use of personal or distributed learning environments to mediate their activities. The research focus was on the technological parts of the PLEs and DLEs. Specifically, the formation of a landscape of tools and services and students' perception of technological components were studied. The following research questions were formulated to guide and frame the study:

1. How did students comprehend the concepts of PLEs and DLEs for supporting their activities?
2. What were students' perceptions of the affordances of their PLEs and DLEs?
3. Based on students' perceptions of the affordances and their comprehension of PLEs and DLEs, what changes are needed to make the course design more supportive for learning?

Participants

The research involved 24 Master's-level students and two facilitators from Tallinn University. The ages of the students varied between 20 and 50 years old. Most of them were active secondary school teachers. Some worked in other fields such as industry or public service. Students had different ICT skills, ranging from basic use of e-mail and web browsers to high-level programming skills. Some of the students were familiar with the concept of social media, but only a few of them had used blogs and synchronous communication tools (e.g., Skype, MSN Messenger) outside of formal education. Facilitators of the course were proficient users of social media and had experience in supporting online courses.

Research Context

The study was conducted as part of a Master's-level educational technology course at Tallinn University in Spring 2007. It was presumed that social media tools and services would enable students to compose their own landscape of tools as part of their personal or distributed environments, allowing them to plan learning activities while supporting self-reflection, monitoring, and knowledge retrieval. The bottom-up approach to finding and developing their learning environments was applied, leaving students a large degree of freedom to develop their own meaningful learning activities in personal environments. Furthermore, the course was designed to promote students' active participation in social knowledge construction processes in which they needed to integrate their personal and distributed environments. Such a course design was undertaken to introduce students with more authentic situations and to prepare them to meet the challenges that emerge when they need to learn without access to institutional LMSs.

The overall objectives of the course were to:

- give students authentic, personally meaningful and challenging learning experiences, where they could form and make use of their PLEs and DLEs for mediating activities;
- introduce students to the concept of self-direction in PLEs and DLEs;
- provide students with conceptual tools for visualizing their PLEs and DLEs that mediate self-directed and collaborative knowledge building;
- enable students to schematically represent their activities and PLEs and DLEs as tools for planning and monitoring their self-directed and collaborative knowledge building activities.

The course lasted for eight weeks and included three face-to-face contact days in addition to individual assignments between class meetings. Contact days focused on practical activities, intended to familiarize students with different social media tools and services. The theoretical framework of using social media for individual and collaborative learning was explained on contact days. Students had to complete three assignments during the course:

1. **Individual task:** Choose one activity (preferably an activity that was to be performed their normal study, work, or leisure time) and develop a learning environment that supports this activity. Describe the perceived affordances in your learning environment.
2. **Collaborative task:** Choose one group activity and develop learning environments that support this collaborative activity. Both assignments were discussed and presented during contact days. Describe the perceived affordances in your learning environment.
3. Individual essays about the affordances students perceived in their personal and distributed environments.

Students were free to use different web-based or desktop tools for visualizing activity schemes and learning environments. As Gliffy (http://www.gliffy.com/) and bubbl.us (http://www.bubbl.us/) were introduced on contact days, these applications turned out to be the most popular for drawing schemes. There were no rules for how the schemes had to be drawn and presented. Students' activity schemes and environment schemes represented their understanding of how the components of their environments were linked to each other, and how their chosen activity could be performed through the tools and services in those environments. In addition to visualizing and explaining the activities and environments, students were asked to write an essay in which they were required to describe the affordances they perceived in their personal and distributed environments while performing their chosen activity.

Learning outcomes of the students were assessed by the course facilitators. The assessment scheme took into account the relationship between the activities the students described and the logical suitability of the environment they designed for supporting this particular activity.

Course Environment and Design

Facilitators and students jointly developed the course environment (see Figure 1) using social

Figure 1. Course landscape of tools and services

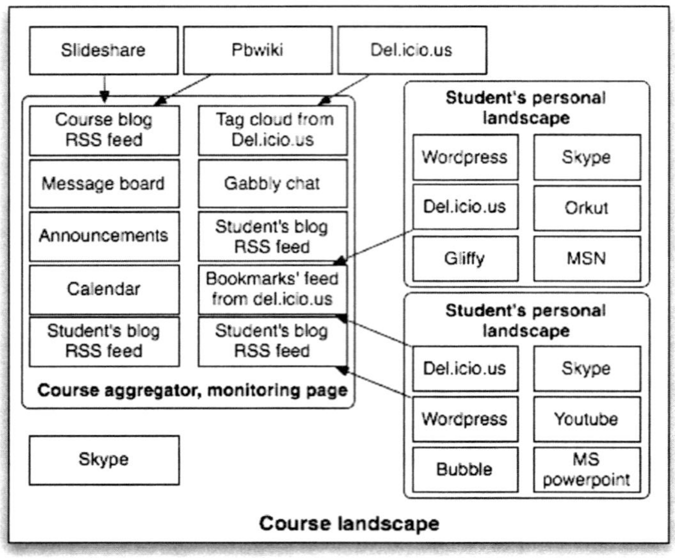

media tools and services including a course blog (using WordPress: see http://www.wordpress.com/), social bookmarking tool (del.icio.us: now known simply as "delicious" at http://www.delicious.com/), slide repository (Slideshare: http://www.slideshare.net/), wiki (Pbwiki: http://www.pbwiki.com/), synchronous communication tools (Gabbly: http://www.gabbly.com/, Skype), and aggregator (Pageflakes: http://www.pageflakes.com/). The social media syndication platform Splashcast (no longer in existence) was also used.

The course blog was maintained by the two facilitators. The primary functions of the blog were to organize learning materials and assignments, and to serve as an information channel between students and facilitators. Learning materials were presented on separate pages of the course blog. Only facilitators had the ability to edit pages in the blog. However, students could contribute to the blog by writing comments. This allowed the facilitators to make additions to the learning materials, if necessary, and adapt them to the students' needs. The feeds from Slideshare and Splashcast were integrated into the learning texts on course blog pages. Learning resources were additionally linked to the sidebar of the course blog. The blog sidebar provided links to a monitoring tool in Pageflakes, a course wiki for collaborative writing hosted on PBwiki, and a collection of social bookmarks for the course in del.icio.us.

The Pageflakes-based course aggregator served as a second central repository for course materials, integrating different media with feed and mashup technologies. The course aggregator brought together feeds from the course blog and students' blogs, enabling mutual monitoring between students and facilitators. Different widgets from Pageflakes enabled the embedding of a public forum that contained a page for announcements, access to a synchronous chat tool (Gabbly), a tag-cloud feed from the social bookmarks site, and the mashed course tag feed from different students' social bookmarking sites. Thus, the aggregator served as a central tool for course management and monitoring for both students and facilitators. Figure 1 demonstrates how the tools and services were bound together in the course environment.

Students were asked to start the course with a set of individual tools and services, including a blog and social bookmarking service. Those who had existing tools were not required to make new ones for the course. Instead they were encouraged to use their existing tools and mark course-specific postings with appropriate tags. This approach was taken to encourage students to use the tools that they had previously used for personal knowledge building and knowledge management, and to expose them to new ways in which these tools could be used to support and enhance their learning. During the course students were asked to present the progress of their assignments and their reflections about their work in personal blogs. This enabled the facilitators to monitor their development between contact days, and give suggestions on how to improve their learning environment to support their chosen activity. On a weekly basis, facilitators provided individual support and feedback to the students by commenting on their blog posts. Students were encouraged to monitor their peers' progress and comment on one another's posts as well.

Each student created a social bookmarking account on del.icio.us, where her or she tagged course-related materials for sharing with peers and facilitators. The facilitators also tagged materials that were relevant to the course with the same course tag. Each student bookmarked the address of his or her own blog on his or her personal del.icio.us site using the common course tag. A social bookmark feed collected all the addresses of students' blogs so they were visible on the course aggregator.

During the course, a comprehensive set of tools and systems for social publishing (e.g., PBwiki, Google Docs and Spreadsheets), synchronous communication (Vyew—http://www.vyew.com/, Gabbly—http://www.gabbly.com/), visual model creation (Gliffy, bubbl.us), knowledge artifact storage and creation (Slideshare, Splashcast, LeMill—http://www.lemill.net/), and aggregation (Pageflakes, Netvibes—http://www.netvibes.com/) were introduced to the students. Several examples of aggregated personal and group environments were described in learning materials.

Data Collection and Analysis

The following types of qualitative data were collected from students' blogs:

1. Activity schemes with explanations of how learning activities were managed in their PLEs and DLEs;
2. Environment schemes that illustrated the various components (human and material resources, tools and services) in the students' PLEs and DLEs;
3. Reflections about the affordances students perceived in their PLEs and DLEs.

These data sources were combined. Two researchers analyzed students' activity and environmental schemes within their PLEs and DLEs and their reflections about the perceived affordances of these environements. The first research question was to investigate the sequential occurrence of affordances along a timeline in students' blog posts—the purpose here was to find out whether and how students' perception of affordances changed over time. Secondly, a sequential analysis of every student's schemes of PLE and DLE along the timeline was carried out from the perspective of evidence of the student as an active agent/designer in the environment and pertaining to connections between different components in PLE and DLE, for example, how the tools and systems were connected to each other in their PLEs and DLEs (e.g., feed pulling, information workflows, tag clouds). In addition, reflections about affordances were used as supporting data, where students' opinions about their development and progress were captured.

The second research question investigated what kind of tools and services students' PLEs consisted of and analysed the types of tools and services they used for forming their DLEs. The third research question investigated the affordances perceived by the students in relation to every tool and service in their PLEs and DLEs.

As students expressed their perceived affordances in various ways, affordances were categorized according to their similarity and semantics into nine types: *affordances related to self-tutoring*; *individual creative assignments*; *collaborative creative assignments*; *assessment and evaluation*; *learning environment assembly*; *community formation and grouping*; *lecturing and presenting*; *information filtering and regulation*; and *monitoring and support.*

Affordances related to *self-tutoring* refers to the concept of self (e.g., self-management, self-assessment, personal scheduling and time management). The second type as *individual creative assignments* indicates creating, sharing, and presenting artifacts individually. *Collaborative creative assignments* focus on the same activities, but in a collaborative context. *Assessment and evaluation* refers to feedback to students, provided not only by facilitators, but also by other students. Activities like finding, selecting, using, and evaluating tools and services are affordances related to *learning environment assembly*. Privacy and rights management issues were added to this type, as they influence the selection and use of tools and services. *Community formation and grouping* refers to activities that support group formation and tasks division between group members. Affordances related to *lecturing and presenting* include publishing artifacts, presenting information in different media formats, and posting news by facilitators and students. *Information filtering* means managing and understanding any kind of information. Some examples are tagging information or content flows, filtering blogs and news feeds, and collecting, aggregating, and mashing different feeds. *Regulation, monitoring, and support* refers to encouraging learner motivation, providing support and supervision, questioning, and monitoring facilitators' and students' activities. This categorization enabled the researchers to count how often students perceived certain affordance types with respect to each tool and service. It also allowed for comparison of the social media tools and services used in the course from a pedagogical perspective.

With respect to the third research question, conclusions were made based on the analysis of affordance categorization, their occurrence in students' PLEs and DLEs, as well as sequential changes in students' schemes of PLEs and DLEs.

RESULTS AND DISCUSSION

Research Question 1: How Did Students Comprehend the Concepts of PLEs and DLEs for Supporting Their Activities?

Schemes of students' learning environments appeared to be an important strategy for students to shape their comprehension about their personal and distributed learning environments. The changes in the schemes of PLEs and DLEs could be observed from sequential posts in students' blogs. Blogs offered data on how students acquired a more complex understanding of environmental functions and how the different components of the environment can be connected by continuously changing workflows and mashed feeds. Such changes occurred for most of the students. Students' initial understanding of the landscape of tools and services in their PLEs and DLEs are illustrated in Figure 2.

Figure 2 shows that students' initial understanding of their personal and distributed environments was centralized, and that they placed themselves in the static center of the group of tools and services they were using. At first students, did not acknowledge that the center of their environments changed from moment to moment according to their actions performed in these environments. Students' understanding of

Figure 2. Students' initial understanding of the landscape of tools and services in their personal and distributed learning environments

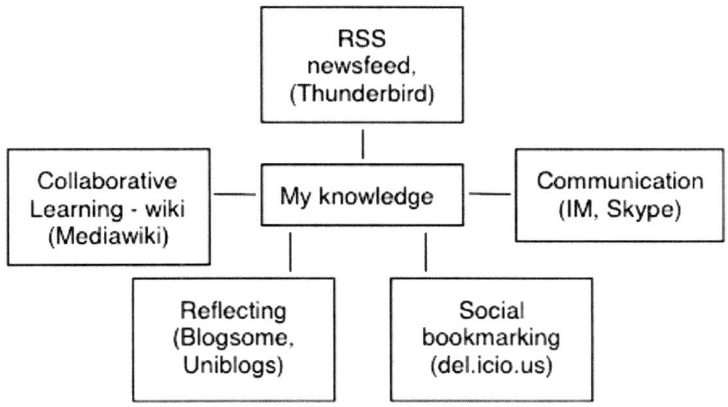

their PLEs and DLEs changed during the course as they were asked to schematically envision their landscape of tools and services from various perspectives (Figure 3). The assignments of the course required students to think of their activities in connection with potential tools and services, and discover the functional purpose of these in relation to their own learning. Gradually students started to understand the information and content flows between tools and services, which caused constant changes in the center of their PLEs and DLEs. They then started to distribute themselves and their activities between the tools and services in their environments.

Research Question 2: What were Students' Perceptions of the Affordances of Their PLEs and DLEs?

The following provides an overview of the perceived affordances that students related to social media tools and services. Figure 4 represents the nine affordance types in relation to four tools that were the most popular in students' PLEs and DLEs. It demonstrates the number of affordances students perceived in personal and distributed learning environments with respect to particular tools and services. However, since not all students made use of these tools, the affordances presented in the figure do not represent the perceptions of every student in the course.

Students' Perceptions of Affordances Related to Blogs

Students perceived blogs as the tool with the widest range of potentials for action (see Table 1). One of the reasons for this result might be the fact that blogs were obligatory tools for all students in the course, so there was a higher likelihood of spending more time to become familiar with this tool.

Students found several affordances that could be classified as supporting *individual creative assignments* (see Figure 4): "getting tasks," "browsing thematic information," "reflecting on artifacts in the blog," and "revising information." However, students also perceived a high number of affordances that involved/implied interaction with other students' artifacts, such as "commenting on the posts," "sharing files" and "giving feedback to peer's work." This indicated an emerging paradigm change: commenting on and sharing each other's assignments shifted the

Figure 3. Students' advanced understanding of the landscape of tools and services in their personal and distributed environments

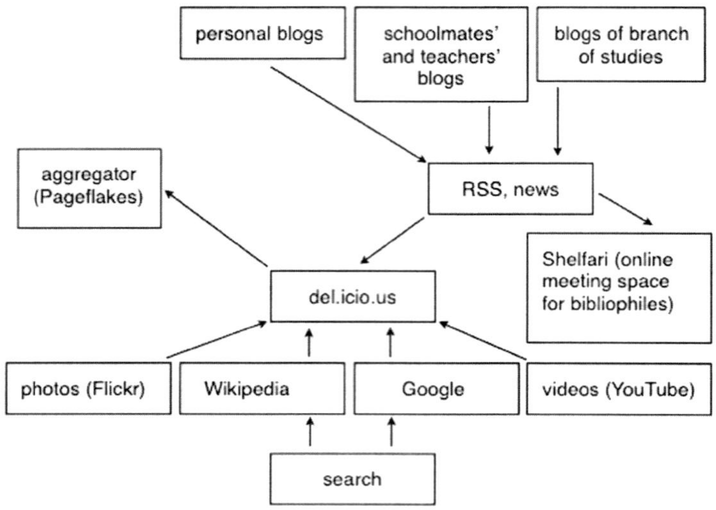

Figure 4. Students' perception of affordances related to social media tools and services, and affordance types

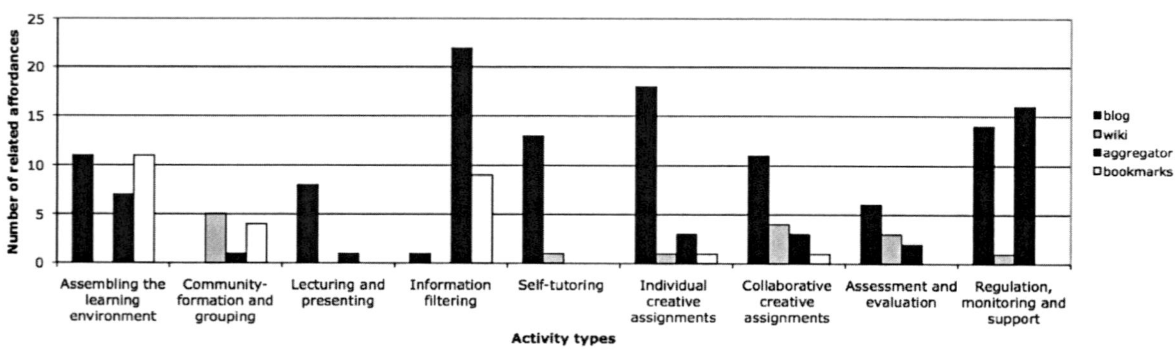

emphasis from outcome-related assignments, where students must produce a final artifact only, towards increased attention to the learning process itself, in which students develop and dynamically change their knowledge.

A number of affordances could be classified as supporting the affordance of *self-tutoring*. Affordances such as "self-reflection," "self-analysis," and "self-evaluation" were perceived as part of blog-related actions. This suggests that blogs could be used actively in educational contexts. Other affordances mentioned by students were "creating time-tables and action plans" and "doing homework."

One of the students mentioned the affordances of "relating blogs with other mediating environments," indicating that indeed such affordances are perceived due to their interrelations with other tools. On the other hand, students did not mention any affordances related to *community-formation*

Table 1. Frequency of instances of the perceived affordances in relation to the tools and services

	Blog	Wiki	Aggregator	Bookmarks
Assembling the learning environment	11	0	7	11
Community formation and grouping	0	5	1	4
Lecturing and presenting	8	0	1	0
Information filtering	1	0	22	9
Self-tutoring	13	1	0	0
Individual creative assignments	18	1	3	1
Collaborative creative assignments	11	4	3	1
Assessment and evaluation	6	3	2	0
Regulation, monitoring, and support	14	1	16	0

activity. This was surprising because it is commonly argued that blogs are effective tools for social networking (Downes, 2006). As a result of this finding, it was decided that subsequent courses should include more activities that are related to social networking and community building, using new social media tools.

The most frequent affordances related to *lecturing and presenting* were "giving tasks" and "presenting information to the students." The fact that students could perceive those task-related affordances is promising for educators who would like to use blogs as primary teaching tools. Some students, however, generalized this affordance and did not mention task-specific actions. The affordances they perceived—"creating information" and "publishing artifacts"—are the most general functions commonly related to blogs.

Only one affordance was classified as supporting the *information filtering* activity type: "understanding the information given by the facilitator." However, this affordance still indicated cognitive information filtering, rather than information retrieval through technical features of social media tools and services. Blogs allow several means of information filtering by tags, keywords, incoming RSS feeds, and tag feeds. The course facilitators concluded that it may be necessary to provide more opportunities to use social information retrieval in the course activities in order to increase students' awareness of various affordances related to information filtering.

Students perceived various affordances supporting *collaborative creative assignments*, including "communication with peers and the facilitator," "sharing and exchanging information with students," "collecting the results from the group activity," and "coordinating the information among the group of students." However, it was evident that students did not yet perceive all the possibilities that social media allows. For instance, there was little awareness of mashing feeds, retrieving information using tags, and social browsing.

Affordances related to *assessment and evaluation* were "evaluation of students' new knowledge," "getting feedback," and "learning from the result of group activities." It is noteworthy that the latter two were related to the aspects that students can gain from assessment activities. Students were not able to point out many different affordances that blogs might offer for evaluation. This indicated that facilitators should develop a bigger variety of assessment methods that originate from the blog functions. It was considered important that assessment and evaluation procedures should increase students' motivation to learn, and not operate merely as grading instruments.

Finally, affordances related to enhancing *regulation, monitoring, and support* were mentioned by students. These included "facilitators monitoring student's action and reflection," "supervising students," "giving feedback and supporting," "recognizing students," and "giving enthusiasm."

Students' Perceptions of Affordances Related to the Aggregator

The majority of aggregator-related affordances perceived by students belonged to activities such as *assembling the learning environment*, *filtering information*, and *regulation, monitoring, and support* (see Table 1 and Figure 4). Though aggregators are commonly introduced as personal tools, in this course they were used as a group tool. Thus, it is understandable that students perceived mainly affordances related to *monitoring and filtering information*. Since an aggregator was one of the central tools for students to monitor each other's blog feeds and offer feedback, this strongly influenced students' perception of aggregators in general. However, students did not pay much attention to the mashed bookmark feeds and bookmark tag cloud, which were also accessible from the aggregation page. The widgets supporting asynchronous and synchronous discussions were part of the group aggregator. Therefore, aggregators were also perceived as a medium for supporting community-formation activities.

Affordances enhancing *information filtering* activities with an aggregator included "social aggregation of tags/feeds/artifacts/information," "collecting friends'/community's feeds," and "creating personal filtering for the feeds." It was notable that, while some students perceived information as feeds, others saw it as an artifact or blog posting. It may be assumed that this represents two types of thinking: technological (feeds, tags) and information-related (artifacts, blog posts). The perceived affordances related to the aggregator clearly expressed students' new technological understanding of social media, as terms like "feed," "social tag," "aggregation," and "filtering" appeared in most of their responses.

Affordances related to *regulation, monitoring, and support* were "getting the instructions," "monitoring students' feeds/artifacts," "aggregating feeds," and "sharing personal feeds." Students used similar expressions for naming affordances as interactions by facilitators and peers regarding regulation, monitoring, and support activities. This indicated that the learning environment of the course narrowed the gap between the facilitators' and students' roles.

Affordances belonging to the *self-tutoring* activity were entirely absent, while *individual creative assignments* were supported by a few affordances (e.g., "collecting information," "reading feeds," and "selecting information"). *Collaborative creative assignments* with an aggregator were expressed mainly by the affordances of "collaborative monitoring the feeds of peers." Again, two distinct perceptions—technological (feed) and student-related (peer, student)—were observed. *Assessment-related affordances* were "evaluating feeds" and "getting feedback." Students saw two aspects of evaluation as similar to blog affordances, namely "facilitator does the evaluation" and "students get benefit from the evaluation." The only affordance supporting *lecturing and presenting* activity was "publishing feeds."

Students' Perceptions of Affordances Related to Wikis

As a wiki tool was not represented very intensively in students' environments, and it was hardly used in the course, the perception of its potential for action remained moderate (see Figure 4 and Table 1).

Affordances that students perceived for wikis could be categorized mostly under activities related to *collaborative creative assignments* such as "joint writing," "analysis of completed community tasks," and "analysis of an action plan made for group." These results were not surprising, because students used wikis mainly for collaborative tasks, and less for individual purposes. In addition, some students perceived wiki-related affordances of *community formation and grouping* (e.g., "supporting the development of group," "creating the work group," "making agreement on tools," and "dividing the tasks in group").

Activities related to *assessment and evaluation* were mentioned frequently in relation to wikis. Affordances like "learning from joint writing," "analysis of thesis structure," and "giving feedback" were mentioned. Among the activities supporting *individual creative assignments* with wikis, only one affordance was mentioned by students—"correction of given information"—suggesting that students used wikis individually for text editing. "Monitoring feedback" was the only affordance mentioned in connection with *regulation, monitoring, and support* activity. Clearly, students found that if they worked and learned together in a group, wikis would be most suitable tool for monitoring feedback from peers and facilitators.

No affordances were mentioned that could be related to the activities of *lecturing and presenting*, *information filtering*, or *assembling the learning environment.* Since wikis could be easily used for presenting assignments, the fact that students did not perceive wikis as a presentation tool was notable. However, there is a need to design more specific tasks that would trigger students to perceive additional hidden or specific learning affordances that are novel and particularly relevant to using social media tools and services in active learning.

Students' Perceptions of Affordances Related to Social Bookmarking

Students shared their blog addresses by tagging them with a specified course tag via a social bookmarking tool (see Figure 4 and Table 2). This tool was another compulsory component of the course. Social bookmarking could offer opportunities of finding and selecting tools and services by subscribing to others' tags. Such tags and comments added to bookmarks about tools might have increased students' awareness of the experiences that other students have had with different tools, broadening their perspective of possible affordances. It was found that a large number of affordances related to the social bookmarking tool could be categorized under the activity of *assembling the learning environment.* This was obviously influenced by the required activities students had to perform with this tool. Similarly, the influence of the learning activities of the course on the awareness of *community formation and grouping* affordances was clearly demonstrated.

The students' perception of *information filtering* was the most frequently mentioned affordance for social bookmarking tools. "Tagging important information, despite the medium used for presenting the information" was the main affordance that students perceived. The affordances supporting *collaborative and individual creative assignment* were seldom mentioned. Only "sharing information" and "saving artifacts" were perceived, which was expected.

Students cited no affordances for social bookmarking tools relating to the activity types *lecturing and presenting*, *self-tutoring*, *assessment and evaluation*, or *regulation, monitoring, and support.* This points to the necessity of making changes in how social bookmarking tools are presented and used in subsequent iterations of the course.

Research Question 3: Based on Students' Perceptions of the Affordances and Their Comprehension of PLEs and DLEs, What Changes are Needed to Make the Course Design More Supportive for Students' Learning?

The dynamic changes in students' perception of the learning environment must also be considered when designing a course. Obvious changes in students' schemes of PLE and DLE show the need for more vizualisation tasks in the course, which help students to understand their learning environment and its affordances as well as their own position within the environment. Students' ongoing perception of additional affordances can be seen as a result of the contiguous practice of using different tools and services for building up one's learning environment, ongoing conversation with peer students and facilitators about the perceived affordances, and ongoing demonstration of tools and services by facilitators. Personal freedom as well as interest and desire to try out various tools and services for one's own purposes plays a crucial role here. This implies the need to give students more opportunities for advancing their competencies with respect to self-direction in terms of giving them not only the freedom to set up their own goals and strategies, but also to choose resources and create their own personal environments for supporting their learning activities.

However, the facilitators' perception of affordances can be different from the students' perception, which makes the choice of the "right" or ideal media and environment a challenging task. Relating affordances for particular activities together and establishing peers as facilitators becomes an essential element of a successful learning environment. Students and facilitators must develop a common understanding of the affordances of a given tool or service to make effective performance possible in the learning environment. The similar use of the tools and services and distribution of labor to support the realization of learning objectives in the environment can be realized when there is communication and joint understanding. Facilitators can attempt to anticipate (but cannot predefine) the affordances of the learning environment. Thus, the learning environment is not complete or fixed when learning starts; it evolves as part of the learning process. The dynamic changes in the students' perception of the learning environment must also be considered when designing a course. Iterative cycles of evaluation among students and facilitators about the components of the environment must be conducted.

IMPLICATIONS AND CONCLUSION

The purpose of this research was to determine how to improve the design of a Web 2.0 technology course in a way that it would take into account students' perceptions of the learning environment. The course provided students with challenging situations and encouraged them to form personal and distributed learning environments supported by a range of social media tools and services. Changes in the students' perception of their PLEs and DLEs were monitored. Applying the concept of affordances in the students' assignments helped to supply insight into how students perceived their environments and therefore facilitated the evaluation of the course.

The study shows that instructional designers and facilitators should take into account students' perceptions and expectations of the learning environment as an important aspect of course design. Furthermore, students should be encouraged and challenged to develop skills and confidence in the selection, application, and use of tools and services for personalized learning. Thus, there is a need for educators to continue to investigate new pedagogical approaches and models that place students at the center and enhance a student's ability to organize and customize his or her own learning environment.

Changes in students' perception of the affordances of their PLEs and DLEs suggest the need to refine the facilitator's role in student-centered, social-media-based courses. Students' differing perceptions of social media as personal learning, knowledge-building, and management tools highlight additional issues and considerations for student-centered course design.

In closing, course design should therefore promote activities that:

- enhance social networking;
- allow commenting and sharing of work, stressing the process instead of the outcome;
- advance self-direction and self-awareness in personal and distributed learning environments;
- enable community and group formation;
- support social information retrieval and the filtering and mashing of feeds;
- allow a greater variety of assessment methods;
- enhance both technological and information-related thinking.

ACKNOWLEDGMENT

This study was funded by Estonian SF grant 7663 and MER targeted research 0130159s08.

REFERENCES

Albrechtsen, H., Andersen, H. H. K., Bødker, S., & Pejtersen, A. M. (2001). *Affordances in activity theory and cognitive systems engineering*. Roskilde, Denmark: Risø National Laboratory.

Arenas, E. (2008). Personal learning environments: Implications and challenges. In D. Orr, P. A. Danaher, G. Danaher, & R. E. Harreveld (Eds.), *Lifelong learning: Reflecting on successes and framing futures. Keynote and refereed papers from the Fifth International Lifelong Learning Conference* (pp. 54–59). Rockhampton, Australia: Central Queensland University Press.

Attwell, G. (2007). Personal learning environments—the future of elearning? *eLearning Papers, 2*. Retrieved July 20, 2008, from http://www.elearningeuropa.info/files/media/media11561.pdf

Barab, S. A., & Roth, W.-M. (2006). Intentionally-bound systems and curricular-based ecosystems: An ecological perspective on knowing. *Educational Researcher, 35*(5), 3–13. doi:10.3102/0013189X035005003

Barnwal, R. (2007, January 21). Web 2.0 is all about understanding the economic value of social interaction. *AlooTechie*. Retrieved July 20, 2008, from http://www.alootechie.com/news/1977.asp

Candy, P. (2002). *Information literacy and lifelong learning* [White paper]. Prague, The Czech Republic: UNESCO.

Chemero, A. (2003). An outline of a theory of affordances. *Ecological Psychology, 15*(2), 181–195. doi:10.1207/S15326969ECO1502_5

Converso, J. A., Schaffer, S. P., & Guerra, I. J. (1999). *Distributed learning environment: Major functions, implementation, and continuous improvement*. Tallahassee, FL: Learning Systems Institute, Florida State University.

Creswell, J. W. (2002). *Educational research: Planning, conducting, and evaluating quantitative and qualitative research*. Upper Saddle River, NJ: Pearson Education.

Dalsgaard, C. (2006). Social software: E-learning beyond learning management systems. *European Journal of Open, Distance and E-Learning, 9*(2). Retrieved April 15, 2008, from http://www.eurodl.org/materials/contrib/2006/Christian_Dalsgaard.htm

Dede, C. (1996). Emerging technologies and distributed learning. *American Journal of Distance Education, 10*(2), 4–36. doi:10.1080/08923649609526919

Downes, S. (2005, October). E-learning 2.0. *eLearn Magazine*. Retrieved July 20, 2008, from http://www.elearnmag.org/subpage.cfm?section=articles&article=29-1

Downes, S. (2006). *Learning networks and connective knowledge*. Retrieved March 12, 2008, from http://it.coe.uga.edu/itforum/paper92/paper92.html

Dron, J., & Bhattacharya, M. (2007). Lost in the Web 2.0 jungle. In J. M. Spector, D. G. Sampson, T. Okamoto, Kinshuk, S. A. Cerri, M. Ueno, & A. Kashihara (Eds.), *Proceedings of the Seventh International Conference on Advanced Learning Technologies* (pp. 895–896). Los Alamitos, CA: IEEE Computer Society.

Entwistle, N., & Tait, H. (1990). Approaches to learning, evaluations of teaching, and preferences for contrasting academic environments. *Higher Education*, *19*(2), 169–194. doi:10.1007/BF00137106

Fiedler, S., & Kieslinger, B. (2006). Adapting to changing landscapes in education. In T. Hug, M. Lindner, & P. A. Bruck (Eds.), *Micromedia & E-learning 2.0: Gaining the big picture. Proceedings of Microlearning Conference 2006* (pp. 78–89). Innsbruck, Austria: Innsbruck University Press.

Fiedler, S., & Pata, K. (2009). Distributed learning environments and social software: In search for a framework of design. In Hatzipanagos, S., & Warburton, S. (Eds.), *Handbook of research on social software and developing community ontologies* (pp. 151–164). Hershey, PA: Information Science Reference. doi:10.4018/978-1-60566-208-4.ch011

Garrison, D. R., & Kanuka, H. (2004). Blended learning: Uncovering its transformative potential in higher education. *The Internet and Higher Education*, *7*(2), 95–105. doi:10.1016/j.iheduc.2004.02.001

Gaver, W. W. (1996). Situating Action II: Affordances for interaction: The social is material for design. *Ecological Psychology*, *8*(2), 111–129. doi:10.1207/s15326969eco0802_2

Gibson, J. J. (1979). *The ecological approach to visual perception*. Boston: Houghton Mifflin.

Gonella, L., & Pantò, E. (2008). Didactic architectures and organization models: A process of mutual adaptation. *eLearning Papers, 9*. Retrieved July 20, 2008, from http://www.elearningeuropa.info/files/media/media15973.pdf

Greeno, J. G. (1994). Gibson's affordances. *Psychological Review*, *101*(2), 236–342. doi:10.1037/0033-295X.101.2.336

Henri, F., Charlier, B., & Limpens, F. (2008). Understanding PLE as an essential component of the learning process. In J. Luca & E. Weippl (Eds.), *Proceedings of World Conference on Educational Multimedia, Hypermedia and Telecommunications 2008* (pp. 3766–3770). Chesapeake, VA: Association for the Advancement of Computers in Education.

Johnson, M., Hollins, P., Wilson, S., & Liber, O. (2006). Towards a reference model for the personal learning environment. In L. Markauskaite, P. Goodyear, & P. Reimann (Eds.), *Who's learning? Whose technology? Proceedings of the 23rd Australasian Society for Computers in Learning in Tertiary Education (ASCILITE) Conference* (pp. 385–389). Sydney: University of Sydney.

Johnson, M., & Liber, O. (2008). The personal learning environment and the human condition: From theory to teaching practice. *Interactive Learning Environments*, *16*(1), 3–15. doi:10.1080/10494820701772652

Jones, D. (2008). PLEs: Framing one future for lifelong learning, e-learning and universities. In D. Orr, P. A. Danaher, G. Danaher, & R. E. Harreveld (Eds.), *Lifelong learning: Reflecting on successes and framing futures. Keynote and refereed papers from the Fifth International Lifelong Learning Conference* (pp. 231–236). Rockhampton, Australia: Central Queensland University Press.

Kolas, L., & Staupe, A. (2007). The PLExus Prototype: A PLE realized as topic maps. In J. M. Spector, D. G. Sampson, T. Okamoto, Kinshuk, S. A. Cerri, M. Ueno, & A. Kashihara (Eds.), *Proceedings of the Seventh International Conference on Advanced Learning Technologies* (pp. 750–752). Los Alamitos, CA: IEEE Computer Society.

Könings, K. D., Brand-Gruwel, S., van Merriënboer, J. J. G., & Broers, N. (2006). Does a new learning environment come up to students' expectations? A longitudinal study. *Journal of Educational Psychology*, *100*(3), 535–548. doi:10.1037/0022-0663.100.3.535

Kreijns, K., Kirschner, P. A., & Jochems, W. (2002). The sociability of computer-supported collaborative learning environments. *Journal of Educational Technology & Society*, *5*(1), 8–22.

MacManus, R., & Porter, J. (2005, May 4). Web 2.0 for designers. *Digital Web Magazine*. Retrieved April 15, 2008, from http://www.digital-web.com/articles/web_2_for_designers

Martin, M. (2007). My personal learning environment [Web log post]. *The Bamboo Project Blog*. Retrieved July 17, 2008, from http://michelemartin.typepad.com/thebambooprojectblog/2007/04/my_personal_lea.html

Muldoon, N. (2008). Self-direction and lifelong learning in the information age: Can PLEs help? In D. Orr, P. A. Danaher, G. Danaher, & R. E. Harreveld (Eds.), *Lifelong learning: Reflecting on successes and framing futures. Keynote and refereed papers from the Fifth International Lifelong Learning Conference* (pp. 277–283). Rockhampton, Australia: Central Queensland University Press. Norman, D. O. (1988). *The design of everyday things*. New York: Basic.

Norman, D. (2008, March 5). On the PLE [Web log post]. *D'Arcy Norman dot net*. Retrieved July 12, 2008, from http://www.darcynorman.net/2008/03/05/on-the-ple/

O'Reilly, T. (2005). *What is Web 2.0: Design patterns and business models for the next generation of software*. Retrieved February 27, 2008, from http://www.oreillynet.com/pub/a/oreilly/tim/news/2005/09/30/what-is-web-20.html

Owen, M., Grant, L., Sayers, S., & Facer, K. (2006). *Social software and learning*. Bristol, UK: Futurelab. Retrieved March 14, 2008, from http://www.futurelab.org.uk/resources/documents/opening_education/Social_Software_report.pdf

Pata, K., & Väljataga, T. (2007). Collaborating across national and institutional boundaries in higher education—the decentralized iCamp approach. In C. Montgomerie & J. Seale (Eds.), *Proceedings of World Conference on Educational Multimedia, Hypermedia and Telecommunications 2007* (pp. 353–362). Chesapeake, VA: Association for the Advancement of Computers in Education.

Schaffert, S., & Hilzensauer, W. (2008). On the way towards personal learning environments: Seven crucial aspects. *eLearning Papers, 9*. Retrieved July 22, 2008, from http://www.elearningeuropa.info/files/media/media15971.pdf

Severance, C., Hardin, J., & Whyte, A. (2008). The coming functionality mash-up in personal learning environments. *Interactive Learning Environments*, *16*(1), 47–62. doi:10.1080/10494820701772694

Shepherd, C. (2007, April 17). PLE—what are we talking about here? [Web log post]. *Clive on Learning*. Retrieved July 5, 2008, from http://clive-shepherd.blogspot.com/2007/04/ples-what-are-we-talking-about-here.html

Snowden, D. J., & Boone, M. E. (2007). A leader's framework for decision making. *Harvard Business Review*, *85*(11), 68–76.

Türker, M. A., & Zingel, S. (2008). Formative interfaces for scaffolding self-regulated learning in PLEs. *eLearning Papers, 9*. Retrieved July 22, 2008, from http://www.elearningeuropa.info/files/media/media15975.pdf

Underwood, J., & Banyard, P. E. (2008). Understanding the learning space. *eLearning Papers, 9*. Retrieved July 22, 2008, from http://www.elearningeuropa.info/files/media/media15970.pdf

Väljataga, T., & Fiedler, S. (2008). Competence advancement supported by social media. In M. Kalz, R. Koper, V. Hornung-Prähauser, & M. Luckmann (Eds.), *Proceedings of the First Workshop on Technology Support for Self-Organized Learners (TSSOL08)* (pp. 54–66). Aachen, Germany: Informatik V, RWTH Aachen University. Retrieved July 22, 2008, from http://sunsite.informatik.rwth-aachen.de/Publications/CEUR-WS/Vol-349/vaeljataga.pdf

Väljataga, T., Pata, K., Laanpere, M., & Kaipainen, M. (2007). Theoretical framework of the iCampFolio—new approach to evaluation and comparison of systems and tools for learning purposes. In E. Duval, R. Klamma, & M. Wolpers (Eds.), *Creating new learning experiences on a global scale: Second European Conference on Technology Enhanced Learning, EC-TEL 2007, Crete, Greece, September 2007, Proceedings: Vol. Lecture Notes in Computer Science* (pp. 349–363). Berlin/Heidelberg, Germany: Springer-Verlag.

van Harmelen, M. (2006). Personal learning environments. In Kinshuk, R. Koper, P. Kommers, P. Kirschner, D. Sampson, & W. Didderen (Eds.), *Proceedings of the Sixth International Conference on Advanced Learning Technologies* (pp. 815–816). Los Alamitos, CA: IEEE Computer Society.

van Harmelen, M. (2008). Design trajectories: Four experiments in PLE implementation. *Interactive Learning Environments, 16*(1), 35–46. doi:10.1080/10494820701772686

Wertsch, J. V. (1994). The primacy of mediated action in sociocultural studies. *Mind, Culture, and Activity, 1*(4), 202–208.

Wild, F., Mödritscher, F., & Sigurdarson, S. E. (2008). Designing for change: Mash-up personal learning environments. *eLearning Papers, 9*. Retrieved July 22, 2008, from http://www.elearningeuropa.info/files/media/media15972.pdf

Wilson, S. (2008). Patterns of personal learning environments. *Interactive Learning Environments, 16*(1), 17–34. doi:10.1080/10494820701772660

Wilson, S., Liber, O., Johnson, M., Beauvoir, P., Sharples, P., & Milligan, C. (2007). Personal learning environments: Challenging the dominant design of educational systems. *Journal of e-Learning and Knowledge Society, 3*(2), 27–38. Retrieved July 22, 2008, from http://je-lks.maieutiche.economia.unitn.it/en/07_02/04Art_wilson_inglese.pdf

Zimmerman, B. J. (2000). Attaining self-regulation: A social cognitive perspective. In Boekaerts, M., Pintrich, P. R., & Zeidner, M. (Eds.), *Handbook of self-regulation* (pp. 13–39). San Diego: Academic Press. doi:10.1016/B978-012109890-2/50031-7

KEY TERMS AND DEFINITIONS

Affordances: Individuals' potentials for actions in a particular environment at a given point of time, which are evoked ecologically and changed dynamically in the mutual interplay of person's objectives and task constraints, cultural experiences, previously experienced emotions and performed activities, and the human and material resources actualized from the environment.

Distributed Learning: An ongoing process of learning through interpersonal interactions across networks, communities, distance, and time.

Distributed Learning Environment (DLE): A group-managed environment with some resources and tools from the group members' personal learning environments (PLEs) and some additional components from other contexts that are necessary to carry out particular collaborative tasks.

Personal Learning Environment (PLE): Entails all the instruments, materials, and human resources that a student is aware of and has access to in the context of an educational project at a given point in time.

Social Media: Refers to the landscape of open access web tools and services that support social activities and learning.

Section 2
Towards Best Practice:
Case Studies and Exemplars of Web 2.0-Based Tertiary Teaching and Learning

Chapter 6
Personal Knowledge Management Skills in Web 2.0-Based Learning

Maria Elisabetta Cigognini
University of Florence, Italy

Maria Chiara Pettenati
University of Florence, Italy

Palitha Edirisingha
University of Leicester, UK

ABSTRACT

At present, many Web 2.0 activities are being integrated into the e-learning spaces designed for learners. We need to analyze and learn from these activities to derive insights about their effectiveness, in order to promote the systematic application of technology in post-compulsory educational contexts, from undergraduate to postgraduate levels and also in professional training. This chapter deals with one aspect of "e-learning 2.0" (Downes, 2005) practices, specifically the importance of acquiring and mastering a set of personal knowledge management (PKM) skills to perform successfully in the Web 2.0 environment for learning in tertiary education. The authors first present a PKM skills model based around a division into (1) basic PKM competencies associated with the social software web practices of Create–Organize–Share; and (2) higher-order skills focusing on the advanced management of one's personal knowledge. A learning design model and related examples are presented, aimed at inspiring and guiding tertiary educators in designing and implementing activities consistent with the goal of developing students' PKM skills.

INTRODUCTION

The traditional approaches to e-learning in tertiary education have so far been dominated by the use of virtual learning environments (VLEs), with teaching and learning structured around courses, timetables, and assessments. This approach has been criticized as being mainly driven by the needs of the institution rather than by those of the learner (Wallace, 1999; EDUCAUSE Learn-

DOI: 10.4018/978-1-60566-294-7.ch006

ing Initiative, 2006). Recent developments in web-based technologies offer new opportunities to experiment with e-learning, where formal and informal activities merge and spaces for knowledge management can be created—all drawing on people and their ability to network and learn naturally and informally (McFedries, 2007). Learning is seen as the integration of formal, informal, and non-formal activities occurring in both online and real-world contexts.

The development of "Web 2.0" (O'Reilly, 2005; see also McFedries, 2005) services and technologies is paving the way for a new era of e-learning. Downes (2005) has coined the term "E-learning 2.0" to refer to these new developments, and to describe the increasing use of Web 2.0 tools in e-learning, along with other emerging trends. E-learning 2.0 involves digital learning spaces in which students create content, collaborate with peers to form learning networks for knowledge sharing and exchange, and engage in activities that take advantage of multiple sources of aggregated content, immersing themselves in rich learning experiences that utilize various tools including but not limited to online references, courseware, knowledge management applications, collaborative and search tools. Many innovative Web 2.0 activities are beginning to emerge as e-learning practices evolve and change (Alexander, 2006).

This chapter deals with one aspect of new and emerging e-learning practices, highlighting the need for learners to develop a set of personal knowledge management (PKM) skills (Frand & Hixon, 1999; Avery, Brooks, Brown, Dorsey, & O'Connor, 2000; Barth, 2005; Dorsey, 2001; Wright, 2005; Grey, 2006; Pollard, 2005) in order to perform successfully in the Web 2.0 environment and knowledge society. Learning to use any new technology effectively necessitates acquiring a set of abilities and skills, but in order to help tertiary students fully benefit from the developments in Web 2.0-based tools and services, there is a need to devise strategies to assist them in developing particular skills in the use and application of these digital tools to achieve their own learning outcomes. In this chapter, the authors define such a core set of skills as PKM skills. They also propose an instructional approach to developing resources that support the development of these skills among learners. The chapter provides a list of PKM skills, divided into basic and higher-order PKM skills. It also offers a learning design model conceived to support the acquisition of both types of PKM skills, together with guidelines and scenarios to demonstrate the application of the model.

BACKGROUND

The continuous and radical changes underway as a result of the widespread diffusion of information and communication technologies (ICTs) is affecting the way we come to know and learn using tools, and our social relations and interactions, both as individuals and in groups (Laurillard, 2002). There is a strong case for recognizing PKM skills as a critical asset in today's professions, in which digital/online and face-to-face actions and interactions are inextricably intertwined.

The term "PKM" (Frand & Hixon, 1999; Dorsey, 2001; Sorrentino & Paganelli, 2006) refers to a collection of processes that an individual undertakes to gain and share knowledge in his or her daily activities, and how these processes support work activities and the management of personal knowledge acquired through ICTs. The set of abilities first identified by Dorsey (2001) and Pollard (2005) hinges around seven main competencies: retrieving information, evaluating information, organizing information, analyzing information, presenting information, securing information, and collaborating around information.

PKM skills encompass a multifaceted set of abilities that are somewhat different from digital and information literacy (Martin & Ashworth, 2004; Martin, 2006; Cronje, 2006; Mayes & Fowler, 2006). Social and relational aspects of learning and social interaction, as described by Siemens in his book, *Knowing knowledge* (2006), also include attitudes and a particular mindset. Siemens highlights the fact that that mastering technology is but one aspect of a more complex skill set that entails the acquisition of social, cognitive, and personal attributes and competencies. Acquiring PKM skills is a complex and long-term process that can be facilitated by creating conditions that help people to learn relevant and effective self-management skills, behaviors, and values needed to operate in the knowledge society.

Developing PKM competencies in learning environments supported by Web 2.0 tools can help today's tertiary education learners for life-long learning, enabling them to perform better in a globalized, connected world. Universities and colleges have a responsibility to equip their graduates with the skills necessary for participation in the new forms of lifelong and life-wide learning supported by social media. The term "Lifelong Learning 2.0" is used by the authors of the present chapter to denote the new set of skills needed by the emerging generation of graduates. Educational practitioners and researchers should not be misled by a general assumption that today's tertiary education students are all "digital natives" who have the ability to use Web 2.0 technologies in the most effective way (Pettenati, Cigognini, Guerin, & Mangione, 2009). Contrary to Prensky (2001), who proposed the notion of "digital natives," other researchers (Lohnes & Kinzer, 2007; Kennedy, Judd, Churchward, Gray, & Krause, 2008) argue that the distinction between "digital native" versus "digital immigrant" is not a function of age. Instead, it is a function of attitude, a mindset of experimentation and experience with technology. Siemens (2007) also warns against an uncritical belief in the competencies of so-called "digital natives." He says that although references to digital natives and immigrants abound in the literature, the terms have little merit "beyond a buzz phrase that has outlived the role it initially played in getting educators to think about the different types of learners now entering our classrooms" (para. 3). According to him, "the concept of immigrant/native gained popularity because it expresses emotions/feelings many educators have about next generation students. They are, like every generation before, different" (para. 2). It would also be a mistake to assume that all learners enrolling in and completing tertiary education courses have the knowledge and abilities to use Internet technologies for effective lifelong learning, and therefore the authors of the present chapter argue that there is a case for teaching them PKM skills.

Most Web 2.0 tools and technologies have been developed outside of academia. Their purposes resolve mainly around social networking, creative expression, and sharing of content, among other informal uses. For this reason, using these tools for personal and social ends is quite different from using them for traditional academic or formal learning purposes. Recent studies (Katz & Macklin, 2007; Salaway, Katz, Caruso, Kvavik, & Nelson, 2006; Kvavik, 2005; Warlick, 2004) into how children and young people become competent in using the Internet and other information tools highlight the finding that the information literacy skills of young people have not improved despite widening access to technology; in fact, their apparent familiarity and competency with computers disguises and obscures some worrying problems and skills deficits in key areas of PKM (Lorenzo & Dziuban, 2006). As an example, there is no evidence in the empirically based literature that young people possess greater expertise as searchers, nor that the search skills of young people have improved with time. Research into young people's web-searching behaviors shows that they scroll through web pages quickly and treat the content on them superficially, spending little time evaluating information for accuracy and authority. Faced with a long list of search hits, young people find it difficult to assess the relevance of material presented, and often print off pages with no more than a surface level glance at them. Moreover, young people have a poor understanding of their information needs and thus struggle to develop effective information search and retrieval strategies (Centre for Information Behaviour and the Evaluation of Research [CIBER], 2008). Studies pre-dating the widespread public use of the Internet have reported that young searchers often appear to have difficulty in selecting appropriate search terms, and research into Internet use has consistently pointed to similar difficulties.

Another issue of current interest, and indeed, concern, is the way young people evaluate—or rather, fail to evaluate—information from electronic sources. Here, too, there is little evidence that this has improved over the last 10 to 15 years. Information management and higher-order thinking skills are needed more than ever before, and at more advanced levels if people are to reap the benefits of resources available in the information society. Making an assumption, therefore, that all "Net Generation" learners (Oblinger & Oblinger, 2005) are sufficiently skilled to undertake online formal/informal learning, and to do so proficiently to achieve high-level outcomes, would be a severe misjudgment. Though technologically talented (Kennedy et al., 2008), the "digital natives" may lack critical abilities and ethical knowledge needed to maximize and self-regulate their learning. (See also Chapter 16 in this book.)

The research presented in this chapter is intended to encourage educational institutions to rise to the challenge and address the importance of teaching PKM skills to students through the development of specific interventions and web-based courses.

LIFELONG LEARNING 2.0

In this section, the concept of PKM skills is explained and elaborated on, with reference to the authors' previous studies, dividing them into basic and higher-order skills. The discussion begins with an overview of what is meant by a "Lifelong Learner 2.0" and the skills he or she possesses.

Defining the Lifelong Learner 2.0

What characterizes a Lifelong Learner 2.0? What is the nature of the learning territory that he or she traverses? Building on the authors' previous work, a Lifelong Learner 2.0 may be defined as an individual who makes use of specific skills and knowledge acquired through training and/or experience while intensively using the Internet—especially social networking applications and other Web 2.0 tools—to engage in a self-regulated lifelong learning journey involving continual formal and informal knowledge construction activities. If a lifelong learner is a multifaceted and interconnected figure immersed in the Web 2.0 environment, in order to take advantage of a Web 2.0 learning environment, he or she needs a set of abilities that are equally multifaceted and versatile. This specific set of skills enables the learner to construct meaning and derive understanding from the learning landscape that he or she constantly traverses.

It is argued in this chapter that becoming an effective user of Web 2.0 technologies for tertiary and lifelong learning requires learners to master a set of PKM skills (Pettenati, Cigognini, & Sorrentino, 2007; Pettenati, Cigognini, Mangione, & Guerin, 2007; Cigognini, Mangione, & Pettenati, 2007a, 2007b). As Web 2.0 is relatively new territory for many educators, an innovative learning design, implementation strategy, and evaluation process are proposed for teaching PKM skills in an online learning environment.

Developing PKM Skills

The development of PKM skills is rooted in a complex picture in which individual choices and activities converge with social and technological aspects. Some of the authors who have dealt with this topic (e.g., Frand & Hixon, 1999; Dorsey, 2001; Barth, 2005; Avery et al., 2000; Pollard, 2005; Grey, 2006; Wright, 2005) present a detailed reference framework relating to terms describing a repertoire of skills associated with PKM. These terms point toward some of the specific features of the concept PKM. Comparing PKM to the concept of "literacy," for example, some related, though distinct, skills emerge. According to the United Nations Educational, Scientific and Cultural Organization (UNESCO), "Literacy is the ability to identify, understand, interpret, create, communicate, and compute, using printed and written materials associated with varying contexts. Literacy involves a continuum of learning to enable an individual to achieve his or her goals, to develop his or her knowledge and potential, and to participate fully in the wider society" (2004, p. 13, citing an international expert meeting in June 2003 at UNESCO). Another related concept is "digital competence," which involves the confident and critical use of information systems and technology for work, leisure, and communication. It is underpinned by basic skills in ICTs: the use of computers to retrieve, assess, store, produce, present, and exchange information, and to communicate and participate in collaborative networks via the Internet (European Union, 2006). The European e-Skills Forum, building on the activities of the Career Space initiative, has adopted the term "e-skills" and developed a scheme covering three main categories—ICT practitioner, user, and e-business skills—but this scheme is centered primarily around the use of tools and applications. To define and distinguish PKM skills it is therefore necessary to focus on the more complex concepts of literacy and competence/competencies by adopting a holistic approach that is attuned to the new knowledge-creation processes and learning landscapes enabled by Web 2.0 tools and services (McLoughlin & Lee, 2008).

Based on their own empirical work and other resources cited from the literature, it is the authors' contention that the notion of PKM skills provides a useful concept that encompasses the range of skills required to learn in the information society. The following terms have been identified as being linked to the concept of PKM skills: "information literacy" (Irving & Crawford, 2007), "media/multimedia literacy" (Aviram & Talmi, 2004), "e-skills" (The European e-Skills Forum, 2004; Commission of the European Communities, 2007), "e-literacy" (Martin & Ashworth, 2004; Martin, 2006), "digital literacy", and "digital competencies" (Mayes & Fowler, 2006; Varis, 2005; Midoro, 2007; Tornero, 2004; Buckingham, 2007). However, the authors' vision of PKM skills, which will be detailed in the next section, is focused on an interpretation of a set of skills closer to the concepts of personal knowledge, learning, and management of personal learning within the context of social networking environments (Dorsey, 2001; Sorrentino & Paganelli, 2006; Pettenati, 2009). The communicative, socio-cultural, and management aspects of learning call for a rethinking of the skills required by the lifelong learner to include a complex set of higher-order skills incorporating metacognitive and conceptual knowledge (Martin, 2006; Midoro, 2007; Hilton, 2006).

In this vein, skills such as reflection, learning management, knowledge construction, and networking (Frand & Hixon, 1999; Dorsey, 2001; Pollard, 2005) become key. Such a holistic approach of mindset and skills for the lifelong learner is considered essential for achieving the objectives of the European Commission's Lisbon agenda (Commission of the European Communities, 2007). The remainder of this section outlines and illustrates the process of developing basic and higher-order PKM skills. It also stresses the important role played by three broad-based factors that form the foundation of PKM skills, and three background factors that constitute enabling conditions for the development of PKM skills. In describing their PKM skills model, the authors acknowledge that, at a first glance, one might notice some overlap between the "basic" and "higher-order" PKM skills. In the authors' view, however, the basic PKM skills encompass abilities and skills that can be deliberately learned and applied as direct "know how," while the higher-order PKM skills require more complex thinking, reflection, and experiential processes, which call for mastery of a more elaborate set of competencies and attributes.

PKM Basic Skills

The issue of defining PKM skills required to support lifelong learners in the knowledge society has been treated in previous work by the authors (Pettenati, Cigognini, & Edirisingha, 2007; Pettenati & Cigognini, 2007; Pettenati, 2009; Cigognini et al., 2007a, 2007b). These studies focused on the development of a pedagogical model aimed at identifying and representing the skills that the learner should develop in order to be able to engage more effectively and meaningfully with formal and informal learning processes in an online environment. In previous research, the authors of the present chapter have also attempted to establish a methodological link between PKM skills and learning design. To this end, PKM skills were grouped under the following three macro-competency categories: Create, Organize, and Share. Each macro-competency is interpreted as an umbrella concept or grouping of several, more specific PKM skills, as shown below (Avery et al., 2000; Dorsey, 2001; Sorrentino & Paganelli, 2006):

- *Create:* Editing (e.g., generating and modifying digital content/information in multimedia formats); Integrating (post-processing of recordings, reuse, digital annotations, automatic abstracting, etc.); Correlating (making connections, drawing diagrams, producing mind maps); Managing content security issues (managing privacy, intellectual property rights, digital rights management, etc.).
- *Organize:* Searching and finding (selecting search engines, querying search, etc.); Retrieving (reading, managing cognitive load, etc.); Storing (archiving, considering resource availability and accessibility, etc.); Categorizing/classifying and synthesizing (defining relations among pieces, using taxonomies and folksonomies, etc.); Evaluating (extracting meaning, determining/attributing relevance, effecting trust levels).
- *Share:* Publishing (presenting relevant information, using appropriate publication channels, etc.); Mastering knowledge exchanges (being concise, using appropriate language, taking turns, focusing on topic, etc.); Managing contacts (keeping profiles, contact contexts and social network representation, etc.); Relating (establishing connections, communicating through new media, understanding peers, using different languages, etc.); Collaborating (sharing tasks, working to achieve a common goal, etc.).

A sample process of how to promote acquisition of basic PKM skills is illustrated in a later section of the chapter. It is suggested that the skills are best developed through the use of a scenario, related "e-tivities" (Salmon, 2002), and supporting Web 2.0 tools, and that the learning environment should be designed according to the phases depicted in the PKM learning design model that appears in Figure 1. The basic PKM skills identified are part of a complex set of cognitive skills that individuals need to develop, and that cannot be considered complete without accounting for deeper mastery of skills such as creating and sharing knowledge within a network and using its resources (Cigognini et al., 2007b). This view, supported by the authors' research and teaching experiences, led them to extend the basic model (Cigognini, Pettenati, Paoletti, & Edirisingha, 2008) to include higher-order skills and abilities, elicited through conducting interviews with individuals deemed to be expert Lifelong Learners 2.0 (Pettenati et al., 2009).

Higher-Order PKM Skills (HO PKM Skills)

The set of higher-order skills and competencies are grouped into four main categories, as follows (Pettenati et al., 2009):

1. *Connectedness:* Being connected has emerged as one of the fundamental skills of the Lifelong Learner 2.0. However, this does merely mean being connected in a technological sense through computer networks, mobile communication devices, and the Internet. Rather, it refers to the process of being networked, i.e., developing and exercising skills to collaborate and interact with others for the purpose of establishing, growing, and maintaining social networks. In line with this perspective, the connected person needs to develop specific abilities to communicate effectively on the Internet and to manage his or her online identity, while dealing with the multiplicity of identities and being aware of how his or her online identity and communication sits within a global system.
2. *Ability to balance formal and informal contexts:* This includes the ability to listen to a variety of opinions sensibly; manage time and relations, being driven by what the authors call the "procrastination principle," i.e., "to deal with problems only as they arise—or leave them to other users to deal with;" combining employment, education/training, and leisure tasks to find a balance between the different learning contexts with which the learner can be confronted; engaging and participating as a listener, observer/reader, and author; being open to interdisciplinary working/learning; being methodical, systematic, punctual, and goal oriented; being "spongy," i.e., able to absorb as much as possible, understanding the essence of the interactions with content and relations so as to manage multiple perspectives as necessary.
3. *Critical ability:* The adoption of a critical ability in the use of Internet-based resources (contents and relations) is closely related to the ability to identify the resources relevant to the context of use, i.e., understanding possible uses of such resources and being aware of their limitations. A key part of this skill is being able to integrate the resources identified into a personal resource management style or approach, which is constantly fine tuned by the learner, closely linked to his or her learning objectives.
4. *Creativity:* The process of developing a creative attitude and approach to lifelong learning requires both structured and serendipitous explorations, observation, linking, and association to perceive and/or imagine unexpected and unusual connections between ideas and entities. Developing a creative mindset for lifelong learning provides concrete ways through which to engage in one's knowledge construction path—interpreting, linking, proposing, and experimenting with new knowledge construction strategies.

Gaining proficiency in the basic PKM skills is simply the first step or entry point into a learning journey leading to the mastery of higher-order skills and competencies, hence enabling and preparing students for a true lifelong learning experience. In order to validate their PKM skills model, the authors conducted a set of semi-structured interviews (Cigognini, Pettenati, & Paoletti, 2008) with 23 respondents involved in education (both from private-sector companies and universities, and from multiple disciplines including biology, medicine, and education). An additional goal of the interviews was to assist in the identification of a set of learning strategies for each HO PKM skill.

Figure 1. Instructional design principles and online learning phases (Pettenati, 2009)

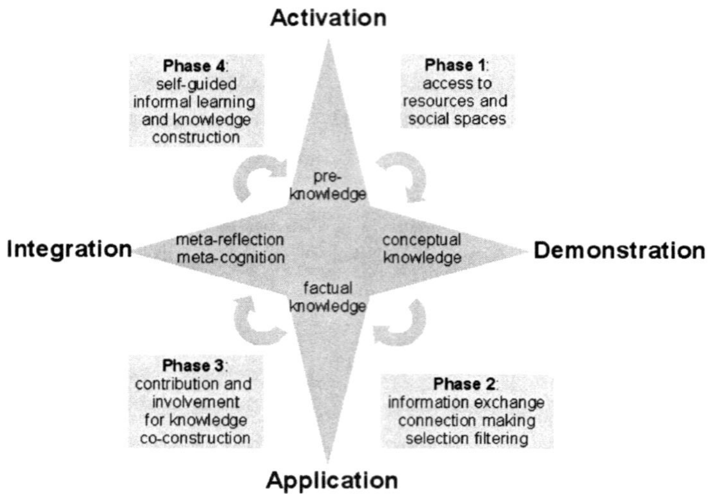

A Learning Design Model for PKM Skills

In order to provide guidance to educators wishing to design e-learning activities targeted at the development of students' PKM skills, the key points of the authors' learning design model are illustrated, highlighting the stages of learning, the enabling conditions, and possible technological tools to be used for the purpose (Pettenati, 2009). The learning design model is presented in Figure 1, Figure 2, and Figure 3, which emphasize the main elements of learning design: Figure 1 and Figure 2 show the instructional design principles and associated phases, and the enabling conditions, competencies, and skills needed for the learning process to occur; Figure 3 depicts the set of environments and tools that can be integrated

Figure 2. Enabling conditions, competencies, and skills needed in the learning process (Pettenati, 2009)

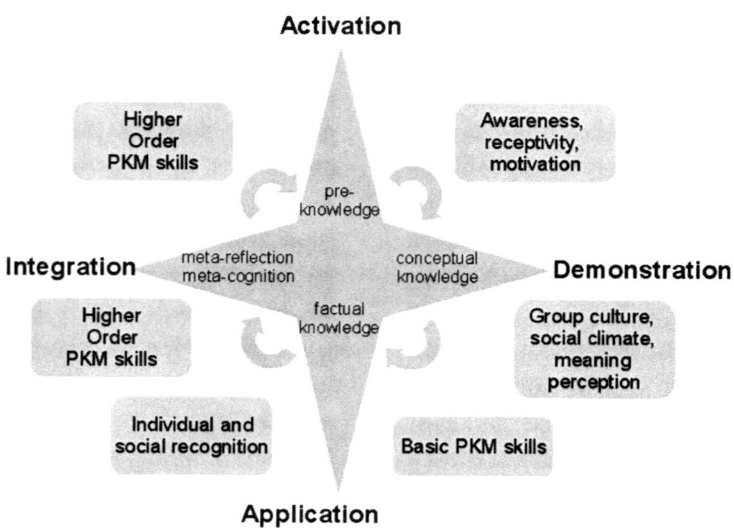

Figure 3. Tools that can be integrated to support and enhance PKM learning processes (Pettenati, 2009)

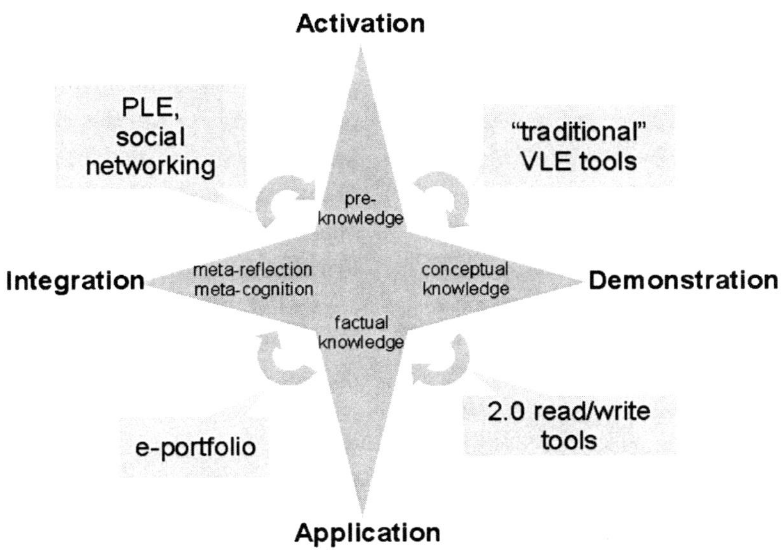

to support and increase the learning processes of knowledge Activation, Integration, Demonstration, and Application. While these figures have been presented as three separate diagrams to draw attention to and clarify the three main elements of learning design mentioned above, all three figures are essentially components of what can be thought of as one large, composite figure. The learning processes depicted in Figure 1, Figure 2, and Figure 3 can be used as a simple model to guide the design of learning activities and environments in different educational contexts.

Figure 1 shows the circular and incremental process, in which three main elements can be identified: the learning design principles (activation, demonstration, application, and integration), similar to those proposed by Merrill (2002), overlapping with stages of knowledge evolution (pre-knowledge, conceptual knowledge, factual knowledge, and reflection/metacognition) adapted from the work of Reigeluth (1999), as well as the phases of online learning experience identified by Calvani (2005), expressed as a sequence of four phases:

1. access to resources and social spaces;
2. information exchange, connection forming, and selection filtering;
3. contribution and involvement for knowledge co-construction;
4. self-guided informal learning and knowledge construction.

Figure 2 shows a set of enabling conditions that are relevant to the development of basic PKM processes. These are awareness, receptivity, and motivation; group culture, social culture, meaning perception; basic PKM skills; individual and social recognition; and higher-order PKM skills. The enabling conditions to support PKM skills acquisition are shown as a cyclical model that progresses from basic skills to higher-order achievements.

The authors believe these enabling conditions are linked to the development of lifelong learning skills, such as self-motivation, goal setting, and self-regulation (Pettenati, 2009). Once such conditions are created and met in an e-learning context, the learner can engage in lifelong learning. However, if such conditions are not met, the educational institution is required to play a central role in guiding and scaffolding effective learning experiences as well as taking steps to increase the learner's skills. The more expert the learner becomes, the less scaffolding, guidance, and structured activities will be required from the educator and educational institution.

Finally, the authors' learning design model advocates thoughtful and systematic use of ICT tools to foster PKM skills. Figure 3 represents a possible setup of Internet tools and services for developing and sustaining the acquisition of PKM skills. These include traditional VLE tools, Web 2.0 tools and services including social networking sites, e-portfolios, and personal learning environments (PLEs)—again, all mapped onto instructional design principles and linked to enabling conditions and the development of the relevant competencies and skills.

The circular process in the figure shows how the learning experience needs to start in a closed and structured environment, gradually moving towards PLEs, and finally to open source tools and social networks as the individual grows in his or her learning experience, maturity, and independence.

Guidelines to Apply the Learning Design Model: Learning Scenario and "E-tivities"

This part of the chapter shows how the phases of the learning design model can be applied to a learning context, and how the conceptual approach presented thus far can be translated into practice. The work presented here is based on real learning experiences—some research has already concluded, with more evaluation still in progress at the time of writing. Most of the learning activities conducted in the skills development modules (SDMs), which are based on the concept of "e-tivities" (Salmon, 2002), were developed from suggestions, experiences, and comments collected through the interviews with the experts alluded to earlier (details are reported in Cigognini, Pettenati, & Paoletti, 2008). The SDMs were developed in the Moodle (http://www.moodle.org/) VLE, which provides integration of and links to Web 2.0 tools, customizable to suit the students' needs and skill levels. An initial questionnaire was constructed to measure and calibrate the instructional design phases around the students and their expected learning outcomes.

In the subsections that follow, each of the four phases of the model is described in terms of its *focus* or position with respect to the circular structure of the model, the targeted *learning outcome* at that phase, and *e-tivities* in the form of possible uses and applications of Web 2.0 tools aimed at supporting the development of the specific PKM skills.

Phase 1: Access to Resources and Social Spaces

This is in the Activation phase, where prior knowledge is recalled. In this stage, individuals become accustomed to "handling information [and knowledge] abundance" (Siemens, 2006, p. 45), and are first confronted with the resources (people and contents) and tools of the new learning environment. Phase 1 can be supported using the following suggestions:

1. *Focus*: This phase is focused on highlighting previous knowledge related to Create–Share–Organize PKM skills and related to balancing formal and informal activities leading to the development of HO PKM skills.
2. *Learning outcome*: Specific learning activities should be designed to leverage already internalized methods for managing personal knowledge.
3. *E-tivities for this phase*:
    a. Use of a "café" forum as a socialization space, with the aim of sharing impressions and expectations on the course;

personalization of user profiles in the VLE.

b. Searching, classifying, and commenting on resources posted in online spaces for the course—for example, documents posted in the Moodle VLE, figures and tables posted on photo-sharing sites (e.g., Flickr—http://www.flickr.com/), introductory audio files posted by the teacher on the course podcasting channel (e.g., using MyPodcast—http://www.mypodcast.com/), video-sharing (e.g., YouTube—http://www.youtube.com/), also using course/subject and e-tivity-specific tags, through a social bookmarking or wiki site. Students rank and comment on the resources to enhance clarity, flag difficulties, make suggestions, and raise questions to ask to the teacher.

Phase 2: Information Exchange, Connection Forming, and Selection Filtering

This is the Demonstration step, in which conceptual knowledge starts to be developed. At this stage individuals begin to use tools and resources to create and form a personal network of resources (people and content). At this point, the learners start to be active in the learning space in terms of consuming or acquiring new resources and tools (Siemens, 2006). Phase 2 can be supported using the following suggestions:

1. *Focus*: Phase 2 is centered around the "Share" PKM basic skill and the "Connectedness" HO PKM skill.
2. *Learning outcomes*: Specific learning activities, designed according to the degree of preconditions realized (ubiquity and being always online), should be created to support the development of social behavior and communication skills used in knowledge exchange through the network.
3. *E-tivities for this phase*:
   a. Each learner studies one of the themes discussed in the Demonstration phase using a wiki (within Moodle or a separate wiki site). The sample wiki page should contain at least three web references—appropriately tagged and classified, shared with the peers—as well as two multimedia resources (images, audio, video). The learners are then invited to comment and reciprocally evaluate the shared wiki-based information and resources.
   b. The learners work in groups, with each group discussing one of the themes from the Demonstration phase using a social networking environment such as Facebook (http://www.facebook.com). Learners create and update their profiles and subscribe to the theme-specific group. Each learner is responsible for collecting two multimedia resources and a web reference, which they comment on and reciprocally rank. Once a group's theme is set up, it allows the other groups to view its resources, thereby enabling knowledge sharing within and across groups.

Phase 3: Contribution and Involvement for Knowledge Co-Construction

This is the Application step, in which the learner begins to actively contribute to the learning network—essentially becoming a "visible node." The learner's active contribution and involvement allow other nodes on the network to acknowledge his or her resources, contributions, and ideas, creating reciprocal relationships and shared understandings (or, if social software technology is used, collaboratively-created understanding). Phase 3 can be supported using the following suggestions:

1. *Focus:* Phase 3 is centered around the "Create" PKM basic skill and the "Creativity" HO PKM skill.
2. *Learning outcomes:* Specific learning activities should be designed to leverage the innovation and experimentation aspects of creativity, encouraging and challenging learners to adapt traditional/existing models and create new models for using technologies.
3. *E-tivities for this phase:* Inside the course space of the social networking environment (Facebook), the learners create a social event, for instance an end-of-course party.
   a. The online event should be linked to the best student's assignments, in order to build a class portfolio and a synthesis of the activities developed through creation of a class journal.
   b. The event should be also documented and narrated online, allowing learners to exercise creativity and initiative. Activities related to coordinating/organizing the event can be supported through various shared calendars and task management utilities, including both those that are internal and external to the VLE (Moodle) and social networking environment (Facebook) spaces.

Phase 4: Self-Guided Informal Learning and Knowledge Construction

This is the Integration step, in which reflection on the knowledge processes and products, self-reflexivity and self-evaluation, as well as meta-cognition (Reigeluth, 1999; Calvani, 2005) play a prominent role. Individuals are actively involved in modifying and rebuilding their own learning networks, acting as network-aware and competent participants. The experience acquired at this stage within the learning network should result in an understanding of the nuances of the space and the knowledge inputs, allowing the subject to both act as a provider of valuable support and help to other networked learners, as well as being capable of accessing just-in-time and personalized knowledge. Phase 4 can be supported using the following suggestions:

1. *Focus*: Phase 4 is centered around the development of "Critical ability" (an HO PKM skill).
2. *Learning outcomes*: Specific learning activities should be designed to address selection, evaluation, synthesis, and development of PKM models, and for reflection and advancement on the learner's progress.
3. *E-tivities for this phase*: The activities relate to the creation of an individual e-portfolio—using a platform such as Elgg (http://www.elgg.org/), for example—describing and documenting the experiences and competencies acquired during the course.
   a. The individual components of the PLE are negotiated and shared with regard to objectives and their meaning. Each phase of the creation of the portfolio includes self-examination and evaluation through Web 2.0 tools that allow comments, ranking, and tagging. The learner's personal blog is used for self and group reflection on the ongoing learning process, building upon teacher and peer feedback.

CURRENT PROGRESS, LIMITATIONS, AND FUTURE WORK

The learning design model presented above was intended to describe an approach to designing teaching and learning interventions aimed at facilitating the development of basic and higher-order PKM skills. One of the most important aspects of the application of what has been presented in this chapter relates to the assessment of learners' acquisition of PKM skills within a broader evaluation framework dealing with the learning experience as a whole (Cigognini et al., 2008a). To this end, a basic SDM was conducted with undergraduate students (studying towards Bachelor degrees) in two different entry cohorts (April/May 2007 and October/November 2007). The first SDM targeted at developing HO PKM skills has been trialled with postgraduate (Master's-level) students, and at the time of writing a second cohort consisting of students from different backgrounds (psychology, economics, mathematics, foreign languages, engineering and educational sciences) is undertaking the HO SDM.

The SDMs are designed and tailored to the skills entry-point level of the students; as mentioned earlier, in each case an initial questionnaire is used to measure and calibrate the instructional design phases around the students and their expected learning outcomes. Overall, three questionnaires are used to evaluate the effectiveness of the SDMs: in addition to the initial questionnaire, one is administered at the end of the course, and another six months after the end of the course. The questionnaires are aimed at assessing the use of Web 2.0 tools as introduced to learners in the SDMs, both with regard to the intended mode of use as well as possible alternative uses adapted and adopted by the learners themselves.

Evaluation Framework and Preliminary Results

The results obtained so far are encouraging. The preliminary results collected from the basic PKM SDM suggest that it was a successful experience. The results attest to the learners' satisfaction and the achievement of favorable learning outcomes (Level 1 in Kirkpatrick's four-level evaluation model—see Kirkpatrick, 2006). They also contain evidence of increased levels of PKM basic skill among the learners. Improvements in abilities (Level 3 in Kirkpatrick's model) and the transfer to the learners' daily practices will continue to be evaluated by the researchers.

The authors have identified some problems with the HO PKM skills development model, leading them to conclude that the experiments require further iterations and refinements. The groups of student participants outlined above have been non-homogeneous in terms of their prior knowledge, and the students have lacked sound and structured background knowledge on HO PKM practices, due in large part to the limited scope and duration of the course (being only a 20-hour blended learning course), in which the Application and Integration phases of the model were only able to be partially developed. In view of this, the authors plan to conduct a further iteration of the study with another cohort of Master's students. The course duration planned for this cohort seems more suitable to allow coverage of all the learning design model phases. Moreover, the group is highly motivated because the course is oriented toward supporting them in writing up their final theses.

Research in this area is still in its infancy, and demands continued attention and dialogue from researchers and practitioners. At the moment, the findings revolve around two main reflections. The first is that both users' attitudes and available technologies are mature enough so that it can be envisaged that each Internet user could easily engage in a personal lifelong learning experience, if properly guided by appropriate methodologies and sustained by pedagogically designed and developed PLEs. The second is related to the development of basic PKM skills. There are some factors that imply they cannot yet be translated into an explicit, coherent, and structured learning design to guide the three stages of content creation, sharing, and delivery. Design of learning activities must be based on the level and motivation of students, and must be grounded in the relevance of PKM abilities for their lifelong learning needs.

Last but not least, it is necessary to highlight the fact that it is crucial to create appropriate learning scenarios with different levels of use and complexity to allow learners to build personal, individualized knowledge construction paths leading to the development of PKM skills.

CONCLUSION

This chapter reported on ongoing research into one important aspect of lifelong learners in the knowledge society: how best to support them to become more effective learners in Web 2.0-based learning environments. This topic is currently a priority of the European educational agenda (Commission of the European Communities, 2000; European Centre for the Development of Vocational Training [CEDEFOP], 2008), and is also receiving similar levels of attention and interest elsewhere around the world. In light of recent developments in web-based technologies and services that hold great potential for learning, the e-learning landscape is changing to incorporate and accommodate Web 2.0. Learners need support, guidance, and pedagogical interventions to make the best possible use of these and other emerging technologies to support their learning goals. The concept of PKM skills was introduced and explored in this chapter, and a model presented for realizing the conditions that maximize the potential of using Web 2.0 technologies for learning.

Research and development in the area of PKM skills faces a number of immediate challenges and issues. Indeed, one of the obstacles that must be overcome is the need to gain acceptance of PKM skills such as those identified in this chapter as a fundamental skill set in tertiary education, and also a mindset to be nurtured in and by each lifelong learner. Successful implementation of the authors' model requires the development of a systemic and integrated approach to teaching and learning PKM skills, with adequate support at the department, institution, and sector levels. Foresight and long-term planning are needed to support these learning outcomes in order to fulfill the ultimate goal of delivering PKM training in a systematic across different academic contexts and disciplines, to help prepare our students to become effective lifelong learners in today's knowledge society. Another issue that must be acknowledged relates to the need for developing sound and practical support to ensure the creation and implementation of appropriate learning designs that translate the ideas and theory into practice. Overcoming these challenges is dependent on continual and ongoing scholarly inquiry into the cognitive, social, and lifelong learning needs of 21st-century students.

REFERENCES

Alexander, B. (2006). Web 2.0: A new wave of innovation for teaching and learning? *EDUCAUSE Review, 41*(2), 32–44. Retrieved November 1, 2008, from http://www.educause.edu/ir/library/pdf/erm0621.pdf

Avery, S., Brooks, R., Brown, J., Dorsey, P., & O'Connor, M. (2001). Personal knowledge management: Framework for integration and partnerships. In P. Smith (Ed.), *Proceedings of the Association of Small Computer Users in Education (ASCUE) Conference* (pp. 29–39). Myrtle Beach, SC: ASCUE.

Aviram, R., & Talmi, D. (2004). *The impact of ICT on education: The three opposed paradigms, the lacking discourse*. Retrieved November 1, 2008, from http://www.elearningeuropa.info/extras/pdf/ict_impact.pdf

Barth, S. (2005, October 1). Personal toolkit: A framework for personal knowledge management tools. *KMWorld*. Retrieved November 1, 2008, from http://www.kmworld.com/Authors/AuthorDetails.aspx?AuthorID=508

Buckingham, D. (2007). Digital media literacies: Rethinking media education in the age of the Internet. *Research in Comparative and International Education, 2*(1), 43–55. doi:10.2304/rcie.2007.2.1.43

Calvani, A. (2005). *Reti, comunità e conoscenza: Costruire e gestire dinamiche collaborative (Networks, community and knowledge: Building and managing dynamic collaboration)*. Trento, Italy: Erickson.

Centre for Information Behaviour and the Evaluation of Research. (2008). *Information behaviour of the researcher of the future*. London: CIBER, University College London. Retrieved November 1, 2008, from http://www.bl.uk/news/pdf/googlegen.pdf

Cigognini, M. E., Mangione, G. R., & Pettenati, M. C. (2007a). E-learning design nell'apprendimento (in)formale (E-learning design for (in)formal learning). *TD: Tecnologie Didattiche, 41*, 16–22. Retrieved November 1, 2008, from http://www.tdmagazine.itd.cnr.it/PDF41/4_Cigognini_Mangione_Pettenati_TD41.pdf

Cigognini, M. E., Mangione, G. R., & Pettenati, M. C. (2007b, September 5–6). *Favouring a critical, creative and ethical use of the network resources through Web 2.0 applications*. Paper presented at the Towards a Social Science of Web 2.0 Conference, York, UK. Retrieved October 24, 2007, from http://www.york.ac.uk/res/siru/web2.0/cigognini.htm

Cigognini, M. E., Pettenati, M. C., & Paoletti, G. (2008). Personal knowledge management skills model for expert lifelong learners: A validation method. In J. M. Nunes & M. A. McPherson (Eds.), *Proceedings of the IADIS International Conference e-Learning 2008* (pp. 215–222). Lisbon: International Association for Development of the Information Society.

Cigognini, M. E., Pettenati, M. C., Paoletti, G., & Edirisingha, P. (2008, June 11–14). *Guiding learners to become knowledgeable Learners 2.0*. Paper presented at the European Distance and E-learning Network (EDEN) 2008 Annual Conference, Lisbon, Portugal.

Commission of the European Communities. (2000). *A memorandum on lifelong learning*. Commission staff working paper. Brussels: European Commission. Retrieved November 1, 2008, from http://www.bologna-berlin2003.de/pdf/MemorandumEng.pdf

Commission of the European Communities. (2007). *e-Skills for the 21st century: Fostering competitiveness, growth and jobs*. Communication from the Commission to the Council, the European Parliament, the European Economic and Social Committee and the Committee of the Regions. Brussels: European Commission. Retrieved November 1, 2008, from http://ec.europa.eu/enterprise/sectors/ict/files/comm_pdf_com_2007_0496_f_en_acte_en.pdf

Cronje, J. (2006). Real learning in virtual environments. In Martin, A., & Madigan, D. (Eds.), *Digital literacies for learning* (pp. 34–41). London: Facet.

Dorsey, P. A. (2001). *Personal knowledge management: educational framework for global business*. Retrieved February 18, 2007, from http://www.millikin.edu/pkm/pkm_istanbul.html

Downes, S. (2005, October). E-learning 2.0. *eLearn Magazine*. Retrieved January 11, 2006, from http://www.elearnmag.org/subpage.cfm?section=articles&article=29-1

EDUCASE Learning Initiative. (2006). *Learner-centered concepts*. Retrieved November 1, 2008, from http://www.educause.edu/content.asp?page_id=940&bhcp=1

European Centre for the Development of Vocational Training. (2008). *European e-Skills 2008 Conference: Implementing a long-term e-skills strategy in Europe*. Retrieved November 1, 2008, from http://eskills.cedefop.europa.eu/conference2008/

European Union. (2006). Recommendation of the European Parliament and of the Council of 18 December 2006 on key competences for lifelong learning (2006/962/EC). *Official Journal of the European Union, 49*(L 394), 10–18. Retrieved November 1, 2008, from http://eur-lex.europa.eu/LexUriServ/LexUriServ.do?uri=OJ:L:2006:394:0010:0018:EN:PDF

Frand, J., & Hixon, C. (1999). *Personal knowledge management: Who, what, why, when, where, how?* Retrieved November 1, 2008, from http://www.anderson.ucla.edu/faculty/jason.frand/researcher/speeches/PKM.htm

Grey, D. (2006, June 21). *Looking at personal knowledge management*. Retrieved November 1, 2008, from http://kmwiki.wikispaces.com/PKM

Hilton, J. (2006). The future for higher education: Sunrise or perfect storm? *EDUCAUSE Review, 41*(2), 58–71. Retrieved November 1, 2008, from http://net.educause.edu/ir/library/pdf/erm0623.pdf

Irving, C., & Crawford, J. (2007). *A National Information Literacy Framework Scotland.* Retrieved November 1, 2008, from http://www.caledonian.ac.uk/ils/framework.html

Katz, I. R., & Macklin, A. S. (2007). Information and communication technology (ICT) literacy: Integration and assessment in higher education. *Systemics, Cybernetics and Informatics, 5*(4), 50–55. Retrieved November 1, 2008, from http://www.iiisci.org/Journal/CV$/sci/pdfs/P890541.pdf

Kennedy, G. E., Judd, T. S., Churchward, A., Gray, K., & Krause, K.-L. (2008). First year students' experiences with technology: Are they really digital natives? *Australasian Journal of Educational Technology, 24*(1), 108–122. Retrieved November 1, 2008, from http://www.ascilite.org.au/ajet/ajet24/kennedy.pdf

Kirkpatrick, D. L. (2006). *Evaluating training programs: The four levels* (3rd ed.). San Francisco: Berrett-Koehler.

Kvavik, R. B. (2005). Convenience, communications, and control: How students use technology. In Oblinger, D. G., & Oblinger, J. L. (Eds.), *Educating the Net Generation* (pp. 7.1–7.20). Boulder, CO: EDUCAUSE.

Laurillard, D. (2002). *Rethinking university teaching: A conversational framework for the effective use of learning technologies* (2nd ed.). London: RoutledgeFalmer. doi:10.4324/9780203304846

Lohnes, S., & Kinzer, C. (2007). Questioning assumptions about students' expectations for technology in college classrooms. *Innovate: Journal of Online Education, 3*(5). Retrieved November 1, 2008, from, http://www.innovateonline.info/index.php?view=article&id=431

Lorenzo, G., & Dziuban, C. (2006). *Ensuring the Net Generation is net savvy*. Boulder, CO: EDUCAUSE. Retrieved November 1, 2008, from http://www.educause.edu/ir/library/pdf/ELI3006.pdf

Martin, A. (2006). Literacies for the digital age: Preview of Part 1. In Martin, A., & Madigan, D. (Eds.), *Digital literacies for learning* (pp. 3–25). London: Facet.

Martin, A., & Ashworth, S. (2004). Welcome to the Journal of eLiteracy! *Journal of eLiteracy, 1*(1), 2–6. Retrieved November 1, 2008, from http://www.jelit.org/archive/00000011/01/JeLit_Editorial.pdf

Mayes, T., & Fowler, C. (2006). Learners, learning literacy and the pedagogy of e-learning. In Martin, A., & Madigan, D. (Eds.), *Digital literacies for learning* (pp. 107–123). London: Facet.

McFedries, P. (2005, December 22). Web 2.0. *Word Spy.* Retrieved November 1, 2008, from http://www.wordspy.com/words/Web2.0.asp

McFedries, P. (2007). Social-isms. *IEEE Spectrum, 44*(4), 56.

McLoughlin, C., & Lee, M. J. W. (2008). Future learning landscapes: Transforming pedagogy through social software. *Innovate: Journal of Online Education, 4*(5). Retrieved November 1, 2008, from http://www.innovateonline.info/index.php?view=article&id=539

Merrill, M. D. (2002). First principles of instruction. *Educational Technology Research and Development, 50*(3), 43–59. doi:10.1007/BF02505024

Midoro, V. (2007). Quale alfabetizzazione per la società della conoscenza (What literacies are needed for the knowledge society)? *TD: Tecnologie Didattiche, 41*, 47–54. Retrieved November 1, 2008, from http://www.itd.cnr.it/tdmagazine/PDF41/8_Midoro_TD41.pdf

O'Reilly, T. (2005). *What is Web 2.0: Design patterns and business models for the next generation of software*. Retrieved November 1, 2008, from http://www.oreillynet.com/pub/a/oreilly/tim/news/2005/09/30/what-is-web-20.html

Oblinger, D. G., & Oblinger, J. L. (Eds.). (2005). *Educating the Net Generation*. Boulder, CO: EDUCAUSE.

Pettenati, M. C. (2009). Social networking theories and tools to support connectivist learning activities. In Zaphiris, P., & Ang, C. S. (Eds.), *Human computer interaction: Concepts, methodologies, tools, and applications* (pp. 961–978). Hershey, PA: Information Science Reference.

Pettenati, M. C., & Cigognini, M. E. (2007). Social networking theories and tools to support connectivist learning activities. *International Journal of Web-Based Learning and Teaching Technologies, 2*(3), 39–57.

Pettenati, M. C., Cigognini, M. E., & Edirisingha, P. (2007). *Educating today's learners to become net savvy.* Retrieved November 1, 2008, from http://ltc.umanitoba.ca/wiki/Oblinger

Pettenati, M. C., Cigognini, M. E., Guerin, E. M. C., & Mangione, G. R. (2009). Personal knowledge management skills for Lifelong-Learners 2.0. In Hatzipanagos, S., & Warburton, S. (Eds.), *Handbook of research on social software and developing community ontologies* (pp. 298–315). Hershey, PA: Information Science Reference.

Pettenati, M. C., Cigognini, M. E., Mangione, G. R., & Guerin, E. (2007). Using social software for personal knowledge management in formal online learning. *Turkish Online Journal of Distance Education, 8*(3), 52–65. Retrieved November 1, 2008, from http://tojde.anadolu.edu.tr/tojde27/pdf/article_3.pdf

Pettenati, M. C., Cigognini, M. E., & Sorrentino, F. (2007, June 13–16). *Methods and tools for developing personal knowledge management skills in the connectivist era.* Paper presented at the European Distance and E-learning Network (EDEN) 2007 Annual Conference, Naples, Italy.

Pollard, D. (2005, November 23). Personal knowledge management (PKM)—an update [Web log post]. *How to Save the World.* Retrieved November 1, 2008, from http://blogs.salon.com/0002007/2005/11/23.html

Prensky, M. (2001). Digital natives, digital immigrants. *Horizon, 9*(5), 1–6. doi:10.1108/10748120110424816

Reigeluth, C. M. (Ed.). (1999). *Instructional-design theories and models: A new paradigm of instructional theory* (*Vol. 2*). Mahwah, NJ: Lawrence Erlbaum.

Salaway, G., Katz, R. N., Caruso, J. B., Kvavik, R. B., & Nelson, M. R. (2006). *The ECAR study of undergraduate students and information technology, 2006.* Boulder, CO: EDUCAUSE Center for Applied Research. Retrieved November 1, 2008, from http://www.educause.edu/ir/library/pdf/ers0607/ERS0607w.pdf

Salmon, G. (2002). *E-tivities: The key to active online learning*. London: Kogan Page.

Siemens, G. (2006). *Knowing knowledge*. Vancouver, BC: Lulu.

Siemens, G. (2007, October 22). Digital natives and immigrants: A concept beyond its best before date [Web log post]. *Connectivism Blog*. Retrieved November 1, 2008, from http://connectivism.ca/blog/2007/10/digital_natives_and_immigrants.html

Sorrentino, F., & Paganelli, F. (2006). *L'intelligenza distribuita—Ambient Intelligence: il futuro delle tecnologie invisibili (Ambient intelligence: The future of invisible technologies)*. Trento, Italy: Erickson.

The European e-Skills Forum. (2004). *e-Skills for Europe: Towards 2010 and beyond.* Brussels: European Commission. Retrieved November 1, 2008, from http://ec.europa.eu/enterprise/sectors/ict/files/e-skills-forum-2004-09-fsr_en.pdf

Tornero, J. M. P. (2004). *Promoting digital literacy, Final report, EAC/76/03: Understanding digital literacy*. Brussels: European Commission. Retrieved November 1, 2008, from http://ec.europa.eu/education/archive/elearning/doc/studies/dig_lit_en.pdf

United Nations Educational, Scientific and Cultural Organization. (2004). *The plurality of literacy and its implications for policies and programmes*. Paris: UNESCO. Retrieved November 1, 2008, from http://unesdoc.unesco.org/images/0013/001362/136246e.pdf

Varis, T. (2005). *New literacies and e-learning competences*. Retrieved November 1, 2008, from http://www.elearningeuropa.info/directory/index.php?doc_id=595&doclng=6&page=doc

Wallace, R. (1999). *Learners as users, users as learners: What's the difference?* Retrieved November 1, 2008, from https://www.msu.edu/~mccrory/pubs/HCIC_LCDboaster.htm

Warlick, D. F. (2004). *Redefining literacy for the 21st century*. Worthington, OH: Linworth.

Wright, K. (2005). Personal knowledge management: Supporting individual knowledge worker performance. *Knowledge Management Research & Practice*, *3*(3), 156–165. doi:10.1057/palgrave.kmrp.8500061

KEY TERMS AND DEFINITIONS

Connectedness: Being networked, being a web connector, collaborating and interacting for the purpose of building, developing, and maintaining social networks.

Creativity: A mental process involving the generation of new ideas or concepts, or new associations between existing ideas or concepts.

Digital Literacy: The ability to read, write, and interact within and across digital social networks.

Lifelong Learner 2.0 (or Learner 2.0): A connected (networked) lifelong learner capable of balancing formal and informal learning contexts, who has the critical ability to evaluate online resources and contacts and to use such resources to empower his or her creativity in his or her PKM.

Personal Knowledge Management (PKM): The act of managing one's personal knowledge through technologies.

PKM Basic Skills: Basic skills related to the use of social software, organized around the three main competencies of Create–Organize–Share, that enable the effective management of one's personal information and knowledge.

PKM Higher-Order Skills: Competencies going far beyond the basic skills of information management, which constitute the distinctive assets in one's PKM: connectedness, ability to balance formal and informal contexts, critical ability, creativity.

Skills and Competencies: The learned capacity or talent to effectively carry out some task to a certain standard / level of performance, and/or to achieve a particular goal/outcome.

Chapter 7
Teaching and Learning Information Technology through the Lens of Web 2.0

Mark Frydenberg
Bentley University, USA

ABSTRACT

Recent advances in Internet technologies, combined with a society that relies upon them, have brought about a new toolset for working and sharing on the World Wide Web. The term "Web 2.0" suggests an updated version of the Web, but really names a new genre of web applications, along with the technologies they rely on and the social content contain. Web 2.0 marks the evolution from a "one-way" Web filled with static content to a dynamic "read/write" Web that has become a platform promoting collaboration and communication, linking people as well as the digital information they share. This chapter applies a connectivist learning approach to creating authentic learning spaces for teaching Web 2.0 concepts in a first-year college information technology course. It suggests best practices for fostering learning by using Web 2.0 tools to create connections with people, ideas, and technology.

INTRODUCTION

Today's "digital natives" grew up with the Internet; they embrace the social networking features that Facebook, MySpace, text messaging, and instant messaging provide (Prensky, 2001; Palfrey & Gasser, 2008; Tapscott, 1998; see also Chapter 16 in this book). Students today are always online, confident with using computers, and able to find what they need on the World Wide Web.

DOI: 10.4018/978-1-60566-294-7.ch007

Advances in technology have changed the way many students learn. Siemens (2005) claims that in recent decades, "technology has reorganized how we live, how we communicate, and how we learn. Learning needs and theories that describe learning principles and processes, should be reflective of underlying social environments" (p. 3).

Many of today's students have the basic media literacy skills required to participate in a Web 2.0 world. What some of them lack, however, is an understanding of the underlying foundations that make their everyday web activities possible.

The simple act of creating and sharing a video on YouTube requires basic skills in editing audio and video, understanding the need for data compression and appropriate file formats, file transfer protocol (FTP), and the notion of a web server to store multimedia on the Internet.

Web 2.0 technologies have changed the way students and their teachers *use* the Web, and they have also impacted how to teach *about* the Web. Drawing on experiences from an introductory information technology (IT) course, *IT 101*, at Bentley University in Waltham, Massachusetts, USA, where a connectivist approach was applied to create a learning space for teaching Web 2.0 concepts, this chapter describes several trends, technologies, and applications and how they may be used to foster student learning both using and about Web 2.0.

CONNECTIVIST LEARNING AND WEB 2.0

Siemens (2005) defines connectivist learning as learning "driven by the understanding that decisions are based on rapidly altering foundations. New information is continually being acquired" (p. 7). It is important to be able to distinguish between what is important and what is not, and understand how changes in information and technology may impact earlier learning and decisions. These are precisely the skills required of tomorrow's knowledge workers. The culture of participation fostered in a rapidly changing Web 2.0-oriented environment supports such a style of learning required in this digital age.

Siemens (2006b) states that a decentralization of knowledge contributes to the enrichment of learning, giving more control to the end-user, so that learning becomes a process of gathering, adapting, and creating knowledge. This results in a challenge to authority, a need to be connected, and ultimately a desire to be able to make change. To fill this gap, Siemens proposes the theory of connectivism, which views learning as occurring in the process of creating connections between new ideas and experiences, an idea that is consistent with and appropriate in a Web 2.0 world.

Siemens (2006b, p. 31) identifies nine principles for connectivist learning:

1. Learning and knowledge require diversity of opinions to present the whole ... and to permit selection of best approach.
2. Learning is a network formation process of connecting specialized nodes or information sources.
3. Knowledge rests in networks.
4. Knowledge may reside in non-human appliances, and learning is enabled / facilitated by technology.
5. Capacity to know more is more critical than what is currently known.
6. Learning and knowing are constant, ongoing processes (not end states or products)
7. Ability to see connections and recognize patterns and make sense between fields, ideas, and concepts is the core skill for individuals today.
8. Currency (accurate, up-to-date knowledge) is the intent of all activities.
9. Decision-making is learning. Choosing what to learn and the meaning of incoming information is seen through the lens of a shifting reality. While there is a right answer now, it may be wrong tomorrow due to alterations in the information climate affecting the decision.

O'Reilly (2005) coined the term "Web 2.0" in recognition of new patterns in the ways people use the World Wide Web. According to him, the Web has become a platform for supporting applications that promote collaboration and sharing, providing rich user experiences on multiple devices. These have become possible because of increased availability of bandwidth and Internet access, advances in networking technologies, and development of new tools and platforms for creating software applications.

Connectivism suggests that knowledge rests in networks and is facilitated by technology. The development and rise in popularity of Web 2.0 applications such as social networks and collaborative tools that work by "harnessing collective intelligence" (O'Reilly, 2005, "Blogging and the wisdom of crowds," para. 10) of users promote and facilitate learning, linking both people and the knowledge they share.

Vossen and Hagemann (2007) attribute the emergence of Web 2.0 to the merging of three independent streams of development: applications, technology, and socialization. New web applications and services have appeared that require little technical background to use. Progress in hardware, networking capabilities, and software tools form the foundation for those applications, and the increased ability for users to participate and interact on the Web through social networking has changed the culture of how people use the Internet. The convergence of these "techniques, technologies, and usage patterns … has received the preliminary and … fancy term 'Web 2.0'" (Vossen & Hagemann, p. 65).

As Web 2.0 software applications are in "perpetual beta" (O'Reilly, 2005, "End of the software release cycle," para. 5), so are Web 2.0 learners—learning is constant, and ongoing. Web 2.0's lightweight programming models allow for information sharing, facilitating the use of technology to enable new learning spaces, activities, and approaches. Harnessing collective intelligence through online collaborative tools such as blogs and wikis encourages the gathering, organization, and discovery of knowledge from many different information sources.

The synergy between both sets of principles is strong, suggesting that a connectivist approach to teaching Web 2.0 concepts using the tools that embody its principles is also in order. The recent shift in how people use web technologies also inspires a shift in how to teach them. The impact of new media on the world is profound. Just as the desktop publishing tools of the mid-1990s spawned the phenomenon of home-grown newsletters, the emergence and acceptance of web publishing tools in the mid-2000s has spawned a "blogosphere" with global reach:

> *Too many educators fail to understand how technology is changing society. While hype words of web 2.0, blogs, wikis, and podcasts are easy to ignore, the change agents driving these tools are not. We communicate differently than we did even ten years ago. We use different tools for learning; we experience knowledge in different formats and at a different pace. We are exposed to an overwhelming amount of information—requiring continually greater levels of specialization in our organizations. It is here—where knowledge growth exceeds our ability to cope—that new theories of knowledge and learning are needed. (Siemens, 2006a, p. 7)*

Given this evolution in how people have come to use the Web, it becomes necessary to teach these tools and technologies in a way that is congruent with current learning styles "influenced … by socialization and technology" (Siemens, 2006a, p. 4). Two main questions emerge, which are addressed in the remainder of this chapter:

- What are core Web 2.0 topics for the IT classroom?
- How might one use Web 2.0 tools to teach these topics in the IT classroom in such a way that models connectivist learning principles and supports collaborative, experiential learning?

INTEGRATING WEB 2.0 INTO THE TERTIARY CURRICULUM

In recent years, an increasing number of students has arrived on campuses of tertiary education institutions with previous computer experience (Palfrey & Gasser, 2008). This is most likely due to greater computer availability and usage at home and in high schools. The popularity of social networking sites such as Facebook and video-sharing sites such as YouTube among college students is perhaps at least partly responsible for their interest in the Web. The traditional computer literacy course required of most first-year college students becomes an important place for teaching not only about these applications and how to use them responsibly, but also how to be literate in a Web 2.0 world.

Integrating Web 2.0 into the tertiary curriculum is becoming more common, as many colleges and universities are offering new courses focused around specific aspects or technologies of Web 2.0. For example, *Create engaging web applications using metrics and learning on Facebook* was offered for the first time at Stanford University in Fall 2007, as an "experiment in how to teach the process of successful software development" using Facebook's open platform (Eldon, 2007, para. 10). In Spring 2008, Matthew J. Hall at Vanderbilt University offered *Beyond the one-way Web: From publishing to participation* as a course concerned with the social impact of new media and technology (see Hall's class blog at http://beyondtheonewayweb.wordpress.com/). Computer Science departments at institutions such as the University of California, Berkeley have offered programming courses using new web technologies such as Ruby on Rails and AJAX. Departments in other schools have introduced Web 2.0 courses that deal with new ways to use the Web for business, marketing, and social media. Executive and business programs teach Web 2.0 from a strategy perspective, discussing trends for transitioning companies to using Web 2.0 techniques and technologies, and the new business opportunities they present (Shuen, 2008).

Another approach is to integrate specific Web 2.0 tools and technologies into existing courses. Alexander (2006) suggests that social writing platforms "appear to be logistically useful tools" (p. 38) in higher education for a variety of purposes such as teaching composition, and suggests that "The rich search possibilities opened up by ... tools [such as Google News and Digg] can further enhance the pedagogy of current events" (p. 40). Students must see the value of the tools they are exposed to in order to continue using them. The adoption of such tools in the classroom will "help student employability by preparing them for teamwork, global audience and peer reviews and in general for the new business model" in which knowledge workers are expected to collaborate (Cubric, 2007, p. 11). Many tertiary teachers have made use of blogs or wikis as a tool for promoting active learning and knowledge creation, or for continuing discussions beyond scheduled class times (Cubric, 2007; Davi, Frydenberg, & Gulati, 2007). Kamel Boulos, Maramba, and Wheeler (2006) cite concerns about monitoring and moderation of open wikis and blog content, especially in the fields of healthcare and medicine, where patient privacy is critical, and note the ease of use of such applications for sharing information.

TEACHING IT THROUGH THE LENS OF WEB 2.0

IT 101 is an introductory technology course at a Bentley University, a leader in business education in the New England region. Students are required to take an introductory technology class in either the first or second semester of the first year in their undergraduate program. The course ensures that all students gain competency in basic IT skills, including using and maintaining their computers, while developing individual skills in creating web pages and spreadsheets, understanding basic Internet protocols and applications, and navigating the Windows operating system.

While the specialized or advanced courses alluded to earlier require specific domain knowledge, this chapter argues that computer literacy and Web 2.0 literacy are both relevant, and surveys common Web 2.0 tools that can be integrated into the curriculum to teach IT concepts. By transforming a traditional, first-year computer literacy course into a relevant, Web 2.0 literacy course, students become active contributors in Web 2.0's "culture of participation," as they use its applications for collaboration and communication, and have an understanding of the technological and social developments that made them possible. The goal of this approach is to teach students traditional IT concepts and current Web 2.0 applications, and show their connections to O'Reilly's (2005) Web 2.0 principles.

Specifically, students in IT 101 interact with Web 2.0 applications in ways that facilitate their development of IT skills and introduce them to the social and business perspectives of Web 2.0. The course aims to achieve the following learning outcomes:

- describe the historical and technological milestones that led up to Web 2.0;
- demonstrate proficiency in using RSS, blogs, live and microblogs, wikis, podcasts, mashups, and other collaborative tools;
- identify characteristics of Web 2.0 applications and apply them in a business context;
- create and participate in social networks and online communities to experience the social impact of Web 2.0 tools.

Authentic Learning: Web 2.0 in the Classroom

Integrating Web 2.0 tools and topics into the IT classroom augments the traditional topics usually found in such a course. Blogs, wikis, podcasts, mashups, tagging, and social networking must all find their way into the syllabus through the creation of real-world scenarios that characterize their use. Collaborating to plan trips, creating podcast videos, writing reflective journals, and developing an online portfolio are among several examples Herrington and Kervin (2007) cite as characteristic of authentic learning enhanced by technology. They provide meaningful activities and contexts for using Web 2.0 tools to create knowledge, and promote reflection to enable abstraction. They place the student at the center, and allow the teacher to play a supporting role as students take the lead role in the learning activities.

One of the main challenges in teaching Web 2.0 concepts in the classroom is designing authentic activities that will engage students as they learn about these technologies. "While blogs, wikis, podcasts, and social bookmarking are receiving much attention, the real point of interest lies not in the tools themselves, but in what the growth of the tools represents and what the tools enable. Primary affordances include: (a) two-way flow, and (b) activities reflective of networked activities of individuals" (Siemens, 2006a, p. 33). Web 2.0 presents a landscape filled with a range of new applications; IT provides a context for examining them as tools for creating opportunities for learning.

Like Siemens, Herrington and Kervin (2007) conclude that teaching technology for its own sake is not sufficient; there must be a clear purpose for including it as part of the learning experience. This puts onus on the teacher to take steps to ensure that students appreciate how introducing technology to solve a problem will improve the process of doing so:

Experiences that put technology into the hands of the students challenge the traditional roles of teachers and students and their associated relationships. It is the teacher's responsibility to ensure that technology experiences are closely associated with the rationale and purpose of an authentic learning experience. Each of these examples highlights the importance of the teacher and students having a clear rationale for completing the task, understanding of the real-life application of the task and appropriate support to complete the task. Technology affords students the opportunity to engage with tasks that could not be completed using traditional paper-based methods. (Herrington & Kervin, 2007, p. 233)

Student Motivation

Anderson (2007) suggests that the participatory nature of the Web 2.0 culture motivates students to learn, and that "the process of learning [will be] more compelling when they are producers as much as consumers" (p. 32) of knowledge. Others argue that Web 2.0 technologies in the classroom are nothing more than a fad that will lose their initial attraction after becoming fully integrated in the classroom.

Pettenati and Cigognini (2007) support the design of effective learning experiences in a networked environment. They find that lifelong learning requires continuously being creative and creating personal learning environments (PLEs), representing the "temporal horizon through which [to] look at the lifelong learning of a subject" (p. 49), which involves both the formal and informal, expected and unexpected learning activities. Teaching Web 2.0 in the IT classroom can contribute to the attainment of such learning goals:

In the emerging social software, "Web 2.0" environment, the production of ideas takes place in a collaborative, participatory mode which breaks down the boundaries between producers and consumers and instead enables all participants to be users and producers of information and knowledge, or what can be described as produsers. These produsers engage not in a traditional form of content production, but are instead involved in produsage—the collaborative and continuous building and extending of existing content in pursuit of further improvement. (Bruns & Humphreys, 2007, p. 2)

Wikis and collaboration tools enable students become co-creators of both knowledge and classroom materials. "All of this blurring of the IT lines portends a further rise in efficiency and productivity as smart managers allow these prosumer/producers to adapt their native tools to fit the demands of their jobs" (Tapscott & Williams, 2006, p. 124). In the classroom, students become teachers and teachers must become students once again, as both engage in a learning partnership.

Technology Advancements Change the Motivation for Teaching Core Concepts

Current Web 2.0 and Internet developments have changed the motivation for teaching many core IT concepts. For example, the main rationale behind teaching the hypertext markup language (HTML) today is different than it was a decade ago, when creating a personal web page by entering HTML tags manually in a plain text editor like Notepad was one of the few common ways to maintain a web presence. Now, one can use blogs, wikis, and web-based web page creation wizards, all of which hide the underlying HTML from the user, to accomplish this task. Hence, the reasons for teaching HTML have to change.

While some students may create personal web pages from scratch, more than half of online teens have profiles on sites like Facebook or MySpace. Along with blogs and other social networks, Facebook has become a place where today's digital natives create true social connections. Text messages and instant messaging are more popular than email as a form of communication (Lenhart, Madden, Rankin Macgill, & Smith, 2007). They need not use HTML to maintain a web presence.

From a learning point of view, today's students learn HTML or XHTML (extensible hypertext markup language) to have the experience of developing an application according to certain rules of syntax to understand the precision that any software or web development task requires. From a practical point of view, today's students also learn to develop web pages in order to gain the basic skills to be able to customize their presence in other places (MySpace, Facebook, etc.) on the Web.

Reasons for understanding the fundamental concepts of computer memory, file sizes, and formats become evident when one looks at the process of downloading multimedia: the smaller the file size, the faster the download. Users also must understand different compressed data formats, recognize those that provide true compressions, those that may lose quality, and when such a loss is permissible. All of these issues come to light when examining the technology through the lens of Web 2.0.

O'Reilly's (2005) principle of "data as the next Intel inside," that the power of one's application today is based on the data it contains, just as the power of the microprocessor defines the power one's personal computer, may best be illustrated by teaching students to create mashups—Web 2.0 constructs that combine and apply data from different sources on the Web. Doing so also reinforces the fundamental concepts of input, output, and processing, the most basic functions of any computing system.

A SURVEY OF WEB 2.0 TOOLS AND TECHNOLOGIES

Blogs and Wikis

Blogs (short for "web logs") and wikis are two specialized web applications for posting or publishing information on the Web, and have varied use in higher education (Davi et al., 2007). Introducing blogs and wikis to the classroom process and requiring students to contribute to them tangibly demonstrates their similarities and their differences: while a blog allows its users to comment on one another's posts, participants cannot change anything that they themselves did not post. Blogs are online journals organized chronologically with new posts at the top, while wikis have a much more open structure, which allows participants to add new pages, or change the content of existing pages. Anyone can post to a blog, but cannot change what is already there. With a wiki, it is possible to change (or delete) existing content. Students also experience being "locked out" of a wiki page when someone else is editing it, and can view the history of the page to see how the wiki tracks all edits and provides the ability to "roll back" to an earlier version. Having mastered the mechanics, students can begin to envisage how they might use these tools as part of their own learning, and in other aspects of their personal and professional lives.

Class blogs have been used across the curriculum in different contexts for students to post topics of discussion for their classmates to answer prior to a class session; doing this lets the students identify the class readings of interest to them (Davi et al., 2007). Some blogging providers such as Blogger (http://www.blogger.com/) support the easy uploading of audio or video files, facilitating the process of having the instructor or students in the class create podcasts or vodcasts based on course sessions. By limiting posting access to only current students, the instructor can easily determine which students participate in the blog. Unrestricted access, on the other hand, allows students to see the benefits of inviting comments from a global audience on the Internet, leveraging the power of the "wisdom of crowds" (Surowiecki, 2004) that epitomizes Web 2.0.

Brownstein and Klein (2006) present several applications for the use of blogging in education: learning, constructing, argument, commentary, chronology, extension, resources, and composition. Individual student blogs support student writing, and give students another presence on the Web without having to master HTML. From a social point of view, bloggers have influence on current events, and have spawned an entire movement of grassroots journalism. This example illustrates the socialization of the Web coupled with advances in technology to support the level of collaboration that many now take for granted. According to Halavais (quoted in "Blogs move student learning beyond the classroom: An interview with Alex Halavais," 2004), blogs support self-regulated learning. Students are more self-directed, as they hold themselves accountable for their own progress and learning.

A wiki is a website whose pages can be added or edited by anyone. Pages are hyperlinked to one another, and little, if any, HTML knowledge is required to create or edit one. Ward Cunningham, who is credited with inventing the wiki, named it after the "quick" shuttle he took between terminals at a Hawaiian airport, to denote the speed and ease with which wiki pages can be created and modified (Cunningham & Leuf, 2001). The term now describes "a freely expandable collection of interlinked webpages … where each page is easily edited by any user with a forms-capable Web browser client" (Cunningham & Leuf, 2001, p. 14).

Wiki software tracks changes as users make them, making it possible to revert back to an earlier version of a page. Because multiple users may modify the same page concurrently, most wikis will prevent ("lock out") others from making changes until the current user has completed his or her updates. While it is possible to host a wiki on a local server, it is more common to register with a free wiki provider. The website WikiMatrix (http://www.wikimatrix.org/) compares the features of several wikis and provides a wizard for determining the platform that best suits one's particular needs.

Wikis have entered the tertiary classroom in many ways, perhaps most notably as a tool to enhance a traditional course management system (CMS). Traditional CMSs are generally used for accessing course materials and student grades. Instructors need to be more creative in their uses of wikis in the classroom, otherwise they are nothing more than "an advanced photocopier, allowing faculty members to deliver course materials to their students with greater ease than was previously possible" (Maloney, 2007, p. B26). A wiki can enhance a traditional content management system, as both students and the teacher may share in the responsibility of creating and posting course materials. A syllabus stored on a wiki page is easy to edit, maintain, and update as the course goes along. Wiki pages also can be used to facilitate students signing up for group projects, or to serve as collaborative workspaces for students working on such projects (Frydenberg, 2008a).

Mindel and Verma (2006) have articulated additional classroom uses for wikis, including collaborative business analysis projects, developing a literature review for research, needs assessment, sharing notes and project summaries, and making materials available for students. Others have adapted or developed specialized Web 2.0 collaborative applications for use in educational settings. Zhang and Su (2007) discuss the development of a new generation of collaborative learning environments to encourage intercultural communications and collaborations in educational scenarios. Their collaborative learning and teaching system "bridges the increasing gap between traditional computing educational systems and the new demands of industrial computing communities" (p. 153). Their extensible system allows students to create additional modules, tag items, and submit and syndicate content.

RSS

RSS (Really Simple Syndication) is the underlying technology that enables sharing of blog posts, podcasts, news headlines, and other content on the Web. The markup scheme was invented by Dave Winer in 1994 as a tool for scripting web content, which later became popular as feeds for blogs and podcasts.

Competing formats, such as Atom and GData, emerged as alternative standards in later years. All syndication mechanisms use a "publish–

subscribe" model, in which the author publishes content, and subscribers use an aggregator program to check the feed periodically and notify them that new content has been posted. RSS syndication and aggregation is possible because the data (originating from blog posts, podcasts, stock tickers, and news headlines, for example) is represented in a standard XML (extensible markup language) format. Such aggregator functionality is now standard in versions of web browsers such as Internet Explorer and Firefox through the use of live bookmarks. A standard RSS feed includes a standard set of XML tags for describing the title, author, publication date, description, and hyperlink for each item in the feed. The RSS feed for a podcast or vodcast contains an additional "enclosure tag" describing the uniform resource locator (URL) for the multimedia, its length in bytes, and content type (audio or video file format).

Mashups

Mashups, the combining of data from multiple sources into a single display, are popular Web 2.0 constructs, often difficult to create without previous programming skills. Mashups are at the heart of the Web 2.0 business revolution, as companies such as Facebook, Google, and Yahoo! make their data available through open APIs (application programming interfaces) for other applications to consume. Web applications that plot landmarks or housing data on maps (e.g., Zillow at http://www.zillow.com/), combine RSS feeds (popurls at http://www.popurls.com/), and graphically display photos from photo-sharing sites (Cooliris at http://www.cooliris.com/) are examples of mashups.

Mashups also introduce the notion of interacting with data, which is a fundamental business problem. Software development has evolved into *application* development, as current approaches to building a complete system entail linking together previously designed core components. The notion of "software as a service" (O'Reilly, 2005, "DoubleClick vs. Overture and AdSense," para. 1) and service-oriented architectures have changed the way in which web-based software is developed and deployed. While some specialized software applications may be necessary, usually off-the-shelf components can be configured to solve common business problems. Web 2.0 shifts the focus from building application software to integrating web applications and services. This promotes the sharing of data between the applications and services. The ability to reuse or remix information becomes significant when resources are open and discoverable, licenses are open and transparent, and formats are open and remixable (Lamb, 2007). Creating mashups introduces students to the API as a core strategy for Web 2.0 companies to share information between software applications, and the importance of XML as the underlying language for representing that information in a manner that permits interoperability.

When teaching about Web 2.0 tools, the task is to empower students to create their own mashups, as the very process of designing a mashup requires an ability to recognize connections between otherwise unrelated objects in the world. In the words of Cronon (1998), "More than anything else, being an educated person means being able to see connections that allow one to make sense of the world and act within it in creative ways" (p. 78), and this also resonates with the aforementioned theory of connectivism. In addition, the process of creating mashups has great educational potential for teaching basic programming constructs and software development and architecture concepts. Because these tools provide access to APIs for many Web 2.0 applications (Flickr, Facebook, and RSS feeds), students learn to interact with data in a new way, and create end products or results that can be shared. Because websites and applications will inevitably change over time, it is important to view each as a potential tool for teaching about mashups. By learning about applications of mashups and what components are needed to create one, as illustrated by using a particular tool, students will be better prepared to adapt in an age of constantly changing software applications.

This approach integrates learning traditional programming concepts using a non-traditional environment that also promotes critical and analytical thinking. These mashup tools reduce the barrier to entry to creating simple Web 2.0 applications, as little or no prior programming experience is required to achieve impressive results. At the same time, the very act of creating a mashup requires students to interact with familiar data in new ways.

Figure 1 shows a mashup created using Popfly, a web-based mashup creation tool from Microsoft. Microsoft supported Popfly from 2007 to 2009. In this example, the Facebook block obtains a list of a user's Facebook friends, and sends the city and state of each to the GeoNames block. The GeoNames block uses a web service to determine the corresponding latitude and longitude. The Virtual Earth block receives that information, along with the friend's first and last name, city and state, and photo, in order to plot each friend's photo on the map in the location of his or her listed city or state. By connecting blocks, students make connections in an information flow that results in solving a problem. They must learn to decompose a larger problem into smaller components, identify the input and output data from each task, and determine how each task fits together to contribute to the larger solution. The key to creating mashups using any application is the ability to access and process data from the Web. Other tools such as Yahoo! Pipes (http://pipes.yahoo.com/) also provide this capability. Their familiar graphical or

Figure 1. Creating a Popfly mashup

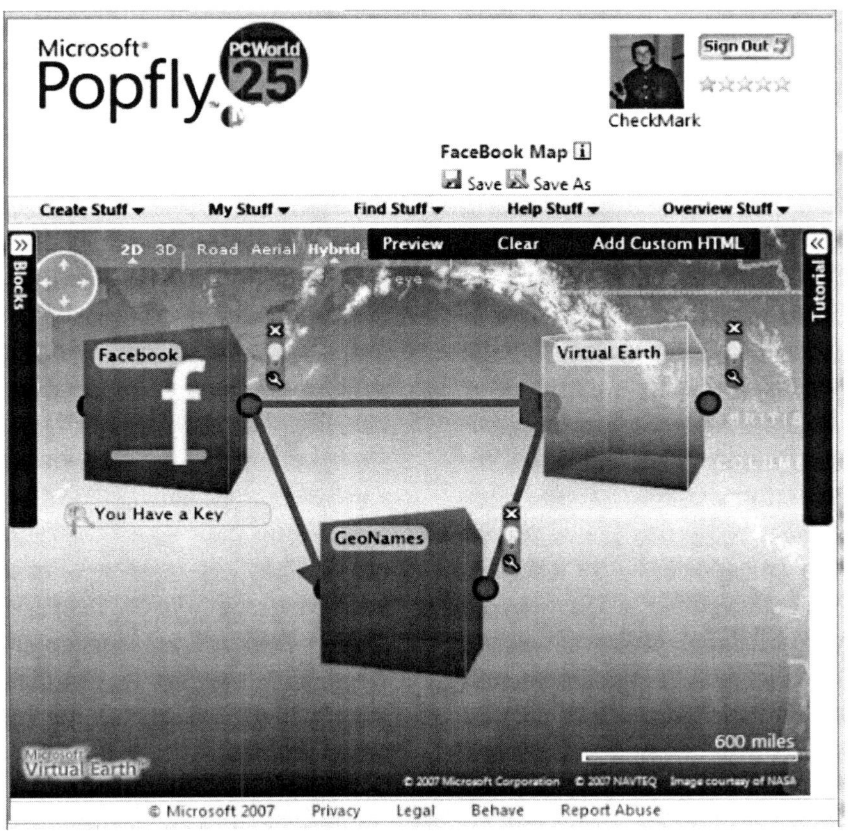

function-based interfaces hide the implementation details that would be of interest to programmers writing code, and enable beginning students to interact with real data to create simple yet useful and interesting applications.

AJAX

O'Reilly (2005) describes a "rich user experience" within the web browser as characteristic of Web 2.0 applications. As such, many Web 2.0 applications sport a rich user interface that has much more of a desktop application "look and feel" than a traditional browser-based application. This is often because such applications are implemented using a combination of web technologies collectively known as AJAX (Asynchronous JavaScript and XML). AJAX has gained popularity as a tool for creating browser-independent, dynamic web pages in which only a portion of the page updates at a time.

While it is outside the scope of an introductory IT course—and beyond the ability level of students with no prior programming experience—to implement even the simplest web-based interfaces in AJAX, it is entirely reasonable to explain the concepts of client-side and server-side processing, and the role of JavaScript, so they might be able to identify an AJAX-enabled page when they see one. Students should recognize this behavior in their web-based Microsoft Outlook client, Google Maps (http://maps.google.com/), and many online travel booking sites. In each case, only the relevant portion of the page changes without reloading the entire page. Relating these concepts to students' own experiences of them while using familiar web applications creates an opportunity for learning.

In AJAX applications, JavaScript function calls run separately (asynchronously) from the loading of a web page. The function calls may invoke web services or other JavaScript methods to acquire new information with which to update the page, and only a portion of the page may be updated without refreshing the whole page. Pages rely on JSON (JavaScript Object Notation), a lightweight data interchange format, for passing structured data across a network in a way that is transparent to the user. As a result, the user's experience is perceived as more interactive. Some ASP.NET AJAX controls obtain input from calls to external web services. Only controls on the page that receive the updated data from a web service call are refreshed, enhancing the experience of using the web application (Frydenberg, 2008b).

Google has introduced several tools for building rich web applications. Google App Engine (http://appengine.google.com/) allows for the production of web applications that run within Google's infrastructure, and Google Gears (http://gears.google.com/) provides open source extensions to add new features to web browsers.

Tagging

Tagging tools are another way to provide for learning by making connections between people and knowledge. Tagging is a fundamental concept in the Web 2.0 world. Students must understand the nature of both physical and digital information to be adequately prepared to manage digital information. Tags are used in applications that extend beyond social bookmarking sites (e.g., delicious at http://www.delicious.com/), Flickr (http://www.flickr.com/-for photo sharing), and Technorati (http://www.technorati.com/-for indexing blogs), which that were the first to use them, and they are now found on websites of all types. According to Bumgardner (2006), "these amorphous clumps of words now appear on a slew of web sites as visual evidence of their membership in the elite corps of 'Web 2.0'" (p. 1). Many sites such as delicious incorporate tag "clouds" in which larger fonts and darker colors indicate more popular topics among those that a user has tagged. Each tag links to a page at delicious containing hyperlinks to the actual articles.

Abbitt (2007) investigated the impact of social content sites such as Digg (http://www.digg.com/)

and delicious in an educational setting. In a pilot study using social content in an undergraduate educational technology course, he examined usage patterns from students who used their customized social content software over the course of a semester. It was found that social content sites were new to most students and many felt that using them helped them to find resources that they believed would be useful later in their careers (Abbitt, 2007).

Microblogging / Social Networking

Twitter (http://www.twitter.com/) is a microblogging application, where users perpetually respond to the simple question, "What are you doing?" Twitter broadcasts and receives short messages to the mobile phones (cellphones) or computers of all those who "subscribe" to another user's broadcast, allowing users to build significant social networks. By signing up to "follow" one another, friends can send and receive messages. Because Twitter messages may be received on mobile phone, the application is highly mobile, which leads to a number of interesting possibilities for classroom use.

Lew (2007) and Parry (2008) summarize several educational applications of Twitter. With its 140-character message limit, Twitter requires students to be concise in their writing. To carry on conversations beyond the classroom, students could sign up to follow each other, posting when they see something that relates to a topic discussed in class. They might view Twitter's Public Timeline (http://twitter.com/public_timeline/) to get a sense of what Twitter subscribers around the world are doing. Twitter can be a research tool as users can track posts containing particular words or phrases and receive updates when any Twitter posts containing those terms are posted. Collaborators can leave short notes for one another as they work on a joint project.

Twitter searches on a current topic give students an instant connection to a network of people with similar interests. There are also several tools for integrating Twitter feeds into a standard RSS format, thus promoting their availability in other applications.

A CONNECTIVIST APPROACH TO TEACHING WEB 2.0 WITH WEB 2.0 TOOLS

This section maps connectivist learning principles to an approach for teaching Web 2.0 concepts in the classroom. Collectively, they all illustrate that gaining up-to-date knowledge of a current technology is the underlying intent of each activity, but more importantly, the process of completing these activities gives students the skills to stay up-to-date by exploring and learning new technologies on their own.

Learning Requires Diversity of Opinions to Present the Whole

An effective way to initiate a conversation with students on Web 2.0 topics and technologies is to show a now-well-known video clip entitled *Web 2.0 ... The machine is us/ing us* (Wesch, 2007b). This short video, available on YouTube, presents a panorama of Web 2.0 technologies, and decisions that must be made about organizing all of the new data brought about by such tools. A major turning point in identifying Web 2.0 as a new phenomenon is Wesch's observation in his video that "The Web is no longer linking information, it is linking people." Through collaborative tools, wikis, blogs, and social networks, people are connected in ways that were not previously possible. The video concludes by raising the issues of ethics, identity, privacy, and copyright that are prevalent as a result of using today's Web 2.0 applications.

The question of how today's students learn and the challenges of surviving in a digital world is the subject of Wesch's (2007a) *A vision of students today* video, also posted on YouTube. This video highlights "some of the most important characteristics of students today—how they learn, what they need to learn, their goals, hopes, dreams, what their lives will be like, and what kinds of changes they will experience in their lifetime." The stark contrast between traditional, frontal teaching and collaborative learning becomes obvious as today's learners multi-task, have a constant need a desire to be connected, spend more time online than in class, and realize that the jobs they may obtain after graduation may not yet exist today.

These two videos present the diversity of opinions and issues related to Web 2.0 and how today's students learn. Asking students to share their opinions of them opens the door to a larger conversation relating to the impact of Web 2.0 tools on the lives of today's students. They need to learn general skills that they can apply in a variety of contexts. "We need to be teaching kids these skills earlier, and in ways that work for them in the digital environment as well as in traditional environments" (Palfrey & Gasser, 2008, p. 183).

Learning Connects Specialized Information Sources

Using social applications is an important step in understanding the impact that one person can have on the web experience of others. Students vote on popular news articles by "digging" (voting for) them at Digg.com, where the stories that receive the largest number of "diggs" (votes) appear on the site's front page. They post to blogs and wikis, upload photos, or tag articles of interest. Performing this activity exposes students' personal and previously private interests and entries to a larger community—be it their classmates, or ultimately the world—all of whom may benefit from their participation.

On a practical level, students experience several advantages to using social bookmarking sites such as delicious over storing bookmarks privately in a browser on their local computer. A user's bookmarks are stored "in the cloud" of the Internet, so they are available from any browser when logged in to the site; bookmarks can be shared; and the same resource can be tagged with multiple keywords. Along with each tag, delicious displays the number of people who tagged the same article along with links to other resources with the same tags. As mentioned earlier, tag clouds visually display more popular tags using variations in font size and color.

Social bookmarking sites are a useful research tool for teaching and learning purposes. Mejias (2006) cites the use of delicious in the classroom by student who contributed articles to pertinent reading list for the class, thereby "creating an effective distributed research community" (p. 2). Students can draw upon the wisdom of crowds to assume that several people tagging a particular article on a topic is an indication that it is probably worth reading for information on that topic. Because tags are assigned by humans rather than programs, they are often a good measure of the quality or usefulness of a resource, and may be more a effective means of locating relevant content than a simple web search engine query based on keywords. This approach blends a "folksonomy" with a more traditional taxonomy for organizing resources on the Web. The application of "social software in this manner supports constructivist pedagogy where students feel empowered to take charge of their own learning" (Mejias, p. 5). For students previously unfamiliar with tagging, the teacher's role is to involve students in a realistic scenario that requires them to organize a large volume of information in a personally meaningful way, and then "evangelize" the use of a social bookmarking tool so students will see its value in making the task at hand manageable. Creating such an authentic learning environment provides a context to reflect the way the knowledge (or tool for classifying it) will be used in real life (Herrington & Kervin, 2007).

Tagging is one of several Web 2.0 tools giving individuals the ability to express and discover their own individuality. Siemens (2006b) notes the tension between privacy and individuality thus:

we know and can be known. We scatter our lives and thoughts across the web. Each question in a forum, each thought in a blog, each podcast, each comment to an article—these distributed pieces are splashed across the internet. They form who we are, how we think (at a certain time), and the things we believe. We are known by what we have done and said, and by what others have said about us. We are laid bare ... Our identities are exposed, revealed for anyone to explore. (p. 72)

After tagging articles related to their interests and favorite activities regularly on delicious, for even a short time, students may notice that their tag clouds begin to form a profile that reveals information about themselves in ways that might otherwise not be so easy to discern.

The strengths and shortcomings of such a "folksonomy" quickly become apparent to students. While users can define their own tags for organizing web content, students quickly find that the same tag may have different interpretations. Students learn that the new "order of order" of Web 2.0 is "changing how we think the world itself is organized, and—perhaps more important—who we think has the authority to tell us so" (Weinberger, 2007, p. 23). Students are empowered when they effectively organize information in ways that make sense to them, thereby creating their own PLEs (Wilson, Liber, Johnson, Beauvoir, Sharples, & Milligan, 2007).

Knowledge Rests in Networks; Learning is Facilitated by Technology

Lippincott (2006) claims that "a social process involving interaction with, and observation of, others is an important component of learning" (p. 169). Fostering communities of learning and practice has long been a model for student engagement across academic disciplines and topic areas. Collaborative Web 2.0 tools extend this notion, as now students can connect with classmates, instructors, and others virtually to share ideas and extend their views.

Requiring every student to contribute to the same wiki page quickly illustrates O'Reilly's (2005) aforementioned notion of harnessing collective intelligence, as students work together to create study materials for themselves and their peers, and improve the quality of the application for other users. Collaboration through Web 2.0 tools shows that students can network with and learn from one another. In one classroom setting, students may collaboratively create a "study sheet" in preparation for an examination. Each student supplies one question and provides the corresponding answer on a wiki page. By doing this, students see how each of their individual questions contribute directly to the production of a joint artifact that is of mutual benefit and value to all students in the class.

Apart from wikis, the use of Twitter and other social networking tools to support collaboration gives students access to a network of individuals with whom they can share their knowledge. Networked collaborative learning is a hallmark of Web 2.0-based tertiary education, and such activities can give rise to increased student engagement, improved student satisfaction, and the development of higher-order thinking skills (Resta & Laferriere, 2007).

Capacity to Know More is More Critical Than What is Currently Known

The ability to model, interact with, and share data is a key idea in a business context but is also relevant in tertiary education. At an introductory level, students interact with data by understanding RSS feeds and what they represent. Showing students the underlying XML data and how it is structured underscores the main difference between XML and HTML: the former is primarily a tool for describing information, while the latter is a tool for displaying (formatting/rendering) information within a web browser.

To reinforce the concept that content is separated from how it is displayed, students interact with RSS feeds in different ways. They subscribe to their feeds within a browser, or use a web-based aggregator such as Google Reader (http://reader.google.com/). In addition, there are several desktop gadgets for displaying information from RSS feeds within a Windows Vista or Google sidebar. Similarly, a web gadget enables the display of the same information on one's blog or website by embedding some HTML code provided to the user when configuring the gadget. Demonstrating these features and/or encouraging students to experiment with them also introduces students to the Web 2.0 concept of a mashup.

Learning and Knowing are Constant, Ongoing Processes; Currency is the Intent of All Activities

Web 2.0 software is in perpetual beta (O'Reilly, 2005), just as its users are in a constant, ongoing process of learning using its tools. Students see new ways to use the Web all semester long and blog several times during the semester about their experiences. Adding content regularly shows that their blogs or websites—like their learning—must remain fresh and current on a continual basis, and chronicle progress throughout the semester. Engaging in such an active approach to learning based on cooperative questioning, conceptual understanding, iterative assessment, and refinement promotes retention and lifelong learning (Wirth, 2007; Nicol, 2007).

Learning Requires an Ability to See Connections and Make Sense of Ideas and Concepts

Interoperability is a major tenet of the Web 2.0 landscape. The ability to use data from different sources in a single application, as well as the ability to use the same application on different platforms, contributes to the openness of this landscape. By relating each of these back to core IT concepts, students are prompted to make connections between Web 2.0 technologies they learn in the classroom and real-world situations they may encounter later in employment or life at large.

For example, in one group assignment on wireless networking, students collaborate by using Google Docs (http://docs.google.com/), a web-based word processing tool with multi-user capabilities, to write their laboratory (lab) reports. This assignment creates an authentic problem scenario for which synchronous collaborative writing is a perfect solution (Herrington & Kervin, 2007). Each student contributes his or her "part" of the assignment to the group's document, editing from a different computer, either at the same or different times as their fellow group members. They must make sense of their own ideas within the context of the same document that their partners are editing at the same time, to determine where in its flow their ideas best belong.

This exercise also introduces students to the benefits and drawbacks of a collaborative desktop application that lives "in the cloud." By requiring their use, students evaluate and master these Web 2.0 tools as part of their regular assignments.

Decision-Making is Learning

Connectivism suggests that an important way in which students learn is by making decisions about their own learning, and choosing what they will learn (Siemens, 2005). One way to learn about Web 2.0 is to select and investigate a collaborative or social media application, and apply O'Reilly's (2005) characteristics to it to determine what "makes" it Web 2.0. Students learn by synthesizing and applying these concepts to a tangible software application, then deciding the best way to present their findings to their classmates through a short video. Students evaluate the application, commenting on its ease of use and how it compares with other similar programs they know about, in addition to suggesting at least one possible enhancement to the functionality of the application.

Students are allowed to present their ideas in groups, where each group's presentation takes 10 to 15 minutes, and includes both a live demonstration and a PowerPoint slide show. Presentations are video recorded so students can later edit the videos and post them to the class pod/vodcast channel for peer critique and comments.

This assignment has several pedagogical benefits. It is one of the first collaborative assignments students complete; they must evaluate an application well enough to demonstrate, comment on, and recommend improvements for it; and they have to apply their understanding of an accepted general model—O'Reilly's (2005) Web 2.0 characteristics—to a specific case, determining which elements of the model are applicable. Finally, they create a collaborative work product to share with their classmates. Students demonstrate their mastery of several technical skills in order to post their videos to the class channel.

Another project introduces the use of the free Voice over Internet Protocol (VoIP) service Skype (http://www.skype.com/) as a new communication tool for collaborative learning and knowledge exchange. Students in IT 101 use Skype to converse with students studying a similar course at a university in another country (Chan, Frydenberg, & Lee, 2007) to produce a collaborative work product in the form of an audio recording. In order to complete the exercise, participants in each team (consisting of members from both countries) use a wiki page as a collaborative workspace to share resources and communicate in between scheduled synchronous conversations. They must decide what the content and format of their recording will be, who will participate, how to delegate responsibilities, and how to generate productive dialogue with peers about a topic with which they are just beginning to gain familiarity. They record and edit their audio conversations, making choices about which clips to share and which to discard, and post the finished products online as podcasts to which others may listen.

Both of these examples show how "the Internet not only makes readily available a vast amount of information and resources but brings people together in a shared environment to exchange ideas, learn and engage in collaborative decision making" (Hamburg, Engert, & Anke, 2008, p. 153). Through collaborative decision making, students not only influence their own learning trajectories, but also those of others who are the audience of their completed presentations.

CHALLENGES OF TEACHING WEB 2.0

Teaching Concepts or Tools?

Teaching IT concepts "through the lens of Web 2.0" requires more than simply integrating blogs, wikis, podcasts, mashups, and social networking applications into the university or college classroom. These tools have found their way in to the digital fabric of students' online experiences. However, the specific tools will change over time; for an IT student the educational value of learning about any Web 2.0 tool is in understanding what it does and why it does it. Developing relevant problem-solving and decision-making skills enables students to make connections between identifying problems and specifying possible solutions, in a way that process of doing so will make an impact on their lifelong learning.

A downside to this approach is that students may become so caught up in the tools or websites they use that they lose sight of the key academic learning objectives—the course could easily fall back into a survey of Web 2.0 sites without looking deeper at their structure, or the impact that they have in on business and/or society. It is particularly important to "keep a balance between literacies and technologies" (Hicks, 2006, p. 51) to develop skills that are transferable. This is crucial in both the K-12 (schools) sector as well as tertiary education. Creating a learning space that enables students to make the connection between the conceptual and the concrete is vital. Siemens (2005) says that participatory tools increase access to a network of people, ideas, and content. In connectivist learning, participatory tools also offer opportunities for conceptual learning through experiential activity that involves a global community.

While the collaborative nature of Web 2.0 encourages assignments that allow students to work together, a network of one does not support connectivist learning. With such a focus on group process, the simple act of assessing an individual's own acquired knowledge as the result of an exercise, rather than his or her contribution to the whole, becomes difficult and problematic. Students no longer live in a "fill-in-the-blank" world. Assessment tasks and evaluation methods need to evolve to ensure that networked, authentic learning is supported and that Web 2.0 tools and strategies are integrated.

Extending the Model

This chapter has discussed techniques for introducing Web 2.0 concepts in an IT classroom through the use of Web 2.0 tools. Certainly, several of the social and collaborative tools mentioned here can be—and have been—applied across the curriculum with success. The trend has been for tools to become so sophisticated that they hide underlying technologies and complexities, to the degree that anyone can create a mashup, web page, or video despite having little technical knowledge or experience. For the non-technical user, such applications open new possibilities in terms of creativity and communication.

What distinguishes the IT classroom from other areas is its focus in cultivating an understanding of the technology *and* experience in using it; in this vein the approach taken in *IT 101* results in a diverse Web 2.0 repertoire or "toolbox" that students can readily apply to all areas of their lives, and that they will hopefully continue to expand and refine well after the conclusion of the course.

CONCLUSION AND FUTURE TRENDS

Web 2.0 is the result of the impact of advances in technology on a changing society constantly connected via the Internet. Portable computers and mobile telephones require software to be developed beyond a single device, necessitating a separation between data access and data presentation. The popularity of software as a service facilitates the move between different devices and platforms.

When considering Web 2.0 tools for classroom administration, tools for content creation must improve to the extent that the process of using them becomes transparent. Much in the same way that student expectations for instructors to post course handouts online prompted the development of automated LMSs such as Blackboard and WebCT in the late 1990s, today's demands for podcasting and participation will see traditional CMS applications integrate additional Web 2.0 functionality for classroom management.

To promote the teaching of Web 2.0 concepts in the classroom, tertiary teachers need to promote the active use of Web 2.0 tools by students. By integrating collaborative and social media applications in authentic learning environments, and creating opportunities for students to become both consumers and producers of classroom materials, students can experience the culture of participation that is central to Web 2.0. In the Web 2.0 classroom, the process is equally as important as the result: by encouraging students to explore, tinker, and experiment with tools they can build competence as well as confidence that will be crucial for continued lifelong and life-wide learning.

Some claim that "Web 3.0," the next stage in the evolution of the Web following Web 2.0, will be the "Semantic Web," where adding meaning to web content will enable machines and humans to both read and understand it. (Berners-Lee, Hendler, & Lassila, 2001; see also Chapter 20 in this book). This is definitely an area open to research, first in development, and second in determining how to make these concepts accessible to students whose major is not in IT.

Tomorrow's university students will continue to embrace Web 2.0 applications, with little knowledge of the developments that led up to them. Incorporating Web 2.0 concepts in the classroom has many possibilities, and empowering students to use Web 2.0 tools to create learning artifacts—podcasts, blog posts, mashups, multimedia objects, tagged resource collections, and so on—and share them is a worthwhile endeavor with many potential educational benefits. A fundamental understanding of the origins and architecture of the Internet, coupled with an awareness of the social and ethical issues related to using the World Wide Web, will be even more crucial for tomorrow's students as they become informed participants and future leaders in a networked, Web 2.0-based society and knowledge economy.

REFERENCES

Abbitt, J. T. (2007). Exploring the educational possibilites for a user-driven social content system in an undergraduate course. [from http://jolt.merlot.org/documents/abbitt.pdf]. *Journal of Online Learning and Teaching*, *3*(4), 437–447. Retrieved November 4, 2008.

Alexander, B. (2006). Web 2.0: A new wave of innovation for teaching and learning? *EDUCAUSE Review, 41*(2), 32–44. Retrieved November 4, 2008, from http://www.educause.edu/ir/library/pdf/erm0621.pdf

Anderson, P. (2007). *What is Web 2.0? Ideas, technologies and implications for education*. Bristol, UK: Joint Information Systems Committee. Retrieved November 4, 2008, from http://www.jisc.ac.uk/media/documents/techwatch/tsw0701b.pdf

Berners-Lee, T., Hendler, J., & Lassila, O. (2001). The Semantic Web. *Scientific American, 284*(5), 29–37. doi:10.1038/scientificamerican0501-34

Blogs move student learning beyond the classroom: An interview with Alex Halavais. (2004, December). *Online Classroom*, 4, 8.

Brownstein, E., & Klein, R. (2006). Blogs: Application in science education. *Journal of College Science Teaching*, *35*(6), 18–22.

Bruns, A., & Humphreys, S. (2007). Building collaborative capacities in learners: The M/cyclopedia project revisited. In A. Désilets & R. Biddle (Eds.), *Proceedings of the 2007 International Symposium on Wikis* (pp. 1–10). New York: Association for Computing Machinery. Retrieved November 4, 2008, from http://www.wikisym.org/ws2007/_publish/Bruns_WikiSym2007_MCyclopedia.pdf

Bumgardner, J. (2006). *Building tag clouds in Perl and PHP*. Cambridge, MA: O'Reilly.

Chan, A., Frydenberg, M., & Lee, M. J. W. (2007). Facilitating cross-cultural learning through collaborative skypecasting. In J. J. Ekstrom (Ed.), *Proceedings of the 2007 ACM Information Technology Education Conference* (pp. 59–66). New York: Association for Computing Machinery.

Cronon, W. (1998). "Only Connect ... " The goals of a liberal education. *The American Scholar*, *67*(4), 73–80.

Cubric, J. (2007). Wiki-based process framework for blended learning. In A. Désilets & R. Biddle (Eds.), *Proceedings of the 2007 International Symposium on Wikis* (pp. 11–24). New York: Association for Computing Machinery. Retrieved November 4, 2008, from http://www.wikisym.org/ws2007/_publish/Cubric_WikiSym2007_BlendedLearningFramework.pdf

Cunningham, W., & Leuf, B. (2001). *The wiki way: Quick collaboration on the Web*. New York: Addison-Wesley.

Davi, A., Frydenberg, M., & Gulati, G. J. (2007). Blogging across the disciplines: Integrating technology to enhance liberal learning. *Journal of Online Learning and Teaching, 3*(3), 222–233. Retrieved November 4, 2008, from http://jolt.merlot.org/vol3no3/frydenberg.pdf

Eldon, E. (2007, September 10). Facebook to take over Stanford classroom [Web log post]. *VentureBeat*. Retrieved November 4, 2008, from http://venturebeat.com/2007/09/10/facebook-to-take-over-stanford-classroom/

Frydenberg, M. (2008a). Wikis as a tool for collaborative course management. *Journal of Online Learning and Teaching, 4*(2), 169–181. Retrieved November 4, 2008, from http://jolt.merlot.org/vol4no2/frydenberg0608.pdf

Frydenberg, M. (2008b). Slickr: A multi-tiered web development capstone project using databases, web services, and AJAX. *Information Systems Education Journal, 6*(37). Retrieved November 4, 2008, from http://isedj.org/6/37/ISEDJ.6(37).Frydenberg.pdf

Hamburg, I., Engert, S., & Anke, P. (2008). Communities of practice and Web 2.0 to support learning in SMEs. In O. Cernian (Ed.), *Proceedings of the Sixth Romanian Educational Network (RoEduNet) International Conference* (pp. 152–155). Craiova, Romania: Faculty of Automation, Computers and Electronics, University of Craiova.

Herrington, J., & Kervin, L. (2007). Authentic learning supported by technology: Ten suggestions and cases of integration in classrooms. *Educational Media International, 44*(3), 219–236. doi:10.1080/09523980701491666

Hicks, T. (2006). Expanding the conversation: A commentary toward revision of Swenson, Rozema, Young, McGrail, and Whitin. *Contemporary Issues in Technology and Teacher Education, 6*(1), 46–55. Retrieved November 4, 2008, from http://www.editlib.org/f/21862

Kamel Boulos, M. N., Maramba, I., & Wheeler, S. (2006). Wikis, blogs and podcasts: A new generation of web-based tools for virtual collaborative clinical practice and education. *BMC Medical Education, 6*(41). Retrieved November 4, 2008, from http://www.biomedcentral.com/1472-6920/6/41

Lamb, B. (2007). Dr. Mashup; or, why educators should learn to stop worrying and love the remix. *EDUCAUSE Review, 42*(4), 12–25. Retrieved November 4, 2008, from http://net.educause.edu/ir/library/pdf/erm0740.pdf

Lenhart, A., Madden, M., Rankin Macgill, A., & Smith, A. (2007). *Teens and social media*. Washington, DC: Pew Internet & American Life Project. Retrieved November 4, 2008, from http://www.pewinternet.org/~/media//Files/Reports/2007/PIP_Teens_Social_Media_Final.pdf.pdf

Lew, A. (2007, August 19). Twitter tweets for higher education [Web log post]. *Web 2.0 Teaching Tools*. Retrieved November 4, 2008, from http://web20teach.blogspot.com/2007/08/twitter-tweets-for-higher-education.html

Lippincott, J. K. (2006). Learning, engagement, and technology. In Gibson, C. (Ed.), *Student engagement and information literacy* (pp. 169–183). Chicago: Association of College and Research Libraries.

Maloney, E. J. (2007, January 5). What Web 2.0 can teach us about learning. *The Chronicle of Higher Education*, B26.

Mejias, U. (2006). Teaching social software with social software. *Innovate: Journal of Online Education, 2*(5). Retrieved February 12, 2010, from http://innovateonline.info/pdf/vol2_issue5/Teaching_Social_Software_with_Social_Software.pdf

Mindel, J. L., & Verma, S. (2006). Wikis for teaching and learning. *Communications of the Association for Information Systems*, *18*(1), 2–38.

Nicol, D. (2007). Laying a foundation for lifelong learning: Case studies of e-assessment in large 1st-year classes. *British Journal of Educational Technology*, *38*(4), 668–678. doi:10.1111/j.1467-8535.2006.00657.x

O'Reilly, T. (2005). *What is Web 2.0: Design patterns and business models for the next generation of software*. Retrieved November 4, 2008, from http://www.oreillynet.com/pub/a/oreilly/tim/news/2005/09/30/what-is-web-20.html

Palfrey, J., & Gasser, U. (2008). *Born digital: Understanding the first generation of digital natives*. New York: Basic.

Parry, D. (2008, January 23). Twitter for academia [Web log post]. *AcademHack*. Retrieved November 4, 2008, from http://academhack.outsidethetext.com/home/2008/twitter-for-academia/

Pettenati, M. C., & Cigognini, M. E. (2007). Social networking theories and tools to support connectivist learning activities. *International Journal of Web-Based Learning and Teaching Technologies*, *2*(3), 42–60.

Prensky, M. (2001). Digital natives, digital immigrants. *Horizon*, *9*(5), 1–2. doi:10.1108/10748120110424816

Resta, P., & Laferriere, T. (2007). Technology in support of collaborative learning. *Educational Psychology Review*, *19*(1), 65–83. doi:10.1007/s10648-007-9042-7

Shuen, A. (2008). *Web 2.0: A strategy guide*. Sebastapol, CA: O'Reilly.

Siemens, G. (2005). Connectivism: A learning theory for the digital age. *International Journal of Instructional Technology and Distance Learning*, *2*(1), 3–10. Retrieved November 4, 2008, from http://www.itdl.org/Journal/Jan_05/Jan_05.pdf

Siemens, G. (2006a). *Connectivism: Learning theory or pastime for the self-amused?* Retrieved November 4, 2008, from http://www.elearnspace.org/Articles/Connectivism_response.doc

Siemens, G. (2006b). *Knowing knowledge*. Vancouver, BC: Lulu.

Surowiecki, J. (2004). *The wisdom of crowds: Why the many are smarter than the few and how collective wisdom shapes business, economies, societies, and nations*. New York: Doubleday.

Tapscott, D. (1998). *Growing up digital: The rise of the Net Generation*. New York: McGraw-Hill.

Tapscott, D., & Williams, A. D. (2006). The prosumers. In *Wikinomics: How mass collaboration changes everything* (pp. 124–150). New York: Penguin.

Vossen, G., & Hagemann, S. (2007). *Unleashing Web 2.0: From concepts to creativity*. San Francisco: Morgan Kaufmann.

Weinberger, D. (2007). *Everything is miscellaneous: The power of the new digital disorder*. New York: Times.

Wesch, M. (2007a, October 12). *A vision of students today* [Video file]. Retrieved November 4, 2008, from http://www.youtube.com/watch?v=dGCJ46vyR9o

Wesch, M. (2007b, March 8). *Web 2.0... The machine is us/ing us* [Video file]. Retrieved November 4, 2008, from http://www.youtube.com/watch?v=6gmP4nk0EOE

Wilson, S., Liber, O., Johnson, M., Beauvoir, P., Sharples, P., & Milligan, C. (2007). Personal learning environments: Challenging the dominant design of educational systems. *Journal of e-Learning and Knowledge Society, 3*(2), 27–38. Retrieved November 4, 2008, from http://je-lks.maieutiche.economia.unitn.it/en/07_02/04Art_wilson_inglese.pdf

Wirth, K. (2007). Teaching for deeper understanding and lifelong learning. *Elements, 3*(2), 107–111. doi:10.2113/gselements.3.2.107

Zhang, H., & Su, H. (2007). Reforming computing education with new web technologies. *Journal of Computing Sciences in Colleges, 23*(2), 150–156.

KEY TERMS AND DEFINITIONS

Application Programming Interface (API): An interface exposed by software to enable programmers of other applications to write code to interact with it and use its services, without the need to understand its inner workings.

Blogs: Web sites on which users can easily post information and comment on one another's posts.

Connectivist Learning: A learning model that suggests learning is an ongoing process that occurs in networks, is facilitated by technology, and connects both people and knowledge.

Mashup: A Web 2.0 application constructed by combining data obtained from two or more other sources on the Web (e.g., an application that displays listings of houses for sale drawn from a real estate website on a map whose data is supplied by Google Maps.)

Social Networking: Web applications that facilitate locating and communicating with people who have similar affinities.

Tagging: The act of assigning keywords to digital artifacts such as images, websites, and videos so they might be easily found and retrieved (by the tagger him/herself and/or others) at a later stage.

Web 2.0: The shift in the use of the World Wide Web from static, "read-only" content to applications that promote collaboration, communication, and user-generated content.

Wikis: Collaborative web applications that enable users to post and edit one another's information.

Chapter 8
University Students' Self-Motivated Blogging and Development of Study Skills and Research Skills

Shailey Minocha
The Open University, UK

Lucinda Kerawalla
The Open University, UK

ABSTRACT

This chapter presents and analyzes an empirically grounded investigation into the self-motivated course-related blogging activities of undergraduate and Master's-level students, and research-related blogging of doctoral students. It focuses on how blogging may help students to develop their study skills and research skills. Analysis of students' blogs and semi-structured interviews with the participants shows that writing in the public domain can encourage networking, commitment to goals, articulation of research ideas, development of confidence in writing, and facilitation of critical and reflective thinking skills. The blog can be a useful repository of ideas and resources, and can be a public platform for the synthesis of ideas. Blogging can facilitate the creation and membership of an online community where academic events are flagged, resources are shared, research is advertised, and ideas and comments are exchanged. The authors conclude with a discussion of the ways in which blogging can support the development of key study and research skills, such as time management, academic writing, and effective communication. It is hoped that the findings will help in guiding students, educators, and institutions considering the use of blogging in university education.

INTRODUCTION AND BACKGROUND

The term Web 2.0 or "social software" covers a wide range of software tools that enable users to interact and share ideas and resources such as photographs and bookmarks, with other users, primarily via the World Wide Web. The Web 2.0 or "read/write" Web is in contrast with the original "read-only" Web (Web 1.0) in which users were

DOI: 10.4018/978-1-60566-294-7.ch008

passive consumers of other people's information (e.g., on websites maintained by an individual, organization, or institution). Blogs, wikis, social networking sites (e.g., Facebook), media-sharing sites (e.g., YouTube, SlideShare, Flickr), and social bookmarking sites (e.g., delicious) are examples of some of the tools that are being used to share and collaborate in educational, social, and business contexts. The key aspect of a social software tool is that it involves wider participation in the creation of information that is shared (e.g., Boyd, 2007, Franklin & van Harmelen, 2007; Leslie & Landon, 2008).

Social software tools allow users to gather and share resources to inform others and receive feedback. In collaborative endeavors using social software tools, the creation of shared content takes place in a networked participatory environment that breaks down the barriers between producers and consumers and instead enables all participants to be users as well as producers of information and knowledge (Bruns, 2008). Bruns refers to the concept of "produser" implying the hybrid role of a participant as producers of content and also using the content or "produsage." Thus, there is a collaborative and continuous building and extending of existing content in pursuit of further improvement.

Social software tools emphasize the importance of interpersonal interaction in groups and can facilitate social equality, collaboration, cooperation, and mutual support. Boyd (in Owen, Grant, Sayers, & Facer, 2006), specifies three types of support provided by social software:

1. Support for conversational interaction between individuals or groups, from real-time instant messaging to asynchronous collaborative teamwork, including blogs;
2. Support for social feedback, in which a group rates the contributions of others, producing a digital reputation for participants;
3. Support for social networks to explicitly create and manage participants' personal relationships and to help them develop new ones.

The ethos of social software tools seems to match well with modern thinking about educational practice. In particular, these tools enable individual learners to be expressive, to be aware of what others are doing, and to engage in collaboration. Social software tools therefore support and encourage individuals to learn together while retaining individual control over their time, space, presence, activity, identity, and relationship (Anderson, 2008). Some of the perceived benefits to the students by using these tools are developing the skills of communication, problem solving, research, and collaborative working, which can equip students well for the world of work (Minocha, Petre, & Roberts, 2008; Minocha, 2009).

Social Software in Education

The underlying pedagogy of social software tools has been considered by Dalsgaard (2006), who argues that social software can support a social constructivist approach to e-learning by providing students with personal tools and engaging them in social networks, thus allowing learners to direct their own problem-solving processes. Social constructivism emphasizes the importance of the learner being actively involved in the learning process and knowledge is constructed in shared endeavors with other learners. Social constructivism is in contrast to traditional educational viewpoints (e.g., instructivist approaches) where the responsibility rests with the educator to deliver knowledge while the learner passively receives it. Felix (2005) proposes the synthesis of cognitive constructivist and social constructivist approaches. In the cognitive constructivist approach, the focus is on cognition that occurs in the mind of the individual, with the learners making intellectual sense of the materials on their own. For example, collaborative writing in a wiki or writing in a blog, and participating in online discussions in forums through peer reviewing and commenting in blogs and wikis, enable knowledge to be constructed individually but mediated socially. In fact, with the advent of social software in education, it is being suggested that the role of an educator is changing to that of a guide, a facilitator, or a mentor as opposed to a "sage on the stage."

A Joint Information Systems Committee (JISC)-funded study (2008–2009) on the effective use of social software in UK further and higher education, led by the first author of the present chapter, has reported that educational institutions are increasingly making use of social software tools (Minocha, 2009). However, this study found that most social software initiatives are small-scale, led by an individual educator, and situated within a single course. Consequently, evidence of the benefits of social software in teaching and learning, as gathered in the JISC study and the literature in general, is rather limited.

In addition, students are adopting tools such as Facebook, Myspace, Twitter, and blogs on their own accord for social and educational purposes. Therefore, there is a need to investigate situations where students have adopted these tools on their own to support their learning and to find out the reasons for adoption of the tool(s), the benefits they perceive, and the challenges they present as learning tools. The empirically grounded findings of students' perceptions and experiences will help to inform institutions, policymakers, and educators who are planning to introduce social software tools into their courses and institutions.

About This Chapter

In this chapter, the focus is on blogs, one of the tools in the Web 2.0 social software toolkit. The chapter discusses a study where blogging was not compulsory and students had adopted blogs of their own free will to support their learning and research. The authors present an analysis of students' experiences and describe the social and educational benefits of blogging in the public domain including the development of students' study and research skills. They also give an analysis of the challenges that students experienced. It is hoped that the findings will help guide students, educators, and institutions considering the use of blogging in higher education. It is noteworthy at this point that the authors' study pertains to blogging in its "macro" sense and not microblogging services such as tweets via Twitter or status messages as on Facebook. Microblogging enables users to send brief opinions, personal status updates, and ephemera, while a blog has a "narrative" and it provides time and space to develop a topic.

The chapter is structured as follows: the next section overviews the usage of blogs in domains such as politics, travel, and business, and considers the motivations for blogging and the concerns of privacy that bloggers may have. To set the context for the study, a literature review of blogging in education is presented—taking into consideration previous research related to self-motivated and Ph.D. research-related blogging—and the research questions of the study are outlined. Following that, the methodology and data analysis are reported, before discussing the implications of the findings and conclusions regarding the significance of self-motivated blogging for facilitating the development of study and research skills. The chapter finishes with a discussion on the limitations of the study and an outline of some ideas for taking the authors' research further.

BLOGS: USAGE IN NON-ACADEMIC DOMAINS

A weblog (or "blog") is a website that allows an author ("blogger") to publish his or her thoughts or diary as a series of "posts." The posts are in a (reverse) chronological order related to the blogger's activities, experiences, and/or thoughts. A blog is an asynchronous publication, in which the blogger posts views or news in his or her own style and rhythm. Sometimes a group of individuals, for example a project team, may set up a group blog where more than one member in the team (depending upon how the "write" permissions are set up) are able to post to the blog. The posts can be "tagged" with appropriate keywords so that related posts can be brought together, or for enabling the blog to be searched. Readers can engage in a discussion about posts by leaving "comments" on the blog. In some blog services, access to posts can be controlled and limited to certain readers, individuals, or to the public. Rettberg (2008) provides an excellent discussion both on the history of blogging and on its future.

Blogs as Social Tools

Blogs provide online space to explore, collaborate, share, and invite others to participate in a "conversation." The major advantage of the blog format is the ability to communicate with an audience in a rapid and casual manner. A blog is, therefore, a social genre. Bloggers (authors) do not simply write "Dear Diary" entries for themselves; they write to the world with the clear expectation of having readers (Rettberg, 2008). Their readership does not necessarily need to be very large. An audience of 15 close friends or 15 people who are generally interested in the blog's content may be quite sufficient. Studies have shown (e.g., Nardi, Schiano, Gumbrecht, & Swartz, 2004; Baker & Moore, 2008) that blogging as a social tool can provide space for catharsis and offer possibilities for social support, friendship, and positive interaction with readers. Readers can respond to blog posts and over a period of time, and, if the blog develops an audience, the blog can provide opportunities for developing communities.

Blogs in Journalism, Politics, Travel, and Business

Journalists and newsreaders are using blogs to express opinions or discuss breaking stories, and to have direct communication with their readership (e.g., http://edition.cnn.com/exchange/blogs/ contains a list of CNN's most active blogs), allowing the audience to participate in discussions via comments. Blogs are also being used in politics for campaigning or for informing the public about the activities of the politicians. Blogging has created a channel of communication through which people can obtain news and political information (Allan, 2006), and this has been perceived as useful for public engagement in democratic processes (Gunter, 2009). Blogging has also enabled the public (who were generally at the receiving end of the media and without professional journalism training) to participate as journalists, and to break stories, post pictures and videos, and analyze news on their blogs. Blogs can also be a means to watch the mainstream media. Bruns (2005) argues that blogs are a means of monitoring and commenting on the traditional "gatekeepers" of information—the mass media (television and newspapers). Blogs are often considered more "independent" and seem to be a "watchdogs" within the media system. The most successful blog in German-speaking Europe, for instance, is *BILDblog* (http://www.bildblog.de/), which "watches" BILD, a German tabloid newspaper. BILDblog writes about all the mistakes, incorrect information, and unfair campaigns by BILD. BILDblog is read by many thousands of readers a day, and many of them may not be typical BILD readers but journalists and other well-informed citizens. Blogs can also be a challenge to press censorship, especially in regimes where human rights such as freedom of speech and freedom of the press are not granted, by providing an opportunity to publish information that would get censored in traditional media.

Blogs are commonly interpreted as online diaries. The chronological order of the blog posts enables temporal structuring of a person's activities, experiences, and/or thoughts, which is the function of traditional diaries. As Gurak and Antonijevic (2008) note, "Unlike personal Web presentations, structured around 'the essence of me,' blogs are structured around 'the process of me.' Unlike chatting, pointed toward 'hear me out at this moment,' blogging is pointed toward 'hear me out throughout time'" (p. 65). Blogging, thus, is a twofold communicative event. On one hand, it is "the event of 'writing oneself' through continuous recording of past and present experiences, just as in the case of traditional diaries" (p. 65), and on the other hand, it is an activity that assumes an audience, and this two-way interactivity with readers leads to revision and reflection.

Travelers use blogs to record, reflect on, and share traveling experiences with their family, friends, and other readers. Travel bloggers can influence the decision making of the blog readers regarding choice of destinations. In fact, travel blogs are an inexpensive means to gather rich, authentic, and unsolicited customer feedback (Pan, MacLaurin, & Crotts, 2007). Such blogs have rich descriptions of every aspect of a visitor's trip, from the overall experience of traveling, the initial booking, anticipation, planning, packing, departure, driving, flying, and reflections on the experience.

The conversational style of blogs, combined with their flexible format, makes them an ideal tool for organizations to communicate the "official" message to their customers in an informal yet credible fashion. Companies such as Coca-Cola, Marriott, and Kodak all have recruited chief bloggers (with or without the actual title) to tell their stories and engage consumers (Bulik, 2008). Bulik reports that just over 11% of Fortune 500 companies have corporate blogs. The number of corporate blogs has risen slowly and steadily since the end of 2005, when only 4% had any kind of blog.

Motivations for Blogging

Since a blog may function as a diary, a collaborative workspace, a marketing or advertising tool, or a political soapbox, bloggers have heterogeneous motivations. Building on the study by Nardi et al. (2004) that investigated motivations for blogging, Huang, Shen, Lin, and Chang (2007) found that there are five motivations for blogging: (1) self-expression (e.g., video blogs on YouTube), (2) life documenting (e.g., personal online diaries), (3) commenting (e.g., political blogging), (4) community forum participation (e.g., project-specific blogs), and (5) information searching (e.g., gathering information through subscription services such as RSS feeds). As all blogging activities revolve around information created and consumed by bloggers, Huang et al. (2007), concluded that there are two primary behavioral motivations for blogging, namely to search for information and to engage in social interaction.

Research by Jones and Alony (2008) revealed the following seven motivations for blogging: (1) need for self-expression, (2) need for recognition, (3) need for social contact, (4) need for introspection, (5) academic needs for knowledge and interests, (6) need for documentation, and (7) need for artistic activity. Luzón (2006) analyzed research group blogs and found that blogs were being used as tools for collaboration, communication, and promotion, such as publicizing the group and the group's research; making available to the public the group's work, usually with the purpose of getting feedback; communicating with other members of the group; and reinforcing the social links between the members of the virtual community. Luzón (2006, 2009) also found that most academics who maintain their own blogs do so for self-presentation, in order to increase their visibility and develop respect and reputation.

Blogs facilitate three processes, which Schmidt (2007) suggests overlap with social software: (1) information management through notes, hyperlinks, and other multimedia resources; (2) identity management as a blog enables presentation of oneself to others by making certain aspects of one's personality, interests, expertise, and so on public; and (3) relationship management as a blog assists the user in articulating, creating, and maintaining social relationships. Needless to say, due to the growth of the blogging genre, by their very nature and proliferation blogs raise a number of privacy issues.

Concerns about Privacy in Blogging

Blogs are easy to produce and disseminate, resulting in large amounts of sometimes personal information being broadcast across the Internet in a persistent and cumulative manner (McCullagh, 2008). Additionally, the collation of posts could easily create an impression of the blogger, and if the blogger's views were presented in a different context, it could pose a privacy risk. Clearly, ideas and opinions can change with time, and when taken out of context, blog posts may be severely misjudged by others. This means that archived posts that are relevant at a particular time may later pose threats to one's career and personal life. Grudin (2001) refers to this "loss of control" as the steady erosion of clearly situated action:

We are losing control and knowledge of the consequences of our actions, because if what we do is represented digitally, it can appear anywhere, and at any time in the future. We no longer control access to anything we disclose. (p. 279)

McCullagh (2008) recommends that organizations should provide blogging guidelines for employers in order to minimize threats to security.

BLOGS IN EDUCATION

Within the education domain, blogs are generally integrated within the virtual learning environment of the institution, or individual course teams may use external blogging services. Blogger (http://www.blogger.com/), Edublogs (http://www.edublogs.org/), and WordPress (http://www.wordpress.org/) are publicly available blogging services that can be used to set up blogs. Educators may decide to keep the access to the blogs restricted to students and tutors on the course, or may make the blogs available to the world.

There have been several papers in recent years that have discussed the role of blogging in education. For example, Downes (2004) has discussed the role of blogs in socialization among students, that is, enabling them to get to know one another better by visiting and reading one another's blogs. Socialization is an antecedent to learning community formation and collaborative learning, particularly in distance or part-time education, where students may not have the opportunity to meet face-to-face (Minocha & Tingle, 2008). Blogging can also help alleviate the feelings of isolation associated with distance learning (Dickey, 2004). The findings of Du and Wagner's (2007) study suggest that the adoption of blogs is likely to enhance individual learning since it integrates the traditional method of (offline) learning logs with online social interaction and reflection. This promotes cognitive knowledge construction along with the sharing of ideas and social networking. Further, blogs help to generate a sustainable knowledge stock, which becomes the community's knowledge asset for all participants to revisit and reuse (Du & Wagner, 2007).

Blogs can be used in creative writing courses, and in courses that require reflective journals and/or e-portfolios (e.g., nursing and teacher education). However, one thing that distinguishes blogs from other forms of reflective journal is the ability to engage with different media in addition to the basic written word (e.g., hyperlinks, images, audio, and video). Fiedler (2004) states that the use of hyperlinks is useful to point to material that is quoted, referred to, critiqued, praised, or that somehow elaborates, illustrates, and enriches the content of a particular blog. Since the students can add hyperlinks in their blogs and comment on one another's blogs, Vygotsky's (1978) notions of social cognition and Wenger's ideas of community of practice (Wenger, McDermott, & Snyder, 2002) are relevant to the blogging genre.

Blogging provides an opportunity for students to collaboratively create knowledge, which can help foster the development of a learning community in which students both support and challenge one another, leading to effective and relevant knowledge construction (see Oravec, 2003). Blogs can be useful for keeping learning journals, as a personal online store with links, excerpts from readings, etc., for self-reflection, for networking with other fellow students in a distance learning environment, and for becoming part of the course community (Kerawalla, Minocha, Kirkup, & Conole, 2008). (For an extensive review of the literature on the role of blogging in education, see Leslie & Murphy, 2008).

Farmer (2006) discusses that online learning has shifted away from the individual with too much emphasis on shared workspaces such as discussion boards or forums. Farmer suggests that online education is facing "a kind of pedagogical crisis" and that blogging can come to the rescue by being inherently student centered, establishing a "social presence" and yet enabling bloggers (learners) to "retain ownership of their writing ... and control in its entirety the space and manner in which the blog is published" (p. 96). Similar to Farmer's views about ownership in a blog, Andreasen (2006), reporting on his study comparing discussion forums with blogs, argues that blogs support development of "individual voices" (p. 86). These individual voices are important to the development of students' independent use of the Web. Andreasen's conclusion is that

The learning potential that can be said to exist in the use of weblogs in relation to a course conducted over the internet relates partly to the increase in the students' opportunities for making their own voice heard, and partly to the active exchange with and reflection on other students' weblogs. (2006, p. 86)

While discussing Andreasen's work Dalsgaard and Mathiasen (2008) suggest that blogs and social software, in general, allow students to form their own "self-organized" networks, which are distinct from participating in public forums. These self-organized networks will facilitate learning that extends beyond the course and curriculum: "Self-organised learning networks provide a base for the establishment of a form of education that goes beyond course and curriculum centric models, and envisions a learner-centred and learner controlled model of lifelong learning" (Koper, 2004, p. 1).

Writing a blog allows students to confront their own opinions and contemplate how their views might be interpreted and reflected upon by others (Lamshed, Berry, & Armstrong, 2002; Mortensen & Walker, 2002). Some students in Lamshed's study mentioned that the process of blogging "forced" them to improve their writing skills because of the need to write for a public audience. The self-directed nature of blogging and yet being open to public scrutiny and support is summarized by Efimova and Fiedler (2004): "A weblog provides its author with personal space for learning that does not impose a communal learning agenda and learning style. At the same time learners are not alienated and can benefit from community feedback, validation and further development of ideas" (p. 4). Efimova and Fielder argue that blogging can support identity development and as bloggers "allow smaller or larger parts of their personality to emerge between her or his words," (p. 3) their blogs are "increasingly becoming online identities for the authors" (p. 3).

However, McCullagh's (2008) study raises the issue of the need to generate policies and guidelines for blogging for both students and educators. In previous research by the authors of the present chapter on blogging practices by students (e.g., Kerawalla et al., 2008), and in the first author's study on effective use of social software in education (Minocha, 2009), it was seen that some students have concerns about their contributions in the public domain. Some students have anxieties about sharing their reflections and ideas with peers. They are worried that other students will steal their ideas for activities associated with formal assessment. Even when the ethos of the social software tools is to be collaborative, individual assessment may create competition among students and undermine the benefits of blogging.

SETTING THE CONTEXT FOR THE STUDY

Much of the previous research into blogging in higher education has tended to focus on course-directed blogging, where students are provided with a blog and directions or suggestions about how to use it to support their learning on a particular course (e.g., Williams & Jacobs, 2004; Kerawalla et al., 2008; Kerawalla, Minocha, Kirkup, & Conole, 2009a). Here, the students share a pedagogical context (their course) and usually have a predefined readership consisting of other students on their course and their instructor/tutor. For example, Williams and Jacobs (2004) tell of an effort to support course-directed blogging by MBA students, where the majority of the students agreed or strongly agreed that blogging facilitated their learning and increased the level of intellectual exchange among the students on the course. Homik and Melis (2006) discuss the use of blogs as learning logs by computer science students; they found that students who blogged regularly felt that their performance was enhanced.

However, the evidence for the uptake of blogging by students and benefits the students perceive is rather limited. For example, Homik and Mellis (2006) report that most students engaged in only a minimum level of blogging to meet assessment requirements. In course-directed blogging, even if it is voluntary and non-assessed, students face several obstacles (Kerawalla et al., 2009a; Kerawalla, Minocha, Kirkup, & Conole, 2009b), for example, not knowing what to blog about, not knowing how to write meaningful reflective accounts, being confused about whether to post in the course forum or on the blog, or being hesitant or lacking in confidence to share their views and thoughts with others.

On the other hand, in the present chapter authors' research they have come across students who engage in *self-motivated* study-related or research-related blogging. These undergraduates, Master's students, and Ph.D. students start blogging about their courses or their research of their own volition, and their institutions do not define their readership. In this chapter, the authors discuss their empirical investigations of such self-motivated blogging activities by these students. Investigated are their motivation for blogging, the benefits they perceive and experience, and the challenges they face. Of particular interest is investigating how blogs (the product) and blogging (the process) may be useful to support the students' learning and research, and the development of their study and research skills.

The research reported in the present chapter is intended to enhance understanding about self-motivated bloggers: what they blog about, what benefits they reap, the relationship between blogging activities and study and research skills, and the challenges experienced by the student bloggers. The outcomes related to self-motivated blogging will help trigger ideas for educators about designing blogging activities in courses, how to enthuse students about the significance of blogging in their learning in terms of the skills gained, and how to cater for some of the perceived challenges faced by participants in the authors' study.

Previous Research on Self-Motivated Student Blogging

Baggetun and Wasson (2006) investigated the role of blogging among self-motivated bloggers on undergraduate and postgraduate programs. However, their data analysis involved using the following predefined categories of self-regulated learning: reflection, motivation, ownership, customization, and categorization. Unlike this purely deductive approach, in the present study the data analysis was not constrained by an *a priori* framework on the benefits of blogging. Instead, a broad but thorough thematic or inductive analysis was conducted of the data obtained from students' blogs and interviews. Consequently, a wide range of social, educational, and organizational factors were uncovered that are seen as influencing, and being a consequence of, students' self-motivated blogging behaviors and activities.

Previous Research on Ph.D. Research-Related Blogging

By drawing on the work by Boud and Lee (2005) and Blood (2000), Ward and West (2008) discuss how blogging may be advantageous for Ph.D. students. They conclude that blogging facilitates socially situated learning, development of communities of practice, co-production of knowledge with a supervisory team and peers, emotional involvement with the student's own research and learning, and development of confidence in writing. However, Ward and West (2008) do not include empirical findings in their publication.

Ferguson, Clough, and Hosein (2007) report on how they (a group of three Ph.D. students) used their individual blogs and a collaborative blog to support their Ph.D. research. In the self-analysis of their blogs, they identified different types of blog post, which included community posts aimed at sharing skills and information, reflective posts containing research questions and ideas, and emotive posts documenting both positive and negative feelings. Ferguson et al. concluded that their blogs were effective in facilitating a community of practice between themselves and the wider research community. Also, they claim that they were able to undertake a broader range of activities in their blogs than they would have been able to do in a traditional research journal. These additional activities included linking to web-based resources, expressing ideas through text as well as images, offering and receiving emotional support, sharing resources, the co-construction of ideas, and having access to and links with the wider academic community.

In another study that was similarly reflexive, Mortensen and Walker (2002) discuss blogging to support their own Ph.D. research. They found that their blogs were a useful place for recording quick ideas and thoughts, which may be either standalone or form a chain of thoughts with other posts. They argue that blogging enabled them to write spontaneously about unformulated ideas and to share ideas with others. These authors also discuss the utility of having an archive of posts that can be drawn upon at any time. They conclude that writing their theses became easier and more focused once they had started blogging.

There may be certain circumstances in which blogging about Ph.D. research might be unwise, and in which the practice may be discouraged by host institutions. Issues of confidentiality within highly competitive subject areas may mean that all research information needs to be carefully guarded. Similarly, Ph.D. research that is being supported by commercial organizations may be politically and commercially sensitive. Butler (2006) reports how blogging within academia can prejudice employment prospects, and Hornyak, Peach, and Fekula (2003) argue that blogging could threaten student research due to the potential for plagiarism, for example.

The research cited above (e.g., Ferguson et al., 2007; Mortensen & Walker, 2002) consists of reports of the personal experiences of Ph.D. students. One set of participants in the empirical study reported in this chapter consisted of self-motivated Ph.D. bloggers. Unlike Ferguson et al. and Mortensen and Walker, the decision was made to objectively analyze the perceptions of the participants in the study rather than discussing the authors' own perceptions or experiences of blogging. An important aspect of the study, as shown by the research questions outlined in the next section, entailed investigating whether blogging supports the development of study skills and research skills.

Blogging and its Role in the Development of Study Skills and Research Skills

There is an extensive body of literature on the development of study skills and research skills in undergraduate and postgraduate study. Fostering these wide-ranging skills is important to ensure students to know how to learn and how to manage their learning. With regard to research skills, Sir Gareth Roberts' (2002) report on the supply of scientists and engineers in the UK, published shortly after the turn of the millennium, emphasized the need to change the way graduate students are prepared for research, suggesting that more attention be paid to enhancing employability through skills training. Subsequently, the *Joint statement of the UK research councils' training requirements for research students* (UK GRAD Programme, 2001) has stressed the importance of developing skills in several areas. However, there appears to be a dearth of empirical research into whether and how self-motivated blogging, within the context of higher education, can help students to develop the necessary study skills and research skills.

The Research Questions

The study sought to investigate two sets of self-motivated bloggers: undergraduate and Master's students involved in part-time distance learning by (taught) coursework, and Ph.D. students engaged in either part-time or full-time research.

The research questions were as follows:

- **RQ1:** Why do self-motivated student bloggers blog in the public domain?
- **RQ2:** What educational and social benefits of blogging do these students perceive?
- **RQ3:** Can self-motivated course or research-related blogging support the development of study skills and research skills?
- **RQ4:** What are the concerns of students about blogging? What are the issues or precautions that the students consider during blogging?

The following section explains the recruitment of participants and the research methods employed, then discusses the approach to conducting the analysis and interpretation of data from multiple sources. The research materials such as consent form, project information sheet, and interview templates were submitted to the Ethics Committee of the authors' University. The Committee subsequently approved the materials and procedures.

METHODOLOGY: PARTICIPANTS AND DATA COLLECTION

The Open University (OU) in the UK currently has around 200,000 students undertaking a range of undergraduate and Master's-level distance learning courses, some of which are wholly online. Most OU students are mature learners and study part time in their own places of residence. They fit their study around other commitments, such as family and work.

As a means of recruiting students for the study, an Internet search was conducted to locate blogs kept by OU students that met the following criteria:

- blogs were initiated and maintained by the student in the absence of any course directions or suggestions;
- blogs were being actively updated or had been in the six months prior to recruitment; and
- blogs included a substantial number and proportion of references to one or more OU courses.

Initially, very few blogs satisfying these criteria were identified, so further blogs were traced by following links from "blogrolls" and from a list of OU bloggers provided by one of the participants. Students were contacted either by email or by leaving a comment on their blog to invite them to participate in the study. Positive replies were received from 10 students whose blogs fulfilled all of the predetermined criteria. Nine of these students were undergraduates and one a Master's student. Their mean age was 45 years and 2 months (range 30 to 56 years), which is representative of the OU student population as a whole.

The students had been studying for varying lengths of time (one to three years). Some students maintained a single blog and continued using it when they started a new course, while others started a new blog with every new course. Consequently, the number of blogs that each student had kept ranged from one to four. There was also variation in whether or not the OU study-related content represented all the content of their blog(s) (two students), most of the content of their blog(s) (three students), or just a part of the blog content (five students).

The students gave varying degrees of consent regarding whether and how quotes from their blogs could be published, depending upon the degree of anonymity they wanted to maintain. When quoting from their blogs in this chapter, acknowledgment to the student by name and/or their blog's URL has been included where appropriate. They all gave consent to the authors to publish anonymous quotes from their interviews. (Where an interview quote has been used in conjunction with a blog excerpt, and the source of the interview quote can be attributed to an identified blog owner, additional consent has been obtained from the relevant participant.)

Ph.D. Students and Their Blogs

Originally, the authors planned to focus their Ph.D. blog research on OU Ph.D. students. Invitation emails were sent out to various OU mailing lists, and notices were posted around the main campus of the University. These efforts identified only a small number of bloggers. This was not surprising, given that acceptance and adoption of e-learning environments by students is a slow process and may require time and persistence. The authors' own experiences with the introduction of new technologies such as wikis, blogs, and three-dimensional virtual worlds (e.g., Second Life) at the OU has shown that it is unlikely that students will make use of these technologies and perform the activities until the activities are situated within the course or study program, with explicit identification of the learning outcomes and links to assessment. Similarly, Kirkwood and Price (2005) found, in their research on the use of information and communications technology (ICT) by students, that "regardless of the media being used, it is very unlikely that students will make use of materials and activities unless they are embedded in the course pedagogy. If materials are not linked to the assessment strategy then the medium is likely to be unused and its potential will remain fallow" (p. 272). In order to recruit more Ph.D. students, searches were carried out on the Internet to find non-OU Ph.D. bloggers. Once again, the students were contacted either by email or by leaving a comment on their blog. In total, positive replies were received from 10 students. Four students were registered with the OU, five at other UK universities, and one in Belgium. Their mean age was 31 years and 5 months (range 23 to 48 years).

There was great diversity among students in terms of research domain (computer science, mathematics, health and social care, art, psychology). Also, they varied in terms of the number of years they had been working towards their Ph.D. and had been engaged in research-related blogging (from six months to five years), whether they were full time (four students) or part time (six students), and with respect to the percentage of their total blog content accounted for by the Ph.D.-related posts.

Semi-structured interviews were conducted with the participants in both the groups. This was done over the phone, except in the case of two undergraduates who preferred epistolary (email) interviews (e.g., Debenham, 2007) due to their busy schedules. The epistolary interviews were carried out over a series of five emails with each student so as not to overwhelm them with too many questions in a single email. Two members of the research team conducted the phone interviews with the remaining participants. Each interview lasted between 45 minutes and one hour.

Analysis of the Students' Interviews

The data from the two participant groups was analyzed separately. To start the process, an independent inductive analysis of the data was undertaken by the research team. This thematic analysis (Braun & Clarke, 2006) involved each of the research team members individually reading the different sociological accounts of the interviews in detail and using the research questions as "lenses" or guides to identify the themes, sub-themes, and any causal interrelationships between the themes.

After this independent data analysis, the team met in a one-day workshop and focused on looking across the data and the team members' independently obtained results to find common and recurring themes. This activity yielded a lengthy list of themes and sub-themes.

Analysis of the Undergraduate/ Master's Students' Blogs

The content of the undergraduate/Master's students' (from this point forward referred to as "U/M students") blogs was analyzed in order to ascertain the different ways in which they were being used in relation to courses. Students gave consent to the researchers to access, read, analyze, and use quotes from their blogs that had been posted prior to the date on which they were first contacted to participate in the study. As with the interview data, an inductive analysis of the blog extracts was conducted to identify themes and sub-themes.

Analysis of the Ph.D. Student Blogs

Analysis of the Ph.D. blogs posed a significant challenge, for two reasons. Firstly, the researchers were not always familiar with the variety of research domains, so it was often difficult or impossible to determine whether and how each post was directly research-related. Secondly, some of the blogs were very large, with several hundred posts over several years, making it impractical to code the whole blog within the timescale of the research project. However, the aim was to gain a general understanding of the types of things that these students included in their blogs, rather than to provide an account of the minutiae of each post.

Consequently, different analytical approaches were adopted to meet this need, depending upon the nature of each blog. Where the blogs were easily understood, the research team coded them (i.e., identifying the themes and sub-themes). Some of these blogs were very extensive, so sample months were randomly selected from each year for coding. Where the students had used tags and categories to organize their posts, these were used as an indication of the content. As before, an inductive analysis of the blog extracts was done to identify the themes and sub-themes.

FINDINGS OF THE STUDY

The themes and sub-themes of the analyzed and synthesized data from the blogs and interviews are presented below, organized around the aforementioned research questions. Included are snippets or vignettes from the interviews and extracts from the blogs to illustrate the various themes and sub-themes.

Motivations for Self-Motivated Blogging

With respect to RQ1, the motivations for students' blogging in the public domain and their educational and social goals were investigated. These motivations (discussed below) are by no means mutually exclusive, and might come into play simultaneously. Furthermore, in the analysis, the boundary between the benefits perceived by the bloggers and their motivations (reasons for blogging) was sometimes blurred. The participants were more inclined to discuss what they were achieving through their blog and by blogging rather than looking back on what made them start blogging in the first place. The students discussed a number of reasons for their blogging, which are covered in turn below.

Sharing Research with the Supervisor and Other Readers

Ph.D. students mentioned that they wanted to make their readers enthused about a new subject area or topic. Two Ph.D. students said that they used their blogs as a way to keep their supervisors informed and up-to-date on their progress, especially if the supervisory team met with the student infrequently. They reported that their supervisors did read their blog. They said:

you're trying to make them see it in a different light, or make it interesting to people

and

there must be people out there who are interested and don't know it yet.

Sharing Resources and Ideas

Five Ph.D. students and four U/M students expressed that they wanted to share personal ideas and resources with the readers of their blogs. One said that *"there are people in [my area] that are interested in seeing what's going on in my mind,"* while another said that he often includes in his blog *"information that I think will be useful to another reader."*

Two Ph.D. students blogged about research ideas that they felt they would not have the time to follow up on, hoping someone else would read the ideas and use them.

Two U/M students created their blogs with the specific aim of the blogs serving as resources for other OU students. One of these students said his blog contained *"what is involved in a particular course."* Both of these students said they felt an obligation to keep their blogs up-to-date. The other student explained that as her course was new, there were teething problems, and she hoped to help students by creating a resource that *"laid it all out"* for them.

Several U/M students included photographs in their blogs. For example, there was a student who was studying Ancient Greek and who, at the time, had no means of typing this alphabet. So, she included photographs of handwritten lettering in her blog. She gave the following reason:

I wanted people to see what Ancient Greek looked like ... [and] thought it might help familiarize my mind with the "look" of Ancient Greek to write things down and post the photos on my blog.

Social Connections with Family and Friends

Two Ph.D. students and four U/M students said that their blog was a way of keeping in contact with their families and friends and letting them know *"what I'm up to."* The students said they had a relatively small audience of family and friends who read their blog to keep up to date with their lives.

Sharing their Lives

Three U/M students talked about blogging in terms of sharing details of their lives with other people. Two said that they were unsure of exactly why they blogged, but that they enjoyed writing about their life. These students' blogs contained a substantial amount of content that was not related to OU study.

A Ph.D. student described how she was inspired to update her blog so as to keep her readers informed about what she was doing. She said:

recently when I was in [X place], I took a photo for the blog. And sometimes I think things [sic] for the blog, to update it, to keep people in the loop of what I'm doing.

For Self-Promotion

Two Ph.D. students and one U/M student said they hoped that the public nature of blogging would help them to promote or advertise themselves. One Ph.D. student had been blogging for only a few months, and so had not seen evidence of this at the time she was interviewed. The other student had several years' experience of personal blogging, and described her Ph.D. blog as being *"a bit like a notice board outside my office, if somebody is wandering past and is interested they can have a look."*

The U/M student was a professional writer and said that her study-related blog was only one of the six blogs she maintained. Also, she runs a website and describes her study blog as *"a marketing tool, another place where I advertise myself and my books."*

Sharing Personal Resolutions with the Readers

Two U/M students said that they blogged to make public commitments. This is similar to making a learning contract (Boud & Sampson, 1996), but in this case the contract is with (known or unknown) readers of the blog. One student posted his work plans and said he was

making a promise to myself that something is going to happen and putting it on the blog and other people reading it makes you stick to things.

The other student posted her assignment marks and set herself the public challenge of doing better next time. She said:

if you write that score [96%] in public it's more humiliating if next time you get fifty ... I compete against myself ... it's a way of putting pressure on myself to study.

Blog as a Personal Resource

For many students, their blog was one of several tools they used to store their resources. One of the Ph.D. students described her blog as

a window on stuff I have got stored elsewhere ... there's a link from my blog to the shared part of my Refworks [bibliographic management software] database.

Blog as a Memory Aid

Two U/M students and one Ph.D. student said that they used their blog for reminders. The Ph.D. student said:

it's nice to open up my blog and see a reminder of where I was, and I've got to get back to doing X ... [also] I go back to my blog to look for inspiration for papers. It's good because I forget about what I had.

The U/M students said they used their blog for work plans and assignments deadlines as they could go back and remind themselves of these.

Keeping a Record of Progress and Planning

Two Ph.D. students said they posted to their blog regularly as it was a good place to record what they had achieved that day. A blog excerpt illustrates this process of progress reporting and planning for the future:

So, here we are again. Ages since I've written ... just such a busy bunny though! The Ph.D. is going fine (I think!), working on first draft of my research proposal at the moment which is all good as the final version isn't due in till about June. I have to send the draft off to my supervisors by Sunday teatime so they can comment on it and I can have version 2 ready for my next supervision. URL: http://www.margomilne.com/wordpress/

Documenting Course and Study Processes

When analyzing the blogs of the U/M students, it was found that the students were primarily writing about their assessment and their workload or work plan. In this blog excerpt, a student is discussing his results from a recent assignment, and is reflecting on his performance and progress while engaging in forward planning and goal setting:

TMA3 results for L120

I've got my TMA (Tutor Marked Assignment) 3 result back, and am quite amazed to see that it's 78%. Why amazed? Well, I'm a LONG way behind on the course, a long way. I'll be relying upon a block of time I have coming to get up to date, but it'll be tough. The TMA was the result of lots of bookwork. The previous pieces scored 90 and 78 with a weighting of 15% each, this one is weighted as 35%. This means that I have 52.5% for my coursework so far (with 35% to play for) The Coursework is worth 50% overall, with 50% coming from the End of Course Assessment in September. URL: http://www.murky.org/blg

The majority of Ph.D. students in the participant group wrote about their research. Eight Ph.D. students' blogs contained some material referring to their research aims and foci, often drawing upon their background materials and considering the direction and focus of their own research. Two students documented their research questions, the rationale for their studies, and the title of their thesis.

The analysis identified different features of the research process that were documented in the content of the Ph.D. students' blogs. These were work plans, thinking and ideas, research progress, supervision meetings, the writing process, and emotional states.

Documenting Research Methodology

Two Ph.D. students' blogs contained posts discussing the ethical issues surrounding their research. Also, three students discussed their research methods, two discussed their study procedures, and one student discussed participant sampling and analysis of data. One student was particularly descriptive of her research methods and analysis. Her methods are discussed in detail and this includes her plans to recruit participants through her blog and conduct her research online:

I've been working on the second part of the measurement instrument for my first experiment. I've already thought about how get at participants' descriptions of the faces, but now I want some method of measuring how they react to them. I'm carrying this experiment out online, so any measurements will be recorded by participants clicking a response or dragging a pointer to indicate agreement/disagreement. I'm not able to take any physiological measurements, and I'm wary of self-reports after using them for my MSc [Master of Science program].

At our planning meeting in February, [my supervisor] suggested that I look at the sorts of scenarios used to explore aversion or attraction. After reading through a lot of examples, I've decided to write some scenarios of my own as nothing I've read it quite close enough to what I want to be reused. I'm not trying to ascertain just whether participants find the uncanny faces attractive, the source of many of the examples, and the scenarios / stimuli from the disgust literature were too extreme for the subtle sense of unease that characterizes the uncanny. URL: http://uncanny-valley.livejournal.com/

As an Events Diary

Eight students documented their daily events, such as what they had read or where they had visited. Nine Ph.D. students reported on workshops and conferences that they had attended. For example, one of the Ph.D. students in the participant group described a talk that he gave at a workshop in this blog, and along with that attached several resources: his presentation, links to related references/materials, and the address of the official website of the workshop. He also discussed his experiences of presenting at the workshop, including the questions he was asked and the answers that he gave.

For Critiquing their Reading Materials

This blog except is from a Master's student's blog. Unlike the undergraduate students in whose cases it was generally found that the course materials were being discussed for clarifying understanding or for making personal notes, the postgraduate students were often providing commentary on and critiquing what they were reading:

Just when you thought it was safe to enter the water ...

Well, in this case a bit more background reading for my assignment (due on Friday!!!). Eric Olson's article Personal Identity looked just up the right street ... until I read it and ... it demolishes lots of the things I thought I could defend. Most worrying is the view that holding to Psychological Continuity really implies that a person is different from a human animal. If so, then what could this difference consist of? Perhaps I just have to adopt the stance of a defence lawyer—I don't want to know if my client is guilty or innocent—I will simply try to prevent the prosecution proving his guilt. One challenge with much of the writing on the subject of personal identity is that it uses thought experiments / cases that are extreme and/or unusual (brain transplants, teleportation, mind transfers etc.). The author usually explains how people would surely react to such scenarios. My problem is that when a scenario that is never encountered in real life is presented then any supposition about how we would react to it is, to my mind, pure speculation. Before organ transplants became commonplace then people had very mixed views about their significance: Would getting someone else's heart make one a different person? We would say "no," but a Middle Ages peasant might take a very different view.

Five Ph.D. students' blogs contained summaries and critiques of material that they had read. Also, four of the blogs contained references to the theories behind the students' research, often accompanied by their own reflections and critiques.

Making Notes of Supervision Meetings

One student reported his experiences in the blog as follows:

I've just had a meeting with [my supervisor]. I began by asking him if he could see/read the test on my sketch map of Clerkenwell. He got really animated at this point and had a go at it methodologically. NOW? I mean I've been talking about this for weeks and about doing this work and only now [he] starts to question the underlying methodology?

To Receive Feedback

Some students, especially from the U/M participant group, were keen to receive feedback from their readers. For example, a student who went on a geology field trip took several photographs of geological features and included these in her blog. Also, she drew geological fault lines onto two of her photographs, and posted the images on her blog with a desire to elicit feedback about whether or not her drawings were correct. This student also said that *"photos help me remember ... the topography of the different landforms that they showed us."*

A Space for Sharing Ideas within a Small Project Team

One Ph.D. student said that he was part of a small, local community of bloggers in his department, who shared a common interest in his domain. He met them in person regularly and said he received comments from them on his blog but would like more interaction this way. He said that his blog had been useful when several people were working on a joint project, as his blog acted as a central location or hub where he could post his ideas and report on his progress without the need to notify people individually by email.

Educational and Social Benefits of Self-Motivated Blogging

In terms of RQ2, the participants discussed the following benefits of blogging.

To Support their Thinking and for Clarifying their Understanding

Seven Ph.D. students and three U/M students said that they consciously set out to explain their domain to their known, potential, or imagined readers, as a way of supporting their thinking and learning. One Ph.D. student said that blogging *"gets me to think through things ... and I get new insights or ways of expressing things;"* another said *"it highlights holes in my thinking ... where I have questions."* Yet another student said:

it was through writing about things in [my blog] that I found my focus was being drawn to things that were unexpected.

On the other hand, the U/M students were likely to focus on improving their understanding and remembering of their course materials. They spoke in terms of *"picking out the salient points,"* to make them *"clearer"* and *"reinforcing information"* so it *"sticks in my head"* and *"helps me to learn."*

One U/M student remarked:

if explaining it is difficult, I then know there's more work to be done to fill the gap between knowing it and explaining it.

This perception is to be expected, as taught program or coursework students such as the U/M students in this study tend to be concerned with assessment and grades.

One U/M student described her coursework, in her own words, to her friends, to help with her understanding and remembering. She posed questions to herself and answered them in her blog as well as including links to external online resources to aid her learning. The following excerpt from her blog shows one of the summaries she wrote:

The role of water in the evolution of the Martian atmosphere

All the terrestrial planets formed from the same stuff so we'd expect their atmosphere to be similar. There are similarities but there are also significant differences in abundance and composition. e.g. carbon dioxide—Earth 0.03%, Venus 96%

Earth stores carbon dioxide in the form of ocean sediments like limestone. When you take that into consideration the abundances are a lot more similar. It is also true for nitrogen.

But the abundance of volatiles on Mars is quite different—why?

If the atmosphere was derived from outgassing it either didn't contain as many volatiles as the other or they did not outgas to the same extent.

The temperature gradient of the solar nebula would mitigate against—there should be plenty of volatiles in Mars' composition—so it seems that less outgassing seems the more likely cause or is it?

The evidence of liquid water suggested that at sometimes the atmosphere had been dense enough for liquid water to form. Perhaps the gas escaped.

Writing as Catharsis

Two Ph.D. students and six U/M students viewed writing for their audience as being cathartic. One Ph.D. student said that he wanted people to know that undertaking a Ph.D. was not *"all sunshine and lollipops"* and that blogging helps *"to make sense of your feelings, and I'm trying to express that in a way that makes sense to other people."* Another said his blog was a place where he could *"whinge [complain] about this and that."*

The U/M students spoke in terms of blogging as enabling them to *"get things off my chest."* They blogged about various course-related issues that stressed or worried them. One student explained how blogging made her feel better:

at the start the course material didn't arrive ... I blogged about that quite a bit 'cos I felt annoyed and stressed out. It just helped me ... I've told the invisible people out there so I can feel a bit better. It was a bit like a confessional.

In this blog excerpt, a Ph.D. student reports his experiences:

Doing research can be a very frustrating experience and when you've spent ages staring at the same bit of work, doing your thinking over and over and praying to the gods to no avail, you soon start to think, "Why do I even care? It's not as though many people care about this. (paraphrased excerpt from anonymous student's blog)

Developing Academic Skills

Three Ph.D. students talked about how writing for an audience helped them to develop both writing and argumentative skills. None of the U/M students discussed this, although one alluded to the fact that blogging had improved her general ICT skills.

Community Building

Six Ph.D. students and five U/M students expressed that they felt part of a geographically dispersed community through blogging. Two Ph.D. bloggers explained how, as their research covered more than one domain, they considered themselves to part of more than one online community.

One of these students was linked to so many other blogs that she said she could no longer keep up with them all. Several of these students gave examples of people they communicated with abroad, who they made contact with by virtue of blogging. One in particular explained how she had made *"cyber friends"* as people had discovered her blog through a search engine.

Networking with other Researchers

One of the Ph.D. students described how complete strangers recognized her name at conferences:

after I put my [name] badge on they were "Oh, I've read your blog." So they knew all about me. People I've never met!

Inviting Participation from the Wider Community

One student's research materials are in the form of online images of uncanny faces, and in one post she invites her readers to help her locate and collect more images:

I'd be very interested in contributions if any of you would like to present images that you find particularly uncanny. (If you'd like to do this, either comment here with a link to the image online, or email it to my email address, details on my userinfo page.) I plan this as an ongoing collection, so there's no particular hurry. URL: http://uncanny-valley.livejournal.com/

Academic Opportunities

A Ph.D. student mentioned that she had been invited to review journal articles and to participate in conferences through recognition of her research as documented in her blog. Another part-time Ph.D. student who was not in close contact with her host institution and the academic network there described how she relied on her blogging community to keep her informed of conferences. Also, she said that she had made contact with a company keen to be involved in her research as a result of them reading her blog and contacting her.

Having a Journal or Diary

Four U/M students saw their blogs as repositories for mementos or souvenirs in the form of text or digital artifacts, or as diaries or records of their experiences. Only the Master's student used his blog as a resource for assignments (he critiqued course-related readings in his blog). However, an undergraduate who had a blog containing voluminous amounts of information, including descriptions, in her own words, of all her course material, said that she had found software that enabled her to convert her blog into a book, and that she found the book to be a useful revision aid for her exams.

Blog as a Repository of Ph.D. Materials

Six Ph.D. students said that their blogs were useful stores of ideas and resources that could be drawn upon to support preparing chapters, papers, literature reviews, talks, and progress reports, as well as to facilitate skill assessments.

Seven Ph.D. students' blogs contained collections or libraries of online resources and background materials. These consisted of links to web pages, journal articles, and other blogs, as well as collections of media (photographs, for example) incorporated into the blog itself. Photographs formed part of the research material for two of these students and consequently featured prominently in their blogs.

One Ph.D. student described how it simplified and assisted the writing process: *"when I start writing a paper I never start from scratch because there's already ideas in my weblog."* Another Ph.D. student had a very large number of posts and remarked that *"if I didn't have my weblog a lot of things would never be written down ... [as] I work in different locations."*

Development of a Personal Voice

Most of the Ph.D. students and all of the U/M students adopted an informed, but not strictly academic, style of writing. Two Ph.D. students said that they enjoyed blogging because the blog was a space in which they could *"have a voice, keep[ing] a balance between being objective and subjective"* and where they could *"get ideas out into the world without having to go through some referee."*

Not surprisingly, none of the U/M students spoke in these terms, probably because they were less engaged with idea generation and innovation, and more focused on their course materials.

Synthesizing Ideas

One of the first-year Ph.D. students said that actively thinking about the existing content of her blog while blogging about new things had enabled her to recognize links and associations between posts, thus helping her to synthesize ideas and begin to make sense of her research field. She said:

I was typing away about [X] and it suddenly dawned on me that [it] was similar to [Y]. I cross reference between posts with common themes. It was like a literature review.

Blog as a Draft of Dissertation

One Ph.D. student described how her blog was like *"a hypertext draft of my dissertation"* as she had created links between her own posts and thus carved out her own research direction.

Reflection of Progress Made

Three Ph.D. students said that their blog was a record of their progress over the months or years that they had been doing their research. One described the benefits thus:

looking through your blog and seeing your progression makes you feel better when you're feeling down. You can see how much you've progressed over the years.

Reflection of One's Understanding

A U/M student described how he revisited his private, (coursework) assignment-related posts to see whether his thoughts at the time of writing were accurate, and whether he needed to address any misunderstandings or misinterpretations.

Ph.D. students wrote about their sense making and gradual improvement of their research ideas and thinking in their blogs. A sample taken from one blog shows that the Ph.D. student here is reflecting on the refining of this thinking related to his research project:

Organizing the main concepts

I've been thinking for a while that I needed to have some kind of clear ordering of the central concepts for my research—that is, what I've seen as the main components of the PHC practitioner experience: aesthetics, ethics, sense making, improvisation, and narrative. This is mostly for communicative reasons. People seem to trip over "aesthetics" and "ethics" when I use them as the organizing principles. The concepts feel too heavyweight. I saw this again in presentations and conversations at the Connections 2007 conference this past weekend. Some clarity also dawned as a result of the conversations with [three people] during the weekend ... I think that narrative, sense making, and improvisation are really the ongoing phenomena in which practitioner aesthetics and ethics—the things I'm trying to characterize and make distinctions about—take place. I'll try to illustrate that below. URL: http://www.knowledgeart.blogspot.com

Study Skills, Research Skills and Self-Motivated Blogging

The findings related to RQ3 are presented in this section. Table 1 contains a synopsis of the main blogging activities discussed by the U/M students, and includes the study skills these activities are believed to have helped develop.

Similarly, the blogging activities of the Ph.D. students helped in the development of a range of research skills. The relevant skill areas that emerged are presented in Table 2, together with the associated blogging activities discussed by the Ph.D. students.

Table 1. Study skills and their associated blogging activities

Study skills	Associated blogging activities and uses of the blog-as-end-product
Active reading and learning (e.g., Rowntree, 1998)	Summarizing and explaining course materials brings clarity, salience, and reinforcement. Helps remembering. Photographs of activities
Dealing with stress (e.g., De Fazio, 2002)	Writing as catharsis: ranting, whinging, sharing experiences with actual or potential readers, celebrating success
Maintaining motivation (e.g., Fry, 2005a, 2005b)	Making public commitments, recording experiences, recording successes
Managing and learning from assignments and exams (e.g., Fry, 2005b)	Mnemonic aid for assignment dates, tutorial times, using your blog as a revision aid
Time management and personal organization (e.g., Fry, 2005a)	Creating work plans, workload, family/work/study commitments, blog as reminder/ place marker
Information management (e.g., Zwier & Mathes, 2005)	URLs of resources, course websites
Critical thinking (e.g., van den Brink-Budgen, 2000)	Summarizing, criticizing, arguing, sharing resources, commenting, community building
Avoiding plagiarism (e.g., Marsh, 2007)	Thinking carefully about posting content of assignments and research, differentiating between personal opinion and substantiated claims

Challenges That Influence Self-Motivated Blogging

With regard to RQ4, the students expressed the following concerns or issues about blogging.

Lack of Community in a Specialized Area

Two Ph.D. students and two U/M students were unhappy as they felt they had not managed to become part of an active, vibrant online community. One Ph.D. student explained how it was difficult

Table 2. Research skills and their associated blogging activities

Research skills	Associated blogging activities and uses of the blog-as-end-product
Networking and giving and receiving feedback Communication skills (e.g., writing skills and contributing to the public understanding of one's research field) Personal effectiveness (e.g., flexibility and open mindedness)	Advertising research, increasing awareness of others about the research project, becoming part of an international/national community, commenting on others' posts/ideas, describing/explaining to an audience, enlightening readers, self-promotion, resource for supervisors, record of work, record of progress
Awareness of the national and international research environment (e.g., context, and justification of research techniques used in one's own research)	Sharing resources, links to other online resources, belonging to a blogging community, national/international networking, awareness of conferences, sharing experiences, writing about methodology
Research skills and techniques (e.g., critical thinking and the application of appropriate methodologies)	Writing for clarifying understanding, articulating ideas, criticizing, discussing methodologies and theories, giving opinions, reflecting
Research management (e.g., the setting of goals and effective information collation)	Creating and documenting research questions, forging a research direction and focus, writing about data collection and analysis, collecting URLs and resources, organizing posts into categories or folders, tagging posts, material for papers/reports etc., work planning, blog as mnemonic aid and progress record

because his research was in a little-known domain with a very limited audience. He said he did not know how to go about finding interested parties. This problem was also discussed by one of the U/M students:

spent hours trying to find people with a common interest ... but people who study [X] tend not to be interested in blogs.

Lack of Comments

Almost all the participants said they would like to receive more comments on their blogs. One Ph.D. student said:

I would like people to comment on my ideas. Whether they're rubbish or good ... just some kind of feedback.

Concerns about Perceptions of Audience

Three Ph.D. students spoke about how they had had to consider the possibility of their readers thinking that their ideas were foolish. One student said:

I went back to my first entry a short while ago and I thought, "Oh my god, how can I have had this as a research question?", because it was awful. But I didn't delete it. Of course I cringe, but I have to live with it because it's me, I've written it ... of course people move on.

However, three Ph.D. students said that they were less concerned, and one said that

for me to put it in a public space accelerates the process, the motivation to write and makes writing much easier.

Issues of Plagiarism, Copyright, and Protection of One's Ideas

Six Ph.D. students and five U/M students discussed the issue of plagiarism and the need to be careful about what they publish in their blog. None of the U/M students discussed or shared the content of their assignments in their blogs.

A Ph.D. student also highlighted how posting draft journal manuscripts can result in problems with the blind-review process and copyright. Two Ph.D. students who blogged prolifically about their research said that they were cautious about how they represented their ideas, being careful to clearly demarcate substantiated claims from unsubstantiated opinions and ideas. One Ph.D. student and one U/M student said they had password-protected posts for material that was too sensitive to make public.

Maintaining Confidentiality and Sensitivity

Two Ph.D. students and seven U/M students said they were careful about publishing the identities of other people in their lives. One Ph.D. student was researching a politically sensitive area and said that she took care not to offend by providing a balanced view of potentially contentious issues.

Blogging or Themselves or for a Small Social Group

Community building may not always be the motivation for blogging. One Ph.D. student and three U/M students said that they did not want to be part of a community. These students primarily blogged for themselves, and to keep in touch with a small group of family and friends. One of these students mentioned that the commenting feature on her blog did not work and she had not rectified this. Another student said that although he received comments, he rarely followed them up as he was *"quite a loner."* Another U/M student said that she read other blogs and felt part of a community that way (i.e., through vicarious participation).

Presentation of the Blog Content

Two Ph.D. students said that they posted about positive events only as they wanted to maintain such a tone for their blog. One said, *"seeing as I am trying to broadcast I'm trying to make it look good."*

All the participants reported checking spelling and grammar, either as they wrote or by using the spell-checking facility of a word processor, before publishing their posts.

IMPLICATIONS OF THE STUDY

The study investigated self-motivated blogging activities by part-time distance education students on OU courses, and doctoral research (Ph.D.) students with the OU and other institutions. It has opened up a useful window of insight into why these students blog and what they blog about. Interviews with the students and analysis of the content of their blogs have revealed that there are several ways in which the students benefited from both the processes and the products of their self-motivated blogging.

The way in which the students utilized the public nature of blogging to their advantage was described earlier. Having an audience inspires many students to write and to describe their thoughts and experiences in a manner that encourages critical reflection and synthesis of ideas. Blogging in the public domain can motivate students to achieve their publicly announced goals and is also a vent for frustrations and emotions. The communicative potential of blogging is beneficial for building communities and sharing experiences and resources. Also, the commenting features of blogs enable the exchange of opinions and ideas. Many students found that the content of their blogs became a useful resource for reports and papers, and that creating links between posts can support the process of synthesizing these materials and facilitate the forging of a research focus and direction.

The chapter has expanded upon the advantages of blogging reported to date in the literature, some of which was reviewed in the early sections. However, it is worth emphasizing that the students in the study were independent, self-motivated bloggers, and while clear educational benefits have been identified, it does not necessarily follow that bringing course-directed blogging into educational programs would generate the same benefits. Nevertheless, when the findings reported here are viewed in terms of the study skills and research skills that students need to develop and apply, it becomes clear that blogging can offer several advantages to students. The findings presented in this chapter and the summaries in Table 1 and Table 2 may inspire students to start blogging, and to consider the challenges and issues highlighted by the participants in the study.

Implications of the Study for Educators

Blogging and Skills Development

Tutors and Ph.D. supervisors may find Table 1 and Table 2 useful for advising students about the role of blogging and the benefits it can provide. The rich variety of content in the students' blogs in this study is an indication of the flexibility of this medium for supporting learning and research. Some of the students did express a certain degree of caution and even apprehension with regards to the potential of plagiarism and the need to maintain a degree of confidentiality and sensitivity, but they all managed to navigate their way through these issues and to find that blogging can offer many advantages that appear to outweigh the problems and risks. The information in Table 1 and Table 2 might also be useful to trigger ideas for blogging activities on courses. Moreover, Educators and students may find it useful to consult the authors' previously published framework (see Kerawalla et al., 2008) to help them consider how they would like to use blogs for educational purposes.

Blogging Literacies

In the research presented in this chapter, the students adopted blogging of their own accord. However, if an educator is planning to introduce blogging as part of a course or program, it is necessary to consider the technical and digital literacy skills of students (including prior blogging experience) and the training required to support the development of these skills.

As noted by Burgess (2006) and also in the first author's social software study (Minocha, 2009), educators often make implicit assumptions that students would already know how to use the technology. However, learning a new technology can be challenging for students. If students are not able to understand the role the technology plays in their learning, or if there is a steep learning curve for the technology or the usability of the tool is poor, they will have an unsatisfying experience and may feel that the technology is "getting in their way."

A Social Genre

Blogging is a social genre and has characteristics of conversation, storytelling, and debate. Writing blog pages and posts is quite different from writing an essay, literature review, or other academic paper. Students who are not used to writing in blogs may face the challenge of maintaining an academic tone in their blog posts but yet having a personal voice for engaging the readers and for having a dialogue or conversation. To "teach" blogging for educational use, an educator may perhaps include guidance on effective public writing and communication.

Peer Reviewing

Just as it is easy to make an assumption that students will know how to use a new technology, students are also expected to know about peer reviewing and commenting on each other's blogs. Students might transfer the mental model of collaborating on a forum to a blog. However, unlike a forum that is everybody's space, a blog is the personal space of an individual and, therefore, there is a need for a different set of norms for peer reviewing and commenting within this personal space.

Students' Personal Connectivity with the Blogging Activity

The study in this chapter has shown that the blogs worked well for the participants as they were blogging of their own accord and were involved in discussing topics that were of direct interest to them. Burgess (2006) also tells us that "Personal research weblogs work best when they focus on the intellectual passions of their creators" (p. 111). In the interest of student engagement in and ownership of the learning process, it is therefore important that blogging activities are designed in ways that allow students to choose topics from the course matching their personal interests and experiences; alternatively, the activities should encourage the students to make connections between the theoretical concepts studied and their own personal and professional lives.

Challenges for Policy Makers in Institutions and for Educators

Policies about Blogging for Students

In the authors' earlier empirical investigations of blogging (e.g., Kerawalla et al., 2008) and in the first author's social software study (Minocha, 2009), no formal institutional policies or guidelines related to blogging were located. The institutions had not advised their students about how course-related or Ph.D.-related blogging should be carried out in the public domain. A student discussing his dissatisfaction with marks, or negative comments about his supervision, for example, may adversely affect the tutor–student (or supervisor–student) and the institution–student relationship.

Further, as discussed earlier, students should be apprised of the inherent privacy risks related to blogging where compilations of posts over a period of time can help the reader to build a detailed impression or "profile" of the blogger. Students should be given advice and guidance on how to negotiate the boundary between public and private by not revealing information about their personal lives, emotions, health, finances, religious beliefs, and political views in the blogs.

Some Ph.D. supervisors may prefer their students to refrain from openly discussing their research in the public domain, particularly if the student's project is a part of a larger research project or program involving other colleagues and students. Further, if the Ph.D. study has been sponsored by funding body or by an industry partner, there might be some restrictions regarding data protection, intellectual property, and copyright.

Training of Educators

With the educator's role becoming more facilitative and in order to help educators become effective moderators, training of the educators is required to impart skills for facilitation of blogs in a course. Further, in order to teach blogging literacies to students, it is important that the educators are themselves trained in a number of aspects: copyright, data protection, and intellectual property issues; how to write and comment effectively in a public space; how to assess online materials; and how to develop blogging activities that are situated within the course but yet allow the students to have some kind of personal ownership of and control over the activities. There is currently little (formal) guidance for educators to assist them with the design and assessment of learning activities involving blogs and for Web 2.0-based social software in general (Minocha, 2009).

CONCLUSION

Unlike the motivations for blogging in other domains discussed earlier in this chapter, which were more focused on community building, social interaction, and on enhancing one's reputation, in the authors' study, blogging activity was more focused on students' personal study and research needs. It can be concluded that the self-motivated student bloggers in the study perceived their blogs as being useful for a variety of study and research-related purposes, including serving as memory aids, for making notes about their reading and research, for keeping a record of their own progress, for project planning, and so on. These blogging behaviors are arguably more self-focused and less community oriented than those of other bloggers. This is not surprising because for these students, the primary motivation for blogging was to support their specific academic programs. Some of the Ph.D. students told the researchers that they found it difficult to find others carrying out research in a similar, relatively narrow area, suggesting that potential readership was small. Likewise, unless other undergraduates on the same course are blogging or aware of their fellow students' blogging, an individual student's blog is unlikely to attract the attention of a wide audience. However, some students did discuss the benefits of receiving comments from others, and some of them mentioned about how blogging was enabling them to gain visibility for their research efforts.

To extend the investigation on how blogs can enhance student learning and engagement, it would be useful to carry out longitudinal studies over a period of time involving both educators and students, with the aim of: (1) capturing the changes in experiences and perceptions of the students and educators over time; (2) observing how the blogs of students change and evolve; (3) determining what the effects are of blogging on students' research output or marks (in a particular course and over their entire program); and (4) identifying the critical factors that help sustain a successful blogging initiative. Eliciting educators' perceptions and experiences would help to provide information about the usefulness of blogs and blogging in their supervision and learning interventions: Are they able to intervene to correct the student's understanding? Does the blog/ blogging help in identifying any gaps in students' research skills? Does writing in the blog in a storytelling style have positive or negative impact on their academic writing?

It would also be useful to speak to the audience of the blogs (e.g., readers who comment on the blog) about their experiences of reading the blogs, how they distinguish between interesting and not-so-interesting blogs or individual blog posts, and whether reading the blog and commenting on the blog posts has benefited them personally. Such feedback would help the educators to emphasize to their students the benefits and challenges of blogging from the perspective of both the authors and the readers.

The coursework (undergraduate and Master's) students who participated in the study reported in this chapter were part-time distance learners. Had the students been full-time and/or campus-based, their experiences and use of blogs for community building and receiving peer feedback could well have been quite different from what was observed in the study. However, the methodology of the study could easily be adapted and applied for investigations with full-time, campus-based students in a range of contexts. Individual, semi-structured interviews or group interviews with educators would also be worthwhile and valuable.

ACKNOWLEDGMENT

The research presented in this chapter was supported by The Open University's Virtual Learning Environment program and the Faculty of Mathematics, Computing and Technology in 2006 to 2008. It is now being supported by the Joint Information Systems Committee (JISC) under the e-learning stream. The authors gratefully acknowledge the funding by JISC and the tremendous support from the JISC program manager, Heather Williamson. The authors would also like to express sincere thanks to all the participants in their research.

REFERENCES

Allan, S. (2006). *Online news: Journalism and the Internet*. Maidenhaid, UK: Open University Press.

Anderson, T. (Ed.). (2008). *The theory and practice of online learning* (2nd ed.). Athabasca, AB: Athabasca University Press. Retrieved April 29, 2010, from http://www.aupress.ca/books/120146/ebook/99Z_Anderson_2008-Theory_and_Practice_of_Online_Learning.pdf

Andreasen, L. B. (2006). Weblogs as forums for discussion—an alternative to the computer conference as a standard in online learning? In Buhl, M., Holm Sørensen, B., & Meyer, B. (Eds.), *Media and ICT—learning potentials* (pp. 71–88). Copenhagen: Danish University of Education Press.

Baggetun, R., & Wasson, B. (2006). Self-regulated learning and open writing. *European Journal of Education*, *41*(3/4), 452–473.

Baker, J. R., & Moore, S. M. (2008). Blogging as a social tool: A psychological examination of the effects of blogging. *Cyberpsychology & Behavior*, *11*(6), 747–749. doi:10.1089/cpb.2008.0053

Blood, R. (2000, September 7). Weblogs: A history and perspective. *Rebecca's Pocket*. Retrieved April 29, 2010, from http://www.rebeccablood.net/essays/weblog_history.html

Boud, D., & Lee, A. (2005). Peer learning as pedagogic discourse for research education. *Studies in Higher Education, 30*(5), 501–516. doi:10.1080/03075070500249138

Boud, D., & Sampson, J. (1996). *Learning contracts: A practical guide*. London: RoutledgeFalmer.

Boyd, D. (2007). The significance of social software. In Burg, T. N., & Schmidt, J. (Eds.), *BlogTalks reloaded: social software research & cases* (pp. 15–30). Norderstedt, Germany: Books on Demand.

Braun, V., & Clarke, V. (2006). Using thematic analysis in psychology. *Qualitative Research in Psychology, 3*(2), 77–101. doi:10.1191/1478088706qp063oa

Bruns, A. (2005). *Gatewatching: Collaborative online news production*. New York: Peter Lang.

Bruns, A. (2008). *Blogs, Wikipedia, Second Life, and beyond: From production to produsage*. New York: Peter Lang.

Bulik, B. S. (2008). Does your company need a chief blogger? *Advertising Age, 79*(15), 24.

Burgess, J. (2006). Blogging to learn, learning to blog. In Bruns, A., & Jacobs, J. (Eds.), *Uses of blogs* (pp. 105–114). New York: Peter Lang.

Butler, C. K. (2006). Blogging their way through academe. *U.S. News & World Report, 140*(13), 48–51.

Dalsgaard, C. (2006). Social software: E-learning beyond learning management systems. *European Journal of Open, Distance and E-Learning, 9*(2). Retrieved April 29, 2010, from http://www.eurodl.org/materials/contrib/2006/Christian_Dalsgaard.htm

Dalsgaard, C., & Mathiasen, H. (2008). Self-organized learning environments and university students' use of social software: A systems theoretical perspective. *International Journal of Instructional Technology and Distance Learning, 5*(2), 3–15. Retrieved April 29, 2010, from http://itdl.org/Journal/Feb_08/Feb_08.pdf

De Fazio, T. (2002). *Studying part-time without stress*. Crows Nest, Australia: Allen & Unwin.

Debenham, M. (2007, February). Epistolary interviews on-line: a novel addition to the researcher's palette. *JISC TechDis*. Retrieved April 29, 2010, from http://www.techdis.ac.uk/index.php?p=3_7_31_1

Dickey, M. D. (2004). The impact of web-logs (blogs) on student perceptions of isolation and alienation in a web-based distance-learning environment. *Open Learning, 19*(3), 279–291. doi:10.1080/0268051042000280138

Downes, S. (2004). Educational blogging. *EDUCAUSE Review, 39*(5), 14–26. Retrieved January 21, 2007, from http://net.educause.edu/ir/library/pdf/ERM0450.pdf

Du, H. S., & Wagner, C. (2007). Leaning with weblogs: Enhancing cognitive and social knowledge construction. *IEEE Transactions on Professional Communication, 15*(1), 1–16. doi:10.1109/TPC.2006.890848

Efimova, L., & Fiedler, S. (2004). Learning webs: Learning in weblog networks. In P. Kommers, P. Isaias, & J. M. Nunes (Eds.), *Proceedings of the IADIS International Conference Web Based Communities 2004* (pp. 490–494). Lisbon: International Association for Development of the Information Society.

Farmer, J. (2006). Blogging to basics: How blogs are bringing online education back from the brink. In Bruns, A., & Jacobs, J. (Eds.), *Uses of blogs* (pp. 91–103). New York: Peter Lang.

Felix, U. (2005). E-learning pedagogy in the third millennium: The need for combining social and cognitive constructivist approaches. *ReCALL, 17*(1), 85–100. doi:10.1017/S0958344005000716

Ferguson, R., Clough, G., & Hosein, A. (2007). Postgraduate blogs: Beyond the ordinary research journal. In S. Wheeler & N. Whitton (Eds.), *Beyond control: Learning technology for the social network generation. Research Proceedings of the 14th Association for Learning Technology Conference* (pp. 179–188). Oxford, UK: ALT.

Fiedler, S. (2004). Personal webpublishing as a reflective conversational tool for self-organized learning. In Burg, T. N. (Ed.), *BlogTalks* (pp. 190–216). Wien, Austria: Libri.

Franklin, T., & van Harmelen, M. (2007). *Web 2.0 for learning and teaching in higher education.* London: The Observatory of Borderless Higher Education. Retrieved April 28, 2008, from http://www.obhe.ac.uk/resources-new/pdf/651.Pdf

Fry, R. (2005a). *Get organised.* New York: Thomson Delmar Learning.

Fry, R. (2005b). *How to study.* New York: Thomson Delmar Learning.

Grudin, J. (2001). Desituating action: Digital representation of context. *Human-Computer Interaction, 16*(2/3), 269–286. doi:10.1207/S15327051HCI16234_10

Gunter, B. (2009). Blogging—private becomes public and public becomes personalized. *Aslib Proceedings: New Information Perspectives, 61*(2), 120–126.

Gurak, L. J., & Antonijevic, S. (2008). The psychology of blogging: You, me, and everyone in between. *The American Behavioral Scientist, 52*(1), 60–68. doi:10.1177/0002764208321341

Homik, M., & Melis, E. (2006). Using blogs for learning logs. In *Proceedings of the Fourth International ePortfolio Conference*. Champlost, France: European Institute for E-Learning. Retrieved April 29, 2010, from http://www.eife-l.org/publications/eportfolio/proceedings2/ep06/ep2006_papers/homik

Hornyak, M., Peach, B., & Fekula, M. (2003). Blogging: A new threat to student research? *Developments in Business Simulation and Experiential Learning, 30*, 131–132. Retrieved April 29, 2010, from http://sbaweb.wayne.edu/~absel/bkl/vol30/30ap.pdf

Huang, C.-Y., Shen, Y.-Z., Lin, H.-X., & Chang, S.-S. (2007). Bloggers' motivations and behaviors: A model. *Journal of Advertising Research, 47*(4), 472–484. doi:10.2501/S0021849907070493

Jones, M., & Alony, I. (2008). Blogs—the new source of data analysis. *Issues in Informing Science and Information Technology, 5*, 433–446. Retrieved April 28, 2010, from http://proceedings.informingscience.org/InSITE2008/IISITv5p433-446Jones530.pdf

Kerawalla, L., Minocha, S., Kirkup, G., & Conole, G. (2008). Characterising the different blogging behaviours of students on an online distance learning course. *Learning, Media and Technology, 33*(1), 21–33. doi:10.1080/17439880701868838

Kerawalla, L., Minocha, S., Kirkup, G., & Conole, G. (2009a). An empirically grounded framework to guide blogging in higher education. *Journal of Computer Assisted Learning, 25*(1), 31–42. doi:10.1111/j.1365-2729.2008.00286.x

Kerawalla, L., Minocha, S., Kirkup, G., & Conole, G. (2009b). Supporting student blogging in higher education. In Hatzipanagos, S., & Warburton, S. (Eds.), *Handbook of research on social software and developing community ontologies* (pp. 222–237). Hershey, PA: Information Science Reference.

Kirkwood, A., & Price, L. (2005). Learners and learning in the 21st century: What do we know about students' attitudes and experiences of ICT that will help us design courses? *Studies in Higher Education, 30*(3), 257–274. doi:10.1080/03075070500095689

Koper, R. (2004). Use of the Semantic Web to solve some basic problems in education: Increase flexible, distributed lifelong learning, decrease teachers' workload. *Journal of Interactive Media in Education*. Retrieved April 29, 2010, from http://www-jime.open.ac.uk/2004/6/koper-2004-6.pdf

Lamshed, R., Berry, M., & Armstrong, L. (2002). *Blogs: Personal e-learning spaces*. Melbourne, Australia: TAFE Frontiers. Retrieved April 29, 2010, from http://www.binaryblue.com.au/docs/blogs.pdf

Leslie, P. H., & Murphy, E. (2008). Post-secondary students' purposes for blogging. *International Review of Research in Open and Distance Learning, 9*(3). Retrieved April 28, 2010, from http://www.irrodl.org/index.php/irrodl/article/view/560/1140

Leslie, S., & Landon, B. (2007). *Social software for learning: What is it, why use it?* London: The Observatory of Borderless Higher Education. Retrieved April 28, 2008, from http://www.obhe.ac.uk/products/reports/pdf/2008-01-01.pdf

Luzón, M. J. (2006). Research group blogs: Sites for self-presentation and collaboration. In *Proceedings of the Fifth Annual Conference of the European Association of Languages for Specific Purposes (AELFE)* (pp. 629–634). Castelló de la Plana, Spain: AELFE. Retrieved April 29, 2010, from http://www.unizar.es/aelfe2006/ALEFE06/5.newtechnologies/87.pdf

Luzón, M. J. (2009). Scholarly hyperwriting: The function of links in academic blogs. *Journal of the American Society for Information Science and Technology, 60*(1), 65–89. doi:10.1002/asi.20937

Marsh, B. (2007). *Plagiarism: Alchemy and remedy in higher education*. Albany, NY: State University of New York Press.

McCullagh, K. (2008). Blogging: Self presentation and privacy. *Information & Communications Technology Law, 17*(1), 3–23. doi:10.1080/13600830801886984

Minocha, S. (2009). *A study on the effective use of social software by further and higher education in the UK to support student learning and engagement*. Bristol, UK: Joint Information Systems Committee. Retrieved April 29, 2010, from http://www.jisc.ac.uk/media/documents/projects/effective-use-of-social-software-in-education-finalreport.pdf

Minocha, S., Petre, M., & Roberts, D. (2008). Using wikis to simulate distributed requirements development in a software engineering course. *International Journal of Engineering Education, 24*(4), 689–704.

Minocha, S., & Tingle, R. (2008). Socialisation and collaborative learning of distance learners in 3-D virtual worlds. In A. Peachey (Ed.), *Proceedings of ReLIVE 08: Researching Learning in Virtual Environments International Conference* (pp. 216–227). Milton Keynes, UK: The Open University. Retrieved April 28, 2010, from http://www.open.ac.uk/relive08/documents/ReLIVE08_conference_proceedings_Lo.pdf

Mortensen, T., & Walker, J. (2002). Blogging thoughts: Personal publication as an online research tool. In Morrison, A. (Ed.), *Researching ICTs in context* (pp. 249–279). Oslo: InterMedia, University of Oslo.

Nardi, B. A., Schiano, D. J., Gumbrecht, M., & Swartz, L. (2004). Why we blog. *Communications of the ACM, 47*(12), 41–46. doi:10.1145/1035134.1035163

Oravec, J. A. (2003). Blending by blogging: Weblogs in blended learning initiatives. *Journal of Educational Media*, *28*(2/3), 225–233.

Owen, M., Grant, L., Sayers, S., & Facer, K. (2006). *Social software and learning*. Bristol, UK: Futurelab. Retrieved April 29, 2010, from http://www.futurelab.org.uk/resources/documents/opening_education/Social_Software_report.pdf

Pan, B., MacLaurin, T., & Crotts, J. C. (2007). Travel blogs and their implications for destination marketing. *Journal of Travel Research*, *46*(1), 35–45. doi:10.1177/0047287507302378

Rettberg, J. W. (2008). *Blogging*. Cambridge, UK: Polity.

Roberts, G. (2002). *SET for success: The supply of people with science, technology, engineering and mathematics skills. The report of Sir Gareth Roberts' review.* London: HM Treasury. Retrieved April 29, 2010, from http://www.hm-treasury.gov.uk/ent_res_roberts.htm

Rowntree, D. (1998). *Learn how to study: A guide for students of all ages* (4th rev. ed.). London: Time Warner.

Schmidt, J. (2007). Social software: Facilitating information-, identity- and relationship management. In Burg, T. N., & Schmidt, J. (Eds.), *BlogTalks reloaded: Social software research & cases* (pp. 31–49). Norderstedt, Germany: Books on Demand.

UK GRAD Programme. (2001). *Joint statement of the UK research councils' training requirements for research students*. Retrieved April 29, 2010, from http://www.grad.ac.uk/downloads/documents/general/Joint%20Skills%20Statement.pdf

van den Brink-Budgen, R. (2000). *Critical thinking for students: Learn the skills of critical assessment and effective argument* (3rd ed.). Oxford, UK: How To Books.

Vygotsky, L. (1978). *Mind in society: The development of higher psychological processes.* Cambridge, MA: Harvard University Press.

Ward, M.-H., & West, S. (2008). Blogging PhD candidature: Revealing the pedagogy. *International Journal of Emerging Technologies and Society, 6*(1), 60–71. Retrieved April 28, 2010, from http://www.swin.edu.au/hosting/ijets/journal/V6N1/pdf/Article4Ward&West.pdf

Wenger, E., McDermott, R., & Snyder, W. M. (2002). *Cultivating communities of practice: A guide to managing knowledge*. Cambridge, MA: Harvard Business School Press.

Williams, J. B., & Jacobs, J. (2004). Exploring the use of blogs as learning spaces in the higher education sector. *Australasian Journal of Educational Technology, 20*(2), 232–247. Retrieved April 28, 2010, from http://www.ascilite.org.au/ajet/ajet20/williams.html

Zwier, L. J., & Mathes, G. (2005). *Study skills for success*. Ann Arbor, MI: University of Michigan Press.

KEY TERMS AND DEFINITIONS

Blog: Short for "web log," this tool allows an author to publish his or her thoughts or diary online. Entries can be "tagged" with appropriate keywords so that related entries or posts can be brought together. In some blog services, the access to entries can be controlled to readers: to certain individuals, or to the public. Other users are typically able to add their own comments to the posts. Blogger, Edublogs, and Wordpress are among the best known publicly available blogging services. "Blog" can also be used as a verb to describe the process of posting, or adding content to, a blog.

Blogger: This term refers to an individual who maintains and posts to a blog.

Research Skills: These skills include organization, reflection, communication, information synthesis, and analysis, all of which are necessary for successful engagement in the research process.

Self-Motivated Blogger: Describes an individual who has decided to blog of their own volition, without encouragement or instruction by an educator or to satisfy the requirements of a program or unit of study.

Social Software: Software that allows people to socialize, interact, and collaborate online. It may also aggregate the actions of networked users. An alternative definition from Anderson (2008) states that social software tools support and encourage individuals to learn together while retaining individual control over their time, space, presence, activity, identity, and relationship. Examples include social networking sites (e.g., Facebook), wikis, blogs, as well as photo- and video-sharing sites such as Flickr and YouTube.

Study Skills: These can be defined as the skills necessary to undertake a period of study, such as time management, critical thinking, and academic writing.

Web 2.0: Web 2.0 is called the 'read/write' Web. Whereas 'Web 1.0' was about making information available, where the owner of a web site publishes information and the user (reader) can view or listen to the content. In Web 2.0, users and readers can also contribute to these web sites. Web 2.0 emphasizes online collaboration and sharing among users, allowing users to build connections between one another.

Chapter 9
Using Wikis in Teacher Education:
Student-Generated Content as Support in Professional Learning

Steve Wheeler
University of Plymouth, UK

ABSTRACT

This chapter reports on the use of online open content software as a learning resource for students enrolled in an initial teacher-training program at a British university. It features a study undertaken to support the development of professional practice in teacher education for undergraduate and postgraduate students using wikis. The 14 cohorts of student teachers in the program (n = 237) approached the activities in blended format, using a wiki as both a repository to store and retrieve their work, and as a discussion space where they could engage in dialogue with their peers and tutors outside of the classroom. Those who responded to the online questionnaire reported on their perceptions of the wiki as a learning environment. The main findings of the study are that students generated a large amount of content in a short space of time using the wiki and enjoyed its collaboration and communication tools, but resented the added time burden of having to complete minimum core tasks online. Students also found initial use of the wiki problematic due to lack of familiarity with the tools and the concept of group editing. The introduction of a series of wiki activities provided useful scaffolding for structured support in professional learning.

THE RISE OF SOCIAL SOFTWARE

Social software, it is claimed, has brought renewed enthusiasm to the use of web-based tools in education (Jones, 2007). Because it relies heavily on user collaboration, social software has been instrumental in restoring the Web, reconciling it to the original vision of a space where all are able to participate (Schaffert, Gruber, & Westenthaler, 2006). The tools and features that contribute to the social Web (or Web 2.0)—for example, blogs, wikis, and social networking sites—have been dubbed the "architecture of participation" (O'Reilly, 2004) because they encourage users to

DOI: 10.4018/978-1-60566-294-7.ch009

move away from passive reception of the contents of web pages toward active involvement and even content generation (Kamel Boulos & Wheeler, 2007; Williams & Jacobs, 2004). Web 2.0 tools offer students the opportunity to create, edit, share, and publish knowledge and information within and across communities of practice and interest (Rudd, Gifford, Morrison, & Facer, 2006). This is, of course, a highly desirable outcome for professional learning in that it fosters reflective learning and encourages engagement within the learning community. One social software tool, in particular, the wiki, is a website that can be edited and expanded by anyone who is a registered user. The wiki idea was first conceived by Ward Cunningham as a means of quick and easy online collaborative text editing (Cunningham & Leuf, 2001) and has rapidly caught on as an online collaborative tool for within education (Wheeler, Yeomans, & Wheeler, 2008). Wikis incorporate a number of content generation support features that enable students to contribute toward a shared online repository of knowledge, including tagging, versioning, hyperlinking, and commenting (Trentin, 2009). Wikis not only create opportunities for students to benefit from the knowledge of others; there is also evidence that users can create their own group consciousness which contributes significantly toward community building (Fuchs-Kittowski & Kohler, 2005) and create their own "knowledge structures," thereby achieving a sense of ownership (McGill, Nicol, Littlejohn, Grierson, Juster, & Ion, 2005).

There is however a caveat: Anyone who enjoys orderliness and clear structure could be uncomfortable when working with wikis. They generally appear to be chaotic and unstructured as they are constantly under development and are invariably a "work in progress." As such they tend to have only a primitive form of navigation, so users must rely on hyperlinking and the use of a search function to locate useful information (Elgort, 2007).

WIKIS IN EDUCATION

Several successful uses of wikis have previously been reported in a number of educational contexts, including compulsory (K-12) education (Richardson, 2006), teacher education (Wheeler et al., 2008), medical and clinical education (Kamel Boulos, Maramba, & Wheeler, 2006), university education (Bruns & Humphreys, 2005), language teaching (Godwin-Jones, 2003), and a host of other learning contexts (Lee, 2005; Parker & Chao, 2007). All the quoted studies share a growing understanding of the collaborative learning potential of wikis and their potential to actively engage students in learning. Previous studies have also shown that some students become aware of a larger audience when creating wiki content, and subsequently write more concisely and accurately (Wheeler et al., 2008).

Wikis also have specific pedagogic functionality. They are useful for creating a record of knowledge accumulation over a period of time, but they cannot and should not be used to generate quick answers or solutions. For iterative work, where students are required to discuss, construct, and negotiate meaning, they are an ideal tool. Most wikis feature a number of collaborative tools, including threaded discussion boards, tagging facilities, and messaging features. Site moderators can gain access to a page history tool that enables them to roll back to a previous version of the page if someone inadvertently deletes important content, or in the event of vandalism. For teachers, the wiki also offers the capability to track changes made on pages, and to view online transactions such as who has done which page edit, complete with a date and time stamp. Wetpaint (http://www.wetpaint.com/), for example, provides images of contributors in a sidebar. Based on the number of contributions a member has made, the size of their picture will grow or shrink correspondingly. Such a feature might prove useful in the context of the assessment of an individual's progress and learning.

However, as has previously been noted, the wiki also has limitations. When users fail to update a wiki on a regular basis, this has a negative effect on the knowledge of the user group as a whole, and can work against productive collaboration (Hodgkinson-Williams, Slay, & Siebörger, 2008). Furthermore, the dynamics of online groups and perceptions of individual users can themselves exert a negative influence on the learning process. If students have an expectation that the learning space will be dynamic and vibrant but few visit the space or contribute to the discussion groups, disillusionment will be a likely outcome (McPherson & Nunes, 2004).

From earlier studies of the implementation of wikis in undergraduate teacher education, it has been observed that students required some semblance of structure in order to maintain their sense of purpose and avoid inertia (Wheeler et al., 2008). It has also been recommended that there should be a real pedagogical purpose and that students should have a defined reason for participation in learning through social software (Kop, 2007). Ebersbach, Glaser, and Heigl (2006) point out that if wikis are not integrated into a regular pattern of learning activity, the result is that one or two people usually do the writing and others merely read. The present study was conducted to investigate how a structured set of activities might enable students to optimize their use of the wiki, both as a collaborative writing tool and as a repository for the storage and retrieval of professional knowledge.

EVOLVING WIKI CULTURE

Despite the doubt and criticism voiced over their effectiveness in presenting relevant and accurate information (Keen, 2007), wikis continue to inspire, and are increasingly used to encourage collaborative learning. Yet beneath the surface, within the social layer of knowledge production, a primal, ruthless potential lurks. Wiki communities can exhibit a feral tendency, particularly if misleading or erroneous content is posted. False, inaccurate, or unsubstantiated wiki content is rarely left for long before someone either removes it or tags it as "needing a quote" or "in dispute," or even deletes it entirely. It is clear then that wiki communities self-regulate both content and the behavior of their members. If contributors are found to be deliberately posting inaccurate, objectionable, or undesirable content to the wiki, they can be excluded from access to editing in future by other members of the group. So although the open nature of wikis creates opportunities for the deliberate sabotage of content, Owen, Grant, Sayers, and Facer (2006) reassure us that there is often a critical mass of users with sufficient ownership of a wiki who will quickly intervene and clean up unwanted postings and recover the site if malicious action occurs.

Within the emerging culture of wiki authoring several practices regulate content. "Mergism," for example, is where the best content from disparate sources is mashed together to create a newer, better item; "deletionism" occurs when all "bad" items are removed to maintain encyclopedic standards; "eventualism" is the long-term view of the wiki where all is a "work in progress" and eventually, over a sufficient period of time, the content will develop into something of true value. This evolutionary metaphor is extended into "Darwikianism," ensuring that only the "fittest"—that is, the most accurate and relevant entries—are allowed to survive and grow, whereas the weaker entries will be identified by community members and deleted or modified (mutated) to make them stronger. This "wisdom of crowds" (Surowiecki, 2004) effect appears to be the most dominant in, for example, Wikipedia, the most visible and well-known wiki site in existence. In evolutionary terms, only the fittest (or in this case most accurate and relevant) content does actually survive.

New wiki pages grow exponentially when a site is first created. The authors and editors work hard to produce useful, relevant, and current information for their pages. Eventually however, most wiki pages seem to "slow down" and eventually reach equilibrium, because there is simply no new material to be added. The evolutionary metaphor used to describe this aspect in the life cycle of a wiki can be useful in another way. When wikis have served their usefulness, they simply become "extinct." In effect, no-one adds any more content, and visitor traffic declines.

WIKI ACTIVITIES: A FRAMEWORK

Wikis are essentially content free shells, so students are confronted with blank spaces when they first log on. This can be a daunting prospect for some. More often than not, students will require some structure and initial content to build upon if they are to start well and exploit this space creatively. "Primer" activities can be devised that not only provide students with that good start; they can also be used to scaffold deeper cognitive engagement and to facilitate progressive involvement in collaborative working. Gunawardena, Lowe, and Anderson (1997) propose a framework for online collaborative learning in which they identify five phases of knowledge construction:

- *Phase 1:* The sharing or comparing of information;
- *Phase 2:* Discovery and exploration of dissonance and inconsistency among ideas, concepts, or statements by different participants;
- *Phase 3:* Negotiation of meaning and co-construction of knowledge;
- *Phase 4:* Testing and modification of proposed synthesis or co-construction;
- *Phase 5:* Phrasing of agreement statement(s) and applications of newly constructed meaning.

This seems to be a useful starting point from which wiki-based activities can be generated. In this study, several activities were devised and tested within the wiki so that trainee teachers could collaborate online. Some are documented below with brief annotation and rationale. It is possible to locate the activities within the phases proposed by Gunawardena and her colleagues.

All About Me

The first simple activity, "All about me," is used primarily as an ice-breaker exercise for new groups, but also as a subtle device to orient students to the topography of the wiki. Students are invited to introduce themselves to the group with a few words about their personal interests and background. To do this they must create a personal space for themselves, which is labeled with their own name and hyperlinked from the main Activity page. They may also be asked to post an image that they think best represents them. A mix of personal portraits, favorite cartoon characters, and images of animals or inanimate objects is usually the result. The "All about me" activity can be identified as a Phase-1 activity in Gunawardena et al.'s (1997) framework, because it involves the sharing of information and has minimal social interchange. To successfully complete the task, students must learn how to enter text into the wiki, create a hyperlink, and upload an image.

Establishing Wikiquette

Another starter activity draws more deeply upon the students' interpersonal skills, tasking them with defining the boundaries of their group activities within the wiki space. Students are asked to decide on what they consider to be the key rules of the space, including what constitutes acceptable and unacceptable behavior on the wiki—this is now popularly referred to as "wikiquette." Wikiquette differs from "netiquette" in that it is generally a set of rules that is agreed on, and imposed by the students themselves, and is therefore also policed by them. Wikiquette rules generally govern not only what is posted onto the wiki, but also the manner in which discussion and editing is conducted. "Establishing wikiquette" is a Phase-2 task, in that it explores differences of opinion and encourages the group to attempt to reach a consensus on how they will behave within the shared online learning space. Discussion tools are the most useful features for use to capture this kind of dialogue, and there is usually also a dedicated wikiquette page on which for students to post their decisions so the entire group can revisit the agreed rules as often as they need/wish.

Gold Mining

One wiki activity has been designed to promote critical engagement by requiring students to find "gold dust" resources online that they consider indispensable to their studies. The students share resources by hyperlinking the URLs on the relevant wiki page. Next to the hyperlink students post an annotated commentary on why the resource is so important to them, while other students are invited to inspect the resource and provide additional or alternative commentary. This represents co-construction of knowledge in the peer group, making it a Phase-3 activity.

The above wiki activities are three of the 20 activities that have so far been devised and applied. They can be seen as a thread of separate but gradually more complex social writing activities. They require the students to engage in individual research, which can lead to increasingly deeper levels of critical reflection and evaluation. As they work their way through the tasks students become more socially and critically aware, working within a community of learning to construct an online "shop window" of their findings over which they must eventually reach some level of consensus. The tasks facilitate collaborative writing and critical thinking within the wiki, and as they progress, deeper levels of critical engagement, co-ordination, and co-operative dialect are achieved.

A FIVE-STAGE WIKI ACTIVITIES MODEL

To categorize the wiki activities, a five-stage model was devised. Reflecting both Gunawardena et al.'s (1997) aforementioned model and Salmon's (2004) five-step e-moderation model, the wiki activities lead students progressively through more complex layers of learning, but the model also depicts a progression of engagement from solo inquiry to group collaboration through increasingly complex skills acquisition and application (modes). Additionally, it captures the journey from superficial technical, social, and academic content through to deeper levels of skill and knowledge construction (activities). The five-stage wiki activities model is depicted in Figure 1.

Although at the time of writing this model has yet to be empirically tested, it nevertheless proves useful as a means of visualizing how the activities can mesh together to provide a coherent learning pathway for students using wikis. There is, of course, a fine balance between providing too much content within an environment that by nature should be "content free," and letting the students loose in an environment where there are no obvious signposts. The author of the present chapter holds the opinion that offering minimal scaffolding in the form of wiki activities can provide useful conceptual frameworks and guidance for students, who will then be well-placed to create their own content and devise their own learning routes thereafter.

METHOD

Data were gathered from three sources. Firstly, student use of the wiki was monitored on a weekly basis and quantitative data gathered to indicate the number of transactions, including page edits, views, and discussion postings (n = 237). Secondly, strategically positioned questions were

Figure 1. Five-stage wiki activity model

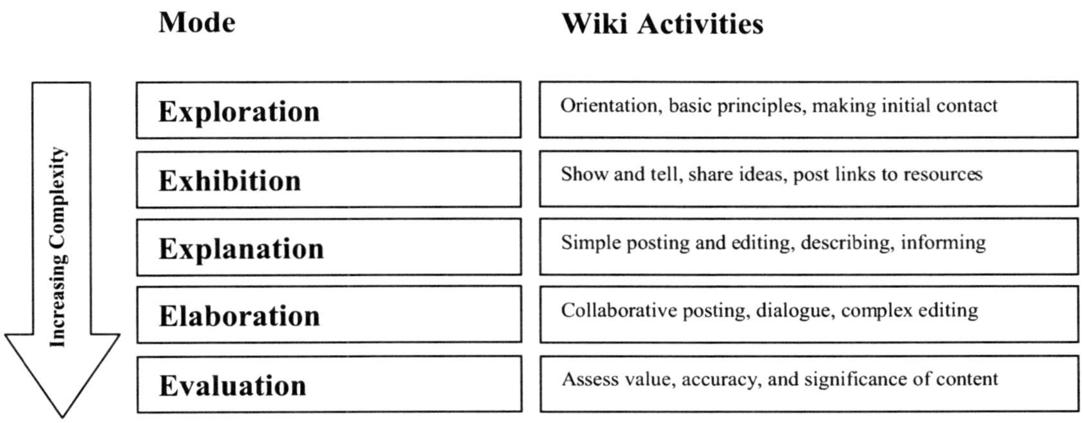

occasionally posted to the discussion board to gain snapshot opinions from the groups. Thirdly, a 22-item, post-experience questionnaire based on a six-point Likert scale was given to students enrolled on the wiki.

Approximately one-third of the students completed and returned their questionnaires (n = 80), a response that was deemed sufficient to provide a representative sample of the activities and opinions of the entire user group. Responses from this questionnaire were coded and entered into a statistical package (SPSS) for further analysis. As space precludes full results from being reported here, the findings from the statistical analysis will be reported in other publications. All responses were anonymous and students participated on the understanding that results would be used solely for research purposes. Students did not receive any course credit or monetary reward for their participation and all did so willingly. The qualitative responses from the questionnaire and online questions form the main data set for analysis in this chapter.

DISCUSSION OF RESULTS

One of the first properties students reported in significant numbers was their sense of ownership over the content they had generated on the wiki. As has previously been discussed, student ownership engenders a positive motivational influence on activities and fosters a sense of group consciousness (Fuchs-Kittowski & Kohler, 2005), which can strengthen group cohesiveness and reinforce group identity. One student was particularly motivated by her own use of the web resources:

I think the usage of an online resource that learners can take ownership of is a good (and can be motivating) thing.

Other observations from some students highlighted an important benefit. Comments were focused on the supportive and collaborative nature of the wiki and its capability to draw the group together:

I think the wiki is a useful tool for consolidating the group—I certainly feel as if I am more in touch with the group than I would do if we did not have the wiki to interact with, particularly as we are only together for two days a week. It feels somehow "supportive".

The main benefit is definitely the immediacy and interactivity and the possibility of sharing and solving problems with an online support group.

Some found the wiki so engaging that they spent considerable proportions of their study time online. The wiki became an always available resource, as can be evidenced by the time stamping of page edits, discussion group postings, and page views around the clock. Usage peaked immediately after taught face-to-face sessions, but instances of access, editing, and posting of discussion comments continued throughout the week, especially on weekends and during the evening hours. Some students adopted the idea and applied it in their own professional practice; at least two trainee teachers reported that they had created their own wikis and were using them, or planning to use them with their own students. One stated:

I think I will certainly consider using wikis in my practice. I feel they will engage students and provide a forum for distribution of information and ideas.

Another was very impressed with the immediacy and interactivity of the wiki, and said:

I love the wiki and it has inspired me to set one up for my family to use. I also think it will be a better, more flexible and interactive VLE [virtual learning environment] for me to offer my yoga teacher training students who currently get info and PDFs off my website. The main benefit is definitely the immediacy and interactivity and the possibility of sharing and solving problems with an online support group.

Technical difficulties became a barrier for some students, but even with access problems, lack of familiarity with navigation, and difficulty in initially coming to terms with the concept of shared collaborative online spaces, students still saw the value of the wiki, and eventually began to reap the benefits of their perseverance. The comment below typifies many that were received from students:

I found the wiki terribly hard to use. I had difficulties logging on, and struggled from thereon in. However, I can see its use and I'm sure as I stick at it, I'll find it easier and more useful.

Although all students participated in the wiki activities, inevitably the levels of participation varied. Some students began to question the meaning of their engagement in the process, particularly the amount of time they perceived as being required of them to successfully complete the wiki activities. One student reflected on her use of the discussion board, questioning the value of her own comments, but accepting that some of the wiki features had a valid collaborative, pedagogical purpose:

I sometimes feel I am making comments for comments sake. I have found collaboration awkward logistically—It is very *time consuming and initially was difficult to access. However, the web links have been useful and it is interesting to read other viewpoints.*

Several students complained that they did not know enough about how to use the wiki effectively, and requested that they be given some training in its use. Evidently, one of the shortcomings of the project was that time and resource constraints prohibited formal initial training in the use of the wiki for some groups. Due to the distributed nature of the groups and the disparate locations they met in, including military bases and prisons, initial training on the wiki was rarely possible, and resourcing was inconsistent. Some groups were therefore disadvantaged and this problem subsequently emerged in the discussion board comments:

This could have been a good resource had we been introduced to it in an IT suite where we could start tasks as a group.

When starting the use it would have been good to have had a computer session in order to get everyone on and started, rather than assuming we know how to do it. I had great difficulties and at the start of a course it is extremely disheartening especially when I view my ICT skills as good.

Lack of knowledge about the open nature of wikis also confused some students. Students often posted content into inappropriate areas of the wiki, or failed to link and signpost correctly to direct other course members to their pages. One student training at a naval (Royal Navy) base made an astute observation about the dangers of students missing information due to their inexperience, lack of wiki use, or the disorganized quality of the wiki content:

The success of how useful it is will be totally dependent on the group members gaining the experience and confidence to be able to make best use of the space. I think at the moment you could quite easily post something onto a wiki page and it be completely missed by the other members of the group. Not because they are not interested but through lack of wiki expertise.

One task required the students to seek out and post a hyperlink to a "gold dust" resource—a website or online learning resource they felt was essential for their studies. They were then tasked to post it to the "Useful resources" space and provide a short annotated commentary on why it was essential. Some enthusiastic students posted more hyperlinks than they were asked, accompanied by copious annotations. Unfortunately, their enthusiastic contributions appeared to cause information overload for some of their peers:

However, the sheer volume of data that appears for any one activity means that I have not had time to investigate, for example, all the gold dust resources posted by my peers. This is a shame as I am sure that many of them are just that—gold dust, but the necessarily contrived nature of the task meant that they have not been given the same consideration as spontaneously posted items.

One of the activities designed as an early collaborative exercise focused on establishing ground rules for use of the wiki. The wikiquette activity yielded some rich data in the form of online conversations between several group members. These discussions took the form of negotiations and decisions across the online communities until consensus was reached about acceptable and unacceptable use of the wiki space. Overwhelmingly, across all the groups, students were uniformly concerned about averting conflict and maintaining respect for each other, including the avoidance of offensive language, bullying, and discrimination, and ensuring confidentiality. Significantly, students in most of the groups unanimously agreed not to edit content posted by others, believing that it transgressed the social boundaries of ownership and intellectual property. One student started the wikiquette activity with this remark:

This is a very obvious one but I do think it's important! Do you think it would be good wikiquette not to (intentionally!) change or delete an entry prior to discussion with that member? Not only will we minimise the risk of upsetting someone and having cyber wars but it also means we can engage in useful discussion as a group.

Another student responded:

I agree with what you've said, but sometimes when something is new to you it's difficult to avoid making mistakes. I suppose the most useful thing to remember is to check before you click that all-important button. That way you won't (intentionally) delete someone else's work. To avoid upsetting anyone in our discussions, certain topics must remain taboo; whilst keeping everything else as democratic and fun as possible. Maybe the best thing is to have a vote on which topics we would avoid.

In another wiki group, one student replied to a rules list posted by another, with a hint of the affordances of online communication:

I completely agree with the rules above. As long as we are all respectful to other people on this site it should work well. Any comments added should be constructive and not offensive to anyone. I don't believe anyone's comments should be deleted, if people believe them to be wrong then it should be discussed not just deleted. This site is a good place to support each other and ask questions that we maybe don't feel we can ask face to face.

It was apparent that wiki activities such as the wikiquette task were valuable for a number of reasons. They eased students into collaborative online working, helped them to orient themselves to the concept of wiki content generation, and encouraged self-organized learning, all within a gradual progression from superficial to deep cognitive engagement. Without the wiki activities, students would have encountered a blank page with no immediate signposts, and may well have floundered more than they actually did. The gradual progression toward group writing enabled them to explore the discussion tools, share the knowledge they accumulated, and critically evaluate and reflect upon their experiences in a manner that was more conducive to professional learning. The following comments place these issues into context:

The whole idea of the wiki space is very good, the resource as an aid to learning is first class. Having a space that is open to the students to do activities and to be able to share information is good. There are only limitations that are put there by the user, as a resource it should be used as what it is a very good means of sharing information.

Finally, it is apparent that some students were looking forward to continued contact with their peers after the course had ended. They saw the wiki as a potential meeting point once their student passwords were rescinded and they could no longer access the online university student portal.

I think the greatest benefit would be when we've left the course and can't use the student portal, it would be good to catch up with each other and discuss latest news, etc.

CONCLUSION

It is clear that the wiki has a number of pragmatic pedagogical uses, particularly in the promotion of collaborative learning, where online tools are required. It is further apparent that students in the study reported in this chapter used the site as a means of communication across the group, and also began to explore the affordances it offered over and above face-to-face contact. Students gained a sense of ownership due mainly to the user-centric character of the wiki, which demanded that they generate their own content. The wiki activity framework appeared to be successful as a form of scaffolding, to provide students with an initial template and guidance in how and what to add to the space. Issues of critical mass such as those cited by McPherson and Nunes (2004) did not appear to exert a noticeable influence on engagement, possibly due to the reasonable group size (average of 18 students per group), and the fact that regular face-to-face sessions supplemented the wiki activities, which served to sustain the impetus of students' use of the wiki. Each time a face-to-face session was conducted, wiki activity subsequently increased. Coupled with the structure and naturally progressive nature of the wiki activities, students were observed to maintain their own momentum, both singularly and collectively. Within the first two terms of the academic year (October 2007 to March 2008), the

14 groups of students between them (n = 237) generated in excess of 65,000 wiki transactions including more than 1,000 message postings and over 3,000 page edits.

One of the chief problems identified during the wiki implementation was lack of initial training on how to access the wiki, create content including hyperlinks, and post comments to the discussion pages. Most students succeeded in overcoming this through trial and error and supporting one another. By far the most trenchant problem for students, however, was the inadvertent deletion or overwriting of someone else's content. Invariably when this occurred, tutor intervention was required to roll back the page to its previous version to restore earlier content. Generally, the conclusion drawn from this study was that the wikis were used successfully to create useful repositories for professional knowledge, and students found them useful and engaging. Most students were reluctant to edit the work of others, but consensus was reached over much of the content they created, using discussion.

Further problems arose when two or more students attempted to edit the same page simultaneously. The software precluded such functionality, and this tended to frustrate students when they had ideas they wished to capture, and could not access the page to complete their work. Issues occurred when students posted haphazardly or produced disorganized content, leading to confusion or information overload. As a collaborative tool, then, the wiki was not completely and directly successful, but due to the use of additional tools such as the discussion group, students were able to collaborate indirectly. The wiki activities were useful as scaffolding tools to encourage students to use the space and maintain impetus throughout their program of study. Some students reported that they wrote more concisely and correctly on the wiki, and further research will ascertain whether these skills are transferable to assessed academic writing. Future use of the wiki in teacher education will take these considerations into account.

REFERENCES

Bruns, A., & Humphreys, S. (2005). Wikis in teaching and assessment: the M/Cyclopedia project. In D. Riehle (Ed.), *Proceedings of the 2005 International Symposium on Wikis* (pp. 25–32). New York: Association for Computing Machinery. Retrieved June 6, 2008, from http://www.wikisym.org/ws2005/proceedings/paper-03.pdf

Cunningham, W., & Leuf, B. (2001). *The wiki way: Quick collaboration on the Web.* New York: Addison-Wesley.

Ebersbach, A., Glaser, M., & Heigl, R. (2006). *Wiki: Web collaboration.* Berlin: Springer-Verlag.

Elgort, I. (2007). Using wikis as a learning tool in higher education. In R. Atkinson & C. McBeath (Eds.), *ICT: Providing choices for learners and learning. Proceedings of the 24th Australasian Society for Computers in Learning in Tertiary Education (ASCILITE) Conference* (pp. 233–238). Singapore: Nanyang Technological University. Retrieved May 3, 2008, from http://www.ascilite.org.au/conferences/singapore07/procs/elgort.pdf

Fuchs-Kittowski, F., & Kohler, J. (2006). Wiki communities in the context of work processes. In D. Riehle (Ed.), *Proceedings of the 2005 International Symposium on Wikis* (pp. 33–39). New York: Association for Computing Machinery. Retrieved June 6, 2008, from http://www.wikisym.org/ws2005/proceedings/paper-04.pdf

Godwin-Jones, R. (2003). Blogs and wikis: Environments for online collaboration. *Language Learning & Technology*, *7*(2), 12–16.

Gunawardena, C. N., Lowe, C. A., & Anderson, T. (1997). Analysis of a global online debate and the development of an interaction analysis model for examining social construction of knowledge in computer conferencing. *Journal of Educational Computing Research*, *17*(4), 395–429.

Hodgkinson-Williams, C., Slay, H., & Siebörger, I. (2008). Developing communities of practice within and outside higher education institutions. *British Journal of Educational Technology*, *39*(3), 433–442. doi:10.1111/j.1467-8535.2008.00841.x

Jones, P. (2007). When a wiki is the way: Exploring the use of a wiki in a constructively aligned learning design. In R. Atkinson & C. McBeath (Eds.), *ICT: Providing choices for learners and learning. Proceedings of the 24th Australasian Society for Computers in Learning in Tertiary Education (ASCILITE) Conference* (pp. 460–467). Singapore: Nanyang Technological University. Retrieved May 3, 2008, from http://www.ascilite.org.au/conferences/singapore07/procs/jones-p.pdf

Kamel Boulos, M. N., Maramba, I., & Wheeler, S. (2006). Wikis, blogs and podcasts: A new generation of web-based tools for virtual collaborative clinical practice and education. *BMC Medical Education, 6*(41). Retrieved November 30, 2006, from http://www.biomedcentral.com/1472-6920/6/41

Kamel Boulos, M. N., & Wheeler, S. (2007). The emerging Web 2.0 social software: An enabling suite of sociable technologies in health and healthcare education. *Health Information and Libraries Journal*, *24*(1), 2–23. doi:10.1111/j.1471-1842.2007.00701.x

Keen, A. (2007). *The cult of the amateur: How today's Internet is killing our culture and assaulting our economy*. London: Nicholas Brealey.

Kop, R. (2007). Blogs and wikis as disruptive technologies: Is it time for a new pedagogy? In Osborne, M., Houston, M., & Toman, N. (Eds.), *The pedagogy of lifelong learning: Understanding effective teaching and learning in diverse contexts* (pp. 192–202). Abingdon, UK: Routledge.

Lee, M. J. W. (2005). New tools for online collaboration: Blogs, wikis, RSS and podcasting. *Training and Development in Australia, 32*(5), 17–20.

McGill, L., Nicol, D., Littlejohn, A., Grierson, H., Juster, N., & Ion, W. J. (2005). Creating an information-rich learning environment to enhance design student learning: Challenges and approaches. *British Journal of Educational Technology*, *36*(4), 629–642. doi:10.1111/j.1467-8535.2005.00540.x

McPherson, M. A., & Nunes, J. M. (2004). The failure of a virtual social space (VSS) designed to create a learning community: Lessons learned. *British Journal of Educational Technology*, *35*(3), 305–321. doi:10.1111/j.0007-1013.2004.00391.x

O'Reilly, T. (2004). *Open source paradigm shift.* Retrieved February 15, 2008, from http://tim.oreilly.com/articles/paradigmshift_0504.html

Owen, M., Grant, L., Sayers, S., & Facer, K. (2006). *Social software and learning*. Bristol, UK: Futurelab. Retrieved November 20, 2006, from http://www.futurelab.org.uk/resources/documents/opening_education/Social_Software_report.pdf

Parker, K. R., & Chao, J. T. (2007). Wiki as a teaching tool. *Interdisciplinary Journal of Knowledge and Learning Objects, 3*, 57–72. Retrieved February 15, 2008, from http://www.ijklo.org/Volume3/IJKLOv3p057-072Parker284.pdf

Richardson, W. (2006). *Blogs, wikis, podcasts, and other powerful tools for classrooms*. Thousand Oaks, CA: Sage.

Rudd, T., Gifford, C., Morrison, J., & Facer, K. (2006). *What if...: Re-imagining learning spaces*. Bristol, UK: Futurelab. Retrieved November 20, 2006, from http://www.futurelab.org.uk/resources/documents/opening_education/Learning_Spaces_report.pdf

Salmon, G. (2004). *E-moderating: The key to teaching and learning online* (2nd ed.). London: Routledge.

Schaffert, S., Gruber, A., & Westenthaler, R. (2006). A semantic wiki for collaborative knowledge formation. In Reich, S., Güntner, G., Pelligrini, T., & Wahler, A. (Eds.), *Semantic Content Engineering: Proceedings of Semantics 2005*. Linz, Austria: Trauner Verlag.

Surowiecki, J. (2004). *The wisdom of crowds: Why the many are smarter than the few and how collective wisdom shapes business, economies, societies, and nations*. New York: Doubleday.

Trentin, G. (2009). Using a wiki to evaluate individual contribution to a collaborative learning project. *Journal of Computer Assisted Learning*, *25*(1), 43–55. doi:10.1111/j.1365-2729.2008.00276.x

Wheeler, S., Yeomans, P., & Wheeler, D. (2008). The good, the bad and the wiki: Evaluating student-generated content for collaborative learning. *British Journal of Educational Technology*, *39*(6), 987–995. doi:10.1111/j.1467-8535.2007.00799.x

Williams, J. B., & Jacobs, J. (2004). Exploring the use of blogs as learning spaces in the higher education sector. *Australasian Journal of Educational Technology, 20*(2), 232–247. Retrieved May 1, 2007, from http://www.ascilite.org.au/ajet/ajet20/williams.html

Chapter 10
Mobile 2.0:
Crossing the Border into Formal Learning?

John Pettit
The Open University, UK

Agnes Kukulska-Hulme
The Open University, UK

ABSTRACT

Many practitioners are looking for ways to bring the vitality of Mobile 2.0—for example, social networking via a mobile phone (cellphone), or photo sharing on a mobile blog—into formal learning and teaching. But they face a complex and even paradoxical challenge: how can they harness that vitality without stifling its most distinctive feature—the fact that it is user led? This chapter begins with an analysis of that paradox as a foundation for understanding the challenges that practitioners face now and in the future. Drawing on data from interviews with six experienced tertiary practitioners, the authors describe and analyze a number of examples that point to the particular power of mobile devices to blur formal and informal activity in people's lives. The aim is to look beyond the hype around innovations in mobile devices and connectivity to focus on the opportunities for practitioners to bend the arc of Mobile 2.0 to the needs of their learners.

INTRODUCTION

The border referred to in the chapter title has the sunny territory of Mobile 2.0 on one side of it. That is where people update their online status while sitting at a café, upload their photos on Flickr while walking by the river, and access Wikipedia from the train. It is where personal interest and enjoyment fuel billions of interactions. It is Web 2.0 on sleek mobile devices.

DOI: 10.4018/978-1-60566-294-7.ch010

On the other side of the border lies the territory of formal learning. At the moment it is not so sunny. Indeed many of its long-term inhabitants—practitioners in colleges and universities—look across the border and wonder whether they can bring some of that energy and vitality over to their side and into formal education. It may not be easy: a 2008 report commissioned by the Joint Information Systems Committee (JISC), based on data from more than 1,000 first-year university students in the UK, found that the rationale for "using social networking sites for *formal teach-*

ing purposes" (Ipsos MORI, 2008, p. 7, emphasis added) was less obvious to these students than was the case with many other information and communications technology (ICT) services. This was despite the fact (or perhaps because of the fact) that over two-thirds of the respondents, who were nearly all aged 18 or 19, used social networking sites "regularly" for their own purposes (Ipsos MORI, 2008, p. 14).

The two opening paragraphs above reveal the dilemma for tertiary practitioners: how can they mobilize the benefits of Web 2.0 and Mobile 2.0 for their teaching without destroying what is most distinctive and interesting about Web 2.0/Mobile 2.0, that is, the fact that it is driven by users? To quote the JISC report again, "Use of social networks … does not feel right when led by the teacher" (Ipsos MORI, 2008, p. 36). That position—even though the authors of the report raise the possibility that it may be more applicable to first-year students than to more advanced students—provides a considerable challenge for practitioners.

Helping to meet such challenges is the key purpose in this chapter, which draws on a wide range of literature to provide pointers and examples, and looks at some of the possible futures for Mobile 2.0. The chapter draws on the authors' own research into practitioners' use of mobile devices to suggest that it is the blending of the personal and the formal—as much as concerns about the distinction between "1.0" and "2.0"—that may hold the key to resolving the dilemma set out above.

OWNERSHIP IN TERTIARY EDUCATION

The metaphor of the two territories with which the chapter opened is, of course, an over-simplification. The differences are not so stark or the border so clear, and this chapter seeks to explore a more nuanced understanding of how Mobile 2.0 can enrich formal learning. Nevertheless, there is a sense that tertiary education has been seriously challenged by the phenomenon of Web 2.0/Mobile 2.0, where users generate and share content and have considerable ownership.

This has happened at a time when mobile devices—whether handhelds, or portables such as laptops—have arrived on campus largely on the learners' own terms. These devices support what one report, based on a study in 2006 of over 400 "technology-savvy" UK students, described as an "underworld of communication and information-sharing invisible to tutors" (Conole & Creanor, 2007, p. 11). The use of "underworld" here is not so much sinister as making the point that these students, who indicate one likely future for tertiary education, use their own devices in their own ways to support their learning.

These trends resonate with Downes' (2006) challenge that "the students own education." How to meet that challenge, or variants of it, is one of the issues at the heart of this book in general, and the present chapter in particular. For many professionals in teaching and learning it is a pressing concern. How, for example, might they harness the power of photo sharing, one of the most vibrant of the participatory practices that can be found within Mobile 2.0? Could they use it in a teaching program on the built environment or ecology, for instance, where students would use their mobile phones (cellphones) to upload images of a building they have just walked past, or of a plant they have found in a meadow? Later in the chapter, some of the issues involved in doing this are considered.

CO-EXISTING PARADIGMS

It is also worth noting how far Web 2.0 and Mobile 2.0 co-exist with earlier but not necessarily inferior paradigms of social and educational communication. A practice with "2.0" in its name seems to assert that it is an evolutionary improvement on its predecessor. However, there is still much to be said about earlier mobile practices such as short message service (SMS) text messaging. SMS is often a straightforward one-to-one communication, and is not one of those services such as Wikipedia or many of the Google applications that harnesses "collective intelligence" (one of the criteria used by Tim O'Reilly when defining Web 2.0, quoted in Linden, 2006). Nevertheless, SMS has extensive application in collaborative mobile learning, and it throws light on the way mobile practices enable learners to cross the border between personal interest and formal learning. Such crossings are crucial if the potential of Mobile 2.0 and Web 2.0 is to be fully realized.

In the present chapter's authors' earlier research with mid-career professionals in education, an interviewee—a teacher of Spanish—illustrated how the crossing might be done. The teacher had asked students to send SMS messages in Spanish as homework while visiting Spain. The teacher reported that students added personal messages asking about the weather and food, and concluded that some "believed it was a personal thing, not homework—somehow they do not link the idea of mobiles with classwork" (reported in Pettit & Kukulska-Hulme, 2007, p. 26).

That merging of formal activity and the "personal thing" also aligns closely with one of the main findings from the interviews carried out by the authors with six practitioners in tertiary education. All of them were experienced users of mobile devices, and several of them were engaged in Mobile 2.0 practices. In addition to commenting on the potential of mobile devices for tertiary education, they spoke about the position of these devices in their professional and personal lives. As reported below, for several interviewees that professional/personal distinction was extremely blurred, even invisible. For one interviewee, the combination of Facebook and mobile phone was important. For another, it was the humblest of mobile devices—the memory stick—that allowed a certain level of nomadism. For a third, it was the personal mobile phone carefully placed on the workdesk that symbolized the dovetailing, rather than total blurring, of professional and private worlds. Even where the practices would not be defined as Mobile 2.0, there was much that was creative and may give pointers to future exploitation of mobile devices.

Overall, then, the emphasis here is on practices—Mobile 2.0, Web 2.0, and earlier practices—rather than on technological innovations. Clearly the latter are important, and reference shall be made to some of them towards the end of the chapter. But the massive publicity they often receive can obscure more important questions—more important, at least, for tertiary practitioners—about the opportunities they offer for learning. If a new paradigm is to emerge in mobile-enabled formal learning, it will ultimately depend on teachers, administrators, researchers, and learners. As Kling (1999) emphasized in his now classic article on social informatics, "technology alone, even good technology alone, is not sufficient to create social or economic value" ("The productivity paradox," para. 10).

MOBILE TECHNOLOGIES IN DAILY LIFE

Those instances of photo sharing and SMS have similarities with the wider aspiration expressed by a number of other researchers. Naismith, Lonsdale, Vavoula, and Sharples (2006), for example, argue that "The challenge will be to discover how to use mobile technologies to transform learning into a seamless part of daily life to the point where it is not recognised as learning at all" (p. 5).

This challenge could be taken in a number of directions. One approach that has brought success is to use mobile devices to enrich participants' visits to museums or heritage sites, to city squares and river banks. As visitors move through the space, their devices present them with information relevant to where they are. Naismith, Sharples, and Ting (2005), for example, evaluated one such case where visitors to a botanic garden used handheld computers that were GPS enabled.

In considering how that most prevalent of mobile devices, the mobile phone, might be used to enable learning, it is worth looking at trends in usage statistics. In the UK, the number of picture and video messages sent from mobile phones showed a year-on-year growth of 9% between 2008 and 2009, and on Christmas Day 2009 more than 4 million picture and video messages were sent by UK consumers (Mobile Data Association, 2009).

These figures suggest there is considerable potential for photo sharing in formal and informal learning. But as stated above, it is also important to explore the potential of "older" mobile practices. The moral basis of that aspiration is massively strengthened by the fact that mobile phones (even if with lower functionality) are also widely used in less-developed areas of the globe. Giridharadas (2010), for example, claims that innovators in developing countries are aiming to "find ever more uses for cheap, basic cellphones" (p. 4)—enabling users to hunt for work, make payments, transmit church sermons, monitor election candidates, and so on. There is, he argues, "a global flowering of innovation on the simple cellphone" (p. 4).

Mobile telephony does not need an infrastructure of cables, which for developing countries would be impossibly expensive in many rural areas, and it offers inhabitants in these countries "a way to bridge the connectivity gap without expanding the networks of fixed lines ... " (United Nations Conference on Trade and Development, 2009, p. 41). The scope to use solar energy to power the base stations adds to the attraction of mobile telephony in these environments (Murray, 2008).

So far in the discussion of mobile phones in the developing world, much of the emphasis has been on their role in economic development. However, Selanikio (2008) is one of those highlighting their educational potential, given the growth in mobile phone use in sub-Saharan Africa, for example. He argues that it is more realistic to focus on mobile phones and mobile telephony than on programs aiming to provide laptops to teachers and schoolchildren. In his view, we need to reconceptualize the mobile phone network as an "international network of wirelessly-connected computers throughout the developing world" (para. 1).

DESIGNING FOR LEARNERS' AGENCY

The thread running through several of the above examples is the attempt to harness activities—some "2.0," some not—that people are already doing for themselves. This is not always as straightforward as it was for the teacher of Spanish alluded to earlier. Thornton and Houser (2005), for example, sent short "mini-lessons" of English language material to 44 Japanese students on their mobile phones. These chunks of material were sent during the day at 9:00 am, 12:30 pm, and 5:00 pm, the intention being that students would learn more if they studied at intervals. Thornton and Houser reported considerable success but noted that over half the students did not engage in this "carefully timed interval study" (p. 222); many of them saved all the chunks for when they were traveling home, since that was the time of day that worked with the grain of their lives. It suited them personally, and it overrode the carefully paced delivery that the educators had designed.

It was reports such as this, combined with the findings of their own research, that led the authors of the present chapter to use "Going with the grain" as the title for their aforementioned 2007 publication (Pettit & Kukulska-Hulme, 2007). It is not necessarily the case that educators should invariably work within the limits of their learners' practices. However, it is arguable that lack of fit between the grain of learners' practices on the one hand, and educators' intentions on the other, is one reason why it may be difficult to design mobile-enabled learning for a group—even when the individuals in that group are very resourceful users of their own mobile devices for their own purposes.

This may be particularly true where educators are attempting to harness Mobile 2.0 activities—where, in the terms of this chapter, they are reaching across the "border." At the heart of this attempt is the question of ownership of these activities:

Outside the boundaries of formal education, there are a number of user-generated activities where mobile devices seem particularly well suited, and where users pull many of the levers themselves; for example, digital storytelling, citizen journalism, blogging, photo sharing and cultural citizenship. (Kukulska-Hulme, Traxler, & Pettit, 2007, p. 58)

The point has similarities with the argument in a wide-ranging paper from Jacobs and Polson (2006). They argue that when educators try to design learning experiences that draw on Web 2.0 practices, they need to give more weight to the "social incentives for participation" (p. 4) and less to entertainment. Like a number of others, the authors also stress the need for learners to retain a sense of ownership of the activity: "The growth of Web 2.0 services such as MySpace, Flickr and user-led information platforms collectively demonstrate a desire among users to have agency over their engagement with ideas" (p. 10). This emphasis on ownership and agency is a clear theme in current discussions about the way educators could harness Mobile 2.0. It also aligns with the point from Heppell (2006), who argues that with the advent of Web 2.0, teachers and administrators need to recognize that there has been a shift of power away from institutions and towards learners.

WHAT DO OUR LEARNERS ACTUALLY DO?

Many in tertiary education acknowledge this argument about the shift of power (even if they are not always certain how to respond). At times, however, this acknowledgment becomes a "homage to the generations"—the "iPod Generation," the "Net Generation," "Gen Y," the "Millennial Generation," the "Google Generation," and so on. It is worth digging below the surface of these claims, not to suggest that there are no inter-generational differences but to learn more about the detail and diversity of students' practices (see also Chapter 16 in this book).

For example, in their study of first-year students' use of ICTs (including mobile devices) at five English universities, Jones, Ramanau, Cross, and Healing (2010) found "a complex picture," and argue that it is "simplistic to describe young first-year students born after 1983 as a single generation" (p. 722). In an earlier study of first-year students at three Australian universities, Kennedy et al. (2007) concluded that students classed as belonging to the Net Generation were not using Web 2.0 technologies to a major extent. The study found that, for example, relatively few students in 2006 were familiar with blogging: 55% had never read a blog, and 73% had not created their own. Kennedy et al. contrast these findings with the assumptions and generalizations that some commentators have made about this generation's appetite for blogging, and warn that "there is a real danger that such commentary will create a vague but pervasive feeling among tertiary educators that every student who enters the higher education system is a blogger" (p. 522).

Kennedy et al. (2007) discuss a number of explanations for the "clear disparity between the proposed and actual technology use of the Net Generation, particularly in the area of Web 2.0" (p. 523). One reason could be that the claims about the Net Generation are derived largely from research in North America; it is possible that "Australian students are not as enamoured with Web 2.0 technologies as American students" (Kennedy et al., p. 523). The authors also tentatively suggest that future intakes of tertiary learners in Australia may be bigger users of Web 2.0.

WEB 2.0 AND MOBILE 2.0: DESIGNING FOR LEARNING

Broadly put, the picture (as presented, for example, by Conole & Creanor, 2007) is one in which many students are adept at using their own mobile devices within tertiary education for seeking information on the Internet, for communicating with other students, for writing assignments, and for storing and transporting electronic media files and documents. A considerable number also participate personally in Web 2.0/Mobile 2.0 activities, although as seen in Jones et al. (2010) and Kennedy et al. (2007), cited above, a single generation is likely to be less homogeneous than some commentators have claimed.

For practitioners, though, there is still much work to be done in realizing the potential of Web 2.0 and Mobile 2.0 for learning. An Open University project in the area of citizen science illustrates one way of doing this. At the Evolution MegaLab (http://www.evolutionmegalab.org/), volunteers from a number of European countries are gathering data related to global warming and evolution. Their task is to search for two common species of land snail, and to report the locations of the snails and the colors and patterns on their shells. Historical records show that there is a tendency for snails in the cooler north of Europe to have darker-colored shells than snails in the south. One aim of the project is to find out whether, with global warming, there is now a higher incidence of lighter-shelled snails in the north.

Variations in the color and patterning (including the number of bands) are also related to differences in the type of predator that the snails need to protect themselves against. As the level of danger changes—for example, if the number of snail-eating birds declines—the camouflage may also change across generations of snails. Another aim of the project, therefore, is to determine whether the camouflage has evolved over time.

When participants upload their report on the Internet, the data "will be automatically compared with historical records from nearby locations, and participants will receive instant feedback on any evolutionary change that may have taken place" (Silvertown, 2008, "Results/Conclusions," para. 1). One longer-term aspiration of a related Open University site, iSpot (http://ispot.org.uk/), is that participants should be able to upload their data using their mobile phones wherever they find any living thing they wish to identify, thus reaping the benefits of using an everyday handheld device.

Participants in Evolution MegaLab can see, in the form of the zoomable map, their own contribution and the collective effort of everyone who has participated thus far. In this way, they are actively taking part in research on the major topics of global warming and evolution, and for some participants this may provide a pathway into formal tertiary study in the biological sciences. This pathway would imply a merging, or at least an overlapping, of informal and formal learning.

The issue of borders and merging is one that was explored in some depth in interviews conducted by the authors of the present chapter with six experienced practitioners at The Open University. This forms the topic of the next section. As will become clear from the accounts below, the blurring of professional concerns and personal interest is one of the strongest themes to emerge, and one where mobile devices and Web 2.0/Mobile 2.0 play a distinctive role.

EXPERIENCED PRACTITIONERS' MOBILE PRACTICES

The six interviewees, three male and three female, were all practitioners in the broad field of digital learning at The Open University. Some were directly involved in writing teaching material, and most were involved in research or projects related to teaching and learning. Their particular interests included mobile-enabled learning, the design of teaching material for small-screen devices, open educational resources, and text-to-audio conversion for learning, among others. The interviews, each of which lasted approximately one hour, were semi-structured and were carried out by the authors in 2007–8. They were conducted face to face, except for one interview that was partially conducted by email. Five of the interviews were audio recorded, and were carried out on the basis that any quotations would be anonymous; the remaining interview was recorded in note form. Interviewees were asked in some depth about a number of issues, and specifically about:

- their use of Mobile 2.0 and Web 2.0 services;
- their use of mobile devices in their professional and their personal lives;
- the boundary (if any) between these spheres, and the way they managed the boundary;
- how, if at all, their use of mobile devices had changed their conceptions of "learning" and "teaching."

For some interviewees, mobile devices supported leisure interests and were in themselves a kind of hobby. The interviews also convey a picture of diversity and highly particular arrangements. Decisions as to what device to use in which location, and for which purpose, were very individualized. At the same time, for any individual there was often device overlap. If for some reason a device did not work, another could often be substituted because most of the interviewees were "device rich," that is, they owned or had access to several devices. Some of these were their own devices; in many cases, interviewees interwove these with the devices provided to them by their employer.

In the article quoted earlier on social informatics, Kling (1999) makes the telling point that "The design and configuration of information systems that work well for people and help support their work, rather than make it more complicated, is a subtle craft" ("Punditry about information technologies and social change," para. 4). It is difficult to see how an institution could design systems down to the level of particularity revealed in the interviews. Rather, the evidence suggests that the interviewees made their own adjustments. They themselves exercised the "subtle craft" within a reasonably flexible institutional framework. Where there was a gap between that framework and their own requirements and preferences, individuals often filled it by buying a device and using it for both professional and personal purposes. This is akin to the practice among many students in the UK (Conole & Creanor, 2007) referred to above: many of them used their own devices within the framework of formal learning provided by the university or college.

Mobile 2.0 and Web 2.0

One interviewee used Flickr when traveling, uploading photographs from a mobile phone and making them available to friends and family. Facebook was increasingly important for this person: *"Now I'm more likely to use Facebook a lot [from the mobile phone] ... If I'm away from home, two or three times a day."* Facebook also plays a role in work: *"Even within the group where I work, we tend to update status at different times [of the day] just to know what other people are doing."* Flickr was used by another interviewee for sharing holiday photos as well as for photo sharing among those attending an academic conference, while yet another preferred to share photos through Facebook. The reasons for choosing a particular service were typically described in terms of convenience and the peer/friendship groups that interviewees were part of, which prompted the selection of one service over another.

OpenLearn (http://openlearn.open.ac.uk/), an Open University site giving free access to learning materials and tools for collaboration, was mentioned as a platform that appears to blur boundaries between formal and informal learning whereas in reality, argued the interviewee, the boundaries may be *"more jagged than blurred"*:

there are social tools on the site that can support informal collaborative learning, but they are not used a great deal. This interviewee maintained that when learners made use of the site as a group, led by a champion who was keen to help them, it seemed they were more likely to benefit from its tools and resources. This highlighted the issue of status or expertise, which might influence participation. Another interviewee stated that device-specific websites, on which users share knowledge about how to get the best out of a particular mobile device, exemplify some of the potential of Web 2.0 and Mobile 2.0.

The social bookmarking service delicious, accessible from anywhere, was a very important Web 2.0 tool for another of the interviewees. He described how his hobby of writing and producing electronic music has gradually merged in with work activity:

I use delicious a lot to keep track, I've got categories of stuff ... for music and for work. I search my delicious bookmarks before searching generally ... I use it all the time, at work and at home ... I did think about having two logins, but that would be more trouble than it was worth.

Some items are *"obviously work,"* some are *"home stuff,"* and some are *"difficult to categorize."* For example, his projects on computer-generated sound are hard to distinguish from his work on the use of audio for learning:

There are some things that are to do with processing, capturing of audio which I may do at home ... that are also relevant to work. Speech synthesizers are something I've been looking at to use in my music, and that's a key feature of turning structured authored texts into talking books and podcasts automatically ... to get everything pronounced correctly.

When interviewees talked about their use of Web 2.0 and Mobile 2.0 services, work and leisure were often mentioned in one breath or without making a clear distinction—a point elaborated on in the next section.

Blurring between the Professional and the Personal

This was perhaps the biggest theme to emerge from the interviews. As one interviewee said,

It's difficult to tell sometimes whether it's work or not ... For me there is no boundary ... I don't know whether I've acquired friends who do what I do, or whether what I do has made me friends ... But the people I write with and teach with are as much friends as colleagues.

This theme of contact with others was particularly important for her: *"wherever you are, and whoever it is, you are assuming they have a mobile phone and you are in text [SMS] contact pretty much when you want to be."* This interviewee also stressed the geographical blurring, through working overseas:

Sometimes I can't tell you whether I was here or there [in the UK or overseas]... It isn't really significant where I was. The fact is that decisions were made, discussions were had, and things were written ... I can barely remember [where].

One of the other interviewees conceptualized the boundary differently: *"the relevant boundary, I would say, is not so much between personal and professional as between different kinds of work."* In an email interview, he explained this in terms of the differences between devices:

I would only use a mobile device for email and maybe editing or note taking (maybe in a library). I couldn't contemplate sustained writing at a mobile device (except maybe a biggish laptop).

For a third interviewee, a single device—a smartphone, for example—might be used for both work and personal interest. The spheres were not clearly separated: *"If I'm thinking about something [to do with] work, that's the thing that's on my mind. So whether I'm at home or at work doesn't really matter too much."* He used the smartphone to capture ideas (about work or personal interest) wherever he was: *"The same device is often being used for both ... It's the fact of having the device there, to record, before you forget them."* He reported being out with friends when *"something occurred to me."* He took out the smartphone and typed in a couple of lines. His friends appeared not to mind this:

People are quite comfortable now with being interrupted by a device ... whether you're sending a text or typing a couple of things ... People are used to me taking notes.

This may appear to illustrate almost complete blurring between personal and professional interests, to the point where they are one and the same thing. While this may be the case for some of our interviewees, this interviewee nevertheless reported using a mobile phone to maintain some boundary at work—placing the phone on the workdesk. He continued,

I don't have to give my work telephone number to [friends and family] because they can reach me on my mobile. I have a personal email and a work email, which I keep distinct as well.

He also reported having two laptops, one of his own and one that was supplied by the employer: he brought the personal laptop into work, and took home the *"work laptop,"* but some distinctions remained: *"My personal laptop comes into work, and vice versa. But they still have a certain degree of autonomy."* This suggests quite subtle use of devices, and near—but not complete—blurring of the boundary.

One interviewee remarked that she no longer shuts the door of her home study as a way of stopping work. The pervasiveness of computers, and being able to work while lounging on the sofa with a laptop, meant that the working day was being stretched, whereas clear boundaries had existed previously.

Perceptions of Learning

How have mobile devices changed perceptions of learning? According to one interviewee,

It was almost immediately accepted that desktop computers were a tool that could be used for learning because they were designed and sold to businesses originally ... So then the move into learning support was kind of smooth, because a lot of education is to get people to move into the workplace. So there is a kind of underlying smoothness of transition there, whereas mobile devices have been consumer devices, and bringing those into use in the classroom seems to be counterintuitive for some practitioners. Not all, but for some. But I see that lessening as the devices become more universal.

An activity like geocaching, popular with another interviewee, could accommodate various types of activity, from playful leisure through to learning:

I go geocaching ... I was on the top of Bodmin Moor, and I got my phone out and went onto the website to read the directions and get the location of the next cache ... People hide and seek caches, and you use GPS coordinates to identify where you've hidden a cache ... it's a hide-and-seek, it's a treasure hunt.

This interviewee mentioned that there are also more overtly educational geocache pursuits, for example, geological geocaches.

Futures for Mobile Learning—Their Own and Others'

Two of the interviewees particularly valued the fact that mobile devices (in one case, a laptop rather than a handheld) enabled them to capture ideas as they came to mind. For example:

I like the idea of having a portable computer with me all the time because ideas are apt to strike me at any time, and I like the idea of being able to capture them on the hoof. I also like the idea of being able to access the Internet on the move. We don't teach students ... specifically about working in this way themselves, although several of our courses now teach something about the technologies that make it possible, such as Wi-Fi, 3G, WiMAX, data transmission, compression, and storage.

This interviewee also saw a role for mobile devices in enabling students to gather material in the early stages of a writing assignment:

They could "research" [the topic] on the train on a portable device, just Googling away, and making clippings of everything that seems relevant, for closer study later ... That's certainly how some of us work on ideas for [writing our teaching material].

Another interviewee spoke of the benefits of using a smartphone for capturing ideas:

When I'm thinking about various things at work ... the ability to have a jotter pad to capture ideas, because I might not necessarily be at my desk ... might be traveling, might be sitting on the sofa at home. So it's handy to have one place where you can put these things in.

He also talked about how he made brief notes about journal articles he was reading. In this case, the fact that it was difficult to input much text was actually seen by him as an advantage in that it *"helps you crystallize your ideas."*

A number of researchers have reported the challenges and constraints of designing for the small screen (e.g., Churchill & Hedberg, 2008). One of the interviewees discussed the implications for teachers of preparing learning material for handheld devices. He argued that the constraints could be an opportunity to find new ways of presenting material: "you really do hone down what you are trying to say." He also highlighted the possibilities of using multimedia technologies such as Flash on mobile devices, for example, to create small, bite-sized chunks or pieces of learning content in physics, music, or mathematics.

As Woukeu, Millard, Tao, and Davis (2005) have pointed out, this type of learning does not necessarily represent a new paradigm in the sense of drawing on the potential of Web 2.0 and Mobile 2.0 participatory practices; it may simply be "providing existing applications on a reduced device" (p. 162). Nevertheless, along with several of the examples in this chapter, it suggests that more conventional mobile-enabled learning still has potential. It also raises the question of the actual difference between Web 2.0 and earlier models. For example, user-generated content—such as information on Wikipedia—is not necessarily pedagogically innovative, even though it may reflect the Web 2.0 practice of harnessing collective intelligence. (Similar questions are explored in a number of other chapters in this book: see, for example, Chapter 2.)

Which Mobile Devices?

The interviewees had evolved certain patterns of technology use, based on experience of what suited them best and what they saw as working to their advantage. For example, *"I only give out this number if I'm supposed to be at work but have to pick up the kids—I use it for my benefit at work"* and *"I have quite a lot of bits of mobile technology for different purposes."* With access to multiple devices in different locations, interviewees were able to find solutions that fitted their needs exactly, such as synchronizing portable devices with computers both at home and at work, or using a large screen to give their eyes a rest. One interviewee described how she would occasionally connect her laptop at home to a 42-inch plasma screen and wireless mouse when her eyes were tired.

As with the findings reported in Pettit and Kukulska-Hulme (2007) on alumni's use of mobile devices, the interviewees reported very strong individual preferences. For one interviewee, she stated *"My life wouldn't work without the mobile phone."* She also relied on a laptop *"That goes pretty much everywhere with me ... My bag is big enough to carry a laptop, I bought it that way ... I don't have holidays from the laptop."* She explained that the laptop was also useful if she needed to find a quiet place to work away from the desktop computer. With the combination of mobile phone and laptop, this interviewee felt no need for a PDA: *"I do what I can on the [mobile] phone, but generally that's too small for me to see ... [The PDA] would give me a bit more screen, but not that much more than the phone."*

For another interviewee, a mobile phone was not important but a memory stick was crucial. Yet another interviewee had owned a succession of mobile phones across a decade. He also reported using a number of other devices including a laptop, smartphone, MP3 player, memory sticks, iPod, digital camera, and PlayStation. For him, a smartphone served the additional function of storing and transferring files; he cited the benefit, compared with a memory stick, of being able to view the files and sort them without needing another device, like a laptop or desktop computer, for this purpose.

Wi-Fi was seen by one interviewee as a motive for a *"step change in the use of the mobile Internet."* She explained:

I see more and more people with devices that they buy for personal use that have Wi-Fi, [so they can] access the Internet wherever there is a Wi-Fi connection ... Lots of people were put off by basically paying a phone company; whereas, given a free connection, they are prepared to pay the device cost but not the connection.

INTRODUCTION TO THE FUTURE

By their nature, interviews are of course partial and incomplete. In any case, these accounts show some of the diverse ways in which Mobile 2.0 is mixed with more conventional practices, and, as with the work from Jones et al. (2010) quoted earlier, they demonstrate the importance of researching how people are actually using technological devices and services. They show the way individuals make creative choices about which devices to use, where, and for what purposes.

This perspective of mixture and choice is important when considering predictions about mobile technologies. Just as Web 2.0 can seem to be the inevitable successor to Web 1.0, so commentators on technological innovation can seem to point the way forward along a single pathway, where people are all going in the same general direction even though some are much further ahead than others. A decade ago, Kling (1999) emphasized the limitations (as well as the attractions) of aspects of commentators' "vivid punditry" ("Punditry about information technologies and social change," para. 1), arguing that it was unlikely to foster a deep understanding of the way communications technologies are affecting our lives. MacManus (2009) also points out the difficulties of making predictions about technological futures: "Twitter came out of left field a couple of years ago ... What New Thing will we be talking about in two years' time?" ("Conclusion," para. 3)

Trends can change. Keegan (2008), for example, quotes Rob Hinchcliffe, UK community manager for qype.com, a review site enabling users to share opinions and feedback on local restaurants, plumbers, and other services. Hinchcliffe describes networks such as Facebook as "time-suck" (quoted in Keegan, para. 4) services. In a similar vein, the issue of "social network fatigue" has been raised by some commentators (see, for example, Weiss, 2009).

Nevertheless, certain trends have been discernible for several years. Faster data transfer is one such, though actual connection speeds and network coverage for mobile broadband have been problematic, at least in countries like the UK (Wray, 2009). The extension of connectivity has been another theme: "Eventually we will blanket the globe in wireless broadband connectivity," in the words of Paul Otellini, Chief Executive Officer of Intel Corporation (quoted in Waters, 2008, para. 6). In that same news report, Otellini predicted an Internet that is "proactive, predictive and context-aware" (para. 4), where our mobile devices pull data from the Internet and deliver information that is relevant to where we happen to be. Increasingly, services that were only available via the desktop are becoming accessible through mobile phones—for example, Google Books (http://books.google.com/) (Sorrel, 2009).

It can be difficult to find a satisfactory position between skepticism and the bland optimism of what Goodyear (2006, p. 84) calls the "dominant techno-romanticist discourse of e-learning," which "asserts that time and space are no longer barriers." In negotiating these assertions in order to develop successful Mobile 2.0 practices, tertiary education will need research that is willing to consider several options for the future.

FUTURE RESEARCH ISSUES

Mobile learning is developing quickly and pulling in several directions, with social aspects gaining ever more prominence. In one device-focused version of the future, individuals will keep acquiring more and better devices and will learn to pick and choose which one is good to use at any given moment, juggling between devices for different purposes and for communicating with different sets of people. It is clear that the devices are acquiring new features (and ever more applications). Evidence from practice such as that gathered through the interviews reported on earlier suggests that user preferences override the fact that a device can, in principle, serve many different purposes.

Thanks to the development of cloud computing, there are increasing numbers of people who are happy to use several different devices, some fixed and some mobile, in the knowledge that they can access storage and processing power anywhere and at any time. At the simplest level, this can be browser access to an application hosted on the Web, but cloud services can deliver more than that: for example, users of Apple's (2008) MobileMe service can synchronize their email, contacts, and photos from anywhere, as long as their device has an Internet connection. (For a further exploration of these issues, see Chapter 21.)

In another version of the future, there will be far less need to own computers or carry personal devices, as it will become more commonplace for anyone to be able to use whatever technology is made available in a given location or mode of transport, for example for the general public to walk up to and use in public spaces. This will easily apply to historical buildings and places where people come to find information or to experience an area of a city (Naismith et al., 2005; Reid, Hull, Cater, & Fleuriot, 2005). Morville (2005) observes that navigation is being taken to a new level, in the form of "Wayfinding 2.0 … [, which] begins with location awareness" (p. 71). This can mean using GPS to determine a device user's location in order to provide relevant content and interaction.

When finally "information processing becomes embedded in the objects and surfaces of everyday life" (Greenfield, 2006, p. 18), we will have a "fundamental alteration in worldview" (p. 16) and will be living in the age of "everyware."

Interpretations of this last scenario include a world of "overlays" where one can specify his or her interests or purposes; the environment he or she is in (or moves through) responds accordingly. From a world filled with portable, networked devices operated by people, we are moving towards "ambient intelligence" in which the networked devices are embedded in the environment and will recognize and anticipate a person's desires and needs, reacting to them as appropriate. These desires and needs might, of course, include learning, or wanting to teach or support other people. (See also Ley, 2007; Lee, 2008.)

All these developments, which are largely driven by technology, call for a great deal of research from human and social perspectives. It is not clear, for example, whether anyone wishes to be in a state of perpetual learning (Lee, 2005; Lee & Chan, 2007). It is also not clear what the implications are of switching attention to learning that takes place outside conventional "learning spaces." For instance, investigations are needed into how people recall what they have learned in non-traditional spaces, and into matters of social etiquette when people unexpectedly shift their attention to learning.

IMPLICATIONS FOR PRACTITIONERS AND RESEARCHERS

Hyped they may be, but Mobile 2.0/Web 2.0 are also phenomena that are encouraging or compelling many practitioners in tertiary education to reconsider and develop their teaching, and are stimulating research of the kind outlined above. Although Mobile 2.0/Web 2.0 have unsavory aspects such as the risk of cyberbullying and the uploading of video clips of violent attacks, there is much about them that appears to be attractive and valuable for learning.

In particular, Mobile 2.0/Web 2.0 involve activities that many learners or potential learners are already engaged in for pleasure. They present rich opportunities for students to contribute to their own and others' learning. And because mobile devices are often highly attractive and woven into the texture of so many lives, Mobile 2.0 gives the possibility—though not the inevitability—of increased motivation to learn, and at times and in places that suit the individual.

However, the evidence from researchers such as Kennedy et al. (2007) and Jones et al. (2010) reminds practitioners of the importance of ascertaining which devices and which "2.0" services, if any, their students already use. Educators and institutions need to find out about their own students rather than simply assuming they are like learners of a similar age elsewhere. The findings of these researchers is also a reminder that:

1. members of a cohort may not all have similar levels of ICT fluency, or similar preferences; and
2. what we discover about our learners is only a snapshot at a given point in time; their needs, desires, and characteristics are dynamic, and our educational decisions and investments need to allow for rapid and constant change.

The authors' own study (Pettit & Kukulska-Hulme, 2007) used a questionnaire and interviews to explore the mobile practices of the alumni of a Master's program, who were mainly mid-career professionals. One key finding was the importance of external factors in influencing which devices they used:

One of the distinctive contributions of the interviews was to illustrate how the participants wove particular devices and practices into their daily lives, especially when travelling. The fit appeared to be intense but provisional, and dependent on factors often outside the control of the individual, and certainly of any educator wishing to design learning around smartphones, PDAs or MP3 players. (Pettit & Kukulska-Hulme, 2007, p. 28)

Another factor to be borne is mind is that, for some students at least, high costs may deter them from accessing Mobile 2.0 services. It is also worth noting the finding from the aforementioned JISC study that some of the participants in that study felt they did not receive enough ICT support from their university, and that in this respect the "proportion is higher amongst arts students" (Ipsos MORI, p. 8). (For further discussion of the role of academic and professional staff in supporting learners, see, for example, Chapters 13 and 21 in this book.)

In addition, where students do not currently envisage the potential of certain "2.0" services for formal learning, this is not the end of the story. Students' attitudes here may well be intertwined with a school-derived, top-down model of teaching (Ipsos MORI, 2008). One possibility, which calls for further research, is that changing learners' conceptions of teaching may increase their openness to the use of Web 2.0/Mobile 2.0 in formal learning.

CONCLUSION

The image of a learner sitting at an outdoor café, enjoying an attractive lifestyle while using a mobile device, has been iconic (or a cliché) for some time. Such an image was used, for example, in a video demonstrating what might become possible at some point in the future if nanotechnology were to be used in "bendable" mobile devices. In the computerized graphics-based video, these devices were unwrapped from the wrist, spread flat for text input, then rewrapped. Wray (2008) wrote that "The developers say the project is based on real research and is not just an aspirational piece of design" (para. 4).

Convenience and connectivity are powerful themes in many of the announcements in this area, but for educators it is important to ask what sort of learning these might encourage. Many of the innovations involve professionally produced content, and/or a model of learning in which the main goal is to connect learners to information. This is not necessarily undesirable, but neither is it necessarily very innovative. It therefore may not exploit the most interesting features of Web 2.0/Mobile 2.0.

This chapter began with a question, asking how far Mobile 2.0 is moving into formal learning. Although there are signs of this happening, there remains the major challenge for practitioners of resolving the dilemma set out at the beginning—namely, that one of the attractions of "2.0" for users is that it is perceived to be theirs, not ours. Returning to the territorial metaphor in the opening sentences of the chapter, can we, as practitioners, find ways to encourage learners to cross that border from "Personal 2.0" to "Tertiary Education 2.0"? And will they still enjoy—and still own—what they find on the other side?

REFERENCES

Apple. (2008). *MobileMe*. Retrieved November 20, 2008, from http://www.apple.com/mobileme/

Churchill, D., & Hedberg, J. (2008). Learning object design considerations for small-screen handheld devices. *Computers & Education*, *50*(3), 881–893. doi:10.1016/j.compedu.2006.09.004

Conole, G., & Creanor, L. (2007). *In their own words: Exploring the learner's perspective on e-learning*. Bristol, UK: Joint Information Systems Committee. Retrieved November 20, 2008, from http://www.jisc.ac.uk/media/documents/programmes/elearningpedagogy/iowfinal.pdf

Downes, S. (2006, June 5). *The students own education*. Presentation delivered at the Vice Chancellor's Forum: Towards a Global Online University, The Open University, Milton Keynes, UK.

Giridharadas, A. (2010, April 18). In many parts of the world, a cellphone is sufficient. *The New York Times/The Observer*.

Goodyear, P. (2006). Technology and the articulation of vocational and academic interests: Reflections on time, space and e-learning. *Studies in Continuing Education*, *28*(2), 83–98. doi:10.1080/01580370600750973

Greenfield, A. (2006). *Everyware: The dawning age of ubiquitous computing*. Berkeley, CA: New Riders.

Heppell, S. (2006, June 5). *It's a new millennium, it's a new century*. Presentation delivered at the Vice Chancellor's Forum: Towards a Global Online University, The Open University, Milton Keynes, UK.

Ipsos, M. O. R. I. (2008). *Great expectations of ICT: How higher education institutions are measuring up*. Bristol, UK: Joint Information Systems Committee. Retrieved November 20, 2008, http://www.jisc.ac.uk/media/documents/publications/jiscgreatexpectationsfinalreportjune08.pdf

Jacobs, J., & Polson, D. (2006, September 26). Mobile learning, social learning. Paper presented at the Online Learning and Teaching Conference 2006, Brisbane, Australia. Retrieved November 20, 2008, from https://olt.qut.edu.au/udf/OLT2006/gen/static/papers/Jacobs_OLT2006_paper.pdf

Jones, C. R., Ramanau, R., Cross, S., & Healing, G. (2010). Net Generation or digital natives: Is there a distinct new generation entering university? *Computers & Education*, *54*(3), 722–732. doi:10.1016/j.compedu.2009.09.022

Keegan, V. (2008, February 14). From global village to a local village. *The Guardian*. Retrieved November 20, 2008, from http://www.guardian.co.uk/technology/2008/feb/14/mobilephones.socialnetworking

Kennedy, G., Dalgarno, B., Gray, K., Judd, T., Waycott, J., & Bennett, S. … Churchward, A. (2007). The Net Generation are not big users of Web 2.0 technologies: Preliminary findings. In R. Atkinson & C. McBeath (Eds.), *ICT: Providing choices for learners and learning. Proceedings of the 24th Australasian Society for Computers in Learning in Tertiary Education (ASCILITE) Conference* (pp. 517–525). Singapore: Nanyang Technological University. Retrieved November 20, 2008, from http://www.ascilite.org.au/conferences/singapore07/procs/kennedy.pdf

Kling, R. (1999). What is social informatics and why does it matter? *D-Lib Magazine, 5*(1). Retrieved November 20, 2008, from http://www.dlib.org/dlib/january99/kling/01kling.html

Kukulska-Hulme, A., Traxler, J., & Pettit, J. (2007). Designed and user-generated activity in the mobile age. *Journal of Learning Design, 2*(1), 52–65. Retrieved November 20, 2008, from http://www.jld.qut.edu.au/publications/vol2no1/documents/designed%20and%20usergenerated.pdf

Lee, M. J. W. (2005). Mobile learning: Should we get a move on? *Training and Development in Australia*, *32*(4), 8–11.

Lee, M. J. W. (2008). Mobile and pervasive technology in education and training: Potential and possibilities, problems and pitfalls. In Godara, V. (Ed.), *Risk assessment and management in pervasive computing: Operational, legal, ethical and financial perspectives* (pp. 73–105). Hershey, PA: Information Science Reference.

Lee, M. J. W., & Chan, A. (2007). Pervasive, lifestyle-integrated mobile learning for distance learners: An analysis and unexpected results from a podcasting study. *Open Learning*, *22*(3), 201–218.

Ley, D. (2007). Ubiquitous computing. In *Emerging technologies for learning* (Vol. 2, pp. 64–79). Coventry, UK: Becta. Retrieved November 30, 2008, from http://partners.becta.org.uk/upload-dir/downloads/page_documents/research/emerging_technologies07.pdf

Linden, G. (2006, May 14). Tim O'Reilly and defining Web 2.0 [Web log post]. *Geeking with Greg*. Retrieved November 20, 2008, from http://glinden.blogspot.com/2006/05/tim-oreilly-and-defining-web-20.html

MacManus, R. (2009, October 21). Emerging Internet trends: An analysis of Mary Meeker's Web 2.0 summit presentation [Web log post]. *ReadWriteWeb*. Retrieved November 20, 2008, from http://www.readwriteweb.com/archives/emerging_internet_trends_meeker_2009.php

Mobile Data Association. (2009). *The Q4 2009 UK mobile trends report*. London: MDA. Retrieved November 20, 2008, from http://www.themda.org/mda-press-releases/the-q4-2009-uk-mobile-trends-report.php

Morville, P. (2005). *Ambient findability: What we find changes who we become*. Cambridge, MA: O'Reilly.

Murray, J. (2008, August 28). Ericsson debuts next generation solar-powered base station. *BusinessGreen*. Retrieved November 20, 2008, from http://www.businessgreen.com/business-green/news/2224857/ericsson-debuts-generation

Naismith, L., Lonsdale, P., Vavoula, G., & Sharples, M. (2006). *Literature review in mobile technologies and learning*. Bristol, UK: Futurelab. Retrieved November 20, 2008, from http://www.futurelab.org.uk/resources/documents/lit_reviews/Mobile_Review.pdf

Naismith, L., Sharples, M., & Ting, J. (2005, October 25–28). *Evaluation of CAERUS: A context-aware mobile guide*. Paper presented at the Fourth World Conference on mLearning (mLearn 2005), Cape Town, South Africa. Retrieved November 20, 2008, from http://www.mlearn.org.za/CD/papers/Naismith.pdf

Pettit, J., & Kukulska-Hulme, A. (2007). Going with the grain: Mobile devices in practice. *Australasian Journal of Educational Technology, 23*(1), 17–33. Retrieved November 20, 2008, from http://www.ascilite.org.au/ajet/ajet23/pettit.html

Reid, J., Hull, R., Cater, K., & Fleuriot, C. (2005, June). Magic moments in situated mediascapes. In S.Z.-Y. Zhou & S. P. Lee (Eds.), *Proceedings of the 2005 ACM SIGCHI International Conference on Advances in Computer Entertainment Technology* (pp. 290–293). New York: Association for Computing Machinery.

Selanikio, J. (2008, January 17). The invisible computer revolution. *BBC News*. Retrieved November 20, 2008, from http://news.bbc.co.uk/1/hi/technology/7106998.stm

Silvertown, J. (2008, August 3–8). *Geographically-referenced teaching and learning (GReTL): Making a virtue out of necessity in distance education and citizen science—the example of the Evolution MegaLab*. Paper presented at 93rd Ecological Society of America Annual Meeting, Milwaukee, WI. Retrieved November 20, 2008, from http://esameetings.allenpress.com/2008/P9955.HTM

Sorrel, C. (2009, February 6). Read Google Books on your iPhone. *Wired.com*. Retrieved November 20, 2008, from http://www.wired.com/gadgetlab/2009/02/read-google-boo/

Thornton, P., & Houser, C. (2005). Using mobile phones in English education in Japan. *Journal of Computer Assisted Learning, 21*(3), 217–228. doi:10.1111/j.1365-2729.2005.00129.x

United Nations Conference on Trade and Development. (2009). *Information economy report 2009: Trends and outlook in turbulent times*. New York and Geneva: UNCTAD. Retrieved November 20, 2008, from http://www.unctad.org/en/docs/ier2009_en.pdf

Waters, D. (2008, January 8). Intel predicts the personal net. *BBC News*. Retrieved November 20, 2008, from http://news.bbc.co.uk/1/hi/technology/7176177.stm

Weiss, S. (2009). Privacy threat model for data portability in social network applications. *International Journal of Information Management, 29*(4), 249–254. doi:10.1016/j.ijinfomgt.2009.03.007

Woukeu, A., Millard, D. E., Tao, F., & Davis, H. C. (2005, November 27–December 1). *Challenges for semantic grid based mobile learning*. Paper presented at First International Conference on Signal-Image Technology and Internet-Based Systems, Yaounde, Cameroon. Retrieved November 20, 2008, from http://www.u-bourgogne.fr/SITIS/05/download/Proceedings/Files/f135.pdf

Wray, R. (2008, February 26). Small and thin—but the phone of the future must bend too. *The Guardian*. Retrieved November 20, 2008, from http://www.guardian.co.uk/business/2008/feb/26/mobilephones

Wray, R. (2009, January 21). Mobile broadband providers promise more clarity over download speeds. *The Guardian*. Retrieved November 20, 2008, from http://www.guardian.co.uk/technology/2009/jan/21/broadband-mobilephones

KEY TERMS AND DEFINITIONS

Cloud Computing: Information is stored in servers on the Internet and can be accessed by users from any computer. For example, Google Apps provides common business applications that can be used directly from a web browser.

Informal Learning: In contrast with formal learning, informal learning is not organized and structured by an institution. It may take place in environments that have some connection with learning, such as museums and art galleries, or anywhere the learner chooses, including the home, workplace, or community.

Multimedia Messaging Service (MMS): A mobile phone standard for sending messages that can include multimedia objects in the form of images, audio, video, and text. The most popular use is for sending photographs.

Mobile 2.0: A term used to refer to services that integrate the social Web with mobility and the use of mobile devices. An example of a popular service is Twitter, which can be used from a web browser on a desktop computer or directly from an Internet-connected mobile device (e.g., a smartphone or PDA).

Pervasive: The aim of pervasive computing is to create a computing infrastructure that permeates the physical environment, that is, chips and sensors are embedded in everyday objects.

Photo Ssharing: The practice of sharing digital photographs with others, on the Web or on mobile devices; facilitated by websites such as Flickr.

Social Bookmarking: Free web services/tools that make it easy for users to save and tag links to web pages that they want to remember or share with others. Delicious is a popular example of a social bookingmarking site/utility.

Social Network Fatigue: The stress or boredom allegedly felt by some users after prolonged participation in social networking sites.

Chapter 11

Meeting at the Wiki: The New Arena for Collaborative Writing in Foreign Language Courses

Ana Oskoz
University of Maryland, Baltimore County, USA

Idoia Elola
Texas Tech University, USA

ABSTRACT

This chapter introduces the use of wikis and written and voice web applications as supporting tools for collaborative writing. It reports on a study examining the processes advanced Spanish foreign language learners engage in while working collaboratively using wikis and chat to complete a writing assignment. Through analysis of students' essays, wiki-based drafts, chat transcripts, and questionnaire responses, it was observed that students maintained an interest in their essays' accuracy as well as a focus on global rather than local aspects. In addition, the combination of wikis and chat provided students with an environment in which to state a clear thesis, provide supporting evidences, and refine the organization of the essay in a manner often missing in individual work. The authors expect that the benefits observed when using social web applications while working collaboratively will provide more evidence for pedagogical shifts that will help students become better writers in their second language.

INTRODUCTION

The burgeoning interest in Web 2.0 technologies such as Flickr, Facebook, blogs, and wikis is indicative of the growth of participatory, collaborative practices in society at large (O'Reilly, 2005). However, within the realm of foreign language (FL) education, the practice of collaboration, in particular collaborative writing—two or more people working together to produce a document with group responsibility for the end product (Bosley, 1989, cited in Ede & Lunsford, 1990, p. 15)—has only been cautiously approached to date. Yet, scholars in first language (L1) and second language (L2) writing have shown that collaborative writing promotes reflective thinking, focuses attention on grammatical accuracy, lexis, and discourse, and encourages a pooling of knowledge about language (Donato, 1994; DiCamilla & Anton, 1997; Hirvela, 1999; Storch, 2005; Swain

DOI: 10.4018/978-1-60566-294-7.ch011

& Lapkin, 1998). The success of a collaborative writing endeavor is evidenced by students being truly involved and engaged in the activity (Forte & Bruckman, 2006; Schaffert, Bischof, Buerger, Gruber, Hilzensauer, & Schaffert, 2006).

Collaborative writing has been recently aligned with Web 2.0-based social software applications such as blogs or wikis (Alexander, 2006). These applications provide for authoring flexibility, content creation, and the generation of new knowledge. The open editing and review structure of wikis makes them the most suitable tool to support collaborative writing (Parker & Chao, 2007). Their collaborative value can be further enhanced when accompanied by the use of web-based audio applications such as *Voice Direct*, a synchronous voice conferencing/chat facility (see University of Maryland Baltimore County, n. d.). This combination of tools can lead to increased levels of interaction and accountability of the participants (Rick, Guzdial, Carroll, Holloway-Attaway, & Walker, 2002). At the same time, however, wikis challenge some of the traditional notions of authorship as understood in Western literary theory in a way that tends to unsettle the student-endorsed model of solitary authorship. Therefore, given the increasing use of social software for L2 educational purposes, there are questions and concerns about its viability in the classroom and the benefits that its use may bring to the L2 writing process.

Within this context the study outlined in this chapter expands upon a growing line of research in education, namely the benefits of using wikis for collaborative writing purposes, but with an emphasis on FL environments. Set in a social constructivist paradigm, the collaborative approach to learning enables students to be connected and participatory in a dynamic, evolving community of practice. This chapter examines FL learners' writing processes while working collaboratively on a task that requires either the discovery of a solution to a given problem, or development of a written text based on a given argument (Trentin, 2009). In particular, it focuses on advanced Spanish second language learners at the tertiary level who were required to use wikis and web-based communication utilities to complete a writing assignment as part of their course. In this process an attempt is made to form a response to the overarching question,

To what extent does students' knowledge about writing in Spanish benefit from the use of wikis and chat?

This is further subdivided into the following, more specific questions:

1. How do these students approach a collaborative writing task (e.g., what writing processes are observed) when using wikis and chat?
2. What are the differences in terms of fluency, accuracy, and complexity between the first and final turn-in drafts when writing collaboratively in wikis?

LITERATURE REVIEW

Wikis

Wikis are collaborative web-based environments consisting of pages that potentially anyone can edit. The most well known wiki, Wikipedia (http://www.wikipedia.org/), is a user-edited online encyclopedia founded in 2001, in which readers elect to write texts and improve the content of existing ones. As modeled in Wikipedia, wikis support collaborative writing in educational settings by providing students the opportunity to co-author a document (Farabaugh, 2007; McLoughlin & Lee, 2007; Parker & Chao, 2007; Trentin, 2009). An important application of wikis for educational purposes is to provide students with both the possibility and accountability to create, transform, and erase their work. At the same time a tracking system allows teachers and researchers to follow the writers' collaborative processes by examining who makes the changes, what changes are made, how often and when.

Because the flexibility of this software facilitates communication among learners and promotes the shaping and sharing of knowledge when working collaboratively, wikis have begun to attract the attention of tertiary educators in distance learning (Augar, Raitman, & Zhou, 2004; Byron, 2005; Tsinakos, 2006) and hybrid or face-to-face courses (Elgort, Smith, & Toland, 2008; Farabaugh, 2007; Farabaugh, Farabaugh, & Freeland, 2005; Hodgkinson-Williams, Slay, & Siebörger, 2008; Trentin, 2009). In particular, within the language learning domain, much interest has been shown in English as second language (ESL) and English rhetoric courses (Chang & Schallert, 2005; Wang et al., 2005), as well as in FL courses (Honegger, 2005). Yet, the use of wikis in L2 contexts for collaborative writing purposes, while growing, is still mostly descriptive and exploratory in nature (Godwin-Jones, 2003; Thorne & Payne, 2005). In one of the first empirical studies examining the use of wikis in the L2 classroom, Kost (2007) found that, while working collaboratively, students focused not only on grammatical accuracy and lexis, but also on features at the discourse level. This is particularly important in foreign language education at higher levels when considering the need to develop advanced composition skills.

Constructivism and Pedagogy 2.0

A key dimension of Web 2.0 use in tertiary education is the way in which it is able to support a constructivist paradigm, in which knowledge and meaning are seen as constructed rather than provided (Mayer, 1998; Parker & Chao, 2007). Web 2.0 also embraces "Pedagogy 2.0" (McLoughlin & Lee, 2007, 2008; see also Chapter 3 in this book): its applications foster interdependence between ideas, individuals, communities and information networks, supported by information and communication technology (ICT).

In contrast to previous learning paradigms that emphasized a teacher-centered approach, constructivism, in particular social constructivism, focuses on a learner-centered approach in which learners interact to construct knowledge and engage in personal reflection on their experiences to form and refine their internal knowledge structures. Following this paradigm, learning is now understood as (1) active and manipulative; (2) constructive and reflective; (3) intentional; (4) authentic and challenging; and (5) cooperative, collaborative, and conversational (Miers, 2004).

Web 2.0 applications including wikis, while not arising from any radical change in the technical capabilities of the Web, have led to some revolutionary uses (O'Reilly, 2005). The power of these applications for educational purposes stems from their *affordances*—actions that individuals can potentially perform in their environment using a particular tool—of sharing, communicating, and information discovery (McLoughlin & Lee, 2007, see also Chapters 1 and 3 in this book). However, while ICT in general and Web 2.0 or social software in particular offer great possibilities for enhancing student learning, they do not in themselves automatically lead to positive learning outcomes (Lindblom-Ylänne & Pihlajamäki, 2003; see also Chapter 2). In the educational context there is a need to understand the relationship between the properties of the technological tools used to support learning interventions, and exactly how each learner uses the tools to construct and/or acquire knowledge (Kirschner, 2002, cited by McLoughlin & Lee, 2007). It is also imperative that it be recognized that "technologies are intricately related to many other elements of the learning context" (McLoughlin & Lee, 2007, p. 666) such as subject content, curriculum, communication, process, resources, scaffolds, and learning tasks, all of these being dimensions of what McLoughlin and Lee (2007, 2008) term "Pedagogy 2.0."

Though not centered around the technology, Pedagogy 2.0 advocates media-rich communication and collaboration. Through the use of various technology tools and multiple forms of interaction, learners embark on collective and co-creative activity. Wikis, for example, which provide an open editing and review structure, when implemented in conjunction with other communication tools (Kost, 2007; Rick et al., 2002) can provide students with a rich environment that enables them to choose tools that best suit their needs for interconnection and social interaction. Immersion in this rich multimedia environment encourages and empowers students to take active responsibility for their work and their own learning (see also Tutty & Martin, 2009).

Constructivism and Pedagogy 2.0 in L2 Writing

Although recent technological advances in writing software have sparked interest in collaborative learning using these tools (Hirvela, 1999), the question of whether more effective use of the technology can be made in L2 writing continues to linger (Elgort et al., 2008). Often, the original intentions of the software designers/developers and the practical activities conducted in the classroom are at odds. The use of pair or group work is central to a social constructivist view of learning; however, the "monolithic view of writing" (Murray, 1992, p. 114), which reinforces the perception that writing is a solely private, individualistic act, is still strongly rooted in instructors' and students' minds. Even when a collaborative writing approach has been adopted, it is often relegated to peer review practices (de Guerrero & Villamil, 2000; Villamil & de Guerrero, 1996, 1998), which still assume single authorship.

Influenced by social constructivist beliefs about the development of knowledge and discourse practices, writing theorists now understand writing as a socially embedded activity (Hirvela, 1999). This view sees writing not as an individual act, but a social one; even when the composing process is performed alone, the writer communicates with an intended audience, and is therefore performing a social act. The use of wikis and chat for collaborative writing emphasizes the social dimension of writing by allowing students to participate in a more overtly social process when writing (Brown & Adler, 2008). In this way, as Schneider (1990) suggests, writers share the authority to make decisions and understand that knowledge is constructed socially, rather than merely being a fixed entity that is transmitted and received. As students negotiate their writing they start to reshape their knowledge of the subject, ultimately becoming responsible for their own work (Farabaugh, 2007).

METHODOLOGY

Background

The study discussed in this chapter was conducted during the fall semester of 2007, at a mid-sized, commuter east-coast university, with 10 students in a Spanish advanced writing class. The course is an intensive, three-credit-hour course, mandatory for all majors in Spanish; its goal is to move beyond the traditional FL writing pedagogy and allow students to develop Spanish writing skills with the aid of innovative tools and techniques that allow them to experience a more learner-directed pedagogy. In line with Pedagogy 2.0 principles, the instructor created a media-rich environment that supported students in communicating with one another and sharing collectively in creating and revising their essays. This new approach gave students the opportunity to participate in collaborative activities that would not have been possible otherwise.

The instructor used PBwiki (http://www.pbwiki.com/) and formed different chat rooms using the written and voice chat integrated within the university's learning management system. The selection of PBWiki over other free wikis (such as Mediawiki) or alterative collaborative writing tools like Google Docs was based on its ease of use and clear processes in tracking user activities and

Table 1. Schedule of activities

Date	Activities
Tuesday, October 2, 2007	In-class discussion about topic, organization, and structure.
Sunday, October 7, 2007	Students completed the first draft via wikis. Instructor provided comments via wikis within two days.
Tuesday, October 9, 2007	In class, students and instructor commented on selected student essays in terms of both content and form.
Tuesday, October 16, 2007	Students completed writing assignment via their wikis.

created content. Students were trained in the use of the wikis for both oral and written chat. After a period of adapting to these tools, the instructor arranged the pairs to better suit students' needs and language levels.

Procedure

The class met one evening a week for two and a half hours. During class, students worked on grammar exercises, organizational and structural issues regarding different genres, and in-class discussions around the topics of the writing assignments. For the specific writing assignment described in this chapter students, discussed the role of men and women in Latino societies. After brainstorming ideas, pairs of students had five days to complete the first draft of the assignment in their wikis; this allowed them to schedule their working time flexibly. The instructor then provided feedback via the wikis regarding content, organization, and form. During the following class, the instructor and students looked at a few examples of student writing, discussing and revising key points about structure, organization, and form. After this class, students completed the assignment during the following week (see Table 1).

By granting several weeks to complete the assignment, the teacher gave students more opportunity to negotiate and reflect on the topics, and to fully consider essay structure, genre and linguistic issues. Students accessed the wiki from different sites, so to support and augment their collaborative process, they communicated through chat. Three pairs chose written (text-based) chat, while the other two used voice chat. Although students were not obligated to communicate any specific number of times, or to address any specific topics, they were encouraged to discuss essay content, organization, and form in Spanish.

At the start of the semester, the instructor had provided students with a questionnaire about writing skills, covering topics such as use of outlines and gauging level of difficulty writing in Spanish. The questionnaire also sought student perceptions about using wikis and voice/written chat tools for writing purposes. After the completion of the last essay, the instructor issued a similar questionnaire in order to gather data about students' experiences of using wikis and voice/written chat as tools to aid their writing.

Analysis

To discover the extent to which the students' Spanish writing knowledge and skills benefited from the use of wikis and chat, the researchers examined:

1. *Wiki drafts and chat transcripts:* The researchers analyzed every draft that was recorded in the history of the wikis. Given that each pair had different dynamics, the number of drafts differed for each pair. The researchers quantified the number of changes, and codified the changes based on whether students were focusing on vocabulary, content, organization, or grammar. With

regard to the chat transcripts, the researchers conducted content analysis to identify salient categories. To do this, the two researchers began by individually reading one of the transcripts, marked every point that revealed information relevant to the study, and wrote comments. The unit of data examined varied from short sentences to several conversational exchanges between the participants. The researchers then met virtually to share their findings, discuss discrepancies, negotiate agreement, and name some preliminary categories and subcategories. Finally, the researchers individually analyzed the four remaining sets of transcripts, before meeting to compare their results and identified categories, achieving an inter-rater reliability of.94.

2. *Students' writing differences between the first and final turn-in wiki drafts:* The first and second drafts were coded for number of words and number of T-units; this is defined as "one main clause plus a subordinate clause attached to or embedded in it" (Long, 1991, p. 1). They were also coded for fluency, accuracy (judged from the percentage of error-free T-units), and complexity (based on the percentage of subordinate clauses). Both researchers analyzed independently the first and final drafts of the first student pair, and compared the results to ensure they had a common understanding of T-units, subordinate clauses, and accuracy. After discussing doubtful examples, they independently coded the first and second drafts for the other pairs. The inter-rater reliability score for number of words was 1.0, for number of T-units was.97, for number of subordinate clauses was.95, and for number of error-free T-units was.95.
3. *Questionnaires:* The researchers compared student answers from the first and second questionnaires regarding the use of wikis and chat to improve the grammar, content, and structure of their writing. The analysis provided insight and made it possible to document students' reactions about the usefulness of a media-rich environment for collaborative writing.

RESULTS

The results of the analysis of students' wiki-based drafts and of the oral/written chat transcripts showed common patterns exhibited by all the pairs when working collaboratively. However, they also confirmed the differences between pairs and the complexities making each pair unique. The analysis of the drafts also illustrated variations in the students' writing skills, between first and final drafts.

Wiki Drafts

Even though each pair of students differed in the extent of their written wiki drafts, the analysis revealed writing processes, concerns, and preferences for each student.

- *Categories for the cohort:* In terms of the whole student cohort, draft revisions were divided into seven categories: content, organization, structure, grammar, style, use of sources, and editing. The analysis showed that while working on their various drafts the main focus was on content (34%), followed by editing (19%), grammar (16%), organization (10%), vocabulary (9%), style (8%), and sources (4%).
- *Categories for the pairs:* The results (see Table 2) related to the individual pairs also reflected common traits seen in the general analysis of the drafts. However, each pair displayed certain characteristics that were intrinsic to that pair or triggered by one individual, either due to personality or preferred mode of approaching an as-

Table 2. Analysis of the five writing processes most frequently identified in the wiki-based drafts produced by the student pairs

Pair 1	Pair 2	Pair 3	Pair 4	Pair 5
content (29%)	content (43%)	content (23%)	editing (47%)	content (47%)
editing (21%)	grammar (17%)	editing (23%)	content (34%)	editing (24%)
grammar (19%)	style (12%)	vocabulary (18%)	organization (13%)	organization (12%)

signment. The drafts from Pair 1 showed that they paid most attention to the content level (29%), followed by editing (21%) and grammar (19%). They also considered organization (10%) and vocabulary (10%). In Pair 2, student drafts focused most strongly on content (43%), followed by grammar (17%), style (12%), and editing (10%). Pair 3's drafts paid equal attention to content (23%) and editing (23%), followed by vocabulary (18%) and grammar (16%). The drafts from Pair 4 showed most concern with editing (47%), followed by content (34%) and organization (13%). Pair 5's results were similar: major attention paid to content (47%), followed by editing (24%), organization (12%), and vocabulary (11%).

Oral and Written Chat

The analysis of the chat transcripts showed 34 categories (see Appendix A for full details), which illustrated the students' interaction in connection to two main blocks of data: the task (e.g., issues of content) and the ways in which pair members communicated and kept their work progressing (e.g., asking for each others' opinions). When working together, the writers' processes and methods of work depended entirely on their own choices and their varying abilities to complete the assignment.

- *Categories for the cohort:* The cohort results highlighted some significant issues about how students approached their task and also how they "talked" to each other. Although from the chat transcripts it was obvious that many students had already discussed the assignment through other means (e.g., offline), the chat still exposed several key features and characteristics of their collaborative work. In other words, regarding the task, the content of the essay triggered most of the negotiations that occurred in the chat (23%), followed by methods of organizing (8.8%) the information that they had collected. (Note: To understand the percentages for the entire cohort, notice that the highest percentage observed in this set of data was 23%, and the lowest 0.12%. There were a total of 819 meaningful units, which were grouped in 34 categories. Only the highest percentages are commented upon in this chapter.) Interestingly, when the partners communicated, they frequently sought each other's agreement as a means to build a successful working environment. The students tended to show their approval by agreeing (13.6%) and asking each other's opinions (6.4%) while they were working together. In the chat sessions, there was a clear emphasis on planning the task (5%) correctly as a way to move forward in the assignment, because although they were working collaboratively, part of the composing process had to be done individually. Students also expressed concern about following or understanding the instructor or the instructions (3.8%), the type of sources (3.8%), and also issues about composition structure (3.7%).

- *Categories for the pairs:* As mentioned above, despite the existence of many common traits in the way the students approached their collaborative writing task, each pair displayed individual characteristics that appeared to be triggered by personality and work ethics (see Table 3). Pair 1 showed most concern with, first and foremost, content (26%); second, ensuring agreement between the two of them was reached (16%); third, identifying sources for expanding the topic (11%); and fourth, use of grammar (10%). They also engaged in dialogue in which they asked each other for feedback (9%), as well as spending time planning their task (6%) and dividing the work between them (5%). This pair worked effectively, although there were a few moments of confusion (2.5%). Pair 2 paid greater attention to content (28%), and moved the task along by showing their agreement (14%) with each other's work; they also paid attention to task organization (10.5%) and ensured that their writing flowed well. They planned the task (9%) and were careful to follow the teacher's instructions and advice (8%); this led to some moments of disagreement (1%) and even anger towards the assignment (1%). Pair 3 focused on content (24%) and quickly reached agreement (12%) in order to progress with the task. They were also concerned about the organization of the essay (11%) and its structure (5%). This was the only pair that used English to express their ideas; they read aloud information from the Web, which suggested that the majority of their sources (5%) were in English. Pair 4 concentrated mainly on content (21%). They also emphasized reaching agreement (14%) in order to progress the task, and sought each other's opinion (9%), in a relaxed and easy-going interaction. The members of this pair were also concerned about organization (6.5%), the sources (6%) they were using, and took structure (3.5%) into consideration. Pair 5, the final pair, focused on content (20%), followed by organization (13%). They, too, used explicit expressions to confirm their agreement (12%) about the essay's progress. They asked for each other's opinion (10%), and although there were clearly

Table 3. Analysis of the writing processes most frequently identified in the chat transcripts of the student pairs

Pair 1	Pair 2	Pair 3	Pair 4	Pair 5
content (26%)	content (28%)	content (24%)	content (21%)	content (20%)
agreement (16%)	agreement (14%)	agreement (12%)	agreement (14%)	organization (13%)
sources (11%)	organization (10.5%)	organization (11%)	asking for opinion (9%)	agreement (12%)
grammar (10%)	planning task (9%)	structure (5%)	organization (6.5%)	asking for opinion (10%)
feedback (9%)	instruction (8%)	sources (5%)	sources (6%)	polite (6%)

some disagreements, they took care to be very polite (6%) in the way they addressed problems encountered.

Results of the Turned-In Drafts

To understand whether there were significant differences between the first and final drafts of the essays produced by the students in terms of the three dependent variables, namely fluency, accuracy, and complexity, a Kruskal–Wallis test was conducted. The results of this test are shown in Table 4.

The statistical analysis indicated that there were no significant differences for accuracy (X^2 = 1.37, p =.241), fluency (X^2 =.079, p =.778), or syntactic complexity (X^2 =.118, p =.731) for the entire cohort, and consequently, there were no significant differences between the pairs.

Table 4. Results of the Kruskal–Wallis test

	Accuracy	Fluency	Syntactic complexity
Chi-Square	1.375	.079	.118
df	1	1	1
Asymp. Sig. (2-tailed)	.241	.778	.731

Results of the Questionnaires

The initial questionnaire administered prior to the learning activities (see Table 5) revealed that the majority of the students thought the use of the wikis would help them improve their grammar. Most of them also believed that working collaboratively via the wikis would help to improve the content and structure of their essays. Opinions were divided regarding the usefulness of the written/voice chat to improve written grammar. Students did, however, believe that these tools could help develop their writing skills in terms of content and accuracy.

After a semester of using the wikis, student opinions regarding their value for improving their grammar were evenly divided, with half the students believing that using the wiki did help them with grammar, and the other half disagreeing. In the latter group, two of the students felt that they did not correct each other's grammar because they had established "different territories" and because they also had different language proficiency levels. One of the students went so far as to complain about the inability of the wiki to highlight incorrect spelling, as one would expect

Table 5. Student perceptions on the value of wikis and chat for grammar, content, and organization, based on the results of the two questionnaires

Item	Strongly Agree	Agree	Disagree	Strongly Disagree
Using the wiki to work collaboratively with my partner improved my written grammar.	Q1: 10%	Q1: 90% Q2: 50%	Q2: 50%	
Using the wiki to work collaboratively with my partner improved the content of my writing.	Q1: 10% Q2: 10%	Q1: 80% Q2: 90%	Q1: 10%	
Using the wiki to work collaboratively with my partner improved the structure of my writing.	Q1: 10% Q2: 30%	Q1: 90% Q2: 50%	Q2: 20%	
Using the written/voice chat to work collaboratively with my partner improved my written grammar.		Q1: 50% Q2: 30%	Q1: 50% Q2: 70%	
Using the written/voice chat to work collaboratively with my partner improved the content of my writing.	Q2: 10%	Q1: 80% Q2: 90%	Q1: 20%	
Using the written/voice chat to work collaboratively with my partner improved the structure of my writing.		Q1: 70% Q2: 90%	Q1: 30% Q2: 10%	

Q1 = Questionnaire 1, administered before the learning activities Q2 = Questionnaire 2, administered after the learning activities from a word processing package like Microsoft Word. The former group of students held a more positive view of the wiki regarding their grammar, and although sometimes they had felt rushed, with insufficient time to revise and carefully proofread together, these students believed that their partners were able to identify their mistakes and provide solutions to fix them; they therefore recognized that they had in effect two editors: the partner and the instructor.

While there was disagreement about the benefits of using the wiki in terms of improving their grammatical skills, all the students agreed that it helped them improve the content of their writing. Students found that the wiki allowed them to see both their errors and accuracies. An almost unanimous comment was that the wiki-based collaboration allowed students to share and receive ideas from their partners that they would otherwise never have considered. Some students remarked that their partners were able to challenge their thoughts and bring up new points and concepts that they had previously ignored.

Opinions were divided regarding the usefulness of working collaboratively on the wiki to improve writing organization. Half of the students believed that working together in this way helped them observe the positive and negative aspects of their writing, and that it forced them to construct a more detailed outline as part of the planning process. Some students created an outline together before they commenced their writing, and then divided the work between them, developing different paragraphs or ideas on their wiki pages. Two of the students strongly affirmed the usefulness of the wiki in that they felt their partners helped them significantly with their essay organization, thus leading them to change and improve the structure of their composition.

Regarding the written and voice chat, students perceived these tools as a good way to exchange ideas quickly and easily, despite some of them having to overcome technical problems with the voice chat, in particular. In evaluating the use of the written and voice chat for grammar improvement, most of the students felt that when using these tools they were not particularly concerned with grammar. They did feel, however, that the tools allowed them to expand the content of their writing. By communicating via voice or written chat, students were able to discuss the overall direction of the essay, pool and combine their thoughts, and come up with better ideas. The majority of the students also discovered that these tools were instrumental in helping with the organization of the essay—in fact, they arguably supplied the best form of help in this regard. Some students remarked that after discussing the organization and delegating subtasks, they finally produced a more clearly structured essay. Other students felt that although the use of chat assisted them in organizing the overall structure of the essay, it did not help with local revisions. There were also some students who reported that disagreements between them during the chat sessions prolonged the time needed to decide on the organization.

DISCUSSION AND RECOMMENDATIONS

The main purpose of the study was to explore the potential of Web 2.0 tools, in particular wikis, used in conjunction with chat, to support collaboration and improve students' writing skills in the Spanish FL domain. The quantitative and qualitative analyses of the wiki drafts, chat transcripts, and questionnaire responses suggest that the media-rich environment that was created did in fact help students construct knowledge about FL writing (i.e., aspects of the FL language and FL composing processes) and improve their skills in this area. The wikis acted like virtual meeting arenas, allowing students to participate actively and productively in collaborative writing activities. It was also true that, when employed in tandem, wikis and chat aided different aspects of students' writing, facilitating the provision of assistance and peer support in various ways during the completion of the task. The implementation of wikis for FL writing in tertiary education is likely to become more widespread and successful as students at large become better accustomed to the use of Web 2.0 applications in an academic context. As this occurs, it is important that in line with Pedagogy 2.0 principles, learning activities are designed that incorporate appropriate scaffolding, and that engage students in ways that promote critical thinking (Elgort et al., 2008).

The results of the questionnaires demonstrate that, despite encountering some technological problems, students found the combination of writing collaboratively with classmates using the wikis and conversing via voice/written chat to be helpful and effective. The negative comments appearing in the questionnaire data often related to factors extrinsic to the collaborative process, such as difficulty in scheduling meeting times, technical issues with the voice chat, or the inability of the wiki to highlight spelling errors. Although some students still see a need to work individually on occasion, and despite technological caveats, which can indeed adversely affect any collaborative endeavor, students' reflections generally showed that a majority used the capabilities of the wiki and the chat tools successfully, appreciating and enjoying the collaborative and communicative aspects (see Tutty & Martin, 2009). Through the wikis and chat, students, working in their pairs, modified and improved each other's outputs, combined ideas, and organized their essays, while accommodating and taking into consideration their partners' writing. Students treated the wikis and chat as both physical and virtual spaces where they could write and where knowledge was constructed.

Yet, some students did not appear to take full advantage of the flexibility that the wiki brings to the writing process. One of the benefits of wiki use is that, from the comfort of their homes or elsewhere, students can share their work with partners on a document that is constantly updated. However, a few students' comments as found in the questionnaire responses and chat transcripts indicated that they sometimes preferred to meet in the University's language lab to work on their writing assignments. Another advantage of wikis was not always used to its full potential by student pairs: when writing directly in the wiki, both students are able to read each other's writing and respond accordingly, which results in more meaningful collaboration; however, a few students constructed the different parts of their essays individually, in a Word document, and then "copied and pasted" into the wikis. This highlights the need for adequate training to show students how to use wikis effectively and appropriately for collaborative writing. Such training could include examples of collaborative FL writing practices to illustrate how students interact, negotiate, and co-construct knowledge during a task to create a dynamic community of writers.

Notwithstanding the fact that students did not always take full advantage of the wiki's features and affordances, their collaborative processes were observed in the different uses they made of the wikis and chat facilities when approaching the writing task. The results of the study suggest that the students did take control and assume responsibility for their own learning. The students themselves decided how and when to engage in personally meaningful tasks. The wikis and chat, through the inclusion of communication, dialogue, and shared activity, provided the impetus for an inquiry-based approach and collaboration among participants. First, using the chat, students worked together to present a clear thesis in the introduction, to obtain adequate supporting evidence, and to organize the essay in accordance with a pre-established genre (i.e., argumentative). Second, students worked individually when researching about the content, writing their assigned parts on the wikis, often adding paragraphs without much initial connection between them, and attending to grammatical issues. Third, via chat, students reconsidered their ideas and then manipulated them in the wikis until the two opposing positions of the argument began to take shape and materialize. It was at this stage of deliberation and revision that students brought cohesiveness and coherence to their essay, and then paid more attention to grammatical aspects. Fourth, students revised their work, often individually, on the wiki pages. Therefore, contrary to a more traditional perspective of FL writers' revision processes, which generally tend to address local problems (grammatical accuracy) rather than global (content and organization), the participants in this study concentrated on global issues first and grammar issues later. Prioritizing global problems over local ones illustrates clearly the impact of the Web 2.0 tools on the students' writing practices. Becoming a good writer, regardless of use of L1 or L2, means that students should be able to observe the task from a strategic, overall or global perspective and see writing as a multifaceted, iterative process. A significant aspect of their collaborative work is that students in this study were able to move beyond their ordinary practices by co-creating and editing joint writing artifacts. Thus, incorporating wikis and chat in FL courses has the potential to help student writers negotiate both the content and the manner in which it is expressed, becoming better critical evaluators or judges of their work and scaffolding the task for each other along the way.

The collaborative work of student pairs often resembled a piecemeal design in which the different pieces were woven together through the two writers' common efforts during the chat sessions. In spite of certain commonalities in the use of wikis and chat, students demonstrated distinct features and patterns in terms of the ways in which they collaborated. Some pairs approached this social practice by attempting to jointly address most aspects of the essay, whereas others felt more comfortable meeting less frequently and using their synchronous sessions to target only specific issues (e.g., title, main thesis, or sources). Possible reasons for the different attitudes towards the task appear to be related to students' personal characteristics (e.g., politeness, work ethic, assertiveness), L2 proficiency, writing ability, and scheduling (i.e., finding the time to set up their chat sessions). Moreover, the different approaches to the task appear to be related to students' individual preferences and concerns. For example, during the sessions some students forced their partners to focus on areas that were connected to prior class instruction as a means to improve their essays. In their repeated and meaningful negotiations they drew on their personal opinions and knowledge both of the essay topic and of writing methodology, in order to progress towards completion of the task. Furthermore, students' interactions during the activities in the study resembled other practices observed in the classroom, but in the absence of instructor intervention. In this learner-centered environment, students took control over their own writing, and collaboratively gained new experiences of and insights into the FL writing process.

Clearly, the collaborative writing processes involved in revising the drafts spawned more focused revisions. Although it was initially disappointing to learn that the statistical analysis of the essays in terms of fluency, accuracy, and syntactic complexity did not yield any significant differences, this may possibly be attributed to several constraints related to the design and nature of the assignment. First, the imposition of a word limit (500 words) restricted the length of the text and number of T-units produced in the final draft. Second, although students were able to correct and revise the first draft, they were also adding new content/information when producing the final draft, and in doing so introduced new problems. Still, despite these changes, students did not produce more grammatical errors than those occurring in the first draft. Third, the provision of only one week between the first turn-in draft and the final turn-in draft allowed for only a relatively short time in which to see improvements in the students' writing complexity (Elola, 2005). More evidently, students did demonstrate overall improvement in the final drafts in relation to content (which became much more detailed) and organization. Although it is arguable as to whether the written products were reflective of and aligned with the maximum capabilities of the students, the final essay drafts showed indications of deeper exploration and examination of their theses. Detailed inspection of the wiki drafts and chat transcripts revealed that most instructor feedback (e.g., regarding grammatical issues, content, and organization) had been addressed and corrected, and redundant text had been modified or deleted as needed. To maximize the likelihood of contributing to significant improvements in students' writing, FL courses should integrate technological applications in ways that allow students to grow as writers in a systematic, progressive manner. Steps should be taken to ensure that collaborative work is not an isolated practice, and becomes an integral part of the FL curriculum.

CHALLENGES AND FUTURE TRENDS

There is no doubt that Web 2.0 applications will increasingly be used in tertiary teaching. To ensure that their adoption does not follow erratic and halting patterns (Lamb, 2004), there is a need for studies that examine the extent to which these emergent technologies support the educational process, and to identify the ways in which they can best be used to enhance student learning. The present chapter has shed some light on how wikis, in particular, can be used in the domain of FL writing. There remain many questions and concerns, however, including those pertaining to the role of the instructor, the notion of authorship, and assessment of student participation in collaborative writing.

The innovative use of wikis and chat to support students' collaborative writing processes as seen in the study discussed in this chapter is representative of the shift from teacher-centered to learner-centered pedagogies, and brings into focus the principles of Pedagogy 2.0, along with its implications for the role of the instructor (see Chapter 2 in this book). It is clear that the instructor must take full advantage of the possibilities that Web 2.0 technologies bring to the tertiary classroom, to engage students as active producers of ideas and knowledge as opposed to them merely being passive consumers or recipients of transmitted information (McGee & Diaz, 2007). In order for the promise of Web 2.0 applications for education to be fully realized, instructors need to constantly assess the value of technological tools and their supporting functions. They need to consider the contemporary range of teaching and learning strategies and experiences, and identify those applications that best suit the chosen instructional and learning practices (see Chapter 21 in this book). Equally important is the need for instructors to convey to learners the value of Web 2.0 applications in an educational context, and to assist them in using the tools for learning in ways that transcend socialization (albeit embedded in a social context), so that they collaborate effectively to expand their individual and collective knowledge (see Chapters 6 and 7 in this book).

As illustrated in Wikipedia, the educational uses of group- or pair-written wikis imply a redefinition of the notion of authorship (Thorne, 2008). Although different from wikis that are open to the general public on the Internet, in which there is no distinction between "author" and "audience" since any reader can become a potential author (Thorne), educationally contextualized wikis are understood as spaces in which individual contributions are merged, leading to a final product where the whole is greater than the sum of its parts. Embracing Web 2.0 applications to their full extent implies acknowledging and accepting the social, collaborative aspects of learning amplified to a new level in which groups become the new author. Finally, despite the potential and increasing use of wikis, their rules and norms are still emergent and subject to constant scrutiny and revision. In conjunction with research that investigates students' use of this medium for group work, studies are also required that examine student performance and ways of assessing it fairly and reliably (Trentin, 2009).

CONCLUSION

It is hoped that the present study, together with the numerous other studies and examples included throughout this book, will make a contribution to the burgeoning research in Web 2.0 applications. This chapter has focused specifically on the use of wikis and chat in the FL classroom at a university level. The aim of the reported study was to observe and document the ways in and extent to which students' knowledge about and skills in Spanish writing benefited from the adopted tools and learning design. The overall picture emerging from the data illustrates that students did benefit from their negotiations and interactions. In general, the students' conversations allowed them to reflect on their writing processes (i.e., planning, generating, and organizing ideas) and critically consider the ways in which they could express created content in their FL, advancing their mastery of grammar, vocabulary, and style. Even though statistical differences in accuracy, fluency, and syntactic complexity were not apparent, possibly due at least in part to the short period of time between drafts, students acknowledged, in their questionnaire responses, that the wiki and chat tools had helped them to better grasp the material and the writing/learning process. While close examination of wiki drafts and chat revealed more detailed essay content and better organization of ideas, there is also scope to apply other measures to gain a more accurate picture of the intricate interchange taking place between students as they collaborate.

While the results are encouraging overall, and both students and instructor saw the benefits of using wikis as a collaborative tool, this study did have several limitations, including the small number of participants, the examination of only one writing task, the word count restriction, the short period of time between turned-in drafts, and the lack of comparison with individual writing assignments. The results, therefore, cannot be generalized. However, analysis of the data provides a valuable perspective on how the participants used wikis and chat; it gives insight into how these can impact on students' FL writing while composing an argumentative essay.

Through the creative and innovative use of Web 2.0 and social software, the writing process can be transformed from an individual act to an intensely social, collaborative activity, enabling and encouraging student interactions around content, organization, and, perhaps to a lesser extent, grammar. This fits well with a curricular shift towards a student-centered approach within a constructivist or social constructivist framework. New pedagogical insights such as those offered by Pedagogy 2.0 will inform us further about novel ways in which to use Web 2.0 to foster collaborative work and learning, leading to a better understanding and awareness of the benefits and possibilities presented for FL education.

REFERENCES

Alexander, B. (2006). Web 2.0: A new wave of innovation for teaching and learning? *EDUCAUSE Review, 41*(2), 33–44. Retrieved June 5, 2008, from http://www.educause.edu/ir/library/pdf/ERM0621.pdf

Augar, N., Raitman, R., & Zhou, W. (2004). Teaching and learning online with wikis. In R. Atkinson, C. McBeath, D. Jonas-Dwyer, & R. Phillips (Eds.), *Beyond the comfort zone: Proceedings of the 21st Australasian Society for Computers in Learning in Tertiary Education (ASCILITE) Conference* (pp. 95–104). Perth, Australia: The University of Western Australia. Retrieved February 10, 2008, from http://www.ascilite.org.au/conferences/perth04/procs/augar.html

Brown, S., & Adler, R. P. (2008). Minds on fire: Open education, the long tail, and Learning 2.0. *EDUCAUSE Review, 43*(1), 16–32. Retrieved February 10, 2008, from http://net.educause.edu/ir/library/pdf/ERM0811.pdf

Byron, M. (2005). Teaching with Tiki. *Teaching Philosophy*, *28*(2), 108–113.

Chang, Y.-F., & Schallert, D. L. (2005). The design for a collaborative system of English as foreign language composition writing of senior high school students in Taiwan. In P. Goodyear, D. Sampson, D. J.-T. Yang, Kinshuk, T. Okamoto, R. Hartley, & N.-S. Chen (Eds.), *Proceedings of the Fifth IEEE International Conference on Advanced Learning Technologies* (pp. 774–775). Los Alamitos, CA: IEEE Computer Society.

de Guerrero, M. C. M., & Villamil, O. S. (2000). Activating the ZPD: Mutual scaffolding in L2 peer revision. *Modern Language Journal*, *84*(1), 51–68. doi:10.1111/0026-7902.00052

DiCamilla, F., & Antón, M. (1997). Repetition in the collaborative discourse of L2 learners: A Vygotskian perspective. *Canadian Modern Language Review*, *53*(4), 609–633.

Donato, R. (1994). Collective scaffolding on second language learning. In Lantolf, J., & Appel, G. (Eds.), *Vygotskian approaches to second language research* (pp. 33–56). Westport, CT: Ablex.

Ede, L., & Lunsford, A. (1990). *Singular texts / plural authors*. Carbondale, IL: Southern Illinois University Press.

Elgort, I., Smith, A. G., & Toland, J. (2008). Is wiki an effective platform for group work? *Australian Journal of Educational Technology, 24*(2), 189–210. Retrieved June 5, 2008, from http://www.ascilite.org.au/ajet/ajet24/elgort.pdf

Elola, I. (2005). *The complexity of revision in an intermediate-level Spanish language classroom and the creation of a foreign language revision model*. Unpublished Ph.D. dissertation, The University of Iowa, Iowa City, IA.

Farabaugh, P., Farabaugh, R., & Freeland, S. (2005, November 7). *Using wikis in teaching and learning*. Workshop delivered as part of the University of Maryland Baltimore Country Teaching, Learning and Technology Brown Bag workshop series, Baltimore, MD. Retrieved June 5, 2008, from http://www.umbc.edu/studio/videos/qtdetail?ID=380

Farabaugh, R. (2007). "The isle is full of noises": Using wiki software to establish a discourse community in a Shakespeare classroom. *Language Awareness*, *16*(1), 41–56. doi:10.2167/la428.0

Forte, A., & Bruckman, A. (2006). From Wikipedia to the classroom: Exploring online publication and learning. In S. A. Barab, K. E. Hay, & D. T. Hickey (Eds.), *Proceedings of the Seventh International Conference on Learning Sciences* (pp. 182–188). Atlanta, GA: International Society of the Learning Sciences.

Godwin-Jones, R. (2003). Blogs and wikis: Environments for on-line collaboration. *Language Learning & Technology, 7*(2), 12–16. Retrieved January 10, 2008, from http://llt.msu.edu/vol-7num2/pdf/emerging.pdf

Hirvela, A. (1999). Collaborative writing: Instruction and communities of readers and writers. *TESOL Journal*, *8*(2), 7–12.

Hodgkinson-Williams, C., Slay, H., & Siebörger, I. (2008). Developing communities of practice within and outside higher education institutions. *British Journal of Educational Technology*, *39*(3), 433–442. doi:10.1111/j.1467-8535.2008.00841.x

Honegger, B. D. (2005). Wikis—a rapidly growing phenomenon in the German-speaking school community. In D. Riehle (Ed.), *Proceedings of the 2005 International Symposium on Wikis* (pp. 113–116). New York: Association for Computing Machinery. Retrieved June 6, 2008, from http://www.wikisym.org/ws2005/proceedings/paper-10.pdf

Kost, C. (2007, May 24–26). *Using wikis for a collaborative writing project*. Paper presented at the Computer Assisted Language Instruction Consortium (CALICO) Conference, San Marcos, TX.

Lamb, B. (2004). Wide open spaces: Wikis, ready or not. *EDUCAUSE Review, 39*(5), 36–46. Retrieved November 30, 2007, from http://www.educause.edu/ir/library/pdf/erm0452.pdf

Lindblom-Ylänne, S., & Pihlajamäki, H. (2003). Can a collaborative network environment enhance essay-writing processes? *British Journal of Educational Technology*, *34*(1), 17–30. doi:10.1111/1467-8535.00301

Long, M. H. (1991). *Measuring classroom language change*. Unpublished manuscript, University of Hawai`i, Manoa, HI.

Mayer, R. E. (1998). Cognitive theory for education: What teachers need to know. In Lambert, N. M., & McCombs, B. L. (Eds.), *How students learn: Reforming schools through learner-centered education* (pp. 353–377). Washington, DC: American Psychological Association. doi:10.1037/10258-013

McGee, P., & Diaz, V. (2007). Wikis and podcasts and blogs! Oh, my! What is a faculty member supposed to do? *EDUCAUSE Review, 42*(5), 28–41. Retrieved November 30, 2007, from http://www.educause.edu/ir/library/pdf/erm0452.pdf

McLoughlin, C., & Lee, M. J. W. (2007). Social software and participatory learning: Pedagogical choices with technology affordances in the Web 2.0 era. In *ICT: Providing choices for learners and learning. Proceedings of the 24th Australasian Society for Computers in Learning in Tertiary Education (ASCILITE) Conference* (pp. 664–675). Singapore: Nanyang Technological University. Retrieved June 6, 2008, from http://www.ascilite.org.au/conferences/singapore07/procs/mcloughlin.pdf

McLoughlin, C., & Lee, M. J. W. (2008). Future learning landscapes: Transforming pedagogy through social software. *Innovate: Journal of Online Education, 4*(5). Retrieved July 6, 2008, from http://www.innovateonline.info/index.php?view=article&id=539.

Miers, J. (2004). *BELTS or braces?* Retrieved June 5, 2007, from http://www.tsof.edu.au/research/Reports04/miers.asp

Murray, D. E. (1992). Collaborative learning as literary event: Implications for ESL instruction. In Nunan, D. (Ed.), *Collaborative language learning and teaching* (pp. 100–117). Cambridge, UK: Cambridge University Press.

O'Reilly, T. (2005). *What is Web 2.0: Design patterns and business models for the next generation of software*. Retrieved May 30, 2008, from http://www.oreillynet.com/pub/a/oreilly/tim/news/2005/09/30/what-is-web-20.html

Parker, K. R., & Chao, J. T. (2007). Wiki as a teaching tool. *Interdisciplinary Journal of Knowledge and Learning Objects, 3*, 57–72. Retrieved May 30, 2008, from http://www.ijello.org/Volume3/IJKLOv3p057-072Parker284.pdf

Rick, J., Guzdial, M., Carroll, K., Holloway-Attaway, L., & Walker, B. (2002). Collaborative learning at low cost: CoWeb use in English composition. In G. Stahl (Ed.), *Proceedings of the Conference on Computer Support for Collaborative Learning: Foundations for a CSCL Community* (pp. 435–442). Atlanta, GA: International Society of the Learning Sciences.

Schaffert, S., Bischof, D., Buerger, T., Gruber, A., Hilzensauer, W., & Schaffert, S. (2006). Learning with semantic wikis. In M. Völkel & S. Schaffert (Eds.), *Proceedings of the First Workshop on Semantic Wikis: From wiki to semantics* (pp. 109–123). Aachen, Germany: Informatik V, RWTH Aachen University. Retrieved June 5, 2007, from http://sunsite.informatik.rwth-aachen.de/Publications/CEUR-WS/Vol-206/paper9.pdf

Schneider, M. L. (1990). Collaborative learning: A concept in search of a definition. *Issues in Writing, 3*(1), 26–39.

Storch, N. (2005). Collaborative writing: Product, process, and students' reflections. *Journal of Second Language Writing, 14*(3), 153–173. doi:10.1016/j.jslw.2005.05.002

Swain, M., & Lapkin, S. (1998). Interaction and second language learning: Two adolescent French immersion students working together. *Modern Language Journal, 82*(3), 320–337. doi:10.2307/329959

Thorne, S. L. (2008). Mediating technologies and second language learning. In Coiro, J., Knobel, M., Lankshear, C., & Leu, D. J. (Eds.), *Handbook of research on new literacies* (pp. 417–449). Mahwah, NJ: Lawrence Erlbaum.

Thorne, S. L., & Payne, S. (2005). Evolutionary trajectories, Internet-mediated expression, and language education. *CALICO Journal, 22*(3), 371–397. Retrieved February 10, 2008, from https://calico.org/html/article_137.pdf

Trentin, G. (2009). Using a wiki to evaluate individual contribution to a collaborative learning project. *Journal of Computer Assisted Learning, 25*(1), 43–55. doi:10.1111/j.1365-2729.2008.00276.x

Tsinakos, A. A. (2006). Collaborative student modeling: A new perspective using wiki. *WSEAS Transactions on Advances in Engineering Education, 6*(3), 475–481.

Tutty, J. I., & Martin, F. (2009). User generated design: Teaching and learning with Web 2.0. In Kidd, T. T., & Chen, I. L. (Eds.), *Wired for learning: An educator's guide to Web 2.0* (pp. 43–58). Charlotte, NC: Information Age.

University of Maryland Baltimore County. (n. d.). *Student use of Voice Direct*. Retrieved June 5, 2008, from http://www.umbc.edu/oit/newmedia/blackboard/help/VoiceDirect_student.pdf

Villamil, O. S., & de Guerrero, M. C. M. (1996). Peer revision in the L2 classroom: Social-cognitive activities, mediating strategies, and aspects of social behavior. *Journal of Second Language Writing, 5*(1), 51–75. doi:10.1016/S1060-3743(96)90015-6

Villamil, O. S., & de Guerrero, M. C. M. (1998). Assessing the impact of peer revision on L2 writing. *Applied Linguistics, 19*(4), 491–514. doi:10.1093/applin/19.4.491

Wang, H.-C., Lu, C.-H., Yang, J.-Y., Hu, H.-W., Chiou, G.-F., Chiang, Y.-T., & Hsu, W.-L. (2005). An empirical exploration of using wiki in an English as a second language course. In P. Goodyear, D. Sampson, D. J.-T. Yang, Kinshuk, T. Okamoto, R. Hartley, & N.-S. Chen (Eds.), *Proceedings of the Fifth IEEE International Conference on Advanced Learning Technologies* (pp. 155–157). Los Alamitos, CA: IEEE Computer Society.

KEY TERMS AND DEFINITIONS

Chat: Written or oral computer mediated communication that occurs synchronously (i.e., in real time).

Collaborative Writing: Two or more people working together to produce a text, with joint responsibility for the final product.

Constructivism: A psychological theory of knowledge that focuses on how we learn rather than on what we learn.

FL Education: Foreign language education. Education that focuses on the teaching and learning of foreign languages.

L1 Writing: Writing in the learner's first language.

L2 Writing: Writing in the learner's second language.

Pedagogy 2.0: A pedagogical model or framework proposed by McLoughlin and Lee (2007, 2008; see also Chapter 3 in this book) that is partly inspired by and based on the principles of Web 2.0. It advocates the use of technology to support the interdependence between ideas, individuals, communities, and information networks.

Web 2.0: A term that refers to a second generation (or apparent second generation) of web-based services such as social networking sites, blogs, wikis, and folksonomies, which emphasize online collaboration, sharing, and content generation by users.

Wikis: A website in which potentially anyone can add, remove, and edit available content. These features make wikis an effective tool for collaborative authoring.

APPENDIX A. CHAT CATEGORIES

Categories	Percentages
Negotiating the content of the essay	23.00%
Showing agreement	13.60%
Organization of the essay	8.80%
Asking for an opinion	6.47%
Planning task	5.00%
Mentioning sources	3.80%
Mentioning the instructor/instruction	3.80%
Negotiating the structure of the essay	3.70%
Dividing their work	3.30%
Asking for specific feedback	3.00%
Feeling confusion	3.00%
Grammar	3.00%
Use of politeness	2.50%
Supporting evidence	2.32%
Reference to previous work (in class, email)	1.90%
Using phone/email for communication	1.60%
Planning time for completing the work	1.58%
Greetings	1.50%
Negotiating style	1.50%
Mentioning the wiki	1.33%
Awareness of the reader	1.00%
Technical problems	0.73%
Connecting to voice chat	0.70%
Using English	0.70%
Having problems with the assignment	0.50%
Creating a working environment	0.36%
Negotiating vocabulary	0.36%
Checking their own work	0.24%
Expressing anger	0.24%
Getting lost in the task	0.24%
Getting on track with the task	0.24%
Disagreeing	0.12%
Issues of self-esteem	0.12%
Setting time for the sessions	0.12%
Total	100.00%

Chapter 12
Podcasting in Distance Learning:
True Pedagogical Innovation or Just More of the Same?

Mark J. W. Lee
Charles Sturt University, Australia

Catherine McLoughlin
Australian Catholic University, Australia

Belinda Tynan
University of New England, Australia

ABSTRACT

This chapter explores how podcasting can be used to support and enhance the student experience, with a focus on tertiary-level distance education contexts. It begins with a review of the rationale behind the use of podcasting and digital audio for distance teaching and learning, including a consideration of the unique features and attributes of podcasting that differentiate it from older or pre-existing educational technologies. The authors then showcase a number of examples involving the use of podcasting in distance e-learning and blended learning, drawn from the exemplary practices of educators across the globe. Discussion of these exemplars centers around four major themes: increasing learner motivation and engagement; facilitating and enhancing learning outcomes; impacting on mobility and lifestyle learning; and fostering a sense of community, with the aim of contributing to the establishment of an evidence-based case about the benefits of podcasting in relation to addressing the needs of distance education students, as well as illuminating some of the problems and barriers that exist. The chapter concludes with a number of recommendations for distance educators.

DOI: 10.4018/978-1-60566-294-7.ch012

INTRODUCTION

Podcasting, alongside other Web 2.0 tools and technologies, is attracting intense interest and investment from administrators and teachers at universities and colleges worldwide. In the field of distance learning, the use of podcasting as a distribution mechanism for digital audio content is believed by educators, for example, to hold tremendous potential to assist in addressing many of the issues and challenges traditionally faced by students studying remotely from their instructors and classmates (Lee & Chan, 2007; Essex, 2006).

The main focus of this chapter is on how podcasting can be used and is being used by tertiary educators to support and enhance teaching and learning in a range of distance education and hybrid or blended contexts. Applications of the technology, as well as claims that have been made about the unique learning benefits afforded, are critically examined, while keeping in perspective other audio-based technologies and tools that have been used in distance education for several decades. The authors present a number of international exemplars from the literature involving the use of podcasting in distance and blended learning, and discuss a number of prominent themes pertaining to the potential, problems, and pitfalls of educational podcasting, before proposing a framework to guide the design of educational podcasts and podcast-based learning activities.

BACKGROUND: THE USE OF AUDIO TECHNOLOGIES IN DISTANCE LEARNING

Amid the current excitement and hype, Schlosser and Burmeister (2006) remind us that "The use of audio in education is not new, but is experiencing a renaissance fuelled by the ubiquity of portable audio players, broadband Internet, and software tools that allow the relatively easy creation and distribution of audio files" (sec. 2, para. 1). Research in open, flexible, and distance learning pre-dating the World Wide Web showed that "As compared with a written text, the spoken word can influence both cognition (adding clarity and meaning) and motivation (by conveying directly a sense of the person creating those words)" (Durbridge, 1984), which presents many valuable affordances for teaching at a distance. With the advent of web-based virtual learning environments (VLEs) in the 1990s, however, there appears to have been a regression into focusing on text-based modes of presentation and communication, using course web pages, email, discussion boards, and chat (Barnes, 1995).

Radio has been used in distance education for many decades, arguably since its early beginnings in mail/post-based "correspondence courses" (Bates, 1981). In combination with tutorials, print materials, local listening groups, and face-to-face meetings, it has been used to teach a wide range of subjects at various levels. Audiocassette tapes, and more recently, compact discs (CDs), have been used as a solution where the ephemeral nature and fixed transmission times characteristic of radio broadcasts (World Bank, 2000) pose a problem, where learners are geographically spread over too large an area, or where radio air time is simply not readily available. Learners see cassettes and CDs as more personal and informal than radio, and cassettes have also been found to be more appropriate than radio for controlled, didactic teaching (Power, 1990, citing Bates, 1981). Kates (1998) proposes the use of voice recordings, distributed on audiotape cassette, to provide feedback to students on their assignments, and discusses the benefits of this method over the traditional, written form.

Laaser (1986, "Introduction," para. 1) summarizes the advantages of using audiocassettes in distance education as follows:

- they can be produced with variable duration (playing time);

- they can be listened to at any time of the day;
- they allow for other activities during the listening (e.g., notetaking, carrying out experiments);
- they can be dispatched easily together with print material;
- they can be addressed directly to the individual student;
- the required equipment is usually easily accessible to students;
- cassettes can be repeated or interrupted at any time;
- control of production on behalf of the distance educator is easy, and requires relatively little technical knowledge;
- production and duplication are inexpensive and not very time consuming.

Podcasting offers "the best of both worlds" by combining the benefits of the broadcast nature of radio with the flexibility, learner control, and personalization made possible by audio recorded on audiocassettes and CDs.

WHAT ARE THE UNIQUE BENEFITS OF PODCASTING FOR DISTANCE LEARNING?

The Scottish Council for Educational Technology (SCET, 1994) provides a useful outline of the relative strengths and weaknesses of audio technologies for learning and teaching (Table 1). Audio has been found to be an extremely powerful medium for conveying feelings, attitudes, and atmosphere. It is also excellent for conveying general opinions and arguments. The shortcomings of this format appear to fall primarily in its unsuitability as a sole medium for imparting detailed or complex information that needs to be heavily processed and/or logically deconstructed, for providing facts and figures that need to be committed to memory, and for presenting learning material that otherwise requires a high level of mental concentration.

Although the SCET's focus at the time of writing was primarily on audiotapes, the strengths and weaknesses identified also seem to apply to newer digital audio media such as podcasts. With the above in mind, Lee (2007) asks the question, "What's new?," in relation to the use of podcasting in education and training. In other words,

Table 1. Strengths and weaknesses of educational audio (SCET, 1994)

Strengths of audio	Weaknesses of audio
• The equipment is cheap and robust. It is also widespread and familiar. • Audiotapes are easy, quick, and cheap to produce and update. As a result there is a high degree of author control. Tapes are also cheap to distribute and store. • They are interesting, personal, and intimate. They can be used to provide human contact and advice. • They can be used to incorporate sounds and music and can be a powerful stimulus to the imagination. • They can be used more effectively than print to talk learners through a passage and to document discussions, case studies, and language pronunciation at work. • They are convenient to use. There is a large degree of learner control. • They can be recorded on by the learner and returned to the tutor to provide feedback.	• Access to a player is necessary, restricting portability. • Complex branching and routing is difficult. • The information conveyed is intangible and, as a result, learners require concentration to absorb facts. • It is difficult to absorb complex information, e.g. a logical argument may be hard to follow and will need confirmation from print or another visual medium for maximum effect. • It can be difficult to find the relevant point of a tape. They cannot necessarily be used everywhere without headphones, e.g. in a library.

he highlights the need to carefully consider the distinct pedagogical capabilities and advantages that accrue from the use of podcasting that were not previously available with other, more mature predecessor technologies. The aforementioned psycho-acoustic benefits clearly have been possible with technologies that have been available for many years; additionally, perhaps due to the media popularization of the term "podcast," (see for example, Oxford University Press, 2005; Skiba, 2006; Pollock, 2006) many people tend to use it extremely loosely to refer to any MPEG Layer 3 (MP3)-based audio recording that can be transferred to and consumed on a portable playback device such as Apple's iPod. One definition that remains true and accurate to the use of the word by its originator, Adam Curry (2004), is that given by Dixon and Greeson (2006), who list three key features of podcasting:

1. It uses *file-based downloads*. Unlike with streaming media (in which the media content is played while it downloads), podcast files are downloaded in their entirety before playback commences.
2. It is *subscription based*. Podcasting is based on Really Simple Syndication (RSS), a technical standard or format used to publish feeds of text data summarizing the content of frequently-updated websites. The user configures a software application called an aggregator to periodically poll one or more feeds for updates and deliver new content to his or her desktop. Podcasting involves the use of a feature of RSS version 2.0 (RSS Advisory Board, 2005) known as enclosures. This feature allows feeds to contain URL references to media files (e.g., MP3 files) that are to be automatically downloaded by the aggregator, which in this case is called a "podcatcher."
3. The content may be consumed on *portable devices*, such as dedicated music players (including but not limited to iPods), as well as a variety of mobile phones and personal digital assistants (PDAs) with MP3 playback capabilities. This presents fertile opportunities for mobile learning (m-learning).

The file- and subscription-based download processes used in podcasting made possible by RSS have much to offer in the way of simplicity, convenience, and time savings for busy distance learners, since with these processes in place, they do not have to laboriously search a plethora of sites for relevant content, nor is there a need for them to engage in the even more tedious process of continually monitoring these sites for updates. As new podcast files become available on the user's subscribed feeds, they are automatically downloaded, with no user intervention beyond the initial configuration of the podcatcher software. By having a computer continuously connected to the Internet, the content can be "dripped in" and made available when ready, so that the "click and wait" situation commonly experienced in streaming is effectively eliminated, even over slow connections (Curry, 2004).

In line with the third point above, following the download of podcast files to the user's computer, they can optionally be transferred to a portable device for listening "on the move." For the millennial distance learner, learning is combined with a myriad of other activities in his or her personal and/or professional life. While the mobility aspects are not entirely novel or unique to podcasting, given the fact that portable audio devices like the Walkman and Discman became commercially available many years ago, the large built-in storage capacities of modern portable electronic devices now permit learners to carry substantial personal "libraries" of digital media content in their pockets for spontaneous and convenient access while on the move, or for "just-in-time" learning in preparation for a task in the workplace or in the field. These devices also represent a technological advance over their predecessors in terms of their decreasing weights and sizes. It is noteworthy at this point that although the portability of other digital forms of media is becoming increasingly viable with portable video players, handheld gaming consoles, 3G mobile phones, and smart phones, with these media types, true mobility is severely restricted due to the need for visual fixation on a screen. This is not the case with listening to audio podcasts, which "frees eyes and hands" (Clark & Walsh, 2004, p. 8) to concurrently perform other physical tasks.

INTERNATIONAL EXEMPLARS OF PODCASTING IN DISTANCE LEARNING

Table 2 presents a number of exemplars of the use of podcasting in distance and blended contexts at higher education institutions worldwide. In the subsections that follow, the various examples are examined through the lens of four major themes that emerged from an analysis of two institutional case studies involving the use of podcasting to support distance learning in Australia (see Lee & Tynan, 2008): increasing learner motivation and engagement; facilitating and enhancing learning outcomes; impacting on mobility and lifestyle learning; fostering a sense of community. The primary aim here is to address current and future directions of educational podcasting in distance and blended learning settings, with reference to the latest work in the field and building on this through the lens of the four aforementioned themes.

Increasing Learner Motivation and Engagement

Podcasting can be used to enable the creation of learning settings that interest and engage students studying at a distance, supporting the motivational and other affective elements of effective learning. As reported by a number of researchers (see for example Tynan & Colbran, 2006; McLoughlin, Lee, & Chan, 2007), the ability to hear what lecturers or peers are discussing can be highly motivating for distance students. Podcasts can also add variety to the distance learning experience (Schlosser & Burmeister, 2006). As such, students may be more receptive to audio than text alone; they may feel more engaged when listening to a podcast as opposed to consuming material delivered solely in the form of printed or online readings. This is especially the case if podcasts are designed to enable students to construct their own understanding of material rather than simply commit it to memory or learn it by rote (Evans, 2008).

As was the case in many of the distance and blended learning scenarios depicted in Table 2, increased engagement with the topic at hand through multiple modalities and perspectives is often perceived by students as one of the key motivating aspects of listening to instructor-supplied educational podcasts. However, podcast creation by students for sharing with peers and a wider Internet audience can also yield considerable learning benefits, and this type of application is congruent with the philosophy and ethos of Web 2.0 (see Chapters 1 and 2 of this book). For example, Frydenberg (2006) tells of how students in his *IT Intensive* course at Bentley College (now Bentley University) purchase Pocket PCs instead of textbooks, which they use to explore technology concepts through an active, hands-on approach. Participants form pairs or groups and work together in a self-directed manner to plan and produce video podcasts (vodcasts). Each pair or group creates a vodcast based on one of the topics in the course schedule, for sharing with the rest of the class. This represents a novel form of peer and reciprocal teaching, and is an excellent example of how empowering students to create multimedia learner-generated content can serve as a powerful catalyst for motivation, engagement, and self-regulated learning in a blended learning setting.

Table 2. Examples of the use of podcasting in distance and blended learning

Institution	Academic discipline	Description	Salient pedagogical features	Literature reference(s)
Georgia College & State University, USA	Various	Since 2002, various courses, including a number of study abroad courses, have been "iPod enhanced" to include a diverse range of audio material ranging from lectures and audio books to language study material and music.	Blending of formal and informal learning; resource-based learning; distributed intelligence approach	Georgia College & State University, 2005
Charles Sturt University, Australia	Information Technology	First-year undergraduate students studying an introductory Information Technology unit listen to weekly talkback radio-style podcasts produced by second-year students who previously completed the unit.	Learner-centered instruction; peer and reciprocal teaching; use of podcasts to foster social presence and sense of community	Lee & Chan, 2007; McLoughlin, Lee, & Chan, 2007
Bentley College, USA	Information Technology	Students in an Information Technology course work in pairs or groups and produce vodcasts to teach topics based on the course lecture materials to their peers.	Peer teaching; reciprocal learning; learner-generated content	Frydenberg, 2006
University of New England, Australia	Law	During 2006, 1,244 students enrolled in six undergraduate Law units, including both on-campus and distance education students, began using audio podcasts of lectures as a complementary strategy for learning, alongside their printed study guides, texts, and unit websites. Many students transcribed the podcasts and used them similarly to a face-to-face lecture and took notes while listening.	Podcasts for revision and reinforcement; resource-based learning; use of podcasts to foster social presence and sense of community	Tynan & Colbran, 2006
Deakin University, Australia	Law	Senior Lecturer John Carmichael records "fireside chats," delivered as podcasts, to support a fully online course in Competition Law. Each week, he produces a 15-minute "chat" reviewing what happened in the online class for the course during the week, summarizing the key issues discussed, questions that arose, as well as relevant cases that may have appeared in the news media. The podcasts supply context and topical references to the enduring concerns of competition law, as well as assisting in the integration of learning into students' daily lives.	Contextual/ situated learning; use of podcasts as supplementary/ enrichment material; authentic learning	Carmichael, 2005; Meister, 2006
University of Leicester, UK	Engineering	Electrical Engineering students studying in blended learning mode make use of "profcasts," material designed to support learning distinct from that which is facilitated through structured on-campus or e-learning processes alone. The instructor releases weekly profcasts to supplement online teaching through updated information and guidance on the weekly activities, and to motivate students by incorporating relevant anecdotes, news items, and jokes. In addition, the podcasts are used to engage students in online activities based on Salmon's (2002) "e-tivities" model.	Active learning in a blended setting; podcasts for enrichment and extension activities; personalization of learning content	Edirisingha, Salmon, & Fothergill, 2006, 2007

continued on the following page

Table 2. continued

Institution	Academic discipline	Description	Salient pedagogical features	Literature reference(s)
Open University, UK	Modern/Foreign Languages	Students studying German and Spanish courses in distance education mode use digital voice recorders and mini camcorders to record interviews with other students and with native speakers, as well as to create audio-visual tours (podcasts and vodcasts) for sharing with their peers.	Learner-generated content; peer-to-peer learning and knowledge sharing	Kukulska-Hulme, 2005
Kingston University, UK	Engish Language and Communication	Podcasts are used as a support strategy for developing students' academic skills in a Level 1 Communication module. Six 10-minute-long podcasts are delivered via the university's Blackboard VLE on a fortnightly basis. Each podcast consists of one or more of the following: summaries of key concepts by the tutors; interviews with students; discussions and conversations on assessment tasks between students, student mentors, and tutors; hints and tips on presentation and research skills given by mentors; references to additional resources to aid the students' self-study and personal development.	Learner choice and flexibility; informal learning; access to tacit knowledge though discussions; blending of face-to-face and online learning; peer mentoring; blending of peer and instructor-led teaching and learning	Edirisingha, Rizzi, Nie, & Rothwell, 2007
University of Regina, Canada	Teacher Education	In-service student teachers studying a fully online graduate course on Information and Communication Technology Curriculum Integration are introduced to podcasting through a combination of synchronous online workshops and self-paced web tutorials. They are immersed in and experience firsthand the roles of both consumers and producers of podcasts—In addition to subscribing and listening to sample podcasts containing material pertaining to the course they are studying, they plan and produce podcasts for use in their own classroom (i.e., with their own students), and critically reflect on both the opportunities and challenges of the technology from a practical and pedagogical standpoint. Throughout the exercise, they critically reflect on their experiences by posting written comments on a class blog in response to various stimulus questions.	Use of both learner-generated and teacher-generated content	Parashar Panday & Lee, 2007
Australian Catholic University, Australia	Teacher Education	Pre-service teachers studying secondary teaching courses use podcasting and blogs to engage in peer mentoring with their classmates while undertaking their teaching practicum, during which they are assigned to geographically dispersed schools. Through their text and voice-based discourse, they share experiences, stories, and anecdotes, as well as offering support, feedback, and encouragement to one another.	Peer-to-peer e-mentoring and support; authentic/work-based learning; community of learning	McLoughlin, Brady, Lee, & Russell, 2007; McLoughlin, Lee, & Brady, 2008

Facilitating and Enhancing Learning Outcomes

Educational podcasting can assist in the achievement of discipline or subject-specific learning objectives, as well as the development of academic skills (Edirisingha, Rizzi, Nie, & Rothwell, 2007) and other generic abilities such as problem solving, teamwork, and communication (see for example Chan, Frydenberg, & Lee, 2007). The authors of many of the studies cited in Table 2 claim to have found that distance students' study habits altered due to interaction with the podcasts in their respective cases, and that the students viewed the podcasts as effective tools that were complementary to other learning resources and activities. For example, students reported using the podcasts to mentally prepare themselves for study sessions, and to supplement other activities undertaken by them in their preparation for formative and summative assessment tasks. In at least one case (Tynan & Colbran, 2006), students claimed to use the lecture podcasts to revisit ideas, and in performing the task of writing notes while listening to the podcasts explored the subject matter in different ways. Podcasts can also be used by distance students to obtain "reinforcement and backup of, and a different perspective on, information and concepts" (Lee & Chan, 2007, p. 96).

The examples individually and collectively suggest that through the use of podcasts, improved student learning outcomes may be possible. Students resoundingly acknowledge that the ability to hear what their lecturers, peers, and in some cases, subject matter experts external to the institution have to say improves their appreciation for and comprehension of the subject material. The ability of podcasting to cater to a range of learning styles and preferences has also been demonstrated, as has its ability to empower students to determine how they go about their study and what tools, strategies, and resources best support their learning. While proponents of active learning may argue that "Listening to audio is] not learning … [because it] is not synonymous with comprehension and action" (Walsh, 2004, p. 25), and although there tends to be a belief or perception that podcasting fails to cater for the needs of all but the auditory learners, strong evidence is mounting that attests to the benefits of learner-generated podcast creation (e.g., Lee, Chan, & McLoughlin, 2006b; Lee, McLoughlin, & Chan, 2008; Frydenberg, 2006; Nie, Cashmore, & Cane, 2008), as well as of designing instructional podcasts to provide supplementary or enrichment material as opposed to material intended as a substitute for lectures (e.g., Carmichael, 2005; Meister, 2006; Edirisingha, Salmon, & Fothergill, 2006, 2007). Even in teacher-driven audio podcasts, learners may be stimulated to think by being asked to respond silently to questions, make mental notes, and/or summarize. Active learning and accommodation of visual and kinesthetic/tactile learning styles, as well as of a range of multiple intelligences (Gardner, 1983, 1993, 2000; Armstrong, 1994), can also be achieved in creative and innovative ways by encouraging learners to engage in online, written, and other activities while listening or after listening to the audio. These tasks may be undertaken individually by students or collaboratively with their peers, and may call for them to refer to text-based and/or visual materials, interpret facts and make connections between those facts, transfer and apply knowledge to new situations, relate knowledge to real life, solve problems, and draw inferences (Gachuhi & Matiru, 1987; see also Edirisingha, Salmon, & Fothergill, 2006, 2007).

Mobility and Lifestyle Learning

As noted earlier, for the 21st-century distance learner, learning is often intermingled with a multitude of activities and competes with numerous other priorities and demands in his or her personal and professional life. If we accept the premise that many students who enroll in distance learning courses do so largely for reasons of convenience (Galusha, 1997), an m-learning application of the use of podcasts would seem to be a natural and logical fit. By allowing learners to consume learning content in parallel with other tasks, "iPod-learning" (Clark & Walsh, 2004) is thought to hold considerable promise in terms of paving the way for pervasive, lifestyle-integrated m-learning. In this sense, it may have the potential to cater to the unique work-style requirements of the mobile workforce, who now form a large proportion of current and potential distance learners (Yuen & Wang, 2004).

In fact, the ability for podcasting to be used as a tool to support m-learning is one of the most commonly cited reasons to justify the use of this technology in education (McGarr, 2009). However, the results of research in Australia at Charles Sturt University (Lee, Chan, & McLoughlin, 2006a; Lee & Chan, 2007), the University of Ballarat (Newnham & Miller, 2007), and the University of New England (Tynan & Colbran, 2006), as well as in the UK at the University of Southampton (Copley, 2007), the University of Leicester (Edirisingha & Salmon, 2007), and Brunel Business School (Evans, 2008) suggest that students may prefer to listen to podcasts at home using a desktop/laptop computer, and to set aside dedicated time to do so rather than multitasking their listening with other activities. These unanticipated findings should prompt researchers and practitioners to be wary of making assumptions based solely on extrapolations of how students' day-to-day uses of technology like mobile devices for work and leisure will carry over into formal learning environments and settings. (For further coverage of the intersection between Web 2.0 and m-learning in tertiary teaching, please refer to Chapter 13.)

Fostering a Sense of Community

As with other social software technologies born of the Web 2.0 era, podcasting has at its heart the ability to promote connectivity and collaboration among users. It is clear from the examples in Table 2 that well-designed learning activities involving the consumption and/or production of podcasts by students in various ways can give rise to rich forms of cooperative and collaborative learning, which have traditionally been difficult to achieve in text-based distance education. In addition, many of the examples in the table show that podcasting may form part of a practical solution to mitigate issues that result from distance learners' physical separation from their instructors, classmates, and university. This was particularly apparent in the cases at the University of New England (Tynan & Colbran, 2006) and Charles Sturt University (Lee & Chan, 2007), especially in the latter, where the talkback radio-style podcasts were used to alleviate isolation-induced anxiety experienced by distance learners.

Lee (2006) advocates the use of podcast-enhanced collaborative blogs to allow students to share their oral presentations with their instructors and peers, as well as to act as a vehicle for feedback and peer evaluation. Using such tools, it is also possible for teachers and learners to become active producers and consumers of asynchronous, voice-based discourse in an online community. In a project facilitated by McLoughlin and colleagues (McLoughlin, Brady, Lee, & Russell, 2007; McLoughlin, Lee, & Brady, 2008) at the Australian Catholic University, Canberra, pre-service teachers studying secondary teaching courses used podcasting and blogs to engage in peer mentoring with their classmates while undertaking their teaching practicum, during which they were assigned to geographically dispersed schools and thus separated from their lecturers and peers for the first time in their study program. They shared experiences, stories, and anecdotes as well as offering support, feedback, and encouragement to one another via podcasting. By engaging with one another, tuning in to each other's experiences, and sharing expertise, the student teachers became active members of an online community of learning and practice, and at the same time had opportunities to critically reflect on and refine their own skills.

Therefore, if used appropriately, podcasting can play an assistive role in "reintegrating" (Keegan, 1996) the teacher–learner transaction in distance education, as well as facilitating peer-to-peer interaction and exchange to foster a sense of belonging to and involvement in an academic learning community. Based on reported student experiences, it appears that there is considerable scope to "close the gap" for distance learners. This points to the possibilities that podcasting offers for creating an inclusive learning environment that morphs the difference between an on-campus and distance education cohort (see also Beldarrain, 2006).

Figure 1. Dimensions of planning for educational podcasting

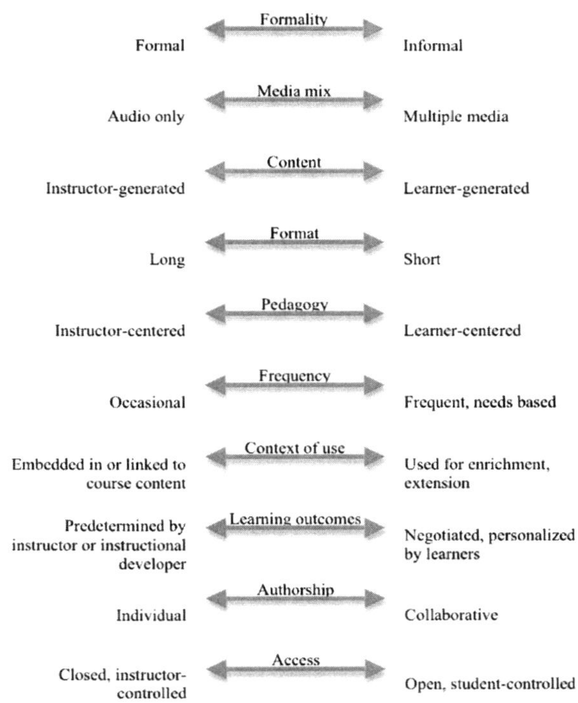

A FRAMEWORK FOR THE DESIGN OF PODCASTS TO SUPPORT DISTANCE AND BLENDED LEARNING

Figure 1, which is based partially on a model developed as part of the UK-based Informal Mobile Podcasting and Learning Adaptation (IMPALA, 2007) project, provides an overview of selected dimensions of design features of educational podcasts. It shows that multiple learning scenarios can be assembled from a range of features that form continua. The list of possibilities is endless, and the ultimate decision on which dimensions to include or exclude is influenced by learner needs, as well as by institutional and curricular priorities. These dimensions can provide a framework for the choices that distance educators and instructional designers need to make prior to embedding podcasts in their teaching.

The various dimensions may be viewed as choices that need to be made in order to generate a range of podcasts that will meet diverse learning needs across a range of distance education and blended learning contexts. Each dimension involves one or more design decisions that can each lead to a particular type of podcast, and the entire decision matrix needs to be considered when commencing the design process:

- *Formality:* Podcast episodes can be formal, lecture-type resources, replicating didactic teaching carried out in face-to-face classes, or informal episodes involving commentary, questioning, or reflections.
- *Media mix:* Podcasts may simply be audio files, or include video (vodcasts), still images (enhanced podcasts—see Apple, 2008), or a combination of media.
- *Content:* The content of podcasts may be created by instructors, learners, or both, according to the desired learning outcomes and pedagogy adopted.

- *Format:* Podcasts may vary in duration from long (over 20 minutes) to short (up to three minutes), with the ideal length depending on the purpose and nature of the learning material and associated task(s).
- *Pedagogy:* The adoption and use of podcasts in any educational setting needs to be driven by a clear rationale and underpinned by a sound pedagogical model/framework. Learner-centered pedagogies include self-directed learning, inquiry-based learning, and problem-based learning, where students are actively engaged in active discovery, exploration, research, and knowledge creation. Several of the examples in Table 2 provide instances of podcasting integration within learning settings where innovative pedagogies are used.
- *Frequency:* The use of podcasts in learning environments may be frequent (i.e., used as a regular part of student learning) or occasional, depending on needs, pedagogies adopted, and nature of tasks. In any case, students need to be clear on when and how podcasts will be used, along with the associated rationale.
- *Context of use:* The podcasts can be embedded in the course (for example, used to deliver core concepts, content, and key ideas) or used as enrichment and extension of prescribed course content and activities.
- *Learning outcomes:* Teachers need to ensure that podcasting activities are clearly linked to learning outcomes, and that learning outcomes are supported by the pedagogies chosen. For example, in Table 2, peer collaboration and reflection on professional practice were the desired learning outcomes of the initiative facilitated by McLoughlin and her colleagues (McLoughlin, Brady, Lee, & Russell, 2007; McLoughlin, Lee, & Brady, 2008), and to achieve these objectives, a learner-centered pedagogy was adopted in which students created podcast episodes reflecting on professional practice.
- *Authorship:* Podcasts may have single or multiple authors or creators, again depending on the learning context and desired learning goals. Instructor-created podcasts can present essential course material, expert ideas, or questions, as in the "profcast" approach proposed by Edirisingha, Salmon, and Fothergill (2007). Alternatively, podcasts can be generated by individual students or groups of students (see for example Lee et al., 2006b).
- *Access:* Educational podcasts can be accessed by students in variety of ways, for example via a VLE or learning management system (LMS). There are also various syndication protocols available to facilitate automatic downloads via subscription, the most common being RSS, Atom, and Outline Processor Markup Language (OPML).

CONCLUSION AND IMPLICATIONS FOR PRACTICE

Although it is unlikely that digital audio will completely replace online lectures/tutorials, textbooks, and printed or electronic study guides in distance education courses, podcasting can augment these forms of activity, while adding yet another modality and increasing the portability and accessibility of resources for learning "on the go." Furthermore, the pedagogic applications showcased in this chapter provide promising examples of how podcasting and other web technologies are being used in ways that represent a shift away from didactic modes of teaching and transmission of content, toward the enablement of greater learner agency in the learning process, increased recognition that student-generated resources are valuable as primary sources of educational content, and the development of peer-to-peer learning in online communities that transcend the walls of organizations and institutions. This is very much in line with the Web 2.0 movement, which emphasizes collaboration, connectivity, and the creation and sharing of user-generated content in the form of social media or "we media" (McFedries, 2007). Arguably, it is this community-building value of podcasting and its ability to serve as a vehicle for disseminating learner-generated content to peers and a wider Internet audience wherein the true pedagogical potential of this technology lies, and which effectively set it apart from older audio-based distance education technologies.

The historical purpose of teaching and learning models traditionally used in higher education was to maximize efficiency and capitalize on economies of scale (Sheely, 2006; Rogers, Liddle, Chan, Doxey, & Isom, 2007); distance learning and e-learning efforts and implementations have tended to replicate these traditional models. This "industrialized" form of education, in which pre-packaged content, lectures, and teacher-controlled syllabi dominate, is highly incongruent with the needs and values prevalent in the Web 2.0 era (see Chapter 3). The podcasting examples presented in this chapter, along with the many other examples contained in other chapters within this book, provide compelling evidence of how Web 2.0 and social software tools and technologies, if used in conjunction with appropriate pedagogical strategies, can lead to individual empowerment of learners through designs that focus on collaborative, networked communication and interaction. Moreover, today's students desire and demand authentic learning experiences that are personally meaningful and relevant to them. This is especially so with distance learners who already have substantial professional and life experience, and therefore correspondingly high levels of needs and expectations. Educators need to capitalize on the interests and competencies that learners already have, while at the same time taking steps to equip them with the additional skills, attributes, and capabilities they need to be successful in the digital economy and networked society.

It is also imperative that educators and institutions constantly remain socially sensitive to the needs of students, and take steps to minimize the risk of creating or widening "digital divides," by ensuring that all learners have equitable access to tools and infrastructure with consistent capabilities and connectivity options, and by making available to them appropriate types and levels of technical and learning/academic support. Despite the ubiquity of the multimedia PC and of broadband network access in most developed nations today, as well as the widespread popularity of the notion of the so-called "digital native" or "Net Generation" student (see Chapter 16), assumptions cannot and must not be made about students' access to, use of, and proficiency with particular technologies and tools. This is especially the case in the Internet-mediated distance education classroom, in which students are not physically present in a single place, in which their locations typically span multiple geographical and political boundaries, and in which social inequalities may be difficult to accurately identify and define as a result. When introducing the use of Web 2.0 technologies, including podcasting, for teaching, learning, and assessment purposes, care must be taken to minimize the risk of exacerbating existing inequalities across the student population, and also of producing new ones.

In closing, the notion that learning environments can be controlled by students is at once both empowering and fraught with inevitable error and risk. As argued earlier in Chapter 3, in Web 2.0-based e-learning, there is still a need for gatekeepers and quality assurance/control measures, for scaffolded learning experiences, for structured learning resources, and for evaluation and feedback. The shift toward open-ended and discovery learning, learner-generated content, and heutagogical (Hase & Kenyon, 2000) approaches in general is not tantamount to acknowledgement that the role of the teacher in higher education has diminished, but rather simply that the "closed classroom" and "sage on the stage" model of centuries past needs to be carefully reconsidered in contemporary face-to-face, online, and blended learning contexts. While the authors concur with Atkinson (2006) in his observation that "The emerging developmental and research direction seems ... to be learning through *creating* podcasts and similar, in contrast to learning *from* podcasts" (p. 21, author's emphasis), the ways in which educational podcasting applications continue to evolve and in which tertiary educators in general and distance educators in particular leverage the medium of digital audio will depend heavily on student needs, availability of technological infrastructure, and teacher confidence with new media. In the words of McGarr (2009):

> *the ultimate use of podcasting [in higher education] ... may not be determined by the potential of the technology, but rather by the way in which it is perceived within the institution, by both teachers and students. Its use will be strongly influenced by the dominant pedagogies employed in these contexts. (p. 319–320)*

Podcasting, as part of the raft of Web 2.0 technologies, can simply be used to reinforce existing didactic pedagogies and transmissive approaches to content delivery, but this would not maximise its potential to support and enhance learning. Instead, creative and pedagogically informed applications of podcasting may be used to bring about a substantive change in tertiary teaching and learning, to support genuine knowledge building and learner creativity as the examples in Table 2 demonstrate.

REFERENCES

Apple. (2008). *Podcasting Frequently Asked Questions (FAQ)*. Retrieved October 29, 2008, from http://support.apple.com/kb/HT1597

Armstrong, T. (1994). *Multiple intelligences in the classroom*. Alexandria, VA: Association for Supervision and Curriculum Development.

Atkinson, R. (2006). Podcasting: Do you really need to know? *HERDSA News*, *28*(2), 20–22.

Barnes, J. M. (1995, April 18–22). *Embodiment, hermeneutic, alterity, and background relations on the Internet*. Paper presented at the Annual Meeting of the American Educational Research Association, San Francisco.

Bates, A. W. (1981). Radio: The forgotten medium? Studies in the use of radio programming and audio-cassettes in Open University courses. In *Papers on broadcasting, No. 185*. Milton Keynes, UK: Institute of Educational Technology, The Open University.

Beldarrain, Y. (2006). Distance education trends: Integrating new technologies to foster student interaction and collaboration. *Distance Education*, *27*(2), 139–153. doi:10.1080/01587910600789498

Carmichael, J. (2005, November 3). A new deal for fireside chats? *Teachers College Record*. Retrieved December 29, 2008, from http://www.tcrecord.org/Content.asp?ContentId=12231

Chan, A., Frydenberg, M., & Lee, M. J. W. (2007). Facilitating cross-cultural learning through collaborative Skypecasting. In J. J. Ekstrom (Ed.), *Proceedings of the 2007 ACM Information Technology Education Conference* (pp. 59–66). New York: Association for Computing Machinery.

Clark, D., & Walsh, S. (2004). *iPod-learning*. Brighton, UK: Epic Group.

Copley, J. (2007). Audio and video podcasts of lectures for campus-based students: Production and evaluation of student use. *Innovations in Education and Teaching International*, *44*(4), 387–399. doi:10.1080/14703290701602805

Curry, A. (2004). *iPodder—A brief history*. Retrieved April 23, 2005, from http://www.ipodder.org/history

Dixon, C., & Greeson, M. (2006). *Recasting the concept of podcasting (Part I)*. Retrieved September 20, 2006, from http://news.digitaltrends.com/talkback109.html

Durbridge, N. (1984). Media in course design, No. 9, audio cassettes. In Bates, A. W. (Ed.), *The role of technology in distance education*. Kent, UK: Croom Helm.

Edirisingha, P., Rizzi, C., Nie, M., & Rothwell, L. (2007). Podcasting to provide teaching and learning support for an undergraduate module on English language and communication. *Turkish Online Journal of Distance Education, 8*(3), 87–107. Retrieved December 14, 2007, from http://tojde.anadolu.edu.tr/tojde27/pdf/article_6.pdf

Edirisingha, P., & Salmon, G. (2007). *Pedagogical models for podcasts in higher education*. Retrieved May 27, 2008, from http://hdl.handle.net/2381/405

Edirisingha, P., Salmon, G., & Fothergill, J. (2006, June 15). *Enriching a blended learning environment with podcasts and e-tivities: A case study*. Paper presented at the First International Blended Learning Conference: Promoting dialogue in innovation and practice, Hatfield, UK.

Edirisingha, P., Salmon, G., & Fothergill, J. (2007). Profcasting—a pilot study and guidelines for integrating podcasts in a blended learning environment. In U. Bernath & A. Sangrà (Eds.), *Research on competence development in online distance education and e-learning: Selected papers from the 4th EDEN Research Workshop in Castelldefels/Spain, October 25–28, 2006* (pp. 127–137). Oldenberg, Germany: BIS-Verlag der Carl von Ossietzky Universität Oldenburg.

Essex, C. (2006). Podcasting: A new medium for distance learning. In M. R. Simonson & M. Crawford (Eds.), *Proceedings of the 2006 Association for Educational Communications and Technology (AECT) International Convention* (pp. 136–139). North Miami Beach, FL: Nova Southeastern University.

Evans, C. (2008). The effectiveness of m-learning in the form of podcast revision lectures in higher education. *Computers & Education, 50*(2), 491–498. doi:10.1016/j.compedu.2007.09.016

Frydenberg, M. (2006). Principles and pedagogy: The two P's of podcasting in the information technology classroom. In D. Colton, W. J. Tastle, M. Hensel, & A. A. Abdullat (Eds.), *Proceedings of ISECON 2006* (§3354). Chicago, IL: Association of Information Technology Professionals. Retrieved November 27, 2006, from http://isedj.org/isecon/2006/3354/ISECON.2006.Frydenberg.pdf

Gachuhi, D., & Matiru, B. (1987). Active learning. In *Distance Education—By Design Symposium '87 Papers* (pp. 1–21). Barrhead, AB: Alberta Correspondence School.

Galusha, J. M. (1997). *Barriers to learning in distance education*. Retrieved June 19, 2008, from http://www.infrastruction.com/barriers.htm

Gardner, H. (1983). *Frames of mind: The theory of multiple intelligences*. New York: Basic.

Gardner, H. (1993). *Multiple intelligences: The theory in practice*. New York: Basic.

Gardner, H. (2000). *Intelligence reframed: Multiple intelligences for the 21st century*. New York: Basic.

Georgia College & State University. (2005). *The iPod at GC&SU: A pocketful of learning*. Retrieved March 2, 2006, from http://ipod.gcsu.edu

Hase, S., & Kenyon, C. (2000). From Andragogy to Heutagogy. *ultiBASE, 5*(3). Retrieved July 12, 2008, from http://ultibase.rmit.edu.au/Articles/dec00/hase1.pdf

Informal Mobile Podcasting and Learning Adaptation. (2007). *A framework for developing your podcasts*. Retrieved June 29, 2008, from http://www2.le.ac.uk/projects/impala/documents/resources-and-tools-for-creating-podcasts/PodcastChoiceFramework

Kates, R. (1998). Tape recorders and the commuter student: Bypassing the red pen. *Teaching English in the Two-Year College*, *25*(1), 21–24.

Keegan, D. (1996). *Foundations of distance education* (3rd ed.). London: Routledge.

Kukulska-Hulme, A. (2005, May 11–12). *The mobile language learner—now and in the future*. Paper presented at Fran Vision till Praktik (Language Learning and ICT Symposium), Umeå, Sweden. Retrieved February 3, 2006, from http://www2.humlab.umu.se/video/Praktikvision/agnes.ram

Laaser, W. (1986). Some didactic aspects of audio-cassettes in distance education. *Distance Education*, *7*(1), 143–152. doi:10.1080/0158791860070110

Lee, M. J. W. (2006, October). Using blogs and podcasting to facilitate delivery and self/peer evaluation of oral presentation assessments. *Learning Technology*, 28–30. Retrieved May 2, 2007, from http://lttf.ieee.org/learn_tech/issues/october2006/lt_october2006.pdf

Lee, M. J. W. (2007). Podcasting and digital audio in L&D: Time to hand over the microphone! *Training and Development in Australia*, *34*(3), 28–29.

Lee, M. J. W., & Chan, A. (2007). Reducing the effects of isolation and promoting inclusivity for distance learners through podcasting. *Turkish Online Journal of Distance Education, 8*(1), 85–104. Retrieved December 14, 2007, from http://tojde.anadolu.edu.tr/tojde25/pdf/article_7.pdf

Lee, M. J. W., Chan, A., & McLoughlin, C. (2006a). Educational podcasting using the Charles Sturt University Flexible Publishing platform. In T. Reeves & S. Yamashita (Eds.), *Proceedings of World Conference on E-Learning in Corporate, Government, Healthcare, and Higher Education 2006* (pp. 2894–2901). Chesapeake, VA: Association for the Advancement of Computers in Education.

Lee, M. J. W., Chan, A., & McLoughlin, C. (2006b). Students as producers: Second year students' experiences as podcasters of content for first year undergraduates. In *Proceedings of the Seventh Conference on Information Technology Based Higher Education and Training* (pp. 832–841). Broadway, Australia: University of Technology, Sydney.

Lee, M. J. W., McLoughlin, C., & Chan, A. (2008). Talk the talk: Learner-generated podcasts as catalysts for knowledge creation. *British Journal of Educational Technology*, *39*(3), 501–521. doi:10.1111/j.1467-8535.2007.00746.x

Lee, M. J. W., & Tynan, B. (2008). Podcasts and distance learning. In Salmon, G., & Edirisingha, P. (Eds.), *Podcasting for learning in universities* (pp. 92–102). London: McGraw-Hill.

McFedries, P. (2007). Social-isms. *IEEE Spectrum*, *44*(4), 56.

McGarr, O. (2009). A review of podcasting in higher education: Its influence on the traditional lecture. *Australasian Journal of Educational Technology, 25*(3), 309–321. Retrieved August 10, 2009, from http://www.ascilite.org.au/ajet/ajet25/mcgarr.pdf

McLoughlin, C., Brady, J., Lee, M. J. W., & Russell, R. (2007, November 25–29). *Peer-to-peer: An e-mentoring approach to facilitating reflection on professional experience for novice teachers.* Paper presented at the 2007 Australian Association for Research in Education Conference, Fremantle, Australia. Retrieved January 17, 2009, from http://www.aare.edu.au/07pap/mcl07393.pdf

McLoughlin, C., Lee, M. J. W., & Brady, J. (2008). A learning architecture framework (LAF) for developing community, engagement and professional identity for pre-service teachers. In I. Olney, G. Lefoe, J. Mantei, & J. Herrington (Eds.), *Proceedings of the Emerging Technologies Conference 2008* (pp. 147–157). Wollongong, Australia: University of Wollongong. Retrieved January 17, 2009, from http://ro.uow.edu.au/cgi/viewcontent.cgi?article=1016&context=etc08

McLoughlin, C., Lee, M. J. W., & Chan, A. (2007). Promoting engagement and motivation for distance learners through podcasting. In *New Learning 2.0? Emerging digital territories, developing continuities, new divides: Proceedings of the European Distance Education and E-Learning Network (EDEN) Annual Conference 2007*. Budapest, Hungary: EDEN.

Meister, J. C. (2006). Keeping learners engaged: Certifying and supporting online instructors. *Chief Learning Officer*, *5*(2), 66.

Newnham, L., & Miller, C. (2007). Student perceptions of podcasting to enhance learning and teaching in an information systems course. In S. Wheeler & N. Whitton (Eds.), *Beyond control: Learning technology for the social network generation. Research Proceedings of the 14th Association for Learning Technology Conference* (pp. 104–115). Oxford, UK: ALT.

Nie, M., Cashmore, A., & Cane, C. (2008). The educational value of student-generated podcasts. In N. Whitton & M. McPherson (Eds.), *Rethinking the digital divide. Research Proceedings of the 15th Association for Learning Technology Conference* (pp. 116–128). Oxford, UK: ALT.

Oxford University Press. (2005). *All hail "podcasting": More also-rans for the 2005 WOTY*. Retrieved July 3, 2006, from http://blog.oup.com/oupblog/2005/12/podcasting_is_t.html

Parashar Panday, P., & Lee, M. J. W. (2007). Graduate education students' perceptions of podcasting as teachers and learners. In T. J. Bastiaens & S. Carliner (Eds.), *Proceedings of World Conference on E-Learning in Corporate, Government, Healthcare, and Higher Education 2007* (pp. 7313–7318). Chesapeake, VA: Association for the Advancement of Computers in Education.

Pollock, J. (2006). Suddenly, it's the podcast era. *Des Moines Business Record*, *24*(16), 1–12.

Power, D. J. (1990). The use of audio in distance education. In Timmers, S. (Ed.), *Training needs in the use of media for distance education* (pp. 43–60). Singapore: Asian Mass Communication Research and Information Centre.

Rogers, P. C., Liddle, S. W., Chan, P., Doxey, A., & Isom, B. (2007). Web 2.0 learning platform: Harnessing collective intelligence. *Turkish Online Journal of Distance Education, 8*(3), 16–33. Retrieved December 14, 2007, http://tojde.anadolu.edu.tr/tojde27/pdf/article_1.pdf

RSS Advisory Board. (2005). *Really Simple Syndication: RSS 2.0.1 Specification (revision 6)*. Retrieved March 2, 2006, from http://www.rssboard.org/rss-2-0-1-rv-6

Salmon, G. (2002). *E-tivities: The key to active online learning*. London: Kogan Page.

Schlosser, C. A., & Burmeister, M. L. (2006, October 10–13). Audio in online courses: Beyond podcasting. Paper presented at the World Conference on E-Learning in Corporate, Government, Healthcare, and Higher Education 2006, Honolulu, HI. Retrieved October 20, 2006, from http://www.nova.edu/~burmeist/audio_online.html

Scottish Council for Educational Technology. (1994). Audio. In *Technologies in learning*. Glasgow: Scottish Council for Educational Technology.

Sheely, S. (2006). Persistent technologies: Why can't we stop lecturing online? In L. Markauskaite, P. Goodyear, & P. Reimann (Eds.), *Who's learning? Whose technology? Proceedings of the 23rd Australasian Society for Computers in Learning in Tertiary Education (ASCILITE) Conference* (pp. 769–774). Sydney: University of Sydney. Retrieved January 12, 2008, from http://www.ascilite.org.au/conferences/sydney06/proceeding/pdf_papers/p167.pdf

Skiba, D. J. (2006). The 2005 word of the year: Podcast. *Nursing Education Perspectives*, *27*(1), 54–55.

Tynan, B., & Colbran, S. (2006). Podcasting, student learning and expectations. In L. Markauskaite, P. Goodyear, & P. Reimann (Eds.), *Who's learning? Whose technology? Proceedings of the 23rd Australasian Society for Computers in Learning in Tertiary Education (ASCILITE) Conference* (pp. 825–832). Sydney: University of Sydney. Retrieved January 12, 2008, from http://www.ascilite.org.au/conferences/sydney06/proceeding/pdf_papers/p132.pdf

Walsh, S. (2004). Appendix: IPod, therefore I learn. In *iPod-learning* (pp. 23–29). Brighton, UK: Epic Group.

World Bank. (2000). *Technology—Broadcast and computer-based: Radio*. Retrieved May 31, 2005, from http://www1.worldbank.org/disted/Technology/broadcast/broad_radio.html

Yuen, S., & Wang, S. (2004). M-learning: Mobility in learning. In G. Richards (Ed.), *Proceedings of World Conference on E-Learning in Corporate, Government, Healthcare, and Higher Education 2004* (pp. 2248–2252). Chesapeake, VA: Association for the Advancement of Computers in Education.

KEY TERMS AND DEFINITIONS

Authentic Learning: Learning that encourages learners to engage in real-world problems and projects that are meaningful and interesting to them, and that have relevance beyond the walls of the classroom.

Blended Learning: A learning delivery approach in which core learning activities are undertaken online via the Internet as well as in traditional, face-to-face settings, as distinct from the practice of simply supplementing face-to-face instruction with online resources and materials, for example, through a course website. Sometimes also referred to as "hybrid learning."

Enhanced Podcasting: An enhanced podcast is an (audio) podcast synchronized with static images such as artwork, photos, or slides. It is not to be confused with a vodcast, which contains video content. Apple's (2008) proprietary MP4a format is typically used, which also allows the inclusion of chapter marks (used to divide a lengthy podcast into sections) and clickable hyperlinks. See also podcasting, vodcasting.

Flexible Learning: A broad term used to describe the design and delivery of programs, courses, and learning interventions in such a way as to cater for student demands for variety, access, recognition of diverse learning styles, and student control over and customizability of the learning experience. It is often incorrectly used in an interchangeable manner with other terms such as "open learning," "distance learning," "work-based learning," as well as "e-learning," which are all instances or forms of flexible learning in that they provide flexibility to the student in terms of time/pace, place, access, content, and/or delivery mode.

Inquiry-Based Learning: A term used to describe a range of instructional strategies based on premises that are centered around the need for learners to ask questions, then actively seek out answers to those questions. It is commonly used in the teaching of science. The teacher takes on the role of a "facilitator," who supports learners rather than simply giving them the answers, encouraging them to take responsibility for their learning through active exploration, discovery, and reflection. See also problem-based learning.

Learning Management System (LMS): An integrated suite of software tools designed to manage learning interventions. Commercial examples are Blackboard and WebCT, although many open-source alternatives, such as Moodle and Sakai, exist. In addition to the provision of online learning content and activities and the facilitation of online assessment, LMSs typically support a range of administrative functions including learner enrollment, workflow, records management (e.g., reporting of assessment results/outcomes), and resource management (e.g., facilities, equipment).

Learner-Generated Content: Content that is produced by students, often for sharing with peers or a wider audience on the Internet, as distinct from instructor-supplied content such as course notes and textbooks. It is arguable that the main benefits to be gained from learner-generated content lie in engagement in the processes of content creation and knowledge construction, as opposed to the tangible end products themselves. Sometimes referred to as "learner-created content" or "student-generated content." See also user-generated content.

Mobile Learning (m-Learning): A form of e-learning and distance education that involves learning through the use of mobile or portable devices, which gives rise to the benefit of being able to undertake learning activities "anytime, anyplace." Proponents of this paradigm believe the flexibility afforded opens up rich opportunities for informal and lifelong learning, as well as learning that is linked to authentic work contexts. See also flexible learning, authentic learning.

MPEG Layer 3 (MP3): A digital audio encoding format that makes use of a lossy compression algorithm, which sacrifices the fidelity of the audio to reduce the amount of data required to represent the audio recording, thereby resulting a file size that is suitable for transmission over the Internet. Since the compression works by reducing the accuracy of certain parts of sound that are deemed beyond the auditory resolution ability of most people, for most listeners, an MP3 file sounds like a faithful reproduction of the original audio. MP3 is commonly used format for consumer audio storage, as well as a de facto standard for the transfer and playback of music on digital audio players. Most podcasts are produced in MP3 format. See also podcasting.

Podcasting: A portmanteau that combines the words "iPod" (the name of Apple Computer's popular portable music player) and "broadcast." It refers to the distribution of digital audio files, typically in MPEG Layer 3 (MP3) format, through a syndication protocol such as RSS. The user subscribes to one or more feeds or channels of his or her choice using a podcast aggregation program, which periodically polls the feeds for new audio files and downloads them automatically to the user's hard disk as they become available. Podcasts may transferred to an iPod or similar device for mobile listening, but users who do not have access to such devices can simply listen to the content on their PCs. See also RSS, MP3.

Podcatcher: An RSS aggregator program that is capable of downloading podcast files (most commonly MP3 files included in an RSS feed as RSS 2.0 enclosures). See also RSS, podcasting, MP3.

Problem-Based Learning: A form of authentic, inquiry-based learning in which students learn by working collaboratively in groups to solve problems, and reflecting on their experiences. The problems are typically challenging and open ended. They mirror problems in the real world in that they are often ill structured and do not result in neat, convergent outcomes. See also inquiry-based learning.

RSS: Really Simple Syndication (also Rich Site Summary, RDF Site Summary). A technology originally designed to facilitate the publication of text summaries of additions to frequently updated websites, such as news sites and web logs (blogs). The user subscribes to the feed(s) of one or more RSS-enabled websites by configuring an aggregator program (sometimes also known as a news reader) installed on his or her computer with the URL(s) of the eXtensible Markup Language (XML) file(s) that comprise the feed. The program periodically checks the feed for new content and downloads it as it becomes available. RSS 2.0 feeds permit the inclusion of enclosures, which permit multimedia files (such as MP3 files in the case of podcasting) to be referenced in the feed. See also podcasting.

User-Generated Content: A term that refers to web-based content created by ordinary people or users, for example, pictures posted on Flickr or encyclopedia entries written in Wikipedia. Such "read-and-write" applications are key characteristic of the Web 2.0 movement, which encourages the publishing of one's own content and commenting on or augmenting other people's. It differs from the "read-only" model of Web 1.0, in which websites were created and maintained by an elite few.

Vodcasting: The publishing/distribution of video files instead of audio files using the same technology (i.e., syndication through a protocol like RSS) as podcasting. See also podcasting, enhanced podcasting, RSS.

Chapter 13

Using Web 2.0 Tools to Enhance the Student Experience in Non-Teaching Areas of the University

Lisa Cluett
The University of Western Australia, Australia

Judy Skene
The University of Western Australia, Australia

ABSTRACT

This chapter aims to provide an overview of the nexus between student learning and student engagement outside the classroom, and to highlight the importance of non-teaching units in contributing to student satisfaction. It discusses the role of non-teaching units (such as libraries, guilds, student services departments, and other bodies) in creating online communities using Web 2.0 tools. The chapter uses the NODE project hosted by the University of Western Australia as a case study to demonstrate how some of these principles can be put into action. The significance of non-teaching units is confirmed, in addition to providing recommendations for fostering greater collaboration between staff and advice on setting up a Web 2.0-based online community in a university.

INTRODUCTION

It is now widely recognized that tertiary students learn both inside the classroom and outside of it (Krause, 2005b, 2007; Light, 2001), examples of the latter being when students engage together in discussion, peer study groups, and other co-curricular activities. While disciplinary content teaching conducted by academic faculties and schools may typically be seen to constitute the bulk of a university's "core business," the contribution made by areas such as libraries, student guilds and societies, transition programs, and academic skills advisors is integral to the way students engage with and connect to their institution. These functions, collectively identified here as non-teaching units, complement academic content and instructional delivery, enhancing and enriching the student learning experience through provision of a wide range of services and programs. Web 2.0 tools offer options to improve communication between students and staff in non-teaching units, supple-

DOI: 10.4018/978-1-60566-294-7.ch013

ment teaching and learning-support activities, and facilitate social networking between groups of students in ways that aid their engagement with institutional and campus culture.

Challenges exist for non-teaching units in that they often do not have a defined student cohort in the same way the lecturer of a subject or unit might. The staff of such units also do not always have access to online learning management systems (LMSs) such as Blackboard or Moodle, and they may have fewer opportunities to develop ongoing relationships with students. Yet the prospects for non-teaching units to engage with students are also considerable. For example, units such as those providing academic skills development have contact with significant numbers of students, often from across the range of teaching disciplines, via face-to-face service delivery in workshops, presentations, consultations, and drop-in sessions. Other services may engage with the students in a more casual, less formal relationship, away from the pressures of assessment, and they are able to supply students with key skills and information, often at the point of need, thus providing a key component of the learning experience. These programs have the scope to use information and communication technologies (ICTs), and particularly, social networking tools, to enhance their service delivery.

The use of technologies in enhancing the student learning experience is, in some ways, neither new nor revolutionary. Students have long used email, mobile phones, and online learning environments to communicate with their instructors and peers, to administer various aspects of their university lives, and to manage their course-related information and study content. However, the growing use of Web 2.0 tools in learning environments that allow users to create and contribute content has generated much discussion about how students learn and interact, the skills they need in order to engage with the tools effectively, and the extent to which this engagement contributes to learning and the quality of the student experience.

This chapter therefore aims to:

- provide an overview of the nexus between student learning and student engagement outside the classroom;
- highlight the importance of non-teaching units in developing the student learning–engagement nexus and its contribution to student satisfaction;
- discuss the role of non-teaching units in creating online communities using Web 2.0 tools;
- use the NODE project at the University of Western Australia (UWA) as a case study to demonstrate how some of these principles can be put into action.

BACKGROUND

Student Engagement

We begin by considering the notion of, and issues surrounding, student engagement. Universities worldwide recognize the importance of students being satisfied with their student experience. Student satisfaction with the quality of their learning outcomes, their graduate opportunities, and their overall experience is reflected in the results of international ranking exercises, and therefore these are important measures that can be used as benchmarks and marketing tools for universities operating in a competitive global environment (Marginson, 2007). University leaders and administrators are keenly aware of the elements of the student experience: quality teaching and relevant curricula are central, but so too are state-of-the-art information technology (IT) infrastructure, comprehensive support services, library resources and a welcoming campus climate (Krause, 2005a). Most university leaders place a high emphasis on the overall richness of the student experience, encouraging students to use every opportunity to expand their personal networks and challenge themselves beyond the demands of their courses and classrooms—recognizing, as Astin (1985) argued, that students learn by getting involved.

As universities intensify their competition to attract and retain high-performing students, awareness of the complexities of current students' experiences come into focus. Students' lives are subject to more pressures than ever before, and their relationship with campus life, their peers, and university staff has changed from what is was just a decade ago. The importance of student engagement has motivated the adoption of instruments to measure dimensions of engagement, such as the National Survey of Student Engagement (NSSE, 2008), first piloted in 1999 and now used by a range of institutions in the United States (Kuh, Cruce, Shoup, Kinzie, & Gonyea, 2007). Other variations now include the Community College Survey of Student Engagement (CCSSE) in the U.S., and an Australian adaptation, AUSSE (AUstralasian Survey of Student Engagement). A recent report summarizing the first five years of CCSSE (2007) data noted that "the more actively engaged students are—with college faculty and staff, with other students, and with the subject matter they study—the more likely they are to learn, to stick with their studies, and to attain their academic goals" (p. 4).

These instruments provide rich data on many aspects of engagement, and allow comparisons on individual measures that can identify strategies for success from institutions scoring well on those measures. They also highlight ways in which students' patterns of behavior are changing. In most western countries, students are working more hours in paid employment away from campus, and many no longer have time to "hang out" in the library coffee shop and swap notes, or to join student activities and extend their peer networks. Krause's (2005b) research in Australia identifies "engagement" for many students as an appointment in their busy diaries, along with work, social activities, and family responsibilities. For others, the term may have a hostile connotation, as they engage in a battle to survive. In attempting to come to terms with the social changes affecting student engagement, the importance of considering the influence of ICT is paramount.

Online technologies have had a positive impact on learning through offering students flexibility to study via distance education modes and through the provision of a vast array of online resources via libraries, for instance, that students can access. Much of the recent research on ICT focuses on distance education or blended learning environments developed in response to the rapid expansion of higher education during the past three decades, enabled by digital technology innovations. At first, many had doubts as to whether these distance learning environments could replicate the benefits of face-to-face teaching modes—the interaction was reduced in most instances to one between lecturer and solitary student, via email, telephone, and print. Distance education students missed out on synchronous (real-time) group discussions and the social interactions that enrich the university experience. The flexibility afforded by online delivery and communication modes offsets some of these disadvantages, but now, emerging technologies can truly begin to address these concerns and support the creation of additional learning opportunities in traditional settings by offering multiple tools to generate content, foster collaborative learning options, and build communities online (Dziuban, Moskal, & Hartman, 2003). The potential of Web 2.0 tools, in particular, to expand and enrich the learning experience of students in the classroom has been argued by supporters in recent years (Millea, Green, & Putland, 2005; Anderson, 2007; McLoughlin & Lee, 2007; Owen, Grant, Sayers, & Facer, 2006). The interactive, participatory nature of Web 2.0 also extends options for student engagement outside the classroom through building networks and communities, including support networks of professional and academic staff.

While educators are contemplating and exploring the potential of Web 2.0 tools, for many students under the age of 25, these tools are integral to their lives to varying degrees. Many "Gen Y" students (born 1982–2000) do not consider devices like mobile phones and MP3 players as "technology." However, Gen Y students do expect that the tools with which they are familiar will be used to enrich their learning environment, and this expectation demands recognition and response (Ipsos MORI, 2007; Conole & Creanor, 2007; White, 2007; Barnes & Tynan, 2007). Although there is extensive literature on generational differences that focuses on the impact of growing up with technology and how this influences behavior and learning (Tapscott, 1998; Howe & Strauss, 2000), it is written largely by those educators whom Prensky (2001) termed "digital immigrants" because they did not have access to ICTs during their formative years. The continuing relevance of the terms "digital immigrant" and "digital native" has been the subject of much debate in the blogosphere (Jenkins, 2008; Baer, 2007; see also Chapter 16 in this book), yet there is some agreement that these terms spark recognition of differing generational attitudes and approaches to ICT that need to be taken into account in framing strategies and policies. The majority of university leaders and administrators responsible for establishing policy directions for teaching and learning and for ICT infrastructure are digital immigrants, and many are challenged by how to respond to the rapidly changing environment of Web 2.0 (the social Web), with further innovation already named as "Web 3.0" (see Chapter 20) already on our horizon. Some defend traditional practices; others explore how students' digital literacy skills influence their learning styles (Hartman, Moskal, & Dziuban, 2005). Whatever one's response, technology is unquestionably giving rise to changes in how we communicate, manage information, make decisions, and interact, in ways that cannot be ignored.

Another key characteristic of Gen Y students is the value they place on their peer group and being constantly in communication. Peer pressure has long been a feature of youth culture, but it appears to have strengthened in this generation's capacity to be in constant contact via ICTs. Authors have also observed that Gen Ys believe some of their most powerful learning experiences occur informally, outside the classroom, when they are interacting with their peers (Markwell, 2007; Light, 2001). Students make use of social networking sites such as Facebook to facilitate the setting up of meetings to progress joint projects, exchange resources, and share ideas. Blogs, wikis, and synchronous collaborative-writing tools provide rich environments for students to write, critique, publish, and comment (Crowe & Tonkin, 2006; Chan & McLoughlin, 2007). Mobile phones and personal digital assistants, with their personal information management and mobile messaging and collaboration tools, are important means by which students coordinate and organize their busy timetables, among other things. In observing their students' use of ICT, many university staff wonder if there is a role for these tools in their own communication with their students. The final report for the JISC *Learner Experience of e-Learning* (LEX) study states that "Effective learners tend to be highly skilled networkers and often use the technology to pull in support when needed" (Creanor, Trinder, Gowan, & Howells, 2006, p. 11), suggesting a need for support services to have flexible delivery (including online) options. Krause (2005b) recommends that universities use online learning environments to capitalize on the community-building capacities available. While some students resist what they see as an invasion by universities into their social space through use of their more informal communication media (Ipsos MORI, 2007), others welcome the advantages of the flexibility that the tools offer and see the benefits of adopting aspects in their university work (Ipsos MORI, 2007; Conole & Creanor, 2007).

The 2008 *Horizon report* (New Media Consortium, 2008) identifies the challenge of bridging the digital divide in expertise between staff and students—where the students are the experts—as a critical challenge for higher education in the next five years. Marc Prensky is among those who advocate consulting students about their digital preferences when devising learning strategies. His view on engagement is that "Our kids *do* know what engagement is: Outside school, they are fully engaged by their 21st century digital lives" (Prensky, 2005/2006, p. 9, emphasis in original) and that if we don't "engage" them, we will "enrage" them (Prensky, 2005, p. 60). The boundaries between teachers and students become blurred when access to information from a seemingly endless variety of sources is widely available, as is the capacity to create content collaboratively. The technical skills, preferences, and practices of Gen Y students are driving change within the higher education sector in many ways, and universities will need visionary leadership to keep apace of the constant evolution of the technologies that their students adopt (Millea, Green, & Putland, 2005; New Media Consortium, 2008).

The definition of the student experience has expanded, then, to recognize that valuable and significant learning occurs beyond the walls of the classroom, and so it becomes even more important to encourage students to become involved in out-of-class activities that will strengthen their engagement with their institution (Krause, 2005b, 2007; Light, 2001). Not much attention has been paid, however, to how centralized services and departments of the university, such as the Library, Student Services, etc., can enhance student learning via online communities, or what possibilities exist for them to facilitate engagement (Cluett & Skene, 2007; Skene, Cluett, & Hogan, 2007). The potential of these non-teaching units to leverage the power of Web 2.0 in the interest of student engagement is therefore explored, with reference to various examples, in the next subsection.

Non-Teaching Units and Web 2.0-Based Online Communities

While academic achievement and graduate employability have long been the indicators of university success, there has been a relatively recent broadening of the definition of success to include a high level of student satisfaction. This has been widely reflected and embraced internationally, nationally, and locally in many countries through participation in surveys and ranking exercises, and through localized support through funding initiatives to improve rankings. This change in the collective mindset has included a growing appreciation that the student experience is made up of components from across—and beyond—the institution. The term "outside the classroom," employed by Richard Light (2001, p. 1) in his book about student experiences at Harvard, is representative of the now commonly accepted view that non-teaching units play a central role in student engagement, student satisfaction, and student learning.

It is useful to note here that non-teaching units have typically always thought of their programs and services as being key to student success and engagement. The "student experience" has long been a driver for the development of projects and initiatives in library services, transition programs, mentoring schemes, academic skills training, and the vast suite of other services distinct from school- or faculty-based instruction/teaching of content. The principles behind these face-to-face services are often centered around social constructivism (with staff providing scaffolding for students to work with one another and take charge of their own learning), communities of inquiry (students collaborating towards achievement of joint learning goals while also interacting socially), and a participatory culture (Jenkins, 2006) often seen in workshop scenarios where students produce content together. All of these aspects of service delivery are well aligned to the principles of Web 2.0 tools, which essentially use relational computing and social informatics to connect and engage users online (Garrison & Anderson, 2003; Garrison, 2007).

While the issue of ICT skills in educational institutions has received some attention and recognition at the broadest scale—as reflected, for example, in the United Nations Educational, Scientific and Cultural Organization (UNESCO, 2008) and Australian Flexible Learning Framework (AFLF, 2007) reports that promote professional development for educators—the incorporation to date of Web 2.0 in non-teaching areas of many universities worldwide may be described as "enthusiastic yet variable." A range of examples is provided here to show how Web 2.0 tools are beginning to be embedded and integrated into university programs by non-teaching units, in an effort to scaffold engagement with students. Links to the websites pertaining to these institutional examples are provided in the "Resources" section at the end of the chapter.

Podcasting has seen a significant growth in the last five years, with universities using it as a medium for sharing everything from course materials to news items, interviews, speeches, transition help, and student testimonials. It is almost difficult to find a university in the U.S., UK, or Australia that does not in some way provide a podcasting service with, many now moving into video podcasting (vodcasting) and syndication of both audio and video material through services such as iTunesU. Non-teaching units play a noteworthy role in the provision of podcasts, as seen in initiatives by libraries (e.g., Newcastle University and the University of Glasgow in the UK, and in Australia, Curtin University of Technology, RMIT University, and James Cook University), counseling teams (e.g., Australian institutions RMIT University and the University of New England, and UK institution the University of Warwick), careers advisors (in the U.S., University of Miami and North Carolina State University; in Australia, The University of Sydney; in the UK, University of Exeter), and academic skills advisors (in Australia, UWA and The Australian National University; in the UK, the University of Leeds).

Blogs are also increasingly viewed by institutions as a way to engage students, by either providing an internally-hosted blogging platform for use by staff and/or students (e.g., in Australia, The University of Sydney and Victoria University; in the U.S., Princeton University and the University of Chicago's School of Law) or by blogging themselves as one of their strategies for disseminating news stories to students and alumni (e.g., Harvard University and the Jonathan Edwards Center at Yale University in the U.S.; Oxford University in the UK; in Australia, Monash University's Faculty of Arts). In some cases senior university staff have their own blog (e.g., the Vice-Chancellors of Macquarie and Griffith Universities in Australia). Libraries are often at the forefront of communicating with students via a blog (Australian universities Curtin and La Trobe, for example). A number of Australian universities also provide and share tips from peers on topics including but not limited to careers (e.g., La Trobe University, The University of Sydney), learning skills (e.g., Murdoch University), accommodation (e.g., The University of Queensland), and the transition to university (e.g., The University of Melbourne, UWA).

Wiki spaces are also either maintained and supported internally by institutions (e.g., in Australia, The University of Adelaide and Monash University; in the U.S., Duke and Brown Universities) for collaborative writing and knowledge exchange, or, in other cases, public wiki sites used to encourage content co-creation, sharing, and revision with and for a global audience. Worldwide, institutions are making the most of the opportunities provided by Wikipedia as the most widely known and accessed wiki available.

It is perhaps in the arena of *social networking* that universities are creating the most flexible ways for students to engage with their institutions. Many institutions are increasingly harnessing the power of social networking sites for building communities and maintaining links between students and the university, via Facebook, LinkedIn, MySpace, Twitter, and Bebo (e.g., in the UK, the University of Aberdeen and the University of Bath; in the U.S., Drake university, the University of Michigan, and Yale University). Other institutions are preferring to establish their own members-only alumni networks based on internally-hosted software packages (as seen in the case of The University of Adelaide and UWA), or to encourage the development of communities via environments such as Ning (as have smaller institutions such as Norwich University and the University of Essex's International Office in the UK, and Texas Southern University in the U.S.).

While blogs, wikis, podcasts, and more recently, social networking sites play the dominant role in universities' Web 2.0 engagement with students and alumni, examples of the use of other tools and applications are increasingly common. These include, to name a few, the establishment of institutional YouTube channels (e.g., Macquarie University), students contacting professors via Short Message Service (SMS) during live help sessions (e.g., Harvard University), virtual campus tours (e.g., Columbia University), and the use of animated online characters to "personalize" material delivery and encourage interaction (e.g.. UWA's Study Smarter team).

A CASE STUDY FROM AN AUSTRALIAN UNIVERSITY: THE NODE PROJECT

Background

To date, little research has been conducted in Australian universities into what impact a technologically-savvy student population will have, specifically in terms of their expectations of services and their preferred methods of communication. Many academics are considering the relationship between ICT-competent students and pedagogy, with varying degrees of disquiet. Some see potential for creativity, flexibility, and innovation (Pesce, 2007) whereas others are concerned about lack of critical rigor and query whether the different learning modes and pathways really entail a lowering of standards (Brabazon, 2002). The question of whether students want, or see the benefits of, using the ICTs from their day-to-day lives in an academic context is also raised (Conole & Creanor, 2007).

Justification for the NODE Project

The NODE (Networking Online to Diversify Engagement) project at UWA aimed to investigate how an online community could be used by any and/or all non-teaching units to add a further layer of service to students, and thus improve student engagement, satisfaction, and learning. The project started by surveying students' access to, experiences with, and expectations of ICT, as well as attempting to elicit information on the understanding possessed by staff on how to use Web 2.0 tools, and to identify ways of developing them professionally in this regard.

UWA has more first-year undergraduate students entering university straight from school than any other tertiary institution in Australia, with approximately 80% of its commencing undergraduates in most years being school leavers. Students have access to a centrally run suite of support services (such as librarians, transition services, learning skills advisors, Internet support, timetabling, English language training), which may be provided by (and funded through) a number of different units.

The underlying pedagogy for the NODE project meant that the project team had the overall aim of using Web 2.0 tools to enhance existing communities (which may have already been established around particular groups of students or particular types of service) and to facilitate the creation of new ones. The project offered the opportunity to cross boundaries between disciplines and enrollment types (i.e., postgraduate/undergraduate/extension), and to apply tools such as wikis, blogs, and discussion forums to the challenges of creating meaningful community among students.

Motivation for the UWA NODE Survey

The huge popularity of social networking sites such as Facebook, MySpace, and Bebo (for younger users) underscores the importance of connectedness and ease of exchange of information, for the principal users of these sites: those born post-1980. The assumption is often made that Gen Y students are technologically competent and well equipped with the latest tools (see Chapter 16). The project team thus set out to test this assumption by surveying the first-year students about their access to ICT, their experiences, and their expectations. It was hoped the results would provide a clearer picture of what students currently do and what they want/expect from the IT environment at university.

Survey Instrument Design and Development

The survey was made up of four sections:

1. Demographic data (date of birth, gender, faculty, domestic or international, and residential postcode);
2. Logistics (relating to ownership of and access to ICT tools);
3. Experiences (with various tools, resources, and processes);
4. Expectations (about what the university could/should provide in terms of ICT to students).

The aim was to obtain useful and reliable data about students' access to computers (at home and on campus), the Internet, printing, laptops, mobile phones, and wireless devices, rather than relying on anecdotal evidence or assumptions about the mostly (purportedly) Gen Y cohort. Students were asked about their experiences with Web 2.0 tools including blogs, wikis, forums, Really Simple Syndication (RSS) feeds, social networking sites, Flickr, podcasts, and YouTube, as well as their use of lecture recordings (especially those produced using the centrally managed Lectopia [http://www.lectopia.com.au] system, formerly iLecture, which was originally developed at UWA), online shopping, email, and chat.

Responses enabled the identification of trends within and differences between various groups, including males and females, different faculties, international and domestic students, and segments of the Gen Y age group. Students were also asked about their expectations of ICT on campus, in areas ranging from Internet access and file storage to the use of Web 2.0 in teaching.

Survey Findings

The survey was administered to UWA students who had successfully attained at least half of the credit points required to complete first year. It received a response rate of 17% (n=643) respondents, of whom 93.5% were born in 1982 or later. More female students completed the survey than males: 61.4% of respondents were females, while 38.6% were male. International students accounted for 14.7% of all respondents.

Similar surveys have been carried out at other Australian universities (for example at the University of Melbourne by Kennedy, Judd, Churchward, Gray, & Krause, 2008 and at Curtin University of Technology by Oliver & Goerke, 2007), and across institutions in the U.S. and UK (e.g., Anderson, 2007; Ipsos MORI, 2007; Conole & Creanor, 2007). A subset of the UWA survey data is presented here.

Laptop ownership across all respondents was reported at 57% (see Table 1), with higher figures reported for international students (75% indicated ownership) and students aged 25 years and over

Table 1. Survey results showing ownership of ICT devices

	Yes (%)	No (%)
Do you own a laptop?	57.1	42.9
Do you own a mobile phone?	98.3	1.7
Do you own a mobile phone with Internet capabilities?	42.0	58.0

(62%). The most common use for laptops was writing assignments (85% of students who owned laptops claimed to use them for this activity), followed by accessing the Internet (68%) and checking email (65%), with approximately half of the laptop owners using them to take lecture notes (51%). Students aged 25 and over were found to be more likely to use their laptops to write assignments (and less likely to play games).

According to the survey data, ownership of mobile phones is almost universal among students, providing an opportunity to use text and multimedia messaging to contact students easily and opening the possibility of adopting tools (e.g., Votapedia—see http://www.urvoting.com) that let students use their phones to vote or respond to questions in real time during conferences or large classes. In the survey data from 2007–08, only 42% of students had Internet capabilities on their phones. It will be interesting to track this statistic in subsequent years as the iPhone and its competitors continue to capture the market, and to consider applications for student communication and engagement.

Of the Web 2.0 tools, blogs and IM were the applications most familiar to the survey respondents. Only 7% of total respondents had never heard of blogs, while 18% had their own blog and 6% were confident enough to train others in the use of this technology (see Table 2). International students were found to be more likely to have a blog than domestic students (31% compared to 15%) and their awareness of blogs was also generally higher (only 3% had never heard of them, compared to 8% of domestic students). A slightly higher proportion of females reported writing their own blogs (19%, compared to 16% of males), although males were more likely to read others' blogs (42% of males indicated they did this, compared to 35% of females). Students aged 25 or older were found to be slightly less likely to have heard of blogs (10%, compared to 7% for those under 25), although these figures do not necessarily indicate a significant difference in blog use between the two age groups.

Only 4% of the total respondent group had not heard of a wiki, with 73% accessing information in wikis (including Wikipedia), 3% writing entries, and a further 4% confident enough to train others. Use of wikis by international and domestic students displayed very similar patterns: 21% of domestic students did not use wikis at all, compared to 19% of international students. Males were found to be more likely to use wikis than

Table 2. Survey results showing student use of Web 2.0 tools and technologies

	No idea what this is (%)	Heard of but not used (%)	I read/view others (%)	I have created my own content (%)	Confident enough to train others (%)
Blogs	7.0	31.6	37.8	17.9	5.8
IM	3.3	18.1	-	41.0	37.7
MySpace	5.0	53.7	12.9	21.2	7.3
RSS	55.0	35.1	8.6	0.0	1.4
Podcasts	14.3	59.5	22.7	0.6	2.9
Wikis	4.2	16.5	72.5	3.2	3.6

Table 3. Survey results showing frequency of Internet, email, and IM access

	More than twice a day (%)	Once a day (%)	Once every few days (%)	Once a week (%)	Less than once a week (%)	I don't use this tool (%)
Frequency of Internet use	60.8	30.2	7.8	0.8	0.5	0.0
Frequency of email use	22.0	46.7	19.4	4.5	4.4	3.0
Frequency of IM use	27.99	19.06	23.3	6.35	8.32	14.98

females (76% of males accessed wikis, compared to 71% of females), as well as being more likely to contribute to a wiki (6% compared to 1%) or to have the confidence to train others in using wikis (5% compared to 3%). Students aged 25 or over were notably less likely to access wikis (52%, compared to 75% of those under 25), possibly indicating the relative newness of this tool to students in the older age group.

Students' use of podcasts and RSS as revealed by the survey was much less frequent than that of the more established tools of blogs and wikis. Moreover, it appears that students' engagement with these syndication technologies is very much as consumers rather than producers, with no students reporting syndicating material via an RSS feed and only 0.6% reporting having produced a podcast for others.

Communicating information to students presents a significant challenge. Most universities now have email as their official communication mechanism, and the difficulty in ensuring that students actually read official correspondence and other required messages is well known by administrators. Students indicated in the survey that personal email accounts were checked at least once a day by 69% of students, although international students reported checking their personal email more frequently (75% check personal email at least once a day compared to 67% of domestic students). However, only 45% of students checked their UWA student email daily, indicating that alternative communication channels external to the institution may be more effective.

A sizeable proportion of students reported accessing the Internet more than twice a day (61%), with a further 30% using the Internet once a day, making a total of 91% of respondents who use the Internet at least once a day (see Table 3). IM was more popular than email, lending weight to Prensky's (2007, p. 46, quoting Carnevale, 2006) claim that "e-mail is for old people": 85% of all respondents stated that they used IM, of whom 48% used it at least once a day. An overwhelming 94% of all international students who responded to the survey reported using IM to communicate, with 67% of them doing so at least once a day. A larger number of students aged 25 or over said they never used IM (40%), and those who said they did accessed it less frequently (only 30% reported using it daily).

node.live Website

The node.live website was launched as a pilot in response to evidence yielded by the UWA student survey and surveys elsewhere that attest to students' strong expectations for universities to use technology to enhance learning, provide flexibility, and be responsive to their IT/ICT needs. Surveys also reveal that many students (Gen Y and older) are enthusiastic adopters of ICT and desire extension of their skills, even if the ways in which technology aid their learning have not yet been explored in depth.

The philosophy and ethos of Web 2.0 and the functionality of the tools it provides to create online communities resonate with the mission of non-teaching units such as UWA Student Services to generate opportunities, wherever possible, to offer flexible services and enhance engagement and learning. The challenging task of exploring the possibilities of an interactive website hosted by a central team with responsibilities across the entire student cohort was judged a worthy investment of time and resources.

The node.live website was therefore developed to address student needs and institutional context as highlighted in the survey findings. The site hosts blogs, wikis, and discussion forums that are populated primarily by students, and occasionally, by staff. This university-hosted community allows and encourages all students to share advice, ideas, and experiences with one another on a diverse range of topics. It is viewable by anyone, although only UWA staff and students can register to add content. In this way, it creates a "community across boundaries" in that international and domestic, undergraduate and postgraduate students, staff, and users from all areas of the university can belong to and contribute to the community.

Uses at the time of writing of the present chapter have included:

- transition blog/vlog (video blog) on settling into first year;
- blogs about moving to Perth (the state's capital city, in which the University is based) from regional Western Australia, living in college, making friends, starting a new course, and balancing commitments;
- wikis on using and troubleshooting Endnote (software tool used for bibliographic/reference management);
- student/staff advice on making the most of campus services, finding the best coffee, etc.;
- forum-based discussions on study techniques such as referencing, public speaking, and avoiding procrastination;
- international friendship program (UniLink) for students from overseas to communicate with local students pre-departure.

It is possible for registered users to modify the look and content of pages and contribute content as they need and desire. The site is a genuinely shared space based on user-generated content—a central tenet of Web 2.0—unlike the models adopted by some other Australian universities, which involve recruiting a restricted number of bloggers/authors and allowing others only to read or comment. Users agree to a set of rules or protocols when they register on the node.live website, and content is not moderated before it is posted. Instead, fellow users can "report abuse" should they consider content to be offensive or contrary to the agreed protocols (this happens very rarely). At a time when some tertiary institutions are moving to limit students' access to Web 2.0 and social networking sites such as Facebook, the node.live website is somewhat unique.

Lessons Learned and Ways Forward

A major challenge in developing the node.live website was to create and capture content while the site was under development and had not yet been widely promoted. A certain level or "critical mass" of content and traffic is needed before promotion, because potential users will not be attracted to an empty site. Those familiar with public Web 2.0 websites such as Facebook may not see any real value in using a university-based social computing site that has some limitations, especially that colleagues, friends, and acquaintances not affiliated with the university cannot use the site. So the challenge becomes promoting the site in such a way that its potential to add value is obvious and significant.

The NODE project has developed incrementally since its inception. Stage 1 lasted one year, in which the main activities were gaining initial funding, surveying staff about their level of ICT knowledge, and surveying students. The staff survey raised awareness of ICT and social computing, and was useful in terms of recruiting a core group of supporters among staff who could promote the website to their own user groups within the student body. The development of the website forms only one aspect of the overall project, albeit the largest component. The NODE project also explored ways in which individual teams within Student Services could adopt ICT; outcomes of that part of the project are reported elsewhere (Cluett, Skene, & Hogan, 2007). The website became the focus as the strong potential and possibilities that it offered became apparent.

Design of the website was an initial hurdle. Once the design was established, the site was promoted to key stakeholders within the university community. With one of the project coordinators being a learning skills advisor, node.live became an additional tool for forums based on workshop topics offered, and for peer learning groups in this area. Due to the other coordinator's focus on transition of first-year students to university, these students became a target group, and they were invited to visit and explore the node.live site via emails and through rigorous promotion during enrollment and orientation. The first-year students have been the most consistent users and as content has built around transition themes, the node.live site has gained a reputation as a valuable resource for commencing students. This potential is being extended with initiatives to link current student mentors with new/prospective students before they arrive on campus, and direct the prospective students to blogs and other resources on node.live.

The NODE project continues under the umbrella of the Online Student Journey (OSJ at http://www.studentservices.uwa.edu.au/ss/learning/networking_smarter/llrs_projects/osj_project) project, funded by a government teaching and learning grant distributed internally by the University. The node.live site is being energetically promoted to commencing undergraduate students as the home of the UWA transition blog. This tool will be joined by other projects across the Student Services Division as the OSJ project aims to initiate and integrate Web 2.0 tools into the work and activities of the Division, and to train staff in applying these and other emerging technologies in their programs.

SOLUTIONS AND RECOMMENDATIONS

The challenge of building and maintaining vibrant Web 2.0-based online communities should not be taken lightly. An online community, like any worthwhile relationship, needs nurturing and frequent attention. While the goal is to make it self-sustaining, at least in the early stages (and perhaps at all stages), the community needs attention paid to it so that there is frequently changing, fresh content and lively debate. It is easy to underestimate the amount of time demanded, and university staff contemplating establishing an online community should be prepared for a long-term commitment, where the membership evolves and fluctuates over time (Haughey, 2007).

The issues and challenges were managed in the NODE project in a number of ways. Firstly, initial content creation was fuelled by recruiting a small team of interested students and encouraging them to upload text and multimedia (e.g., video) content on the site regularly, to "seed" discussions and knowledge building/exchange. In addition, existing communities were encouraged to make use of the website, through explicit offers of training and support. Secondly, a focus was placed on promoting the site to staff and students in a broad and prolonged marketing campaign, which was then followed up by monitoring presence on the site. Commencing students were a particular target group, as much of the content in the early stages was either from first-year students or had a transition focus and was thus most relevant to them. Thirdly, the research basis to the project (i.e., surveys of staff and student experience with ICT) garnered attention and interest within the institution.

When considering the logistics, principles, and management of online communities in general and Web 2.0-based communities in particular, it may be worth applying what has been learned about student group work. When students are completing a collaborative task online, the same principles apply as with traditional or face-to-face group work, if students are to have an educationally purposeful experience. Like their face-to-face counterparts, online teams, workgroups, and communities in higher education need to be managed with clear guidelines, a defined level of student autonomy, and appropriate oversight from responsible staff members (Caspersz, Skene, & Wu, 2006). When assessment is linked to participation online, students are more inclined to take part, and this may be a good way to introduce those who are not confident at communicating and publishing online to acquire the confidence and competence required. Alternatively, a platform like node.live offers the chance to experiment with or "try out" content creation without any pressure of assessment judgment.

There is no doubt, then, that Web 2.0-based online communities are more robust and have greatest potential to be maintained over time when they stem from communities that exist face-to-face. In the case of communities fostered by non-teaching units of a university, they may be most effective where members can extend relationships with peers and/or staff initiated in person during on-campus meetings or programs. Nevertheless, it is possible—not to mention beneficial, important, and future focused, as argued here—to develop online communities of members that may not have met face-to-face, provided that they derive some genuine benefit from participation. After all, some of the most successful communities on the Internet are composed of individuals who have by and large never met in person.

CONCLUSION AND FUTURE TRENDS

Emerging technologies are having a significant impact on all aspects of learning and teaching, and demand re-evaluation of the services and resources that today's students need and expect. Web 2.0 tools enable new forms of work and scholarly activity that are interdisciplinary, collectively authored, and draw on a variety of new media forms (New Media Consortium, 2007). Developing expertise to teach the skills to create meaningful digital content, assessing the learning outcomes of collaborative efforts, ensuring equal access to resources, and meeting the continuing demand for flexible services are just some of the many issues arising from adoption of the new tools. But student uptake of Web 2.0 in their own lives leaves no option for university staff to do anything less than keep pace, sometimes leading but also learning from students, as the potential and pitfalls of emerging personal and collaborative technologies are explored.

Non-teaching units have a vital role to play at the interface between faculty teaching, support services, internal university communities, and external communities. Their position at the nexus between student learning and student engagement allows them to explore possibilities of ICT in enhancing learning and engagement. Initiatives like the NODE project discussed in this chapter are a first step in creating communities online: there is much that can be done to extend such efforts as technological and social innovations and changes continue to unfold. University leaders, administrators, and teachers must constantly challenge themselves and their students to keep exploring options offered by emerging technologies. Those who fail to do so will stagnate and struggle to remain leaders in knowledge creation and dissemination, and in the quest to stay relevant to the life experiences of their students.

Social networking and personal publishing/broadcasting offer opportunities to engage students and expand the university community beyond the physical boundaries of the campus. This can create a virtual, worldwide community and connect students, staff, prospective students, and other users (e.g., employers, subject matter experts, members of other institutions) as desired. A number of positive trends for the successful establishment of online communities by non-teaching units can be identified from experiences such as the NODE project. First and foremost, closer relationships between academic and professional staff are being developed in order to explore the intersection between use of ICT within and beyond the classroom and flexible delivery of services. Secondly, best practices and guidelines are being devised for adopting shared content, including assessment and the potential for team teaching through integrating learning support with subject curricula in online components of units. Thirdly, students continue to be challenged to discover ways of using their technical skills to facilitate learning. There exist opportunities to "teach the teachers," but teachers will also need to work to reduce the growing ICT skills gap between themselves and their students (see Chapter 19). Fourthly, there is a need for more coordination between central, non-teaching units to provide cohesive services, to avoid competition and overlap, and to improve collaboration (Berg, Berquam, & Christoph, 2007; Krause, 2005a; Wager, 2005). Staff of these units need to be alert to the opportunities for online engagement, particularly in environments where the focus is on content teaching by faculties. Last but not least, there is growing recognition that the skills used by students to engage in online communities are more than technological and social "extra-curricular" abilities. It is likely that these skills will increasingly be required of graduates by employers, and universities must find ways of more formally including them in course structures.

In closing, "Web 3.0" is already on the immediate horizon (see Chapter 20), and may be thought of and referred to either as the "Semantic Web" or the "geo-spatial Web;" both options raise interesting new opportunities to create ever-increasingly more sophisticated virtual communities and networks in all areas of higher education.

RESOURCES

These resources last verified in December 2008. The list is not meant as an exhaustive list of the use of Web 2.0 in higher education, but rather is intended to represent the wide range of tools being used in various contexts across the world. Of course, this field of knowledge is fast paced and new examples emerge every day. Readers are urged to seek fresh examples as well as reviewing the ones listed in this chapter.

Podcasting

- The University of Glasgow—Library (UK): http://www.lib.gla.ac.uk/podcasts/index_podcasts.html
- Curtin University of Technology—Library (Australia): http://library.curtin.edu.au/research_and_information_skills/online_tutorials/podcasts/
- Newcastle University—Library (UK): http://www.ncl.ac.uk/library/podcasts/
- RMIT University—Library (Australia): http://www.rmit.edu.au/browse/Our%20Organisation%2FRMIT%20University%20Library%2FInformation%20and%20Services%2FPodcasts%20and%20vodcasts/
- James Cook University—Library (Australia): http://www.library.jcu.edu.au/InfoHelp/Training/
- RMIT University—Counseling (Australia): http://emedia.rmit.edu.au/communication/content/7_Rss/00_intro.htm
- University of Warwick—Counseling (UK): http://www2.warwick.ac.uk/services/tutors/counselling/
- University of New England—Counseling (Australia): http://www.une.edu.au/counselling/self-help.php
- Miami University—Careers (USA): http://www.units.muohio.edu/careers/students/podcast/

- North Carolina State University—Careers (USA): http://www.ncsu.edu/career/careertalk/index.php
- The University of Sydney—Arts careers (Australia): http://www2.arts.usyd.edu.au/podcast/podcastdirectory.cfm?po_id=4
- University of Exeter—Careers (UK): http://www.exeter.ac.uk/employability/students/podcasts/podcasts.php?id=4
- The Australian National University—Academic skills (Australia): https://academicskills.anu.edu.au/podcasts.php
- The University of Western Australia—Academic skills (Australia): http://www.studentservices.uwa.edu.au/ss/learning/studying_smarter/podcasts
- University of Leeds—Academic skills, hosted by the Library (UK): http://skills.library.leeds.ac.uk/podcasts.php?PodcastEpisode=1

Blogs

- Princeton University (USA): http://blogs.princeton.edu/main/
- La Trobe University—Library (Australia): http://www.lib.latrobe.edu.au/blog/index.php?entry=entry081119-143535
- Macquarie University—Vice-Chancellor's blog (Australia): http://www.vc.mq.edu.au/blog/
- Harvard University (USA): http://harvard-university.biz/2007/11/14/harvard-university/
- Griffith University—Vice-Chancellor's blog (Australia): http://app.griffith.edu.au/03/vcblog/
- University of Chicago—Law School (USA): http://uchicagolaw.typepad.com/
- University of Oxford—Science (UK): http://www.ox.ac.uk/media/science_blog/
- Victoria University (Australia): http://wcf.vu.edu.au/studentsblog/
- The University of Sydney (Australia): http://blogs.usyd.edu.au/support/
- The University of Melbourne—Transition/first year (Australia): http://transition-blogs.unimelb.edu.au/first_year/
- The University of Western Australia—Transition (Australia): http://www.node.uwa.edu.au/
- Yale University—John Edwards Center (USA): http://www.jonathanedwardscenter.blogspot.com/
- Monash University— Faculty of Arts (Australia): http://arts.monash.edu.au/blogs/
- Curtin University of Technology—Library (Australia): http://apps.library.curtin.edu.au/blogs/public/
- La Trobe University—Careers (Australia): http://www.latrobe.edu.au/blogs/careerschat/
- The University of Sydney—Careers (Australia): http://www.usyd.edu.au/fstudent/careers/communicate/may06/blog.shtml
- Murdoch University—Learning skills (Australia): http://blogs.murdoch.edu.au/juliah/
- The University of Queensland—Accommodation (Australia): http://www.educations.com/The_University_of_Queensland__b3397.html

Wikis

- Duke University (USA): http://www.duiki.com/wiki/Main_Page
- Brown University (USA): https://wiki.brown.edu/confluence/dashboard.action
- University of Bath (UK): http://wiki.bath.ac.uk/
- Monash University (Australia): http://wiki.monash.edu.au/
- The University of Adelaide (Australia): https://wiki.adelaide.edu.au/index.php?title=Main_Page

Social Networking

- Drake University (USA): http://www.drake.edu/alumni/socialnetworking.php
- Yale University—Science Library (USA): http://www.library.yale.edu/science/socialnetworking.html
- University of Aberdeen (UK): http://www.abdn.ac.uk/central/social-networking.shtml
- University of Bath (UK): http://www.facebook.com/group.php?gid=20383853395
- University of Michigan (USA): http://alumni.umich.edu/networking-tools/social-networking
- The University of Adelaide—Alumni (Australia): http://www.alumni.adelaide.edu.au/s/923/start.aspx
- University of Essex—International students (UK): http://essexinternational.ning.com/
- Texas Southern University (USA): http://texassouthernlivenetwork.ning.com/

Other Tools

- Macquarie University—YouTube channel (Australia): http://www.youtube.com/macquarieuniversity
- Columbia University—Virtual campus tours (USA): http://www.columbia.edu/about_columbia/tour/
- The University of Western Australia—Study Smarter vokis (Australia): http://www.studentservices.uwa.edu.au/ss/learning/studying_smarter/online_tutorials
- Harvard University—SMS service (USA): http://www.usatoday.com/news/education/2008-01-07-virtual-office-hours_N.htm?csp=tech

REFERENCES

Anderson, P. (2007). *What is Web 2.0? Ideas, technologies and implications for education*. Bristol, UK: Joint Information Systems Committee. Retrieved November 28, 2008, from http://www.jisc.ac.uk/media/documents/techwatch/tsw0701b.pdf

Astin, A. (1985). *Achieving educational excellence: A critical assessment of priorities and practices in higher education*. San Francisco: Jossey-Bass.

Australian Flexible Learning Framework. (2007). *"PUT THE HARD WORD ON 'EM" campaign report*. Brisbane, Australia: AFLF. Retrieved December 15, 2007, from http://pre2009.flexiblelearning.net.au/flx/webdav/shared/NCP/HARD_WORD.pdf

Baer, J. (2007, December 19). "Digital natives" under attack! (as a metaphor) [Web log post]. *Digital Natives Blog*. Retrieved December 3, 2008, from http://blogs.law.harvard.edu/digitalnatives/2007/12/19/digital-natives-under-attack-as-a-metaphor/

Barnes, C., & Tynan, B. (2007). The adventures of Miranda in the brave new world: Learning in a Web 2.0 millennium. *ALT-J Research in Learning Technology*, *15*(3), 189–200.

Berg, J. E., Berquam, L., & Christoph, K. (2007). Social networking technologies: A "poke" for campus services. *EDUCAUSE Review, 42*(2), 32–44. Retrieved December 13, 2007, from http://www.educause.edu/ir/library/pdf/ERM0721.pdf

Brabazon, T. (2002). Point, click and graduate: Student motivation in the information age. In *Digital hemlock: Internet education and the poisoning of teaching* (pp. 128–152). Sydney: University of New South Wales Press.

Caspersz, D., Skene, J., & Wu, M. T. W. (2006). Managing cultural diversity in student teams: A proposed conceptual framework. In A. Bunker & I. Vardi (Eds.), *Critical visions: Thinking, learning and researching in Higher Education. Proceedings of the 29th Higher Education Research and Development Society of Australasia (HERDSA) Annual Conference* (pp. 73–80). Milperra, Australia: HERDSA. Retrieved December 13, 2007, from http://www.herdsa.org.au/wp-content/uploads/conference/2006/Caspersz.PDF

Chan, A., & McLoughlin, C. (2007). Choice, communication and learner autonomy: The development of social competence skills using podcasting technologies. In R. Atkinson & C. McBeath (Eds.), *ICT: Providing choices for learners and learning. Proceedings of the 24th Australasian Society for Computers in Learning in Tertiary Education (ASCILITE) Conference* (pp. 132–134). Singapore: Nanyang Technological University. Retrieved April 23, 2008, from http://www.ascilite.org.au/conferences/singapore07/procs/chan-poster.pdf

Cluett, L., & Skene, J. (2007). A new(er) dimension to online learning communities: Using web tools to engage students. In R. Atkinson & C. McBeath (Eds.), *Student engagement: Proceedings of the 16th Annual Teaching Learning Forum*. Perth, Australia: The University of Western Australia. Retrieved April 23, 2008, from http://lsn.curtin.edu.au/tlf/tlf2007/refereed/cluett.html

Cluett, L., Skene, J., & Hogan, J. (2007). *The NODE summary report: Findings of a 2006–07 survey into UWA students' experiences with, access to and expectations of ICT*. Perth, Australia: Univesity of Western Australia. Retrieved April 23, 2008, from http://www.studentservices.uwa.edu.au/ss/learning/networking_smarter/llrs_projects/publications?f=249629

Community College Survey of Student Engagement. (2007). *Committing to student engagement: Reflections on CCSSE's first five years. 2007 findings*. Austin, TX: Community College Leadership Program, The University of Texas at Austin. Retrieved December 6, 2008, from http://www.ccsse.org/publications/2007NatlRpt-final.pdf

Conole, G., & Creanor, L. (2007). *In their own words: Exploring the learner's perspective on e-learning*. Bristol, UK: Joint Information Systems Committee. Retrieved December 6, 2008, from http://www.jisc.ac.uk/media/documents/programmes/elearningpedagogy/iowfinal.pdf

Creanor, L., Trinder, K., Gowan, D., & Howells, C. (2006). *LEX: The Learner Experience of e-Learning—Final project report*. Bristol, UK: Joint Information Systems Committee. Retrieved December 3, 2008, from http://www.jisc.ac.uk/uploaded_documents/LEX%20Final%20Report_August06.pdf

Crowe, C., & Tonkin, J. (2006). Fifteen megabytes of fame blogging, learning and assessment. *Synergy,* 24. Retrieved December 20, 2006, from http://www.itl.usyd.edu.au/synergy/article.cfm?articleID=287

Dziuban, C., Moskal, P., & Hartman, J. (2003). Higher education, blended learning and the generations: Knowledge is power—no more. In Bourne, J., & Moore, J. C. (Eds.), *Elements of quality online education: Engaging communities* (pp. 85–100). Needham, MA: The Sloan Consortium.

Garrison, D. R. (2007). Online community of inquiry review: Social, cognitive and teaching presence issues. *Journal of Asynchronous Learning Networks*, *11*(1), 61–72.

Garrison, D. R., & Anderson, T. (2003). Community of inquiry. In *E-learning in the 21st century: A framework for research and practice* (pp. 22–31). London: RoutledgeFalmer. doi:10.4324/9780203166093

Hartman, J., Moskal, P., & Dziuban, C. (2005). Preparing the academy of today for the learner of tomorrow. In Oblinger, D. G., & Oblinger, J. L. (Eds.), *Educating the Net Generation* (pp. 6.1–6.15). Boulder, CO: EDUCAUSE.

Haughey, M. (2007, May 14). Some community tips for 2007: Seven tips on how to run a successful community [Web log post]. *Fortuitious*. Retrieved December 10, 2007, from http://fortuito.us/2007/05/some_community_tips_for_2007

Howe, N., & Strauss, W. (2000). *Millennials rising: The next great generation*. New York: Random House.

Ipsos, M. O. R. I. (2007). *Student expectations study: Key findings from online research and discussion evenings held in June 2007 for the Joint Information Systems Committee*. London: JISC. Retrieved August 15, 2007, from http://www.jisc.ac.uk/media/documents/publications/studentexpectations.pdf

Jenkins, H. (2006). *Convergence culture: Where old and new media collide*. New York: New York University Press.

Jenkins, H. (2008, November 21). "Hanging out, messing around, geeking out": A conversation with the Digital Youth Project (Part Two) [Web log post]. *Confessions of an Aca-Fan: The Official Weblog of Henry Jenkins*. Retrieved December 4, 2008, from http://henryjenkins.org/2008/11/hanging_out_messing_around_gee.html

Kennedy, G. E., Judd, T. S., Churchward, A., Gray, K., & Krause, K.-L. (2008). First year students' experiences with technology: Are they really digital natives? *Australasian Journal of Educational Technology, 24*(1), 108–122. Retrieved December 4, 2008, from http://www.ascilite.org.au/ajet/ajet24/kennedy.pdf

Krause, K.-L. (2005a, September 5–7). The changing student experience: Who's driving it and where is it going? Keynote paper presented at the Student Experience Conference, Wagga Wagga, Australia. Retrieved April 23, 2008, from http://www.csu.edu.au/division/studserv/sec/papers/krause.pdf

Krause, K.-L. (2005b). *Understanding and promoting student engagement in university learning communities*. Melbourne, Australia: Centre for the Study of Higher Education, The University of Melbourne. Retrieved August 11, 2006, from http://www.cshe.unimelb.edu.au/pdfs/Stud_eng.pdf

Krause, K.-L. (2007). Who is the e-generation and how are they faring in higher education? In Lockhard, J., & Pegrum, M. (Eds.), *Brave new classrooms: Educational democracy and the Internet* (pp. 125–139). New York: Peter Lang.

Kuh, G. D., Cruce, T., Shoup, R., Kinzie, J., & Gonyea, R. M. (2007, April 9–13). *Unmasking the effects of student engagement on college grades and persistence*. Paper presented at the 2007 Annual Meeting of the American Educational Research Association (AERA), Chicago. Retrieved December 4, 2008, from http://nsse.iub.edu/uploads/AERA_2007_Kuh_et_al.pdf

Light, R. J. (2001). *Making the most of college: Students speak their minds*. Cambridge, MA: Harvard University Press.

Marginson, S. (2007, August 8–10). *Rankings: Marketing mana or menace?* Paper presented at the 16th Annual New Zealand International Education Conference, Christchurch, New Zealand. Retrieved December 4, 2008, from http://www.cshe.unimelb.edu.au/people/staff_pages/Marginson?KeyMar8-10Aug07.pdf

Markwell, D. (2007). *A large and liberal education: Higher education for the 21st century*. Melbourne, Australia: Australian Scholarly Publishing.

McLoughlin, C., & Lee, M. J. W. (2007). Social software and participatory learning: Pedagogical choices with technology affordances in the Web 2.0 era. In *ICT: Providing choices for learners and learning. Proceedings of the 24th Australasian Society for Computers in Learning in Tertiary Education (ASCILITE) Conference* (pp. 664–675). Singapore: Nanyang Technological University. Retrieved April 23, 2008, from http://www.ascilite.org.au/conferences/singapore07/procs/mcloughlin.pdf

Millea, J. Green. I., & Putland, G. (2005). *Emerging technologies: A framework for thinking.* Adelaide, Australia: Education.au. Retrieved October 23, 2009, from http://www.det.act.gov.au/__data/assets/pdf_file/0010/74485/ACT_EmTech_Report_v1_2.pdf

National Survey of Student Engagement. (2008). *Our origins and potential*. Retrieved October 23, 2009, from http://nsse.iub.edu/html/origins.cfm

New Media Consortium. (2007). *The Horizon Report: 2007 edition.* Austin, TX: NMC. Retrieved December 4, 2008, from http://www.nmc.org/pdf/2007_Horizon_Report.pdf

New Media Consortium. (2008). *The Horizon Report: 2008 edition.* Austin, TX: NMC. Retrieved December 4, 2008, from http://www.nmc.org/pdf/2008-Horizon-Report.pdf

Oliver, B., & Goerke, V. (2007). Australian undergraduates' use and ownership of emerging technologies: Implications and opportunities for creating engaging learning experiences for the Net Generation. *Australasian Journal of Educational Technology, 23*(2), 171–186. Retrieved December 4, 2008, from http://www.ascilite.org.au/ajet/ajet23/oliver.html

Owen, M., Grant, L., Sayers, S., & Facer, K. (2006). *Social software and learning*. Bristol, UK: Futurelab. Retrieved April 23, 2008, from http://www.futurelab.org.uk/resources/documents/opening_education/Social_Software_report.pdf

Pesce, M. (2007). *Challenges and opportunities: Peer-produced knowledge and Australian education.* Adelaide, Australia: Education.au. Retrieved April 23, 2008, from http://api.edna.edu.au/attachment/2150/39455/1/pesce_seminar_report.pdf

Prensky, M. (2001). Digital natives, digital immigrants. *Horizon*, *9*(5), 1–6. doi:10.1108/10748120110424816

Prensky, M. (2005). "Engage me or enrage me": What today's learners demand. *EDUUCAUSE Review, 40*(5), 60–65. Retrieved April 23, 2008, from http://www.educause.edu/ir/library/pdf/ERM0553.pdf

Prensky, M. (2005/2006). Listen to the natives. *Educational Leadership*, *63*(4), 8–13.

Prensky, M. (2007). How to teach with technology: Keeping both teachers and students comfortable in an era of exponential change. In *Emerging technologies for learning* (Vol. 2, pp. 40–46). Coventry, UK: Becta. Retrieved April 23, 2008, from http://partners.becta.org.uk/upload-dir/downloads/page_documents/research/emerging_technologies07_chapter1.pdf.

Skene, J., Cluett, L., & Hogan, J. (2007, July 3–6). *Engaging Gen Y students at university: What web tools do they have, how do they use them and what do they want?* Paper presented at the First Year in Higher Education Conference, Brisbane, Australia. Retrieved December 6, 2008, from http://www.fyhe.com.au/past_papers/papers07/final_papers/pdfs/2b.pdf

Tapscott, D. (1998). *Growing up digital: The rise of the Net Generation*. New York: McGraw-Hill.

United Nations Educational, Scientific and Cultural Organization. (2008). *ICT competency standards for teachers: Competency standards modules*. Paris: UNESCO. Retrieved October 23, 2009, from http://cst.unesco-ci.org/sites/projects/cst/The%20Standards/ICT-CST-Competency%20Standards%20Modules.pdf

Wager, J. J. (2005). Support services for the Net Generation. In Oblinger, D. G., & Oblinger, J. L. (Eds.), *Educating the Net Generation* (pp. 10.1–10.18). Boulder, CO: EDUCAUSE.

White, D. (2007). Some real data on Web 2.0 use [Web log post]. *Tall Blog*. Retrieved April 23, 2008, from http://tallblog.conted.ox.ac.uk/index.php/2007/03/16/some-real-data-on-web-20-use/

Chapter 14
"You Can Lead the Horse to Water, but ... ": Aligning Learning and Teaching in a Web 2.0 Context and Beyond

Henk Huijser
University of Southern Queensland, Australia

Michael Sankey
University of Southern Queensland, Australia

ABSTRACT

This chapter outlines the potential benefits of incorporating Web 2.0 technologies in a contemporary higher education context, and identifies possible ways of doing this, as well as expected challenges. It uses the University of Southern Queensland (USQ), primarily a distance education provider, as the context for many of its case study examples. In particular, it addresses the important role of the allowances of particular learning management systems (LMSs) in pedagogical applications of Web 2.0 technologies. Overall, this chapter argues that the goals and ideals of Web 2.0/Pedagogy 2.0 can be achieved, or at least stimulated, within an institutional LMS environment, as long as the LMS environment is in alignment with such goals and ideals. It uses the implementation of Moodle at USQ as a case study to reinforce this argument and explore which factors potentially influence a shift in thinking about learning and teaching in a Web 2.0 context.

INTRODUCTION

Collectively, Web 2.0 technologies constitute a major conceptual shift in the way the Web is used. Two central concepts within this shift are collective intelligence and user participation, as these have seriously blurred the boundaries between knowledge management and dissemination. From a learning and teaching perspective, Web 2.0 technologies offer a variety of opportunities in terms of what such technologies *could* be used for, and in many cases already *are*, by a new generation of students entering universities. The challenge from a higher education perspective is to align what students are already doing with technologies with how they are being taught, without blurring the boundaries between "private" and

DOI: 10.4018/978-1-60566-294-7.ch014

"educational" spaces to the point where students become disengaged. How students already use Web 2.0 technologies and social software tools, particularly with regards to social networking and user participation, are to an important extent driven by the affordances of the technologies themselves. However, such affordances do not necessarily predict the type of teaching practices that could be adopted by universities to exploit their potential. Aligning learning and teaching in ways that suit a Web 2.0 context implies a major shift in thinking about knowledge creation and dissemination, and thus about pedagogy. It requires a conceptual shift from thinking about the Web as a method of communication, to thinking about it as a method of education, and thus of knowledge creation and dissemination. Almost a decade ago, Dreyfus (2001) pointed out that much of the transformation driven by the Internet in general constitutes a transformation in the "*method of communication*" (p. 30, emphasis added). This in turn led him to question, "What proposed *method of education* generates all this excitement?" (p. 30, emphasis added). Although Web 2.0 technologies have largely developed after Dreyfus posed this question, it is still an urgent question in the current context, and one that directly relates to the types of learning environments we use in contemporary university contexts. While many current learning management systems (LMSs) could be seen as largely text-based (Wuensch, Shahnaz, Ozan, Kishore, & Tabrizi, 2008), and too inflexible to allow for Pedagogy 2.0 (McLoughlin & Lee, 2008; see also Chapter 3 in this book), more recently, LMSs have been developed that are potentially far better equipped to address changing learning needs in a Web 2.0 context. This ability has been further enhanced by the extended functionality that some LMSs provide to extend their core environments with additional, and in some cases, third-party, applications.

Moodle is an example of an LMS that appears to be well suited to address learning and teaching needs in a Web 2.0 context, and affords the potential to think about the Web as a method of education, as it is essentially based on an open source philosophy of co-construction of knowledge. However, feedback to date suggests that many university teachers merely use it as a traditional method of communication, or as a way to disseminate existing content. In this chapter, it is argued that the goals and ideals of Web 2.0/ Pedagogy 2.0 can be achieved, or at least stimulated, within an institutional LMS environment, as long as the LMS environment is in alignment with similar goals and ideals. However, this requires universities to resist the temptation to rigidly close the "wall around the garden," which is a long-established practice to control and manage all aspects of the student experience, and is difficult to change. This chapter uses the implementation of Moodle at the University of Southern Queensland (USQ) as a case study to reinforce this argument and explore which factors potentially influence a shift in thinking about learning and teaching in a Web 2.0 context. The chapter addresses issues of institutional change, and asks, "What would encourage institutions of higher education to adopt Web 2.0 tools and pedagogies?"—or, in other words, "What would make the horse drink?"

WEB 2.0, GENERATION V, AND E-LEARNING

Collectively, Web 2.0 technologies constitute a major shift in the way the Web is used (Boyd, 2008). More importantly, from an educational perspective, Web 2.0 technologies offer major opportunities for the way in which they *could* be used. This is not to say that the technology necessarily drives these changes in a technologically determinist sense, but rather that educators could potentially capitalize on the ways in which these technologies are already being used by Generation Y, and appropriate and guide this usage in particular directions. This is rather different than arguing that Generation Y is completely distinct from previous generations (Prensky, 2001) and therefore needs a completely new approach (see also Chapter 16 in this book). In recent years, much has been written about this generation, which is variously referred to as "Generation Y," the "Net Generation" (Oblinger & Oblinger, 2005), "digital natives" (Prensky, 2001), and "Generation V" (where "v" is for "virtual") (Havenstein, 2007), and which is characterized by having grown up in a "technology-saturated" environment. Particular sets of characteristics are ascribed to such a generation, which in turn makes it tempting to call for a complete overhaul of the way we teach such a generation of students in response to those characteristics. For example, Barnes, Marateo, and Ferris (2007) note that the Net Generation "needs" active, engaged learning experiences (as they get easily bored); self-directed learning opportunities; immediacy; interactivity; experiential learning; and above all, opportunities for social interaction (see also Oblinger & Oblinger, 2005). It is not difficult to see parallels between these perceived "needs" and what a Web 2.0 environment appears to be able to offer. More recently, however, more nuanced critiques have begun to challenge calls for complete and radical transformation into doubt (Kennedy, Judd, Churchward, Gray, & Krause, 2008; Huijser, 2006), while accepting the need to address changing student characteristics.

According to Batson (2008), "The most significant fact about Web 2.0 for educators is that key functions and intelligence have moved or are moving from the desktop to the Web, and by doing so they have changed" (para. 1). He stresses the social implications of this movement: "Those functions and intelligence are no longer just about personal productivity, but about the social context for information—what *other* people think about the information" (para. 1, emphasis in original). de Byl and Taylor (2007) focus on this social context by referring to a "Web 2.0 ethos centering on the idea of a collective intelligence which evolved from hyper-linking, web services, platform-independent software, re-usable and re-mixable content and, above all, user participation" (p. 110). The two central concepts here are collective intelligence and user participation, as these have eroded the boundaries between knowledge management and dissemination. As Batson (2008) states, "If we accept that all learning is social, Web 2.0 may be more in step with learning reality than the book or the PC" (para. 2). Clearly, the development of a Web 2.0 ethos is, to an important extent, driven by the affordances of the technologies themselves. Whether it is a wiki, a blog, or a photo-sharing site like Flickr, the ways in which each of these is structured invites certain uses, which are all social in nature. However, once the technologies are available, the ways in which they will actually be used, and the extent to which they will be used, are firstly not always predictable, and secondly not always desirable from a pedagogical point of view. In other words, it is important to resist the temptation to follow unquestioningly what Generation V (Havenstein, 2007) does, under the guise of "student centeredness," without carefully considering what members of this generation (and others!) *should* be able to do upon completion of their tertiary course or qualification.

Recently, as mentioned above, empirical research is beginning to appear that challenges common assumptions associated with Generation Y, V, or Net (Kvavik, 2005; Kennedy et al., 2008; see also Chapter 16), assumptions that often identify potential Web 2.0 applications and uses from a theoretical perspective rather than an empirical one (Leslie & Murphy, 2008). While such empirical studies confirm that Generation Y has grown up in an environment "saturated" by technology, they also suggest that there is much variation with regards to types of use, associated skills, and preferences for use in education. A recent Australian study by Kennedy et al. (2008, p. 108) shows that "many first year students are highly tech-savvy. However, when one moves beyond entrenched technologies and tools (e.g. computers, mobile phones, email), the patterns of access and use of a range of other technologies show considerable variation." For example, while Kennedy et al. found a significant growth in students' general use of instant messaging, blogs, and podcasting, they also found that the majority of students rarely or never used these technologies for study, and importantly, "the transfer from a social or entertainment technology to a learning technology is neither automatic nor guaranteed" (p. 119). In terms of educational applications, this has significant implications for rural or regional universities such as USQ, with geographically dispersed student populations, many of whom study in distance mode and therefore do not know each other offline.

Overall, then, the onus is on universities to clearly define coherent strategies to align the already existing skills of Generation Y with learning objectives and outcomes based on providing tools for meaningful knowledge creation and dissemination suited to a Web 2.0 context on the road to "Web 3.0" (Alexander, 2008; see also Chapter 20 in this book). The authors of the 2008 *Horizon report* (New Media Consortium, 2008) note that Web 2.0 technologies allow for the creation of "collective knowledge stores" (p. 23), where the "data are not organized in the traditional sense, and indeed it is in part the unstructured nature of collective intelligence which allows it to be created and mined in ways that often lead to multiple levels of new insights" (p. 23). Similarly, Unsworth (2008) argues that what universities should recognize in the emergence of Web 2.0 is "a shift in emphasis from the computer as platform to the network as platform, from hardware to data, from the wisdom of the expert to the wisdom of crowds, and from fixity to remixability" (p. 227). Of course, there is a sense of inevitability in descriptions like these, and a lack of recognition that this is essentially contested territory, which is echoed in a recent report entitled *Harnessing technology* (Chowcat, Phillips, Popham, & Jones, 2008), when the authors argue that "If education does not develop ... [Web 2.0-based] personalized services, others may do so" (p. 26), referring to increasingly closer links between commercial and educational applications of technology. The challenge for universities is therefore twofold: on the one hand they are required to address the question of access, and on the other hand they are required to devise strategies to teach students to engage with these new insights in meaningful ways. To confront this challenge requires experimentation with educational applications of Web 2.0 technologies based on sound pedagogical principles. It is important to keep in mind, however, that this kind of experimentation is difficult "when the technology that is being evaluated goes rapidly out of date" (Chowcat et al., 2008, p. 27). In short, there is a very real danger of "jumping on the bandwagon" and pressure to do so should put the focus back on pedagogical principles and outcomes as a starting point.

McLoughlin and Lee (2008) have made a useful attempt to define such principles under the banner of "Pedagogy 2.0," which they define as follows: "Pedagogy 2.0 integrates Web 2.0 tools that support knowledge sharing, peer-to-peer networking, and access to a global audience with socioconstructivist learning approaches to facilitate greater learner autonomy, agency, and personalization" (para. 2). Importantly, they also identify the main challenge as enabling "self-direction, knowledge building, and learner control by offering flexible options for students to engage in learning that is authentic and relevant to their needs and to those of the networked society *while still providing necessary structure and scaffolding*" ("New forms of participation: How social software tools empower users," para. 3, emphasis added). It is the latter that presents the biggest challenge, and goes to the heart of the discussion in this chapter, because it forces the spotlight on a potential contradiction between "open" (Web 2.0) and "walled" (or "managed") learning systems. In short, it creates unease, because it demands a major shift in the way we think about the role of the teacher or instructor, and indeed about the level of teacher control over the learning process. This, in turn, has implications that impact on every aspect of many traditional organizational structures of universities, according to which the teacher assesses, judges, and evaluates (and thus "controls") student learning outcomes. Ultimately, this is a fundamental way in which individual universities build and maintain their reputations. As Geith (2008) notes, "measuring, valuing, and recognizing learner performance remains an exclusive function inside formal education systems" (p. 224). Pedagogy 2.0, by contrast, increases "the level of collaboration with experts and peer groups and ... [connects] students to an emerging global network or 'architecture of participation' that transcends the walls of the institution" (McLoughlin & Lee, 2008, "Pedagogy 2.0: Teaching and learning for the knowledge age," para. 5). The role of teachers or instructors in this context becomes one of working "collaboratively with learners to review, edit, and apply quality assurance mechanisms to student work while also drawing on input from the wider community outside the classroom or institution" (McLoughlin & Lee, 2008, "Challenges in implementing of Pedagogy 2.0," para. 1). This is therefore the main challenge, and to do it successfully requires a series of adjustments within institutions that have historically been resistant and slow at adapting to major changes (Henshaw, 2008).

CHANGING PRACTICES IN PEDAGOGY AND INSTITUTIONAL USE OF TECHNOLOGIES

The required changes relate to institution-level changes, as well as changes to the ways in which individual teachers conceptualize their function, and ultimately the ways in which they approach knowledge creation and dissemination. To begin with the latter, Geith (2008) identifies the emergence, in a Web 2.0 context, of an abundance of what she calls "credentialing options focused on the performance of the learner outside the walls of formal education" (p. 225). This, in turn, leads to a context where learners and teachers are "freed from constraints imposed by a scarcity of expertise and a scarcity of learning resources" (p. 225). Again, to accept this in principle, as a university teacher, requires a level of comfort with relinquishing control that is likely to take a significant amount of time to develop for a large percentage of those teachers, as it upsets their perceived *raison d'être* in fundamental ways. Furthermore, to negotiate the levels of "outside" and "inside" expertise and integrate these in flexible ways in their teaching necessitates an in-depth understanding of the Web 2.0 environment, as well as continuous updating of such knowledge and perhaps a degree of immersion in such an environment, which is another challenge for an ageing university workforce of "digital immigrants." Mabrito and Medley (2008) note, for example, that "while N-Gens interact with the world through multimedia, online social networking, and routine multitasking, their professors tend to approach learning linearly, one task at a time, and as an individual activity that is centered largely around printed text" ("The challenge of Net-Generation learners," para. 1). To prepare teachers for Pedagogy 2.0 would therefore call for "a tremendous amount of institutional support" (Mabrito & Medley, 2008, "Pedagogy for the N-Gen student," para. 3). Furthermore, it would require a flexible, "whole-of-institution" approach (Taylor, 2001), where universities are traditionally monolithic systems that in practice tend to be "less flexible and ultimately less innovative than the granular and remixable information services now often called Web 2.0" (Unsworth, 2008, p. 229). While this may sound rather fatalistic, it is not to suggest that there are no ways forward. Universities need to find ways and learning systems that allow for a balance between commercial imperatives and pedagogical strategies and outcomes.

There are already many instances of individual teachers taking advantage of the increasing availability of "ubiquitous, free, and efficient online collaboration tools for teaching and learning"

(Hargis & Wilcox, 2008, p. 9), for example through innovative uses of blogs (Bruns & Jacobs, 2006) and by incorporating Web 2.0 environments like Wikiversity (http://en.wikiversity.org/) (Friesen & Hopkins, 2008), social networking sites (Boyd, 2008), or Second Life (SL) (Kelton, 2007), among many others. The emphasis in these instances is on the openness and searchability of such tools and environments, which contrasts sharply with virtual learning environments consisting solely of students and their teacher, which are unable to take advantage of network effects (Alexander, 2008) and thereby risk becoming irrelevant. As noted above, however, empirical evidence is beginning to suggest that the role of the teacher and sound pedagogical principles are vital in such environments for learning to occur. For example, in their study of blogging for instructional purposes, Leslie and Murphy (2008) found that students did not move beyond low-level information sharing, nor engage in knowledge construction, which they attributed to a lack of teacher presence. In short, what students lacked in this context was what teachers traditionally offer: the design of the educational experience, the facilitation of that experience, and subject matter expertise (p. 10). These results are echoed by Reynard (2008), who identifies the "5 most common mistakes in using blogs with students."

What this research suggests is a need for an LMS that is characterized by openness and searchability, but at the same time provides a consistent environment and adequate institutional support for professional development of teachers to allow them to take full advantage of the possibilities that Web 2.0 applications offer, based on sound pedagogical principles. At USQ, Moodle has recently been implemented, based on the expectation that it will deliver an LMS that allows teachers to take advantage of openness and searchability of Web 2.0 tools and environments, while maintaining a level of control and "scaffolded safety" in which to learn how to take full advantage of such an environment.

WEB 2.0, TRADITIONAL LMS, AND OPEN SOURCE (MOODLE)

The more recent generations of LMSs, particularly the open source systems such as Moodle, have begun to recognize the need for the ability to socially engage participants in greater ways than was provided through the use of threaded discussions and email notifications in earlier generations of LMSs. The ability to network, usually with other students, and the development of personal learning environments (PLEs), have now become a much higher priority (Dron & Bhattacharya, 2007). However, universities have struggled with this need to provide equivalent open access, or "freedom," to their Internet-based systems, a freedom individuals are accustomed to when using a private ISP (Internet Service Provider).

This dilemma for universities has primarily been due—and for good reasons—to the security implications of providing access to secure or privileged information, such as information about an individual's identity and copyrighted materials. This is where the newer generations of open source LMSs begin to gain credibility and are seen to be, in part, the answer to this dilemma for the institution. Not only do they, like earlier versions, allow secure access to a particular learning environment, but they also allow the creation, in some cases by using additional applications, of social networking environments (SNEs) and PLEs for students, spaces that can potentially also be shared with the wider world. In many cases these environments also allow students to create quite extensive profiles for themselves, and they allow them to choose how they will receive and distribute a range of communication services. In Moodle, for example, students can, within their profiles, add their own pictures, choose to have communications feeds or syndicated links to other environments, participate in one-on-one or group chat sessions with students online, create personal blogs, link to other online spaces, and choose (within limits) the way their environment will appear. Much of this information within their profile can then also be shared with their more extensive PLE either within the LMS or by using an additional application, like an e-portfolio. (See also Chapters 5, 15, and 16 in this book.)

These PLEs and SNEs are usually housed within the confines of the university but stand separate from the traditional course/subject or program environment, thus providing a level of independence to students to personalize their learning experiences. Attwell (2007) believes that the introduction of PLEs can in fact "bridge the walled gardens of the educational institutions with the worlds outside" (p. 7), tying together a range of context-specific sources of information aggregated or syndicated from other environments, thereby creating a more meaningful learning environment based on the individual's educational needs.

However, while suggesting this "open" approach, this chapter is at the same time advocating, at least in part, the existence of a "walled garden" as the most appropriate place in which to house a formal online learning environment. There are several reasons for this. Firstly, the new-generation LMSs are flexible and more robust than those of previous generations. Secondly, and for reasons already mentioned, sometimes privacy is appropriate, especially in an educational context. As Feldstein (2006) suggests, this is for the same reason we like to have the option of closing the door to a physical classroom. Teaching is about trust, and if we want our students to take risks then we have to be able to provide an environment in which it is initially safe for them to do so. For once outside the wall, "the wilderness contains sites that may reveal or misuse personal details, malicious crackers and hackers, uncredentialled strangers and technologies of uncertain reliability or longevity" (Dron & Bhattacharya, 2007, p. 895).

This is not to suggest that there are not times when we would want our students to take risks in the wider world or "wilderness" beyond the walls of the university, its classrooms and its systems. On the contrary, one of the most important learning objectives in a Pedagogy 2.0 context is precisely to teach students how to negotiate a Web 2.0 environment confidently, productively, and safely. Feldstein (2006, para. 1) also states that

> *A good learning environment should enable faculty to password-protect course content but not require it. Further, it should not favor password-protection, encouraging teachers to explore the spectrum between public and private learning experiences. (emphasis in original)*

Moreover, choosing best practices is about academic freedom, and while the tools are important, they should not dictate this choice. Ultimately, however, the university does require the ability to use copyrighted material legally within their courses at their discretion. Currently, and at least for the foreseeable future, the only legal place it can do this is behind some form of wall, where students can rely upon the resources provided by the teaching staff (Dron & Bhattacharya, 2007) as students "still see faculty knowledge and expertise as the most important element in learning" (Thompson, 2007, p. 2). Moreover, Barnes et al. (2007, "Conclusion," para. 1) link this directly to the responsibilities of educators, by arguing that

> *educators must not abdicate their role as authorities directing the learning experiences of their students. ... [There is] a fine line: Educators should continue to find ways to exploit the skills students develop outside of class without accommodating the habits of instant gratification and shallow thinking.*

The more compelling argument, and the third reason for choosing this approach, is about the enabling aspects of providing such spaces within which for students to learn. This is what we might call an ontological stance—"ontology" in this context meaning that which gives a framework, or seeks to explain why we do what we do in different situations to address diversity within our student cohorts—and it is one that, until recently, has been difficult to adopt and realize, mainly due to the limitations of LMSs. However, this more "closed" approach can now be taken for more pragmatic reasons. Shadbolt, Gibbins, Glaser, Harris, and Schraefel (2004) state that their

choice of a single ontology for the system reduces the amount of translation required. Information from external sources (which may have been expressed in other ontologies) still needs to be translated into the system ontology, creating a "walled garden" in which it is easier to work. (p. 5)

The alternative to this is, as Shadbolt et al. (2004) suggest, is "an open approach that might figuratively be described as a meadow in which many ontologies bloom" (p. 45), leading inevitably to a number of heterogeneous ontologies being used, possibly concurrently, throughout the chosen system or schema, which then potentially leads to a fragmented learning experience. This "open" approach runs the risk of unnecessarily overcomplicating the design of the learning experience, as the implication is that each of the individual components must be either translated, or mediated, between each of the individual systems. In addition, and usually as an unforseen consequence of this, the ontologies associated with each experience may well have mutual inconsistencies, inevitably raising "the cost of deciding upon appropriate mappings between ontologies or ontology fragments" (Shadbolt et al., 2004, p. 45). In practice, this potentially means that a student studying four courses in a semester may be required to negotiate a multiplicity of different environments, potentially having to reorient him or herself and learn to deal with a new way of doing things each semester.

"SAFE" VS. "OPEN" VIRTUAL LEARNING SPACES: PEDAGOGICAL AND INSTITUTIONAL IMPLICATIONS

The main concern with the "open" approach described above is that students, in having to cope with new or different ways of doing things, may be subject to additional and possibly unnecessary cognitive load, as opposed to using this capacity to focus on the actual learning that is required (Dror, 2008). This concern relates primarily to the ontology of Web 2.0 technologies and social software that is "based on the idea of 'small pieces, loosely connected' utilising commonly recognised standards and web services for linking ideas, knowledge and artefacts" (Attwell, 2007, p. 5). This may not be a problem for competent students, but for those who might be considered "on the edge," this strategy can increase the amount of mental stress associated with study (Kalyuga, 2007). Shadbolt et al. (2004) reinforce this when they suggest that in taking this temporal (open) approach, "there is a higher cognitive load on the user to remember the relevant previous information" (p. 46). Thus, this raises a question of whether this load should be scaffolded instead, which would imply a less "open" environment, at least initially. (See also McLoughlin & Lee, 2010.)

The "open" approach may be sustainable where it is employed occasionally and when the context is appropriate, but once it is adopted more widely or for novelty (e.g., to do "something different") serious planning across the program is advised. However, if such an "open" approach can be used in conjunction with, or mediated by, an LMS such as Moodle and/or a PLE, it has the potential to provide a coordinated suite of information allowing users to focus their energies on knowledge building, "rather than on splitting their attention, and hence increasing cognitive load, between remembering which instance was next to another while focusing on the detail of a current selection" (Shadbolt et al., 2004, p. 46). Dror (2008) states that by adopting this approach, "one can considerably reduce cognitive load by tailoring the learning to the architecture of cognition" (p. 218).

Overall, Dron and Bhattacharya (2007) suggest the following 10 considerations when considering going outside the LMS. They are presented here from a USQ-contextualized perspective, and include both pedagogical and institutional considerations:

1. *Technical problems:* These manifest themselves in a number of ways. From a user perspective this may include using environments that use voice and/or video applications requiring plugins and download capabilities greater than some students have access to. Most universities have adequate computing standards to which staff are expected to adhere, but once outside the university's systems there is little or no control over this. From the university's standpoint, security issues can also arise from staff (and students) accessing sites that use protocols unacceptable to the infrastructure, particularly when these are accessed from within the university's systems. This has led USQ to develop a series of "minimum standards" for the delivery of electronic course materials, along with a range of alternative delivery options for those who have access problems/restrictions, or no Internet access at all.
2. *Clashing cultures:* As traditional hierarchies or more "traditional" ways of teaching exist in many courses/subjects, tensions can arise if a "whole-of-program" approach is not adopted for the use of new technologies or "ways of doing things." Particularly at USQ, with its strong distance education focus, staff may come to the university having taught in very different contexts (e.g., primarily in face-to-face mode). This may lead to students becoming dissatisfied with staff and staff being dissatisfied with fellow staff pushing the boundaries in isolation. In other words, consultation to overcome the issue of isolated pockets of innovation is recommended for those wishing to extend their school, department, or discipline in new directions.
3. *Technophobia*: This looms large for both students and staff, as part of a natural resistance to change. In some extreme cases, staff do not even use online discussion forums for their students, which is problematic in USQ's institutional context where 80% of students are never physically on campus. In addition, the high proportion of non-traditional students, many of whom are mature aged people returning to formal study after extended periods of time, means that adopting too many "new ways of doing things" too quickly—particularly with Web 2.0 technologies—can be off putting. However, if these tools can be integrated within the "walled garden" then some monitoring and support can be provided for those who may be struggling. Again a staged, program-focused approach is recommended.
4. *Loss of monitoring:* In many cases the use of Web 2.0 technologies bypasses traditional ways of teaching with students operating outside the gaze of the teacher. In a sense this is not dissimilar to students gathering in a café or other informal setting to talk about their work; however, in the context of USQ, where such a high percentage of students (80%) study at a distance, the lack of ability to adequately monitor students, and the consequent difficulty in diagnosing and addressing problems as they arise, may pose significant issues. Nevertheless, if Web 2.0 tools are being used as part of assessment and are housed within the public domain there can be no effective monitoring of when, how, or by whom these sites are accessed and used. This may be addressed within the design of the course by limiting

the dependence on this aspect for assessment, but that would then limit the uses of assessment for pedagogical purposes.

5. *Loss of control:* In a similar vein to lack of monitoring, when using Web 2.0 tools outside the university's domain there is no assurance for staff or students that those tools will endure, even for the life of a course/subject. This may result in the loss of important data and can potentially affect student outcomes. If Web 2.0-type tools can be employed within the university environment then there is at least a reasonable compromise. This will be demonstrated in the USQ case studies below.
6. *Loss of history:* The main benefit for both staff and students in using an LMS such as Moodle to house Web 2.0-type tools is that there is always a record of practice that can be retrieved or called upon if needed. In most cases systems are backed up on a daily basis and do not run the risk of outsiders corrupting important data. This may not be important for some individual staff members, however at USQ it is a corporate requirement that course materials and interactions be housed in an unchanged and accessible form for at least a year, and that records of previously run courses are held for at least two years.
7. *Assessment woes:* This relates very much to the loss of history and the ability of staff to assess the veracity of work presented by a student for assessment. This is not to suggest these problems do not also exist within "the wall," but there is at least a track of the identities that have logged into the site. This also offers the student a level of security as her or she can, in most cases, track his or her assignment submissions. USQ's introduction of PLEs, allowing for the syndication of external sources, attempts to bridge this divide and provide a minimum level of monitoring based on a common student disclaimer of source materials.
8. *Overwhelming choice:* There are so many choices now in the vast "wilderness" of the Internet that it is impractical for teaching staff at USQ to be conversant with, or have accounts with, all of the possible tools, sites, and environments that could be used for learning and teaching. At a simple level Wikipedia alone, for instance, lists 130 different social networking sites ("List of social networking websites," 2009). Potentially, one teacher uses Facebook, another uses MySpace, while yet another wants to use the university's approach to PLEs. As previously mentioned, the additional cognitive load students (and staff) may be faced with when so much choice is offered can indeed be overwhelming. If the teacher is to be an effective mentor and guide, leading students through a process of learning, universities need to support this by empowering their staff to become more familiar with the diversity of new and emerging digital landscapes. However, the cost of such an approach certainly challenges the will of some department heads, even if their resistance runs the risk of their program and course offerings becoming increasingly irrelevant to students.
9. *Loss of trust:* If Web 2.0 tools can be mediated by a student's PLE, or even housed within the LMS, the student can then trust the integrity of the content being supplied (as discussed above). There is also the sense that the teacher or university can monitor the secured space, thereby protecting students (and staff) from misuse, the threat of hackers, and the unreliability of transient spaces.
10. *Inequalities:* With the large diversity of experience within the USQ non-traditional student base it can be considered inequitable to subject these students to a wide variety of Web 2.0 tools that may simply be used, or trialled, for their novelty value. Solid pedagogical advantage should be discernable prior to particular tools being taken up and

used. Again, this is not to suggest that these spaces should not be used, but rather that a Pedagogy 2.0 approach is preferred if they are to be used, which would include sufficient scaffolding to prevent the privileging of one set of prior skills, or understanding, over another. (Once again, see Chapter 3, as well as McLoughlin & Lee, 2010.)

EFFECTIVE USE OF WEB 2.0 TOOLS

Having highlighted the main considerations in using Web 2.0 technologies the chapter will now provide some examples of how these new technologies can be used effectively in learning and teaching programs, both within and outside of "the wall." The affordances of Web 2.0 technologies have allowed the more traditional (face-to-face) universities to embrace the notion of flexibility in the way they provide opportunities for student learning, which was previously the domain of institutions that focused more on distance and e-learning. On the other hand, institutions that have had a high dependence on providing individualized distance and online learning experiences increasingly need to supplement their materials and methods, to address the changing needs of their increasingly diverse student cohorts. The potentially limitless choice of technologies and approaches for learners and teachers requires great adaptability to changing circumstances and learning needs. For today's digital learner, who moves fluidly through the digital world, this is a limitless learning landscape (Dron & Bhattacharya, 2007). Again, some caution is warranted here, as certain hyperbolic assumptions underlie statements like these: "today's digital learner" presumably belongs to Generation Y, but the "movements" of this generation in the "digital world" are highly varied and not necessarily fluid (Kennedy et al., 2008; see Chapter 16). In other words, what about those who move "less fluidly" or do not move in the digital world at all? In short, despite the exciting opportunities that Web 2.0 technologies offer, it is vital to carefully consider the wide range of student abilities and needs at every step of the design and implementation process.

For USQ the need for more meaningful interaction between staff and students and among students has spawned an emerging dependence on a range of Web 2.0 communication tools embedded within the LMS and PLEs, such as:

- virtual classroom technology;
- synchronous and asynchronous voice and chat applications;
- three-dimensional (3-D) virtual worlds;
- e-portfolios and PLEs;
- blog and wiki spaces allowing for collaboration and reflection.

Brief examples of how these tools are currently being used at USQ are described below. It should be noted that USQ has employed a range of tools in conjunction with its installations of Moodle and Mahara e-portfolio software. The Moodle software has been employed at multiple levels: there is an installation for the student LMS; there is a separate environment for staff professional development and to serve as a playground for trialling new and emerging tools; a further installation for community activities engaging institutions and identities outside of the university's walls; and finally, an OpenCouseWare installation housing courses offered through the International OpenCourseWare Consortium emanating from the Massachusetts Institute of Technology (see http://www.ocwconsortium.org/ and http://ocw.mit.edu/).

Virtual Classroom Technology

The implementation of a campus-wide approach to virtual classrooms (VCs) at USQ in 2008, using the Wimba Collaboration Suite (http://www.wimba.com/products/wimba_collaboration_suite/), has allowed this technology to be embedded into the Moodle LMS. This has facilitated the establishment and contextual use of the VC at both a course/subject level and a university community level. The VC permits the synchronous sharing of voice, video, and presentations as well as application sharing, allowing these sessions to be either instructor or student led. Over the course of 2008, VCs were used in over 61 courses/subjects to host live interactive sessions, both in staff–student interactions and student–student interactions. Once a VC is established within a course, anybody enrolled in that course can access this room at any time. Archives can also be made of specific sessions to allow for recording of particular interactions for later, asynchronous use. This technology feels "natural" to Gen V students and yet is simple and intuitive enough for novices to cope with, and it has allowed many students, particularly distance students, to establish new networks previously unattainable.

As previously discussed, usability issues have been a concern, particularly for an institution with a high proportion of non-traditional learners such as USQ. For those students unable to interact in the online sessions due to bandwidth constraints, each VC can be accessed by telephone link at the cost of a local call. Initially it was not clear how many students would require this functionality; however, within the first 10 months this feature had been used well in excess of 500 times.

Synchronous and Asynchronous Voice and Chat Applications

The use of voice and chat applications has steadily been developing for many years at USQ. In previous years tools such as MSN Messenger (now "Windows Live Messenger") and Skype were used in an ad hoc way. However, the implementation of Moodle has allowed the course/subject and community-based embedding of voice and text-based chat applications. The tools being used are the Wimba Voice Board tool, allowing asynchronous voice and text messaging, and the Wimba Pronto tool, allowing synchronous chat with similar functionality to MSN Messenger. These two tools were not implemented until Semester 2, 2008, and adoption into courses is increasing, with over 1,700 sessions being recorded prior to the end of 2008. The Moodle LMS also allows for asynchronous chat within the individual student profile.

3-D Virtual Worlds

The proliferation of 3-D games environments, particularly over the last three to four years, has opened up new possibilities for creating immersive multi-user learning environments, even if this is problematic for the university from a security perspective. However, the security issue has mostly been resolved by employing and integrating two 3-D environments simultaneously, Second Life (SL) and the open source product Open Simulator (OpenSim). There were occasions where it was considered important for students to be in a wider and more open environment than SL provides, while on other occasions it was necessary to ensure more privacy than SL could offer, or a more secure space for students to interact. This more secure space was achieved by deploying the OpenSim environment "within the walls" but using the interoperability features of that product to take students out to SL when required, and vice versa.

For example, USQ currently has an island in the SL environment called *Terra Incognita*, hosting a range of different activities, including marketing and promotional activities for the university, a careers fair, teaching areas, breakout rooms, a mock law court for hosting moot courts, and a number of social spaces. The only concern with this has been that anyone who can access the USQ island can drop in at any time and observe what may be considered as private. On the other hand, OpenSim embedded in the USQ environment allows for the creation of more discreet spaces. For the most part this has alleviated many of the security concerns, while also providing a controllable level of interoperability with SL. In practice this means that a 3-D course can be set up within "the wall," which then allows teaching staff to send students out and potentially bring information back in.

E-Portfolios and PLEs

The move towards e-portfolios for both students and staff has taken an interesting turn at USQ in recent times. The adoption of the open source Mahara (http://mahara.org/) software has opened up a range of new vistas for teaching staff. Mahara and the integration of this software with the Moodle LMS has allowed the university to provide not just a space for students to create a profile for themselves with some additional features, but also an environment for them which is akin to a PLE. The Mahara environment allows for the creation of multiple views that students can set up for a range of purposes. They can create and upload documents, house a blog, and draw in content from external spaces, making a variety of these available for different people to view, and in some cases interact with (see Figure 1).

For example, education students are using their Mahara-based PLEs to house records of their professional practice while also using them to complete assignments for another course. Final-year accounting students are building up their PLEs with portfolios of their work-integrated learning practice. Visual arts and multimedia students are using their PLEs as a stage from which to link to a range of other environments housing video and audio components while uploading others. These elements then all appear within one or multiple views. Staff undertaking professional development activities are using the PLEs to house and manage artifacts that they can then use towards promotion, while also linking to the University's ePrints (research publications) repository that feeds all their publications into this same environment. Yet all of this is only just scratching the surface of what can be potentially done with PLEs, thanks to the rich affordances of Web 2.0 technologies.

Blog and Wiki Spaces Allowing for Collaboration and Reflection

The final example relates to a series of four work-integrated journalism professional development courses housed in the Faculty of Arts at USQ. The courses use a combination of interactive

Figure 1. The USQ PLE using Mahara

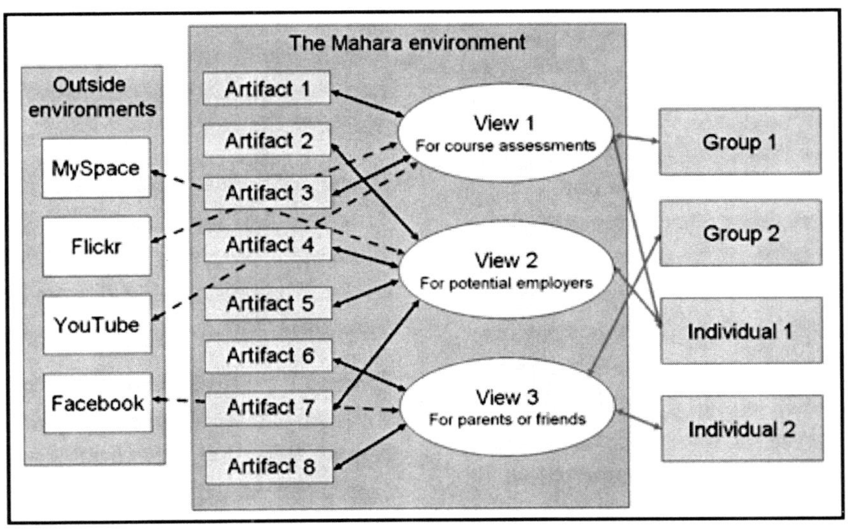

tools integrated into the Moodle LMS. A program website manages how students should negotiate the learning environments and interactive tools, providing information pertinent to the whole program. This site then provides links to the four online multimodal course materials sites, using USQ's Integrated Content Environment (ICE) with integrated multimedia enhancements, and links to each course's blog, wiki, and discussion forum spaces. The use of blogs in assessment enables students to complete story-writing assignments as part of their daily work at the newspaper and, as with the feature assignments for the standard university course, submit the stories as coursework, engaging in critical evaluation of the practices they applied in story composition. Elements such as a newsroom diary, a research record and reflective posts on self-selected stories, a court experience journal, and a story mission statement are built into an e-portfolio-based assessment model.

CONCLUSION

As the examples above suggest, the introduction of Web 2.0 technologies into the online learning and teaching environment at USQ is characterized by a staggered whole-of-institution approach, and deliberately so. This staggered approach is based on the recognition that while the introduction of Web 2.0 technologies in a higher education context has many potential benefits, such benefits are at the same time largely unproven and still highly contested. There are, for example, issues of privacy and ownership of data to consider, as well as ethical issues related to inadequate evaluation of implementation (Chowcat et al., 2008). The staggered approach is thus designed to allow time to work through some of the issues, without putting innovation on hold in the meantime. While the uptake is initially driven by early adopters, the ultimate objective is for staff and students to engage with a Web 2.0 environment and its ever-expanding array of tools, and all the advantages that this would afford. The advantages are roughly twofold: firstly, in a professional context most students will need to be at least comfortable in a Web 2.0 environment upon graduation, and have the ability to quickly adapt to changing circumstances and opportunities in this environment; secondly, moving academic teaching staff towards adopting Pedagogy 2.0 is expected to instill a lifelong learning ethos, and thus the ability to consistently take advantage of the potential of new technologies, while stimulating continuous reflection on pedagogical practices. Both the staggered and whole-of-institution aspects of the approach are designed to provide adequate support and professional development opportunities on the one hand, and on the other hand to provide a safeguard against ad hoc and inconsistent practices across different faculties and even within different faculties. In this way, the approach is designed to not frighten the horses away, but instead to make the water attractive enough to drink.

REFERENCES

Alexander, B. (2008). Social networking in higher education. In Katz, R. N. (Ed.), *The tower and the cloud: Higher education in the age of cloud computing* (pp. 197–201). Boulder, CO: EDUCAUSE.

Attwell, G. (2007). Personal learning environments—the future of elearning? *eLearning Papers, 2*(1). Retrieved November 4, 2008, from http://www.elearningeuropa.info/files/media/media11561.pdf

Barnes, K., Marateo, R., & Ferris, S. (2007). Teaching and learning with the Net Generation. *Innovate: Journal of Online Education, 3*(4). Retrieved December 4, 2008, from http://www.innovateonline.info/index.php?view=article&id=382

Batson, T. (2008, January 16). A new social context for information. *Campus Technology*. Retrieved January 18, 2009, from http://campustechnology.com/articles/2008/01/a-new-social-context-for-information.aspx

Boyd, D. (2008). Why youth (heart) social network sites: The role of networked publics in teenage social life. In Buckingham, D. (Ed.), *Youth, identity, and digital media* (pp. 119–142). Cambridge, MA: MIT Press.

Bruns, A., & Jacobs, J. (Eds.). (2006). *Uses of blogs*. New York: Peter Lang.

Chowcat, I., Phillips, B., Popham, J., & Jones, I. (2008, July) *Harnessing technology: Preliminary identification of trends affecting the use of technology for learning*. Coventry, UK: Becta. Retrieved February 12, 2009, from http://emergingtechnologies.becta.org.uk/upload-dir/downloads/page_documents/partners/ht_trends_july08.pdf

de Byl, P., & Taylor, J. (2007). A Web 2.0/Web3D hybrid platform for engaging students in e-learning environments. *Turkish Online Journal of Distance Education, 8*(3), 108–127. Retrieved December 5, 2008, from http://tojde.anadolu.edu.tr/tojde27/pdf/article_7.pdf

Dreyfus, H. L. (2001). *On the Internet*. London: Routledge.

Dron, J., & Bhattacharya, M. (2007). Lost in the Web 2.0 jungle. In J. M. Spector, D. G. Sampson, T. Okamoto, Kinshuk, S. A. Cerri, M. Ueno, & A. Kashihara (Eds.), *Proceedings of the Seventh International Conference on Advanced Learning Technologies* (pp. 895–896). Los Alamitos, CA: IEEE Computer Society.

Dror, I. E. (2008). Technology enhanced learning: The good, the bad, and the ugly. *Pragmatics & Cognition, 16*(2), 215–223. doi:10.1075/p&c.16.2.02dro

E-learning—the virtual classroom. (2005, October 27). In *M/cyclopedia of new media*. Retrieved January 8, 2009, from http://wiki.media-culture.org.au/index.php/E-Learning_-_The_Virtual_Classroom

Feldstein, M. (2006). In defense of walled gardens [Web log post]. *e-Literate*. Retrieved December 11, 2008, from http://mfeldstein.com/in_defense_of_walled_gardens/

Friesen, N., & Hopkins, J. (2008). Wikiversity; or education meets the free culture movement: An ethnographic investigation. *First Monday, 13*(10). Retrieved October 16, 2008, from http://www.uic.edu/htbin/cgiwrap/bin/ojs/index.php/fm/rt/printerFriendly/2234/2031

Geith, C. (2008). Teaching and learning unleashed with Web 2.0 and open educational resources. In Katz, R. N. (Ed.), *The tower and the cloud: Higher education in the age of cloud computing* (pp. 219–226). Boulder, CO: EDUCAUSE.

Hargis, J., & Wilcox, S. M. (2008). Ubiquitous, free, and efficient online collaboration tools for teaching and learning. *Turkish Online Journal of Distance Education, 9*(4), 9–17. Retrieved December 5, 2008, from http://tojde.anadolu.edu.tr/tojde32/pdf/notes_for_editor_1.pdf

Havenstein, H. (2007, November 14). Forget Generations X and Y: Here comes Generation V. *Computerworld*. Retrieved February 22, 2008, from http://www.computerworld.com/s/article/9046879/Forget_Generations_X_and_Y_Here_comes_Generation_V

Henshaw, R. G. (2008). A singular vision for a disparate future: Technology adoption patterns in higher learning through 2035. *Innovate: Journal of Online Education, 4*(6). Retrieved June 24, 2008, from http://www.innovate.info/index.php?view=article&id=533

Huijser, H. J. (2006). Refocusing multiliteracies for the Net Generation. *International Journal of Pedagogies and Learning, 2*(1), 21–33.

Kalyuga, S. (2007). Enhancing instructional efficiency of interactive e-learning environments: A cognitive load perspective. *Educational Psychology Review, 19*(3), 387–399. doi:10.1007/s10648-007-9051-6

Kelton, A. J. (2007). *Second Life: Reaching into the virtual world for real-world learning*. Boulder, CO: EDUCAUSE. Retrieved December 5, 2008, from http://www.educause.edu/ir/library/pdf/ERB0717.pdf

Kennedy, G. E., Judd, T. S., Churchward, A., Gray, K., & Krause, K.-L. (2008). First year students' experiences with technology: Are they really digital natives? *Australasian Journal of Educational Technology, 24*(1), 108–122. Retrieved December 5, 2008, from http://www.ascilite.org.au/ajet/ajet24/kennedy.pdf

Kvavik, R. B. (2005). Convenience, communications, and control: How students use technology. In Oblinger, D. G., & Oblinger, J. L. (Eds.), *Educating the Net Generation* (pp. 7.1–7.20). Boulder, CO: EDUCAUSE.

Leslie, P. H., & Murphy, E. (2008). Post-secondary students' purposes for blogging. *International Review of Research in Open and Distance Learning, 9*(3). Retrieved October 24, 2008, from http://www.irrodl.org/index.php/irrodl/article/view/560/1140

List of social networking websites. (2009, January 7). In *Wikipedia, the free encyclopedia*. Retrieved January 8, 2009, from http://en.wikipedia.org/wiki/List_of_social_networking_websites

Lubensky, R. (2006, December). The present and future of Personal Learning Environments (PLE) [Web log post]. *Deliberations*. Retrieved January 8, 2009, from http://www.deliberations.com.au/2006/12/present-and-future-of-personal-learning.html

Mabrito, M., & Medley, R. (2008). Why Professor Johnny can't read: Understanding the Net Generation's texts. *Innovate: Journal of Online Education, 4*(6). Retrieved July 20, 2008, from http://www.innovate.info/index.php?view=article&id=510

McLoughlin, C., & Lee, M. J. W. (2008). Future learning landscapes: Transforming pedagogy through social software. *Innovate: Journal of Online Education, 4*(5). Retrieved May 31, 2008, from http://www.innovateonline.info/index.php?view=article&id=539

McLoughlin, C., & Lee, M. J. W. (2010). Personalised and self-regulated learning in the Web 2.0 era: International exemplars of innovative pedagogy using social software. *Australasian Journal of Educational Technology, 26*(1), 28–43. Retrieved February 23, 2010, from http://www.ascilite.org.au/ajet/ajet26/mcloughlin.pdf

New Media Consortium. (2008). *The Horizon Report: 2008 edition*. Austin, TX: NMC. Retrieved December 4, 2008, from http://www.nmc.org/pdf/2008-Horizon-Report.pdf

Oblinger, D. G., & Oblinger, J. L. (2005). Is it age or IT: First steps toward understanding the Net Generation. In Oblinger, D. G., & Oblinger, J. L. (Eds.), *Educating the Net Generation* (pp. 2.1–2.20). Boulder, CO: EDUCAUSE.

Prensky, M. (2001). Digital natives, digital immigrants. *Horizon, 9*(5), 1–6. doi:10.1108/10748120110424816

Pukunui Technology. (2005). *About Moodle*. Retrieved April 24, 2008, from http://moodle.com.au/index.php

Reynard, R. (2008, October 1). Avoiding the 5 most common mistakes in using blogs with students. *Campus Technology*. Retrieved October 16, 2008, from http://www.campustechnology.com/printarticle.aspx?id=68089

Shadbolt, N., Gibbins, N., Glaser, H., Harris, S., & Schraefel, M. C. (2004). CS AKTive Space or how we learned to stop worrying and love the Semantic Web. *IEEE Intelligent Systems, 19*(3), 41–47. doi:10.1109/MIS.2004.8

Taylor, J. C. (2001, April 1–5). *Fifth generation distance education*. Keynote address delivered at the 20th International Council for Open and Distance Education (ICDE) World Conference, Düsseldorf, Germany. Retrieved April 24, 2008, from http://www.usq.edu.au/users/taylorj/publications_presentations/2001ProfessorialLecture.ppt

Thompson, J. (2007). Is Education 1.0 ready for Web 2.0 students? *Innovate: Journal of Online Education, 3*(4). Retrieved April 24, 2008, from http://www.innovateonline.info/index.php?view=article&id=393

Unsworth, J. (2008). University 2.0. In Katz, R. N. (Ed.), *The tower and the cloud: Higher education in the age of cloud computing* (pp. 227–237). Boulder, CO: EDUCAUSE.

Web 2.0. (2009, January 7). In *Wikipedia, the free encyclopedia*. Retrieved January 8, 2009, from http://en.wikipedia.org/wiki/Web_2.0

Wuensch, K. L., Shahnaz, A., Ozan, E., Kishore, M., & Tabrizi, M. H. N. (2008). Pedagogical characteristics of online and face-to-face classes. *International Journal on E-Learning, 7*(3), 523–532.

KEY TERMS AND DEFINITIONS

Generation Y: Also called "digital natives," "Net Generation," "Generation Next," and "Millennials." Refers to a group of individuals, born roughly between 1980 and 1994, who have been characterized by their familiarity with and reliance on ICTs. See also Generation V.

Generation V: "Generation V" (for "virtual") is a concept that removes the specific age bracket from the definition of "Generation Y," to include anyone immersed in virtual environments (Havenstein, 2007). See also Generation Y.

Learning Management System (LMS): Basically software for designing and managing a learning environment. LMSs used by universities facilitate the management of courses and information sharing, and can include Web 2.0 applications such as blogs and wikis.

Moodle: A "software package for producing internet-based courses and web sites ... [and] an ongoing development project designed to support a social constructionist framework of education" (Pukunui Technology, 2005, "Moodle," para. 1). Moodle is provided freely as open source software (under the GNU Public Licence), which means it is copyrighted, but clients have additional freedoms to tailor the software to their specific needs.

Personal Learning Environment (PLE): A "facility for an individual to access, aggregate, configure and manipulate digital artefacts of their ongoing learning experiences" (Lubensky, 2006, "Towards a definition," para. 1). PLEs are directly related to the affordances of Web 2.0, and an example of a PLE is an e-portfolio as outlined in this chapter.

Social Networking Environment (SNE): Broadly refers to various Web 2.0 applications, each of which depends on social networks. Examples include blogs, wikis, and social networking sites like Facebook.

Virtual Classroom (VC): A "learning environment that exists solely in the form of digital content that is stored, accessed, and exchanged through networked computer and information systems" ("E-learning—the virtual classroom," 2005, para. 1). Examples include Wimba and Elluminate, each of which allows for multiple forms of synchronous interaction, in the form of chat, voice, and video.

Web 2.0: Refers to a perceived second generation of web development and design, that aims to facilitate communication, secure information sharing, interoperability, and collaboration on the World Wide Web ("Web 2.0," 2009). Some of the Web 2.0 applications include social networking sites, blogs, and wikis.

Chapter 15
Facebook or Faceblock:
Cautionary Tales Exploring the Rise of Social Networking within Tertiary Education

Peter Duffy
The Hong Kong Polytechnic University, Hong Kong

ABSTRACT

This chapter presents an introduction to an overview of the rise of social networking platforms, systems, and tools within tertiary education, through an analysis and exploration of one such platform, namely the popular social networking website Facebook. Social networking sites, like other Web 2.0 services, emphasize online socialization, collaboration, user-driven content generation, and sharing among users. They enable different forms of pedagogy equally as they disable and challenge more traditional teaching and learning approaches within tertiary education. In this chapter, various criticisms, challenges, and concerns in relation to the incorporation of the new tools within the student learning experience are explored. The chapter seeks to illuminate some of the educational possibilities of incorporating Web 2.0 social network structures provided by websites such as Facebook into academic courses, and to offer suggestions for effectively leveraging these emergent social networks to enhance the student learning experience.

INTRODUCTION

Educators have widely acknowledged the value of community building and social interaction with and among students, in both face-to-face and online classes (Palloff & Pratt, 2007; Chickering & Gamson, 1987). With the emergence of Web 2.0-based social networking sites such as Facebook (http://www.facebook.com/), learners have developed a social world that is parallel to and often interlinked with their everyday work and study activities. The deep penetration of web technologies into the lives of students has been highlighted by a number of researchers (e.g., Conole, de Laat, Dillon, & Darby, 2006; Green & Hannon, 2007; Kamel Boulos & Wheeler, 2007) and their immersion in digital technology is argued to have influenced the interests, attitudes, and aptitudes of

DOI: 10.4018/978-1-60566-294-7.ch015

students in ways significant for education. Multiple studies and authors (see Frand, 2000; Oblinger & Oblinger, 2005a; Tapscott, 1999) suggest that the digital generation learns differently compared with preceding generations of students. Many researchers see Web 2.0 as having the potential to transform e-learning and traditional teaching methods (Lytras & Naeve, 2006; Owen, Grant, Sayers, & Facer, 2006; Kohut, Parker, Keeter, Doherty, & Dimock, 2007), and current research shows a growing interest in ways of harnessing the new opportunities offered to improve the student learning experience (Kamel Boulos & Wheeler, 2007; Anderson, 2007). Suggested is that Web 2.0 tools, including social networking sites, offer possibilities to assist in a move from paradigms of teacher-centered, "sage on the stage" delivery of instruction in which learners are passive recipients, towards the facilitation of active, participatory, co-collaborative interactions that transcend traditional classroom boundaries.

Student use of Web 2.0-based social networks (e.g., Facebook and MySpace) has provoked a variety of responses from teachers and educational institutions (refer to Huijser, 2008 and also to later sections within this chapter dealing with specific strategies as well as challenges). Some schools in the USA have explicitly banned these sites and blocked them from being accessed on campus (Cameron & Fox, 2007), while many educators' blogs anecdotally expound the pedagogic benefits of these tools and advocate their use to enhance teaching, learning, and assessment. Regardless of the policies and views of teachers and institutions, students are virally immersing themselves into online social networks. Successful realization of the potential and possibilities of Web 2.0-based social networking requires a thorough understanding of the potential barriers influencing acceptance of these technologies by educators and learners alike. The capabilities of the current wave of online spaces for social networking and their application in tertiary education raise a range of questions connected to copyright, content ownership, privacy and identity online, content reuse, and the role/place of the educator in these social networks.

The objectives of this chapter are to provide an overview of social networking sites, and, through an exploration of one illustrative example, Facebook, explore some of the educational possibilities, challenges, and cautionary tales relating to the rise of social networks within tertiary education. Some specific strategies and considerations are provided for the reader to ponder in relation to the pedagogic adoption of Facebook appropriate to a tertiary education context.

ONLINE SOCIAL NETWORKING

Lenhart and Madden (2007), in their report for the Pew Internet and American Life Project, state that social networking use has quadrupled in the last three years among adults in the U.S., and that roughly 35% of adults now have profiles on social networking sites. However, it is arguable that the Internet has been used for social networking since its early days, even before the genesis of the World Wide Web. Early adopters engaged in online interactions through newsgroups, listservs, and discussion forums, and participated in communities comprised of individuals who possessed the ability to access and technical competence to make use of these forms of online communication.

In the late 1990s and early 2000s, online social networking became more proliferate with the emergence of sites like Friendster and MySpace. These sites allow people to create personal profiles and build networks of connections with others. More recently, Facebook, incorporating ease of use and ability to connect with others of shared interests, moved social networking from the domain of early adopters into the mainstream. Stutzman (2007) offers the following depiction of the capabilities of and user experience offered by sites such as MySpace and Facebook:

There is something essentially placeful about online social networks; as I log in, I am engaged by a cross-section of my social relationships. In an instant, information is revealed, opportunities are discovered, and a website becomes a social nexus—from which I can derive a sense of gratification, meaning and identity. (p. 1)

Since their introduction, social networking sites such as MySpace, Facebook, Cyworld, and Bebo have attracted millions of users, many of whom have integrated these sites into their daily routines and practices. Presently, there are hundreds of social networking sites, incorporating various technological affordances and capable of supporting a wide range of interests and practices. While their key technological features are fairly consistent, the cultures that emerge around the sites are varied. Table 1 contains an attempt to capture and encapsulate the multifaceted perspectives of what social networking sites involve.

Web 2.0-based social networking sites such as Facebook are challenging existing learning theories and paradigms that were developed at a time when immersive online communication between people was not as prevalent as it is today. Mason and Rennie (2008) support this view, citing Siemens' (2005) claim that Web 2.0 technologies have changed the learning landscape. These changes are captured, at least in part, by Siemens' notion of connectivism, which he describes as "a learning theory for the digital age" (p. 3), arguing

Table 1. Perspectives on social networking site features/functions

Feature/function	Explanations/perspectives of what is enabled
Establish a personal profile	• Construction of a public or semi-public profile within a bounded system (Boyd & Ellison, 2007) • Construction of an online identity through an online space where one can "type oneself into being" (Sundén, 2003, p. 3) • Maintenance of a certain level of visibility of the profile within the site, which may differ depending on the site and according to user discretion (Note: Structural variations around visibility and access are one of the primary ways in which social networking sites differentiate themselves from one another.)
Identify "friends"	• Articulation of a list of other users with whom one shares a connection or affiliation (which may or may not extend to the offline world), i.e. "friends"—this term can be misleading, because the connection does not necessarily equate to friendship in the everyday sense (Boyd, 2004) • Incorporation of friendships in social networks that often began offline and later migrated online (Lampe, Ellison, & Steinfield, 2006)
Establish/indicate connections	• Showing of "public displays of connection" (Donath & Boyd, 2004, p. 71); these can serve as important identity signals to help navigate the networked social world, and may assist in the validation of information presented in profiles • Viewing and traversing one's connections and those made by others within the community or system (Boyd & Ellison, 2007) • Finding others (strangers) with shared interests, political views, and/or activities • Supporting the maintenance of pre-existing social networks
Share content and collaborate	• Incorporation of user-generated content, including the co-creation, co-editing, co-construction, and sharing of ideas and knowledge artifacts, often reflecting the collective intelligence of users • Integration (to varying degrees, depending on the site) of new information and communication tools and applications, e.g., mobile connectivity, blogging, photo/video sharing • Fostering of a "gift culture" in which users contribute as much as they take on the Web (Mason & Rennie, 2008, p. 4)
Join/establish communities and groups	• Establishment of communities of practice (Lave & Wenger, 1991; Wenger, 1998) • Application of Lave and Wenger's (1991) concept of legitimate peripheral participation as users progress from being newcomers to fully participating in the community • Facilitation of regular communication and interaction between "latent ties" (Haythornthwaite, 2005, p. 136) who share some offline or online connection • Creation of formal connections to people one is acquainted or familiar with, and/or with whom one communicates and shares views/preferences/interests (Mason & Rennie, 2008)

that we derive our knowledge and competence through establishing connections. This stands in contrast to the view adopted by constructivism, which sees learners as attempting to foster individual understanding by meaning-making tasks and experience. In connectivism, this "meaning making" is reframed as the perception/recognition of patterns and the formation of links both within and between specialized communities and information/knowledge architectures. Connectivism is proposed as a new theoretical framework that recognizes the limitations of behaviorism, cognitivism, and constructivism, and extends our understanding of knowledge and learning to reflect and explain the dimensions of social interactions enabled by new connective technologies, including but not limited to those of the Web 2.0 movement.

INTRODUCING FACEBOOK

Facebook was founded in 2004 by Mark Zuckerberg with his fellow computer science classmates at Harvard. It is a social networking site that allows members to participate in an online social community, creating profiles, forming connections with others, and engaging in discussion and information/media exchange. Although Facebook is by no means the only social networking site in existence (see Sharma, 2007 for a list of 350 other such sites), it was originally intended for and has become increasingly popular with students, drawing massive numbers of them in to an online world where they spend countless hours browsing profiles, meeting new people, building relationships, exchanging information and media, and exploring shared interests. The EDUCAUSE Learning Initiative (2006) suggests that any technology that is able to captivate so many students for so much time not only carries implications for how those students view the world, but also offers rich opportunities for education. In particular, there is scope for educators to identify and analyze the elements of social networking that students find so compelling, and to incorporate those elements into teaching and learning. Some of these elements are discussed and explored in later sections of this chapter.

According to Wikipedia, Facebook is the leading social networking site based on monthly unique visitors, having overtaken its main competitor, MySpace, in April 2008 (*Facebook*, 2009). As of September 2009 there are a reported 250 million active users (Facebook, 2009), with the site widely described as a "viral" phenomenon. One possible explanation as to why students find Facebook so compelling may lie in its "one-stop-shop" nature. For example, it incorporates the ability to create online a "complete" snapshot of the various facets of one's life, inclusive of plans for the weekend, photos from recent outings, messages and updates from friends present and past, access to numerous applications for a variety of purposes, the ability to be part of online communities and maintain membership across a wide range of interests, and news updates ranging from assessment requirements to reviews of the best place to buy coffee.

Social networking sites in general, and Facebook in particular, are being actively investigated across a number of research areas. For example, research has been conducted on identity presentation and privacy concerns in Facebook (Gross & Acquisti, 2005; Stutzman, 2006). In light of the amount of information Facebook members provide about themselves, the relatively public nature of the information, and the lack of privacy controls enacted by members, Gross and Acquisti (2005) argue that users may be putting themselves at risk both offline (e.g., stalking) and online (e.g., identify theft). Other recent Facebook-related studies examine student perceptions of teacher presence and self-disclosure (Hewitt & Forte, 2006; Mazer, Murphy, & Simonds, 2007), temporal patterns of use (Golder, Wilkinson, & Huberman, 2007), and the relationship between profile and friendship articulation (Lampe, Ellison, & Steinfield, 2007). Some exploration of social networking and the benefits of social capital has also been carried out (Ellison, 2007). The term "social capital" here refers to the idea that social networks have value and can affect the productivity of individuals and groups.

EDUCATIONAL BENEFITS OF FACEBOOK

This section broadly situates the potential educational benefits of using online social networking sites such as Facebook, in preparation for the next section, where specific teaching and learning strategies are proposed. The main benefits of Facebook for teaching and learning arise from its ability to enable students to share information, knowledge, and artifacts within a community and co-creative, dynamic network linked through members' personal profiles and the associations between them. The information in these profiles serves as links from which other network members with similar interests, communities, or latent ties can associate. Users can navigate through profiles based on criteria and communicate with others via asynchronous and instant messaging, comments, blogs, and so on. They can add "friends" and gain access to various sorts of semi-public information such as pictures, personal details, and blog entries. Although some concerns about the educational use of social networking sites have been expressed (Anderson, 2007), its benefits are clear, given that learning is a social activity; social networking sites, with their powerful social affordances, have the capability to connect and engage students and to involve both students and teachers within new community and connected pedagogies.

As previously discussed, many students are already using Facebook for their own purposes outside the classroom, and it is already very much integrated into their day-to-day practices. Within the site, they engage in educationally useful and relevant social behaviors such as converting historical associations and weak ties to contextually relevant links, and building on these to grow and strengthen communities. They draw upon shared information and connections to learn about acquaintances based on groupings related to common interests, managing a large network of existing relationships and often resurrecting past relationships—all of which Ellison (2007) suggests relate to the formation and maintenance of social capital. "Social capital" in this context of Facebook use and as adapted from Donath and Boyd (2004) is used to describe the use of technologies in ways that expand one's social network and result in an increase in available information, opportunities, and benefits from this large, heterogeneous network. Educators can tap into this existing behavior to promote higher levels of engagement as well as immersion in authentic learning experiences that take place beyond traditional boundaries.

The use of Facebook's "comments" feature (similar to a multi-user or community blog) aligns with a number of potential educational benefits of Web 2.0 and social software tools as outlined by Richardson (2006) in his book, *Blogs, wikis, podcasts, and other powerful web tools for classrooms*. Richardson suggests that the act of responding to others' postings ("postings" here being a broad term encompassing many forms of visual and textual online discourse) can trigger and promote critical as well as creative, intuitive, and associational thinking. Ellison (2007) also identifies other educational benefits of blogs that may apply to the use of the Facebook "comments" feature. According to her, the posting of online comments by students encourages them to engage with positions divergent from their own; the ability to write for and present to a worldwide audience on the Internet as opposed to an audience of one also engenders greater investment from students in the topic, activities, and tasks at hand.

Broadly speaking, the educational benefits possible within the structure of Facebook allow students to demonstrate critical thinking, take creative risks, and make sophisticated use of language and digital literacy skills. In doing so, the students acquire creative, critical, communicative, and collaborative skills that are useful in both educational and professional contexts. Facebook can facilitate the development of communities of practice (Wenger, 1998) and communities of interest (Fischer, 2001). These communities allow individuals from *spatially*, *temporally*, and *conceptually* distant or disparate areas to work together on a specific educational activity. Spatial distance here refers to the use of Facebook (or more specifically, the "groups" function within Facebook, for example) to support geographically distributed people working together, enabling the sharing of experiences and informed participation (Arias, Eden, Fischer, Gorman, & Scharff, 2000). Temporal distance refers to the creation, over time, of learning artifacts. Finally, conceptual distance relates to the establishment of a shared understanding or common ground (Resnick, 2006) in the fostering of co-creative and collaborative interactions. The growing popularity of Facebook points to the possibility that some of the educational experiences traditionally relegated to a classroom experience may be accomplished under circumstances dramatically different from those typically seen in tertiary education.

In summary, there appear to be three key advantages of social networking technologies for tertiary education. Firstly, they offer a set of affordances relating to the creation of online collaborative activities. Secondly, many students are already using these technologies for socialization and communication, and so may be willing to use them in their learning. Thirdly and lastly, many of the systems and tools are free to use and come without the restrictions found in existing institutional learning management systems (LMSs). Other advantages include the ability to aggregate information, data, and ideas from different places quickly and easily, and the ability for students to maintain access to the material after they have completed their studies, which has implications for lifelong learning. As social networking technology deepens its impact and is increasingly used by the new generation of learners, educators and tertiary education will be under increasing pressure to consider its appropriate use. The next section suggests some specific strategies for using Facebook in tertiary teaching and learning.

STRATEGIES FOR USING FACEBOOK IN TERTIARY TEACHING AND LEARNING

Many claim that today's students approach and use technology as "digital natives" (Prensky, 2001, 2004; see also Chapter 15 for a critical examination of this concept), navigating through online communities in ways that allow them to do what they want, communicate with whom they want, and in ways, times, and places/spaces of their choosing. Easily accessible and user friendly, social networking tools such as Facebook allow students to explore, share, engage, and *connect with people and content* in meaningful ways, a notion that resonates with Siemens' (2005) aforementioned theory of connectivism. From a pedagogical perspective the changing "connection" between the teacher and student mediated through such sites as Facebook can be described as a move from "sage on the stage" to "meddler in the middle" (McWilliam, 2008). McWilliam tells of a shift in the learning landscape in which the teacher and student are positioned as partners or associates in the learning process. She suggests that in the new landscape, the teacher must be a pedagogical expert but may not necessarily be an expert in the knowledge domain and/or the technology, as given the pace at which knowledge is generated and becomes superseded in the digital age, teachers will need to learn continuously with and from their students.

In the next two subsections, some specific, practical strategies are offered that tertiary educators can use to incorporate Facebook into their teaching practice. Then, in the following section, challenges and cautions regarding its use are outlined. It is important to note that the strategies suggested below are intended to be combined into holistic, overall approaches appropriate to the educational context, rather than being taken individually and implemented in isolation.

Building Online Communities through Facebook

Facebook can be used to set up discussion groups and collaboration environments to accommodate and support student project teams, units or courses of study, and even university-wide initiatives. The development of virtual communities in tertiary education has been the subject of analysis and investigation by many authors in recent years (e.g., Luppicini, 2007; Hotrum, 2008), many of whom suggest that continuous learning and pedagogical multiplicity can be encouraged and supported through the effective use of social networking tools and platforms. These tools and platforms also have the potential to promote continuity of the learning process and the community beyond the conclusion of a formal academic program or unit of study.

The following recommendations/strategies relating to the establishment of a community space within Facebook have been adapted from Hotrum (2008):

- Create an informal network space for students and teachers with personal profiles, blogs, and resource repositories. This is especially relevant to courses and cohorts highly reliant on peer support, such as those in which students are enrolled in part-time studies.
- Ask students to locate and join at least one Facebook group pertaining to their discipline or area of study. (See for example the "Educators using Facebook" group at http://www.facebook.com/group.php?gid=7036945291.)
- Design collaborative learning and group work activities within the social networking site as a supplement to activities carried out in other virtual learning environments. Web 2.0-based online spaces like Facebook often provide access to far more extensive toolsets than is available within the "walled garden" of an institutional LMS. The toolsets are also constantly growing, and offer both students and teachers a higher degree of flexibility and customizability.
- Take steps to foster a community culture of continuous learning and knowledge sharing in which students contribute to the ongoing expansion, refinement, and the use of the knowledge base of collaboratively generated content.

Using Facebook Applications in Tertiary Education

As was alluded to in the previous subsection, Facebook contains a large and growing collection of tools. The following list of Facebook applications has been adapted from the article, *The Facebook classroom: 25 Facebook apps that are perfect for online education* (2008), and also draws on the personal experience of the author. This is by no means a definitive list, but it does offer some suggestions regarding applications that may be suitable for adoption in tertiary teaching and learning:

- *JSTOR Search:* Using this application, students can find and access the full text of scholarly research articles.
- *Notely:* An application that assists in organizational activities by providing calendar, notes, and assignment functions.
- *Study Groups:* This tool allows the creation of online spaces for study groups and project teams.
- *Add Courses:* At the time of writing of this chapter, this is the only application with instructor and course management functionality (see http://apps.facebook.

com/courses/). Courses can be used without "friending" students, and teachers can manage specific classes. It also permits the creation of an instructor page, and provides the ability for students to post assignments to the online class space.

- *Make a Quiz:* This is an application that can be used by teachers and students to facilitate the creation of simple online quizzes.
- *Courses 2.0:* Facilitates the sharing of class schedules, work activities, and the formation of study groups. It also enables communication with peers regarding common course challenges and allows multiple settings to control privacy and notifications.
- *Flashcards:* Allows the creation of flashcards to be used in drills/exercises that aid retention and memorization.
- *My Documents:* Allows students and teachers to upload documents for sharing with other users.

Good Practices and Tips/Guidelines

Regardless of whether Facebook is being used for the establishment of an educational community space, in support of a particular pedagogical intent, or for the functionality provided by a particular constituent tool (e.g., the "Courses 2.0" application mentioned above), there are some overarching considerations regarding its adoption and implementation within a tertiary education context. Some of these are discussed below; they have been adapted from the work of Staton (2008) as well as, once again, being informed by the author's personal experience.

One common concern relating to Facebook use by educators is the need to keep the social and personal aspects separate from the professional (academic) aspects. One way of accomplishing this is to create a "teacher" profile separate from one's "personal" profile; this requires the use of two different email accounts. Related to this is are issues arising from the choices students need to make in regards to what information is to be shared with their teachers and the ways in which it is to be shared. If not properly planned and considered, this may lead to a number of problems. It is recommended that students be asked to create a limited profile with controlled settings, "friend" the teacher, and add him or her to the limited profile list. In this way, students need not show teachers their photos, videos, status updates, friends, posts, or notes. "Mini-feed" and "Photo Albums" should also be turned off.

Group work, collaboration, and co-creation within an online space such as Facebook can be facilitated through the establishment of Facebook groups. The group can be set up around a particular topic, assignment, subject, or even a faculty or department. Groups in Facebook allow the administrator as well as group members to manage basic information, memberships, officers, photos, videos, and links, in addition to providing a wall for posting public notices, a facility for uploading documents, as well as the ability to share opinions through the comments feature and schedule events through the calendar.

Rich media sharing within a Facebook group or community space is a powerful way of drawing students into the online environment and associated educational activities. In particular, the sharing of photos and "tagging" students within the community can enhance the sense of belonging to the community. The group or community space can also be used to share examples of student work with instructor feedback or to subject the work to constructive criticism from peers through the comments feature. The use of notes allows students to collaboratively provide more personal feedback to the authors of uploaded work products.

Many students entering tertiary education are likely to be users of Facebook (Golder et al., 2007). Although most of this activity is hidden to educators, it is significant because it is interlaced with studying and more formal teaching and learning structures. The use of Facebook within tertiary education does represent a new, and so far, tentatively explored landscape for learning; however, as with all new and unexplored realms there are some challenges and areas to be avoided or entered with caution.

CHALLENGES, CRITICISMS, AND CAUTIONARY TALES

The previous sections have adopted a largely positive and optimistic view of Facebook in education, discussing its potential benefits and suggesting strategies for its use for tertiary teaching and learning. However, the possible risks and negative aspects of the use of this emergent technology remain to be considered. This section is therefore devoted to discussing some of the challenges and criticisms regarding educational uses of social networking sites and Facebook, from various perspectives. It includes some "cautionary tales" with which to contemplate the appropriateness of Facebook within the reader's context.

Oftentimes, technology is incorporated into pedagogy due to the popularity of the tool or application and its buzz-word status in mainstream, non-educational settings. Adoption is largely based on the rationale or premise that if students are already using the tool outside the classroom, it is possible—and beneficial—to leverage this interest and associated technological skill for teaching and learning. However, it is questionable whether this reasoning can be broadly applied to *all* technologies and learning scenarios. Facebook is a social space, used for informal conversations, building and maintenance of relationships, and the voyeuristic tendency of "profile surfing." While students may use Facebook to create informal networks, study groups, or communication tools for clarifying assignment requirements, for instance, at present its use for formal teaching and learning is relatively unexplored territory and is thus somewhat uncertain.

The use of online social networking sites and their appropriateness to tertiary education *must* be considered from a cautionary point of view. Currently, there are reports that cast a shadow of doubt on the accepted wisdom of whom and how many people use social networking sites, although research indicates that they are growing in popularity worldwide (comScore, 2007). This growth does not necessarily equate with an imperative for educational use. Even outside of the tertiary education arena, questions are being raised regarding the value and usefulness of social networking sites vis-à-vis the dangers and drawbacks. For example, U.S. military soldiers were banned from accessing MySpace (Frosch, 2007); the Canadian government prohibited employees using Facebook (Benzie, 2007); the U.S. Congress proposed legislation to ban youth from accessing social networking sites in schools and libraries through the Deleting Online Predators Act (H. R. 5319, 2006) and the Protecting Children in the 21st Century Act (S. 49, 2007). Ellison (2007), in an EDUCAUSE Center for Applied Research (ECAR) report, lists several concerns related to Facebook, including those relating to accountability to the university in terms of intellectual property, privacy, archiving, and exposure to advertising. Additionally, it is important that educators are aware that they may face resistance from students in their attempts to co-opt Facebook for academic purposes.

Many authors are also beginning to question claims and assumptions regarding "digital native" (Prensky, 2001) and "Net Generation" students, and their use of technology within tertiary education (see Chapter 15). Oblinger and Oblinger (2005b) suggest that students are generally technology savvy but may not be as adept at using the technology effectively for academic or study purposes. Professor Rosemary Luckin of the London Knowledge Lab at the Institute of Education, University of London (quoted in O'Brien, 2008, para. 8) claims that "The worrying view coming through is that students are lacking in reflective awareness ... Technology makes it easy for them to collate information, but not to analyse and understand it. Much of the evidence suggests that what is going on out there is quite superficial."

In the U.S., an ABC news story (Davis, 2009) told of how a Facebook group entitled "For the love of god—don't let parents join Facebook" recruited 5,819 high school and college-aged members, intent on stopping the growing number of parents joining Facebook from "spying" on them. It quoted a comment by a university sophomore, who remarked: "It's really weird that nonstudents and parents use Facebook ... It makes me feel really uncomfortable that my older aunt has Facebook, because she says that she likes to check up on her teenage nieces and nephews and takes our pictures for her own use. That's creepy." (para. 3). An article in the UK publication *The Guardian* (Hoare, 2007) bore the headline, "Students tell universities: Get out of MySpace!" Similar sentiments were echoed in an article that appeared in *The Chronicle of Higher Education*, entitled "When professors create social networks for classes, some students see a 'creepy treehouse'" (Young, 2008).

Chu and Meulemans (2008) provide empirically supported insight into how students are using Facebook and MySpace in academic libraries. Data gathered through a survey and focus group revealed that 67% of surveyed students discussed their schools and professors on these two sites. Students reported a reluctance to communicate with professors via these means and indicated that email was a more appropriate method of communicating with faculty.

Many of the above cautions regarding the use of Facebook are summarized within a comment made by Danah Boyd (2008):

In their current incarnation, social network sites (SNSs) like Facebook and MySpace should not be integrated directly into the classroom... I have yet to hear a compelling argument for why social network sites (or networking ones) should be used in the classroom. Those tools are primarily about socializing, with media and information sharing there to prop up the socialization process (much status is gained from knowing about the cool new thing). I haven't even heard of a good reason why social network site features should be used in the classroom. ("Danah's response to said proposition," paras. 1 & 5)

In spite of the above, however, the final report of the Joint Information Systems Committee (JISC) Learner Experience project (White, 2007) asserts that universities cannot afford to ignore social networking. Despite students wanting to keep their online personae separate, the JISC report maintains that universities and teachers can and should make sensible and considered use of Web 2.0. JISC project manager Lawrie Phipps believes Facebook and MySpace could soon replace the student union bar as a venue for meeting and chatting. According to him, "We're seeing a set of new online literacies emerging but we need to understand how students use those literacies ... The challenge for tertiary education is to learn how to integrate the social networking sites with traditional academic practice and traditional ICT systems" (Hoare, 2007, para. 15). Some universities are taking this consideration on board. McKigney (2007) reports on the establishment of Ithaca College's Facebook Task Force, a committee of faculty members, administrators, and students established to study the Facebook phenomenon and its impact on life at the College. Also, Shepherd (2008) stresses that universities need to review plagiarism policies to catch Facebook cheats. Interestingly it appears as if some institutions are establishing regulatory policies for Web 2.0 and social networking prior to devising institutional strategies for their instructional use. Clearly, deeper and more systemic analysis of the appropriateness of social networking sites like Facebook is needed as it relates specifically to teaching and learning.

In general, the advantages of using of information and communication technology (ICT) for enhancing student learning are well known and accepted, yet widespread adoption by university faculty whereby ICT is embedded transparently and appropriately with a clear pedagogical intent still eludes us (see for example Zemsky & Massy, 2004). Although there have been some successes, overall, tertiary education has yet to convincingly demonstrate that ICT has had a systemic, widespread, or sustained impact on the process of teaching or on student learning outcomes, and still the "potential" of ICT to transform teaching and learning remains. In continuing to explore the use of social networking sites for Web 2.0-based e-learning, it is imperative to establish sound and research-informed pedagogical frameworks with which to underpin instructional/learning design and practice. Suggested broadly is that these frameworks should evolve from the same critical aspects deemed instrumental to the success of e-learning as outlined by Alexander (2001). These frameworks must be based on similar pillars of:

- *University context:* Is the institution ready for social networking technologies? Universities and colleges need to respond by resolving traditional organizational issues surrounding technology, staff and student support, intellectual property and privacy, and appropriateness to context.
- *Teachers' perception and skills:* What teaching philosophy and technical skills frame the effective use of social networking technological systems? This is especially important when considering the use of sites such as Facebook, where the boundary between teachers' personal and professional/academic lives can be affected through the misunderstanding or accidental modification of a profile setting.
- *Instructional planning:* There is a need for careful pedagogical planning oriented towards learning outcomes, not "bolt-on" (Graves, 2005, p. 96) technology development. Also, the careful design and articulation of appropriate assessment strategies, including a consideration of issues such as plagiarism, are required.
- *Teaching strategies:* Learners must be provided with a clear understanding of the learning process and what is expected of them prior to the commencement of activities. The effective use of technology within pedagogical tasks must also be appropriately and adequately scaffolded.

In summary, the following are seven key points for educators seeking to capitalize on the potential of Facebook for tertiary teaching and learning:

1. Establish a clear rationale for the use of a social networking site likes Facebook, supported by a solid pedagogical framework that is aligned with the intended learning outcomes and suitable for the learning context.
2. Acknowledge that part of the benefit of the use of a site like Facebook can come from its novelty and social popularity, and that this can act as a motivating factor for students. However, do not allow this to be the sole driving force.
3. Have a clear understanding of the potential benefits, pitfalls, and challenges specific to the educational context in which social networking is to be integrated.
4. Explore the online space and functions offered by Facebook (i.e., register an account, examine the features, set up a profile, test out / experiment with applications, join relevant groups, etc.) *before* using it with a cohort of students.
5. Create a professional profile in Facebook that is separate from your personal profile, to ensure a clear delineation between the two realms.

6. Clarify your expectations with your students on *why* you are using Facebook within the educational context of your course. In particular, establish clear guidelines and boundaries regarding participation in activities.
7. Support and scaffold learning tasks incorporating Facebook from an assumption that students may *not* be competent or skilled in the use of this medium for educational/academic purposes.

CONCLUSION

What is beyond debate is that social networking technologies have redefined the way in which digital generation students—and the wider community—communicate, collaborate, and share information. Social networking sites like Facebook have the potential to transform the traditional learning lifecycle and extend it well beyond a student's departure from the tertiary education environment or institution. Current LMSs are attempting to integrate social networking features to compete with public social networking sites. However, the centrally controlled, "walled garden" approach to LMSs is at odds with the principles of Web 2.0 (see Chapters 3 and 14), and the fact that LMS-based courses traditionally expire at the end of a semester means that the potential is lost for embedded knowledge and communal learning to last beyond the arbitrary semester timeframe.

Technology and education are sometimes seen as areas which challenge and produce tensions for each other. Some researchers indicate that educators are less technology inquisitive and regard learning new technology as an administrative burden (Laurillard, 2002). It is imperative for learning technologies to be simple and transparent if they are to be embraced with equal effectiveness by both educators and students. Benkler (2008) argues that the networked information economy and society present a new social, technical, and economic environment within which the university functions. McWilliam (2008), in her article entitled "Unlearning how to teach," provides useful observations and insight into how emerging pedagogies inclusive of the use of social networking sites can be considered. She suggests that the move from "sage on the stage" to "guide on the side" (reflecting a shift in focus from teacher-centered to learner-centered pedagogies) needs to be taken one step further to what she portrays as "meddler in the middle." This characterization positions the teacher and student as co-directors and co-editors of their social (and educational) world, challenging models and conceptualizations of traditional teaching in a number of ways. In particular, it situates the student within a learning landscape in which the teacher takes on a number of new roles: a co-worker in the thick of the action; an experimenter and risk taker; a designer, editor, and assembler; and a collaborative critic and authentic evaluator (McWilliam, 2008).

In this chapter the emerging prevalence and influence of social networking sites have been discussed, as applied to Facebook in particular. Some implications and recommendations for the use of this platform in terms of teaching and learning have been described and analyzed. Ultimately, which technologies are used by learners and teachers, and whether such tools will be used at all, will always depend on the specific pedagogical needs of a teaching situation. The growing popularity and use of ICT in general, and the emerging social and community affordances of Web 2.0 in particular, are widely acknowledged. Social networking sites like Facebook offer distributed expression and interaction with an authentic slice-of-life creative opportunity to share, respond to, and collaboratively develop collections of interlinked social knowledge. The specific focus here on Facebook has presented some ideas and illustrative examples whose intention is to prompt discussion and provoke thought in relation to the use of the technology in the reader's own context. Overall, ensuring the alignment of theory, pedagogical approach, learning outcomes, technology, teaching methods, and assessment will make for the best chances of achieving effective learning experiences for students. Suggested is that the use of social networking sites such as Facebook are an emerging field of "cautionary educational possibilities" worthy of further exploration.

REFERENCES

Alexander, S. (2001). E-learning developments and experiences. *Education + Training*, *43*(4/5), 240–248. doi:10.1108/00400910110399247

Anderson, P. (2007). *What is Web 2.0? Ideas, technologies and implications for education*. Bristol, UK: Joint Information Systems Committee. Retrieved January 8, 2009, from http://www.jisc.ac.uk/media/documents/techwatch/tsw0701b.pdf

Arias, E. G., Eden, H., Fischer, G., Gorman, A., & Scharff, E. (2000). Transcending the individual human mind—creating shared understanding through collaborative design. *ACM Transactions on Computer-Human Interaction*, *7*(1), 84–113. doi:10.1145/344949.345015

Benkler, Y. (2008, November/December). The university in the networked economy and society: Challenges and opportunities. *EDUCAUSE Review*, *43*(6), 59–60. Retrieved January 8, 2009, from http://www.educause.edu/ir/library/pdf/ERM0866.pdf

Benzie, R. (2007, May 3). Facebook banned for Ontario staffers. *The Star*. Retrieved July 21, 2007, from http://www.thestar.com/News/article/210014

Boyd, D. (2008, January 16). The Economist debate on social "networking" [Web log post]. *Futurelab*. Retrieved March 3, 2009, from http://blog.futurelab.net/2008/01/the_economist_debate_on_social.html

Boyd, D. M. (2004). Friendster and publicly articulated social networking. In E. Dykstra-Erickson & M. Tscheligi (Eds.), *Proceedings of the SIGCHI Conference on Human Factors in Computing Systems* (pp. 1279–1282). New York: Association for Computing Machinery.

Boyd, D. M., & Ellison, N. B. (2007). Social network sites: Definition, history, and scholarship. *Journal of Computer-Mediated Communication*, *13*(1). Retrieved October 11, 2008, from http://jcmc.indiana.edu/vol13/issue1/boyd.ellison.html

Cameron, M., & Fox, J. (2007, September 4–6). *Whose e-learning is it anyway? A case study exploring the boundaries between social networks and VLE courses*. Paper presented at the 14th Association for Learning Technology Conference, Nottingham, UK.

Chickering, A., & Gamson, Z. (1987). Seven principles for good practice in undergraduate education. *AAHE Bulletin*, *39*(7), 3–7.

Chu, M., & Meulemans, Y. N. (2008). The problems and potential of MySpace and Facebook usage in academic libraries. *Internet Reference Services Quarterly*, *13*(1), 69–85. doi:10.1300/J136v13n01_04

comScore. (2007). *Social networking goes global*. Retrieved March 3, 2009, from http://www.comscore.com/Press_Events/Press_Releases/2007/07/Social_Networking_Goes_Global

Conole, G., de Laat, M., Dillon, T., & Darby, J. (2006). *JISC LXP: Student experiences of technologies. Final report*. Bristol, UK: Joint Information Systems Committee. Retrieved September 23, 2008, from http://www.jisc.ac.uk/media/documents/programmes/elearningpedagogy/lxpprojectfinalreportdec06.pdf

Davis, A. (2009, January 3). Friended by Mom and Dad on Facebook. *ABC News*. Retrieved February 14, 2009, from http://abcnews.go.com/OnCampus/story?id=6555853&page=1

Deleting Online Predators Act of 2006, H. R. 5319, 109th Cong. (2006).

Donath, J., & Boyd, D. (2004). Public displays of connection. *BT Technology Journal, 22*(4), 71–82. doi:10.1023/B:BTTJ.0000047585.06264.cc

EDUCAUSE Learning Initiative. (2006). *7 things you should know about Facebook*. Retrieved January 28, 2009, from http://net.educause.edu/ir/library/pdf/ELI7017.pdf

Ellison, N. (2007, December 5–7). *Facebook use on campus: A social capital perspective on social network sites*. Presentation delivered at the EDUCAUSE Center for Applied Research Symposium, Boca Raton, FL. Retrieved February 14, 2009, from http://www.educause.edu/ir/library/pdf/ECR0713.pdf

Facebook. (2009). In *Wikipedia, the free encyclopedia*. Retrieved April 11, 2009, from http://en.wikipedia.org/wiki/Facebook

Facebook. (2009). *Statistics*. Retrieved April 13, 2009, from http://www.facebook.com/press/info.php?statistics

Fischer, G. (2001, August 11–14). *Communities of interest: Learning through the interaction of multiple knowledge systems*. Paper presented at the 24th Information Systems Research Seminar in Scandinavia, Bergen, Norway. Retrieved July 21, 2007, from http://l3d.cs.colorado.edu/~gerhard/papers/iris24.pdf

Frand, J. L. (2000). The information-age mindset: Changes in students and implications for higher education. *EDUCAUSE Review, 35*(5), 14–24.

Frosch, D. (2007, May 15). Pentagon blocks 13 web sites from military computers. *The New York Times*. Retrieved July 21, 2007, from http://www.nytimes.com/2007/05/15/washington/15block.html

Golder, S. A., Wilkinson, D., & Huberman, B. A. (2007, June). Rhythms of social interaction: Messaging within a massive online network. In C. Steinfield, B. Pentland, M. Ackerman, & N. Contractor (Eds.), *Proceedings of Third International Conference on Communities and Technologies* (pp. 41–66). London: Springer.

Graves, W. H. (2005). Improving institutional performance through IT-enabled innovation. *EDUCAUSE Review, 40*(6), 78–99. Retrieved February 14, 2009, from http://www.educause.edu/ir/library/pdf/ERM0564.pdf

Green, H., & Hannon, C. (2007). *Their space: Education for a digital generation*. London: Demos. Retrieved February 14, 2009, from http://www.demos.co.uk/files/Their%20space%20-%20web.pdf.

Gross, R., & Acquisti, A. (2005). Information revelation and privacy in online social networks. In S. De Capitani di Vimercati & R. Dingledine (Eds.), *Proceedings of the 2005 ACM workshop on Privacy in the Electronic Society* (pp. 71–80). New York: Association for Computing Machinery.

Haythornthwaite, C. (2005). Social networks and Internet connectivity effects. *Information Communication and Society, 8*(2), 125–147. doi:10.1080/13691180500146185

Hewitt, A., & Forte, A. (2006, November 4–8). *Crossing boundaries: Identity management and student/faculty relationships on the Facebook*. Paper presented at the 2006 20th Anniversary Conference on Computer Supported Cooperative Work, Banff, AB.

Hoare, S. (2007, November 5). Students tell universities: Get out of MySpace! *The Guardian*. Retrieved February 21, 2009, from http://www.guardian.co.uk/education/2007/nov/05/link.students

Hotrum, M. (2008, June 20). Personal learning environment and evolutionary pedagogy [Web log post]. *Choice Learning*. Retrieved March 24, 2009, from http://choicelearning.blogspot.com/2008/06/personal-learning-environment-and.html

Huijser, H. J. (2008). Exploring the educational potential of social networking sites: The fine line between exploiting opportunities and unwelcome imposition. *Studies in Learning, Evaluation, Innovation and Development, 5*(3), 45–54. Retrieved June 23, 2009, from http://sleid.cqu.edu.au/include/getdoc.php?id=708&article=199&mode=pdf

Kamel Boulos, M. N., & Wheeler, S. (2007). The emerging Web 2.0 social software: An enabling suite of sociable technologies in health and health care education. *Health Information and Libraries Journal*, *24*(1), 2–23. doi:10.1111/j.1471-1842.2007.00701.x

Kohut, A., Parker, K., Keeter, S., Doherty, C., & Dimock, M. (2007). *How young people view their lives, futures and politics: A portrait of "Generation Next"*. Washington, DC: The Pew Research Center for the People & the Press. Retrieved March 23, 2009 from http://people-press.org/reports/pdf/300.pdf

Lampe, C., Ellison, N., & Steinfield, C. (2006). A Face(book) in the crowd: Social searching vs. social browsing. In *Proceedings of the 2006 20th Anniversary Conference on Computer Supported Cooperative Work* (pp. 167–170). New York: Association for Computing Machinery.

Laurillard, D. (2002). *Rethinking university teaching: A conversational framework for the effective use of learning technologies* (2nd ed.). London: RoutledgeFalmer. doi:10.4324/9780203304846

Lave, J., & Wenger, E. (1991). *Situated learning: Legitimate peripheral participation*. Cambridge, UK: Cambridge University Press.

Lenhart, A., & Madden, M. (2007). *Teens, privacy & online social networks: How teens manage their online identities and personal information in the age of MySpace.* Washington, DC: Pew Internet & American Life Project. Retrieved July 30, 2008, from http://www.pewinternet.org/~/media//Files/Reports/2007/PIP_Teens_Privacy_SNS_Report_Final.pdf.pdf

Luppicini, R. (Ed.). (2007). *Online learning communities*. Charlotte, NC: Information Age.

Lytras, M., & Naeve, A. (2006). Semantic e-learning: Synthesizing fantasies. *British Journal of Educational Technology*, *37*(3), 479–491. doi:10.1111/j.1467-8535.2006.00617.x

Mason, R., & Rennie, F. (2008). *E-learning and social networking handbook: Resources for higher education*. New York: Routledge.

Mazer, J. P., Murphy, R. E., & Simonds, C. J. (2007). I'll see you on "Facebook": The effects of computer-mediated teacher self-disclosure on student motivation, affective learning, and classroom climate. *Communication Education*, *56*(1), 1–17. doi:10.1080/03634520601009710

McKigney, E. (2007, February 15). College forms committee to examine use of Facebook. *The Ithacan Online*. Retrieved July 30, 2008, from http://theithacan.org/am/publish/news/200702_College_forms_committee_to_examine_use_of_Facebook.shtml

McWilliam, E. (2008). Unlearning how to teach. *Innovations in Education and Teaching International*, *45*(3), 263–269. doi:10.1080/14703290802176147

O'Brien, C. (2008). How the Google generation thinks differently. *The Times*, Retrieved January 23, 2009, from http://women.timesonline.co.uk/tol/life_and_style/women/families/article4295414.ece

Oblinger, D. G., & Oblinger, J. L. (Eds.). (2005a). *Educating the Net Generation*. Boulder, CO: EDUCAUSE.

Oblinger, D. G., & Oblinger, J. L. (2005b). Is it age or IT: First steps toward understanding the Net Generation. In Oblinger, D. G., & Oblinger, J. L. (Eds.), *Educating the Net Generation* (pp. 2.1–2.20). Boulder, CO: EDUCAUSE.

Owen, M., Grant, L., Sayers, S., & Facer, K. (2006). *Social software and learning*. Bristol, UK: Futurelab. Retrieved February 14, 2009, from http://www.futurelab.org.uk/resources/documents/opening_education/Social_Software_report.pdf

Palloff, R. M., & Pratt, K. (2007). *Building online learning communities Effective strategies for the virtual classroom*. San Francisco: Jossey-Bass.

Prensky, M. (2001). Digital natives, digital immigrants. *Horizon*, *9*(5), 1–6. doi:10.1108/10748120110424816

Prensky, M. (2004). *Digital game-based learning*. New York: McGraw-Hill.

Protecting Children in the 21st Century Act, S. 49, 110th Cong. (2007).

Resnick, M. (2006). Computer as paintbrush: Technology, play, and the creative society. In Singer, D. G., Golinkoff, R. M., & Hirsh-Pasek, K. (Eds.), *Play = learning: How play motivates and enhances children's cognitive and socio-emotional growth* (pp. 30–37). Oxford, UK: Oxford University Press.

Richardson, W. (2006). *Blogs, wikis, podcasts, and other powerful tools for classrooms*. Thousand Oaks, CA: Sage.

Sharma, D. (2007). *SOCIAL NETWORKING GOD: 350+ social networking sites*. Retrieved April 11, 2009, from http://mashable.com/2007/10/23/social-networking-god/

Shepherd, J. (2008, October 31). Universities review plagiarism policies to catch Facebook cheats. *The Guardian*. Retrieved November 23, 2008, from http://www.guardian.co.uk/education/2008/oct/31/facebook-cheating-plagiarism-cambridge-varsity-wikipedia

Siemens, G. (2005). Connectivism: A learning theory for the digital age. *International Journal of Instructional Technology and Distance Learning, 2*(1), 3–10. Retrieved January 16, 2009, from http://www.itdl.org/Journal/Jan_05/article01.htm

Staton, M. (2008, February 2). *Best practices for educators using Facebook*. Presentation delivered to Classroom 2.0 LIVE. Retrieved February 9, 2009, from http://www.edumorphology.com/wp-content/uploads/2008/02/fb_classroom1.pdf

Stutzman, F. (2006). An evaluation of identity-sharing behavior in social network communities. *International Digital Media and Arts Journal*, *3*(1), 10–18.

Stutzman, F. (2007). *The vibrancy of online social space*. Unpublished manuscript. Retrieved April 11, 2009, from http://fredstutzman.com/papers/MG2008_Stutzman.pdf

Sundén, J. (2003). *Material virtualities: Approaching online textual embodiment*. New York: Peter Lang.

Tapscott, D. (1999). Educating the Net Generation. *Educational Leadership*, *56*(5), 6–11.

The Facebook classroom: 25 Facebook apps that are perfect for online education. (2008). Retrieved March 28, 2009, from http://www.collegedegree.com/library/college-life/15-facebook-apps-perfect-for-online-education

Wenger, E. (1998). *Communities of practice: Learning, meaning, and identity*. Cambridge, UK: Cambridge University Press.

White, D. (2007). *Results and analysis of the Web 2.0 services survey undertaken by the SPIRE project*. Bristol, UK: Joint Information Systems Committee. Retrieved March 28, 2009, from http://www.jisc.ac.uk/media/documents/programmes/digitalrepositories/spiresurvey.pdf

Young, J. (2008, August 18). When professors create social networks for classes, some students see a "creepy treehouse". *The Chronicle of Higher Education*. Retrieved February 9, 2009, from http://chronicle.com/wiredcampus/article/3251/when-professors-create-social-networks-for-classes-some-students-see-a-creepy-treehouse

Zemsky, R., & Massy, W. F. (2004). *Thwarted innovation: What happened to e-learning and why*. Philadelphia, PA: The Learning Alliance at the University of Pennsylvania. Retrieved April 11, 2009, from http://www.irhe.upenn.edu/Docs/Jun2004/ThwartedInnovation.pdf

KEY TERMS AND DEFINITIONS

Web 2.0: The term "Web 2.0" is commonly associated with web applications that facilitate interactive information sharing, interoperability, user-centered design, and collaboration. The term suggests the emergence of a second generation of the World Wide Web, characterized by a movement away from predominantly static web pages to dynamic and shareable content and social networking.

E-Learning: Learning conducted via electronic media, especially the Internet.

Social Networking: The interaction among a group of people who share a common interest.

Social Networking Sites: Any of several websites that provide a virtual online community in which people with shared interests may connect, communicate, and collaborate.

Connectivism: "A learning theory for the digital age," developed by George Siemens and Stephen Downes based on their analysis of the limitations of behaviorism, cognitivism, and constructivism to explain the effect technology has had on how we live, how we communicate, and how we learn.

Facebook: A social networking website that is privately owned and operated by Facebook, Inc. Its target audience is youths, and it was originally intended for university/college students, but it is now open to anyone aged 13 and over.

Social Capital: Represents the active connections between people, including trust, mutual understanding, shared values, and behaviors that bind together the members of groups, networks, and communities and make cooperation possible.

Chapter 16
Catering to the Needs of the "Digital Natives" or Educating the "Net Generation"?

Thomas Ryberg
Aalborg University, Denmark

Lone Dirckinck-Holmfeld
Aalborg University, Denmark

Chris Jones
The Open University, UK

ABSTRACT

In this chapter, the authors explore perspectives on the notion of "digital natives" and present a case in which Web 2.0 technologies were introduced to students. They discuss studies critical of the generational metaphor, and argue that it should not be uncritically assumed that there is a generation of digital natives, but that young people may need to develop skills often associated with the digital natives. The authors present a case reflecting these pedagogical aims, involving an online Web 2.0 learning environment called Ekademia. The findings of the case reflect a gap between the researchers' intentions and the actual outcomes. In particular, the learning environment failed to provide sufficient scaffolding for the students, who needed more support than was assumed. It is therefore suggested that educational use of social software technologies should have stronger connections to curricular activities, involve a more concerted pedagogical effort, and be supported by a higher degree of institutionalization.

INTRODUCTION

In the last 10 to 15 years, the rapid development of the Internet and mobile devices and the increased popularity of computer and video games have created an intense interest in the generation that has grown up with these technologies as part of everyday life. The increased use of information and communication technology (ICT) by children and young people has led to claims about an emerging generational gap between the young, tech-savvy "digital natives" and the older, technologically challenged "digital immigrants" (Prensky, 2001). Furthermore, this has led to calls for educational

DOI: 10.4018/978-1-60566-294-7.ch016

change to accommodate the needs of the new generation of students entering schools and universities. Within an even shorter time span, we have witnessed radical popularization of a range of social computing technologies often referred to as Web 2.0, which has resulted in an explosion of multimedia user-generated content on the World Wide Web. This has further fuelled the notions of digital natives or the "Net Generation," also referred to as "Generation Y," who, it is argued, are part of a collaborative, participatory culture in which creative production, remixing of digital media, and the development of advanced learning capabilities take place through informal use of ICT. Therefore, it has been claimed that we need to fundamentally rethink the entire educational system to accommodate and cater to the needs of students belonging to this new generation (Prensky, 2001). The argument in support of this rests on the supposed advanced skills of Generation Y, and the assertion that they are bored with traditional education and desire learning environments that reflect their rich, varied, and sophisticated use of technology. However, claims about marked generational discontinuities and the need to rethink the entire educational system have been called into question by some researchers, who frame it as a "moral panic" (Bennett, Maton, & Kervin, 2008, p. 776) in academia and contend that the assumptions lack empirical basis. In this chapter, the digital natives and Net Generation Ideas are critically examined and questioned. A case relating to this discussion is presented and used not only to illustrate some the possibilities afforded by Web 2.0 and social software technologies, but also to highlight some of the difficulties associated with their educational use. What is known about contemporary students or "digital natives," their assumed abilities and skills, and the challenges and opportunities brought about by Web 2.0 are also examined.

The chapter therefore begins by considering some of the potential problems with generational labels such as those reflected in the digital natives and Net Generation concepts, along with their ability to inform educational change. In doing so, the chapter highlights and explores the skills and literacies that young people potentially have, or will need to develop, along with the resulting implications and challenges for formal education. The case study is then presented to highlight different aspects of Web 2.0 in higher education. It is based on a small-scale experiment with social networking technologies in a university context, and was carried out by one of the authors in collaboration with local colleagues. The participants were 180 first-year students at a Danish university, who were invited into a web-based environment called Ekademia ("Ecademy") upon commencement of their studies in humanistic informatics in September 2007. The online environment contained features often characterized as social software or Web 2.0, such as blogs, social networking, personal profiles, podcasting, widgets, Really Simple Syndication (RSS) feed integration, tagging, and so forth.

The case is introduced by reviewing and synthesizing some of the current ideas about Web 2.0 in teaching and learning contexts. The pedagogical aims/intentions and design of Ekademia are described and related to the learning outcomes and literacies that were intended to support or strengthen skills among the students. The outcomes of the experiment are then analyzed and discussed by drawing on the empirical data collected through a survey and through participant observation. In the concluding section, the advantages and limitations of such small-scale experiments are briefly covered.

IS THERE REALLY A GENERATION OF HIGHLY ICT-LITERATE "DIGITAL NATIVES"?

"Digital natives" and other similar generational labels, such as the "Net Generation," "Generation Next," and "millennials," have attracted much attention and interest in recent years. These terms suggest that there are marked differences or even gaps between the tech-savvy youth, born in the 1980s and later, and those who belong to former generations. Perhaps most visible and well known in this area is the work of Marc Prensky, who argues that a large discontinuity has emerged, and that there are substantial generational differences between the "digital immigrants" and the younger "digital natives." According to Prensky (2001) the discontinuity does not only concern a change of "slang, clothes, body adornments, or styles" (p. 1); rather, a whole new mindset has come about and it is claimed that digital natives fundamentally *think* and *process* information differently. Likewise, Oblinger and Oblinger (2005b) have suggested the emergence of a particular Net Generation mindset and they argue that the "Net Gens" are characterized by their social openness, preference for team work, multitasking, learning through discovery, and high degree of connectedness (Oblinger & Oblinger, 2005b, pp. 2.5–2.7). There is, however, some variation between the arguments of Prensky and those of Oblinger and Oblinger, as the latter do not view age as necessarily being a determining factor:

Although these trends are described in generational terms, age may be less important than exposure to technology. For example, individuals who are heavy users of IT tend to have characteristics similar to the Net Gen. (Oblinger & Oblinger, 2005b, p. 2.9)

This is particularly noteworthy, since a number of recent studies have questioned and criticized the claims of an entire generation of Internet-savvy, technologically advanced young people, claiming that they are fundamentally different from former generations. Some argue that there seems to be a disparity between claims about an entire generation of digital natives and the evidence available to support such broad claims (Bennett et al., 2008; Kennedy, Judd, Churchward, Gray, & Krause, 2008). This, of course, also casts questions on the call for immediate and necessary rethinking of the entire educational system—what Bennett et al. (2008) describe as constituting "the academic equivalent of a 'moral panic'" (p. 776). They point out that no studies seem to support the idea that an entire generation of students is bored with or alienated by current educational environments. Other studies have found that young people do not necessarily desire extensive use of ICT as part of their education (e.g., in the form of online courses), and that many are reluctant when asked whether educational institutions should adopt social software technologies that young people now regularly use in their day-to-day lives, such as popular social networking sites (Salaway, Caruso, & Nelson, 2008)—a point also made by Oblinger and Oblinger (2005b). Furthermore, empirical research shows that there are great variations and differences within the alleged digital native generation, and it is becoming increasingly evident that young people are not a homogenous group with equal access to digital technologies or capabilities for using these technologies (Facer, Furlong, Furlong, & Sutherland, 2003; Kennedy et al., 2008; Livingstone, 2002; Selwyn, 2008). These studies paint a more complex picture of the purported digital generation than is suggested at face value by the generational labels, but they also indicate that some changes *are* indeed happening, and that education is undeniably facing new challenges and opportunities.

The debates concerning the Net Generation have not affected the general interest in Web 2.0 within educational research. Rather, there has been a growing interest in exploring the potential of these technologies for educational purposes (Dalsgaard, 2006; Hewling, 2006; Jenkins, Purushotma, Clinton, Weigel, & Robison, 2006; Redecker, 2009). While the idea of Web 2.0 has engendered considerable interest within education and many other domains, it is a concept that does not have a distinct or clear definition, and critical voices have questioned assertions about the paradigmatic shift as suggested in the rhetoric surrounding Web 2.0. In spite of the criticism and lack of clarity in definition (or perhaps as a result thereof), Web 2.0 as a concept has spread with an immense force and speed across a number of loosely related domains. This signals that there is, if not a paradigm shift, at least a reconsideration and re-examination of traditional ways of thinking about technologies for sharing, collaborating, participating, and learning, which in turn raises new challenges and opportunities for education. These challenges are perhaps even more pronounced, as universities and colleges may be faced with students with different needs and characteristics, and who bring to the classroom and institution experiences that have been shaped by their interactions with various ICTs and social computing technologies.

Skills and Technology Use: Indicators of a Changing but Complex Landscape

Even though Kennedy et al. (2008) heavily criticize the generational idea of "digital natives," they also state that young people are heavy users of technology, and view networking and social software technologies as an increasingly important, and necessary, part of their studies and learning environments:

Moreover, despite the diversity of technological experience in this sample of first year students, the degree to which they are using some emerging technologies and tools does point to a number of promising opportunities for integrating innovative technologies into university curricula. It cannot be ignored that substantial proportions of incoming university students are using and reading blogs, are taking photos with their mobile phones, are regularly using social networking software such as MySpace, are communicating via web conferencing, and are sharing all sorts of digital files using both their mobile phones and the web. (Kennedy et al., 2008, p. 117)

Likewise, studies by Salaway et al. (2008) and Jones and Ramanau (2009) criticize the digital natives rhetoric and the idea of a Net Generation, while simultaneously pointing to patterns of change among young students in their use of ICT. In particular, these authors highlight the use of social networking technologies by students to communicate and stay connected, and the use of visual media by them as a means to creatively express themselves. Equally, results from a large-scale qualitative study of American youth indicate that participation in networked publics through the use of social networking sites, online games, video-sharing sites, and devices such as iPods and mobile phones is now central to youth culture (Ito et al., 2009). The study also shows that there are several layers of peer and informal learning associated with the use of social software technologies, including, most notably, that youth today prefer to engage in advanced and specialized learning activities through their interest-based networks. Similarly, a number of other studies underline that *some* young people evidently develop advanced skills through their informal use of ICT, and through their engagement in a participatory culture or networked publics (Facer et al., 2003; Sørensen, Olesen, & Audon, 2001; Sørensen, Jessen, & Olesen, 2002; Ito et al., 2009; Jenkins et al., 2006).

While some young people are frequent users of ICT and engage heavily with social media (in particular, for social and informal purposes) it also seems that young people's use of technology and their technological skills are much more diverse than the generational metaphors suggest. Opponents of the generational metaphors essentially argue that they pose the danger of oversimplifying and stereotyping, thereby overshadowing the existence of inequalities and more patterned use of technology. In this way, they lack the ability to account for certain details necessary to make them useful for informing the design of teaching and learning strategies and activities (Jones & Ramanau, 2009). In addition to this, it is questionable as to whether actual or potential capabilities the Net Gens might possess can be readily transferred or translated into skills relevant within academic or educational contexts. This is also highlighted by Oblinger and Oblinger (2005b, p. 2.5), who argue that "their understanding of the technology or source quality may be shallow," and Kvavik (2005), who to his surprise found the following:

We expected students to already possess good IT skills in support of learning. What we found was that many necessary skills had to be learned at the college or university and that the motivation for doing so was very much tied to the requirements of the curriculum. Similarly, the students in our survey had not gained the necessary skills to use technology in support of academic work outside the classroom. We found a significant need for further training in the use of information technology in support of learning and problem-solving skills. (p. 7.17)

Furthermore, Facer et al. (2003) argue that students might not be able to obtain the necessary critical literacies on their own, and Bennett et al. (2008) refer to a number of studies reporting "lack of critical thinking when using Internet-based information sources," which may "imply that "students aren't as net savvy as we might have assumed" (Bennett et al., 2008, p. 781). A general point related to this, which can also be extracted from the book *Educating the Net Generation* (Oblinger & Oblinger, 2005a), is that young people may be tech-savvy and heavy users of ICT, but may not necessarily be comfortable and/or adept with using the technologies for educational or academic purposes. It is important to bear these issues in mind when discussing young people and their use of ICT and social media, particularly in relation to education.

Reasons for Educational Change and Teaching of New Skills

While the critique of claims and assumptions about digital natives and the Net Generation is extremely valid, it is equally arguable that there are compelling reasons for educational institutions to develop and intensify the focus on adopting new technologies and pedagogies apposite to students' current and future needs. Although claims about an entire generation of digital natives might be exaggerated, it should be kept in mind that young people have grown up with Internet and mobile technologies, and it would be unwise to ignore studies showing that young people have well-developed skills and learning capabilities associated with their use of technology. While there might not be an entire generation of highly ICT-literate digital natives with certain learning preferences and learning styles, social media technologies will inevitably become more rather than less important for learners in the years to come. The authors of the present chapter therefore prefer to adopt the stance that young people will still need to develop skills and digital literacies that are *often associated with* the digital natives—and which some young people may develop through their informal use of ICT. Nevertheless, care must be taken not to simply assume that all young people entering higher education institutions have such skills, or that they will automatically acquire such skills through their informal use of the technology.

But what are these skills and literacies that young people, and members of society at large for that matter, might need to develop? It is outside the scope of this chapter to review, synthesize, and compile a list of various skills and literacies that have been suggested, and caution must be exercised in inventing new "skills" or "literacies," that may be meaningless (Buckingham, 2006). However, a well-researched view on the digital literacy skills needed for the 21st century is offered by Jenkins et al. (2006), who outline a relatively broad spectrum of skills:

Play—the capacity to experiment with one's surroundings as a form of problem-solving Performance—the ability to adopt alternative identities for the purpose of improvisation and discovery. Simulation—the ability to interpret and construct dynamic models of real-world processes Appropriation—the ability to meaningfully sample and remix media content Multitasking—the ability to scan one's environment and shift focus as needed to salient details. Distributed Cognition—the ability to interact meaningfully with tools that expand mental capacities Collective Intelligence—the ability to pool knowledge and compare notes with others toward a common goal Judgment—the ability to evaluate the reliability and credibility of different information sources Transmedia Navigation—the ability to follow the flow of stories and information across multiple modalities Networking—the ability to search for, synthesize, and disseminate information Negotiation—the ability to travel across diverse communities, discerning and respecting multiple perspectives, and grasping and following alternative norms (Jenkins et al., 2006, p. 4)

An important thing to note is that, as the authors point out, these skills extend and supplement existing or traditional literacies, such as research skills, technical skills, and critical analysis skills, rather than replacing them. These skills, they suggest, are much in line with more traditional generic skills, typically developed in the classrooms, but have the additional dimension of being developed in digital contexts (see also Facer et al., 2003).

WEB 2.0 IN A BROADER SOCIAL AND EDUCATIONAL PERSPECTIVE

The shift from Web 1.0 to Web 2.0 is often characterized as a movement from a one-way informational media where consumers "read" or consult content published by others, to a two-way, conversational and interactional media where users become co-producers and "writers" of the content (Mayfield, 2008; O'Reilly, 2005). Similar ideas or ideals have surfaced within educational contexts, where it has been argued that Web 2.0 technologies enable students to become active producers of knowledge and to creatively experiment with various multimodal forms of expression, rather than being passive recipients of knowledge. Furthermore, the social, collaborative, and connective features of Web 2.0 have been emphasized as important in relation to educational use.

Many of these ideas or ideals, however, are not particularly new within the realm of learning technologies. Some of the terms often associated with Web 2.0 such as participation, openness, conversation, community, and connectedness (Mayfield, 2008) are very similar to the first wave of thinking in the field of computer-mediated communication (CMC) (see also Chapter 1 in this book). Likewise, the research area of computer-supported collaborative learning (CSCL) has, from its beginning, been occupied with notions of peer learning and collaborative learning (Koschmann, 1996). In this regard, it is worth noting that many of the conceptual ideals linked to Web 2.0, such as a bottom-up approach, user-generated content, democratization, and collaboration have revitalized and strengthened already existing ideals within constructivist and student-centered learning approaches, because they resonate well with these traditions (Dalsgaard, 2006; Downes, 2005).

In a similar vein, the current web trends, it can be argued, reflect or amplify common sociological trends, namely that we are witnessing increased individualization and personalization in the way we live, and in how we (prod)use media and connect to others and various communities or affinity groups. This is what Castells (2001, p. 129) and Wellman (2002, p. 10) term "networked individualism," which refers to the trend that it is increasingly our individual preferences, affinities, and orientations that shape our lives, rather than family traditions, cultural heritage, or geography. These are ideas that have also been articulated by a number of other sociologists, for example Beck and Giddens (cited in Castells, 2001, p. 128). Current social networking technologies are prime examples of this. A central feature of most Web 2.0 sites is the individual profile (Cormode & Krishnamurthy, 2008). However, such "individual" profiles also feature one's relations and connections to the world, whether these are "friends" or various "resources" (e.g., music, favourite blogs, bookmarks, interesting news, or videos). In this sense, while we are witnessing an intensified personalization and individualization, we are simultaneously increasingly connected to and dependent on the knowledge of the collective or network. This does not only apply to social or informal uses of technology, but also to work and education, as noted by Wenger (2006, p. 32), who suggests that we are all "partial knowers":

While the anachronistic "universal knower" à la Leonardo da Vinci is replaced by teams and communities of "partial knowers," we also see individual identity becoming a "project" that occupies center stage in society.

As noted by others apart from Wenger it is increasingly important for learners to be able to connect to and learn from one another in various learning communities or networks. For example, Siemens (2005) argues that an individual's ability to connect and maintain connections to knowledge networks will become increasingly important. These aspects are also reflected in the 21st century literacy skills outlined by Jenkins et al. (2006); in particular, skills such as collective intelligence, transmedia navigation, networking, and negotiation seem to be especially relevant in this regard. As such, the discussions of Web 2.0 within education are not only about employing new technologies, but equally about enabling new types of connections between students, teachers, learning material, and the multiple communities, networks, and resources existing outside the walls of educational institutions. Furthermore, the emergence of large-scale social networks (e.g., Facebook, delicious, YouTube, Twitter) where people connect, share, and produce resources provoke us to think differently about these relations.

Whereas educational research has a long tradition of studying and designing for learning at the level of students in particular classes, study groups, or project teams, learning in or from larger-scale social constellations has not been explored to the same extent. For example, the area of CSCL has been occupied with notions of peer and collaborative learning, but as argued by some authors, the tendency has been to focus on small, tightly-knit groups—a unit of analysis explicitly emphasized in the theory of group cognition (Stahl, 2006). Other researchers, particularly within the area of networked learning, have suggested that we need to better understand learning happening in larger-scale, loosely tied groups and networks with more ill-defined boundaries (Jones, Dirckinck-Holmfeld, & Lindström, 2006; Jones, Ferreday, & Hodgson, 2008; Ryberg & Larsen, 2008). In this regard, the ideas of Dron and Anderson (2007) are useful and interesting, as they argue that emergent forms of social media and technologies enable new types of relations and ways of connecting to both knowledge and people.

Enabling New Connections across Different Levels of Social Aggregation

While current web technologies reflect an increased emphasis on personalization or individualization, they also enable new social constellations or levels of social aggregation (Dron & Anderson, 2007). This has interesting yet profound implications for the educational uptake of the technologies. Dron and Anderson point to three levels or types of social aggregation: the *group*, the *network*, and the *collective*. They describe the group as:

Groups are more or less tightly knit teams of individuals who are committed to each other and usually to a task or tasks. Often the group commits only for a period of time or to undertake a particular task. For example: relatives supporting an invalid, team members assigned to a project at work, or a class of students moving through a program of studies. (Dron & Anderson, 2007, p. 2461)

The network, in contrast, entails more fleeting membership structures and boundaries; also, networks do not necessarily revolve around particular tasks:

Networks connect distributed individuals. People may be connected to other people either directly or indirectly, but may not be immediately aware of all those who form part of the wider network. The shape of the network is emergent, not designed. Notable network behaviours include the groupings that emerge in syndicated blogs of the blogosphere, or through social networking software such as LinkedIn, Elgg or Facebook. (Dron & Anderson, 2007, p. 2461)

Finally, the collective has an even looser and more emergent structure with no sense of conscious membership or belonging:

Collectives are aggregations, sets formed of the actions of individuals who primarily see themselves as neither a part of a group nor connected through a network. Like the Network, the shape of the collective is emergent, not designed. Notable collective behaviours include the formation of tag clouds, the ordering of results in Google, recommendations of collaborative filters or social navigation in various social systems (Dron & Anderson, 2007, p. 2462)

In particular, Web 2.0 technologies have amplified and rendered the latter two levels of social aggregation visible through social networking technologies and systems building on the aggregation of spontaneous, unstructured actions of individuals (e.g., Digg, tag clouds, and various recommendation systems). This is leading to a reconceptualization of the role and form of online learning systems in terms of how they support collaboration between students and teachers and how they offer connections to various external resources (including experts). This is strongly pronounced in current trends of moving the focus from virtual learning environments (VLEs) towards personalized learning environments (PLEs). (See also Chapter 5 in this book.)

In his article, "Social software: E-learning beyond learning management systems," Dalsgaard (2006) argues for increased use of personal and collaborative tools owned and controlled by students themselves. He argues that personal tools can support interaction across different levels of social aggregation, which are very similar to those identified by Dron and Anderson (2007), including networks between people collaborating, networks between people sharing a particular context, and networks between people sharing a field of interest. Broadly speaking, the calls for PLEs and educational uptake of current social software technologies seem to revolve around supporting increased personalization of tools and the learning environment itself, while taking advantage of social constellations not restricted to tightly-knit groups like project teams or classes. These were also some of the reasons for initiating the pilot experiment with Ekademia at AAU, which adopted a social networking environment for learners using Web 2.0 tools.

EKADEMIA: AN ONLINE LEARNING ENVIRONMENT BUILT ON SOCIAL SOFTWARE TECHNOLOGIES

When 180 undergraduate students began their studies in humanistic informatics at AAU in September 2007, they were introduced to Ekademia as a new online learning environment supplementing the existing system, IBM Lotus QuickPlace (http://www.ibm.com/lotus/quickplace/, which has now been superseded by IBM Lotus Quickr at http://www.ibm.com/lotus/quickr). QuickPlace functioned as a more traditional VLE segmented into semesters and course pages with schedules and announcements, whereas the intention was for Ekademia to be more social and interactive. The decision was therefore made to base Ekademia on the open source software Elgg (http://www.elgg.org/), which reflects a social networking or e-portfolio metaphor, and contains a number of Web 2.0 features such as blogs, personal profiles, podcasting, widgets, RSS feed integration, and tagging.

The rationale for using a more Web 2.0 and socially oriented learning environment was theoretically underpinned by the ideas of authors such as Dron and Anderson (2007), Dalsgaard (2006), and Wenger (2006). The intention was to offer students personal tools for construction, presentation, reflection, and collaboration while also enabling and encouraging the sharing and exchange of various resources across different levels of social aggregation (i.e., the group, the network, and the collective), as well as to place the individual learner at the center of the environment by allowing him or her to create and maintain a personal presence. It was hoped that participants, over time, would develop a stronger sense of professional identity as students and future practitioners of humanistic informatics, and that Ekademia would support them in developing their personal, online learning records and portfolios.

The idea of supporting the development of professional identity by engaging with communities at various levels of scale was inspired by Wenger (2006):

Our identities also reflect the heterogeneity of learning systems as we develop relations of participation and non-participation in multiple communities of practice ... Essential to the construction of identity is the ongoing work of reconciling (with various degrees of success) membership in multiple communities and our involvement in multiple relationships into the experience of being one person. (p. 20)

One of the aims was to support each student's shaping and molding of his or her own individual learning trajectory, connecting to communities, networks, and resources of personal interest, while simultaneously belonging to an "interpretative community of practice," which could be helpful in making sense of the many, possibly fragmented, resources and ideas encountered by the individual. Whereas a community of practice is typically a group or network of people with a joint enterprise, shared repertoire, and mutual engagement (Wenger, 1998), it can be argued that an interpretative community of practice is a more weakly tied network, but with strong overlaps in interests and backgrounds. This could involve, for instance, students and researchers on a semester or educational program, who share interests but also have relatively overlapping perspectives and backgrounds in terms of theories, methods, and academic outlook. Thus, it was hoped that Ekademia would encourage students (and instructors) to connect to a multiplicity of resources and simultaneously function as an interpretative community of practice that could act as a stable context in which fragmented and multiple experiences, resources, or ideas could be shared and discussed. In this sense a conscious attempt was made to develop or strengthen a number of the skills described by, for example, Jenkins et al. (2006), Oblinger and Oblinger (2005b), and Siemens (2005), such the ability to search for, synthesize, and disseminate information (networking), pool and share this knowledge (collective intelligence), and evaluate the reliability and credibility of different information sources (judgment). This also encompasses skills such as the ability to follow a flow of stories and information across multiple modalities (transmedia navigation), or being able to travel across diverse communities and appreciate a diverse range of perspectives.

Another important goal was to support the students in their project-based group work. This was very important as the foundational pedagogy for teaching and learning at AAU is a problem-based learning (PBL) approach often termed the "Aalborg model" (Kolmos, Fink, & Krogh, 2004) or "problem-oriented project pedagogy" (POPP) (Dirckinck-Holmfeld, 2002). At AAU, each semester is organized around approximately 50% course work and 50% project work in groups, where students collaboratively work on their semester projects. However, an additional aim in relation to the group work was to enable greater collaboration and transparency *between* the project groups, so that they would be more aware of one another's work and progress.

The Design and Features of Ekademia

To support these intentions each student had a personal profile that he or she could populate with various details, such as name, skills, and interests (see Figure 1). Some of these would serve as tags to find others with similar interests or skills, whom one could then add as "friends." On the profile page, students could create a number of widgets, such as widgets for importing external blog posts, RSS feeds, and delicious bookmarks, or those for displaying recently logged-in friends or YouTube videos. Each student also had access to a blog, a personal file space, a private messaging tool, an RSS aggregator, and a shared discussion forum. Furthermore, the students could freely create groups for their project work or for any other purpose.

The students thus had access to a range of personal tools for producing, presenting, sharing, and reflecting, and the hope was that they would slowly start to blog and incorporate into their profile links, files, and resources that might also be of interest to others (e.g., by importing content from external websites). The aspect of sharing could be achieved through monitoring friends' activities, creating or joining interest groups, communicating in the common forum, or by drawing on material and updates from the front page, where the ten newest blog posts were shown. This stream of information presented on the front page was intended to create transparency among the students and give them awareness of one another's interests and postings.

In this way, the design supported both personalization and individualization, but also enabled multiple connections between people and resources across the three different layers of aggregation. While a community could be used for internal communication and collaboration within a *group* of students (e.g., a project group working on their semester project), it could equally act as a support for a *network* of students (e.g., some students created a support group for Mac users). The level of the *collective* was supported in the sense that students could import and share bookmarks, blog postings, and videos from external sources, some of which could be aggregated through searchable tags or presented as part of the stream on the front page. In addition, there was a built-in RSS reader that made it possible to explore feeds subscribed to by other students. However, these features were not heavily used by participants. Even though some students linked to their private blogs in their profiles, they did not take advantage of the ability to import the posts directly. Likewise, very few students actually subscribed to RSS feeds or imported widgets into their profiles (Clausen & Jacobsen, 2008). So, then, what did the students use Ekademia for?

Communication and Interaction in Ekademia

The online learning environment was evaluated by collecting and analyzing data based on one year of following the students' postings and interactions online, and from a questionnaire created by Clausen and Jacobsen (2008). The questionnaire was distributed to 162 students, but only 36

Figure 1. Example of a profile page (personal images and details have deliberately been blurred)

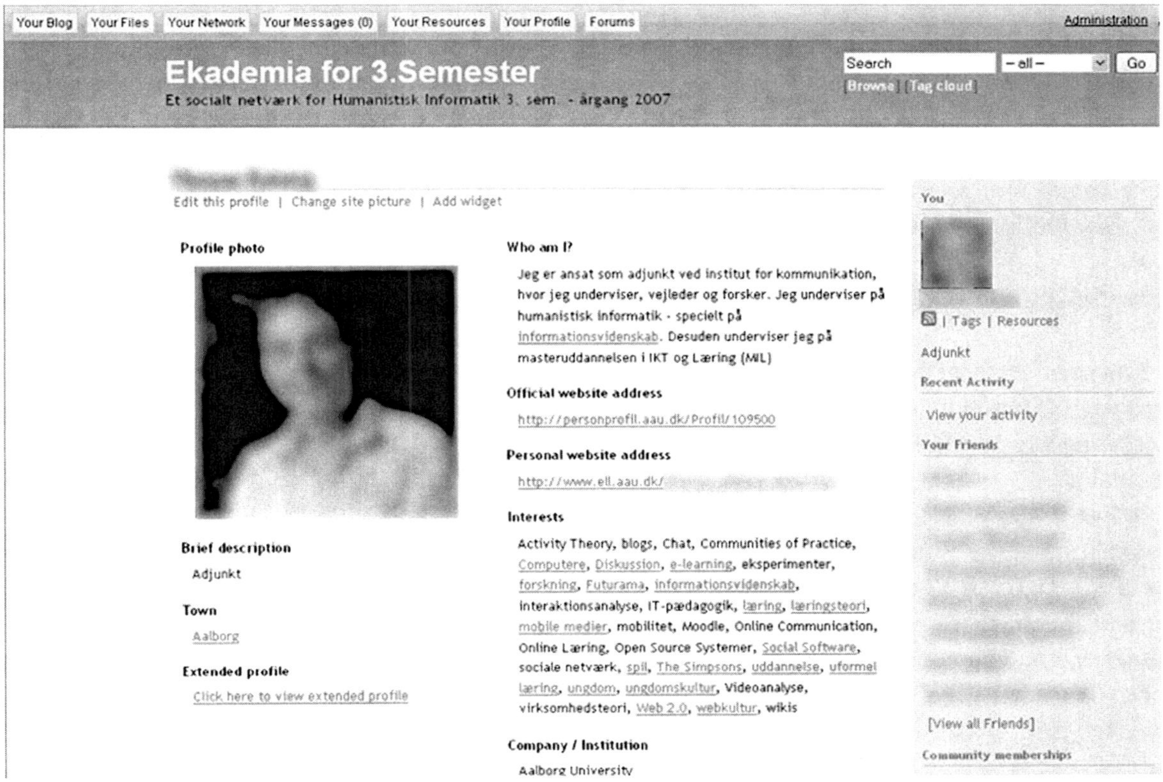

students responded in full, which amounts to a response rate of 22%. Furthermore, the majority of these respondents were active users of Ekademia (logged in once a day), which does not seem to be representative of the general usage pattern of the entire student population. Therefore, the questionnaire was not used as a way of producing broadly generalizable statistical findings or arguments, but rather to simply provide a window of insight into some of the patterns emerging from the quantitative and qualitative data collected.

Based on the questionnaire and observations, it was concluded that the students used Ekademia predominantly for group work in relation to their semester projects. The environment was, however, also used for other purposes, such as social purposes like inviting others for parties, arranging football matches, or for supporting small interest groups like the Mac community. When students were asked about their perceptions of the roles of Ekademia and QuickPlace, several of them indicated that they felt the role and expectations related to the use of Ekademia were not clear from the outset. Most of them commented that they saw Ekademia more as their own platform for group work and as a "social platform," whereas QuickPlace was the more formal space for teachers to upload instructional/learning material and course descriptions, as evident in some of their answers below (Clausen & Jacobsen, 2008, p. 172):

"It is a good alternative to QP [QuickPlace]. I think Ekademia is more user friendly for the students because they can create and administer their groups."

"The groups are gathered through Ekademia."

"QP is the knowledge database for us, that is where we get our information. But it does happen that I look at Ekademia first. Ekademia is more of a social forum in my opinion."

"We use it in the group to send material to each other and to read what the others have written. And then social activities with other students."

(Translated by the authors—original in Danish)

Only a minority of the students were interested in using Ekademia for the "formal" purposes or in creating stronger links between Ekademia and the courses.

While it was of course very positive that the students found the system useful for their group work, it was interesting that this was seen as one of the main functions from the students' perspective. In a sense it may be considered hardly surprising, since the students had to work in groups every semester. Still, it was somewhat unexpected, as one of the aims of using Ekademia was to enable greater communication *between groups* and *among all students* in the semester cohort, rather than being restricted to supporting the more narrow and confined communication within groups (understood as a particular level of social aggregation).

In terms of sharing resources, most postings were directly related to the immediate social context of the semester, apart from occasional postings in which individuals shared links to, for example, YouTube videos or amusing websites. Furthermore, there were very few examples of what would be regarded as traditional blog posts (e.g., personal accounts, opinion pieces, professional observations, or other types of narratively structured and authored postings). The communication and interaction, therefore, were primarily related to the project groups, the various interest groups, and occasional messages to all students (typically announcements of events or questions regarding, for instance, an assignment). In addition, Clausen and Jacobsen (2008) observed that there were few public postings dealing explicitly with purely academic questions, and of those, most were written by teaching staff.

In summary, it seems fair to conclude that there was a gap between the researchers' expectations and intentions and the actual outcomes, which will be explored in the concluding discussion. Even though the learning environment did not evolve as expected, a number of students (20 to 40) are still actively using it for their *group* work, but not as a platform for exchange and sharing as a *network* or *collective*.

CONCLUDING DISCUSSION

The case presented in this chapter, involving the use of the Ekademia learning environment with humanistic informatics students at AAU, has yielded valuable experiences and insights in relation to educational use of social software technologies and the notion of students as "digital natives." The experiment was, like many other educational experiments with emerging technologies, very much a grassroots initiative rather than being implemented at an institutional level. The authors believe that the case represents a valuable illustrative example that highlights the skills demonstrated by students as "digital natives" or members of a "Net Generation." In this concluding section, some of the inherent limitations and shortcomings of the project are considered in light of the results, before critically discussing the researchers' own way of framing and communicating their intentions to the students, and their failure to provide sufficient scaffolding.

The experiment was, as with many other Web 2.0 initiatives (Fischer, Kretschmer, Kugemann, & Cullen, 2008), a small-scale activity involving only a few of the lecturers and supervisors in the relevant semester (although all were invited to participate and contribute). Supervisors could only be *encouraged* to use Ekademia as a way of engaging with student project groups and lecturers to use it as part of their courses. This also meant that the expectations of the students were framed in terms of voluntary activities and opportunities, rather than strict requirements. In relation to one course (Science of Philosophy) it was *suggested* that students could use their individual or group blog to reflect on questions posed by the lecturer—few students, as already indicated, actually did that. Obviously, the researchers' perceived need to rely mostly on voluntary participation also meant that engagement would impose an extra workload for the students without official reward in terms of assessment, grades, or fulfilling requirements of an existing course. The voluntary approach was partly due to the lack of institutionalization, but also, in retrospect, too much confidence was placed in the belief that social, informal activities would in time spawn academically related discussions and collective gathering of resources.

It would be highly unfair to conclude that students did not bother to engage or were not interested or intellectually mature and independent enough to partake in academic discussion and the sharing of resources. This is especially so because there was actually a high level of activity and interaction in the project groups that were established, and also, some of the interest groups were relatively active. A fairer conclusion to draw would be that students were not provided with adequate scaffolding on a number of different levels. First of all, the overall goals and purposes of Ekademia were not made explicit enough, as reflected in the students' feedback in the questionnaire. The theoretical intentions of establishing an emergent and developing *collective* among students were quite abstract and not sufficiently communicated to the students. Although the ideas were presented in a lecture and through blog posts on the site, this was not supported in concrete ways, such as by providing participants with tasks or examples of how monitoring other people's RSS feeds or sharing bookmarks might be useful in relation to their group work or other academic practices during the semester.

In retrospect, there was also an over-reliance on the belief that students were comfortable with similar practices through their existing use of social software technologies, and would be able to, and wanted to, translate these experiences into academic use. Too much confidence may have been placed in the skills of the students, who it was assumed would be familiar with and possess expertise in using RSS feeds, widgets, and embedding various media on web pages. It was expected that many students would be avid readers/writers of blogs, as well as using social bookmarking tools and web-based productivity and collaborative applications such as Google Docs and online calendars. While some of the students were indeed using such tools, the researchers' general observations and experiences were very similar to those of Kvavik (2005), namely that their use of ICT in support of learning and academic purposes was not as advanced as had been expected, and that additional training was needed.

It is not claimed that the researchers' own observations and experiences in the study constitute valid and generalizable evidence in regards to students' skills, but combined with the studies discussed earlier they do seem to indicate that caution should be exercised in assuming that students are necessarily highly ICT-literate or possess advanced skills in relation to social software technologies—particularly for learning and academic purposes. This does not mean that tertiary education should refrain from using and experimenting with such technologies. On the contrary, as the title of this chapter suggests, it can be argued that universities and other educational institutions have an important role to play in developing, supporting, and nurturing their students in acquiring the necessary skills and literacies to support them in making sound academic use of social software technologies.

The range of studies discussed and the authors' own experiences seem to suggest that there is a need for a more concerted pedagogical effort in order to support students in developing digital literacy skills. With reference to the title of the chapter, it is arguable that educators should be wary of focusing narrowly on catering to the needs of an assumed generation of digital natives. At the same time, they should not dismiss the fact that many students are now heavy users of ICT and have valuable experience and skills in using social software technologies that may be able to be leveraged for formal learning purposes. Nevertheless, the students of the Net Generation might need support and guidance in order to unpack and develop their technical skills for use within an academic context. While many students might have extensive experience using social software as part of their everyday life, they may need support in translating these experiences into academically informed practices, including judging the validity of sources, pooling knowledge, and searching, synthesizing, and disseminating information as a collective. Pedagogical aims such as these, and the goal of assisting students in developing stronger professional identities, documenting and reflecting on their own learning, and participating actively in collaborative and interpretative communities calls for more than providing them with a set of technological tools. Some points are therefore outlined below that will inform the researchers' future practice in the use of Web 2.0 and social software in tertiary teaching and learning, as well as hopefully providing useful advice and guidance for others interested in this area.

In light of the discrepancies between the original pedagogical intentions and the actual outcomes in the small experiment using Ekademia, it can be said that there is a need to establish stronger connections between curricular activities and Web 2.0 or social software technologies. It is also necessary to provide clear guidance to students and ensure they understand the value and purpose of the activities, and of using the tools and technologies. The small-scale, grassroots nature of the experiment, in this case, however, made it difficult to implement it widely, integrating it with other courses running during the semester and developing shared tasks such as students writing reflective blogs, sharing notes and resources, or maintaining e-portfolios. In this way the experiment underscores the necessity of a concerted effort and a certain degree of institutionalization (see also Chapter 14 in this book).

Future pedagogical directions could be in the form of training relating to regular courses, where the social software tools' capacities for supporting learning and academic purposes could be rendered visible to the students. This training would not simply be about how to use the tools in general, but rather would involve demonstrating and modeling how the tools can be meaningfully embedded into academic practices, and how they might inform these to the benefit of learners and their learning. If it can be assumed that students need to develop professional, academic identities as lifelong learners who are able to connect and contribute to a variety of formal and informal communities and networks, then more than mere "training sessions" centered around the operational use of tools is required. Many generic skills such as research skills, critical literacy, and academic writing skills are also highly tacit and developed through engaging over time with academic practices through interaction, discussion, and collaboration with other students, lecturers, tutors, and supervisors. This exceeds what can realistically be achieved within the duration of a single semester, and such an enterprise might require the establishment of wider institutional policies and strategies. However, development processes of this magnitude should build on critical, empirical educational research and experiments, rather than assumptions about the student population. In this regard, it is hoped that the case and discussion presented in this chapter, along with those presented elsewhere in this book as a whole, will contribute to critical and reflective use of social software technologies and informed change within higher education.

REFERENCES

Bennett, S., Maton, K., & Kervin, L. (2008). The 'digital natives' debate: A critical review of the evidence. *British Journal of Educational Technology, 39*(5), 775–786. doi:10.1111/j.1467-8535.2007.00793.x

Boyd, D. M., & Ellison, N. B. (2007). Social network sites: Definition, history, and scholarship. *Journal of Computer-Mediated Communication, 13*(1). Retrieved April 3, 2009, from http://jcmc.indiana.edu/vol13/issue1/boyd.ellison.html

Buckingham, D. (2006). Defining digital literacy. *The Nordic Journal of Digital Literacy, 1*(4), 263–276.

Castells, M. (2001). *The Internet galaxy: Reflections on the Internet, business, and society*. New York: Oxford University Press.

Clausen, S. K., & Jacobsen, M. K. (2008). *Læringspotentialer i social software* (Learning potential in social software). Unpublished Master's thesis, Aalborg University, Aalborg, Denmark.

Cormode, G., & Krishnamurthy, B. (2008). Key differences between Web 1.0 and Web 2.0. *First Monday, 13*(6). Retrieved April 30, 2009, from http://www.uic.edu/htbin/cgiwrap/bin/ojs/index.php/fm/article/viewArticle/2125/1972

Dalsgaard, C. (2006). Social software: E-learning beyond learning management systems. *European Journal of Open, Distance and E-Learning, 9*(2). Retrieved December 5, 2008, from http://www.eurodl.org/materials/contrib/2006/Christian_Dalsgaard.htm

Dirckinck-Holmfeld, L. (2002). Designing virtual learning environments based on problem oriented project pedagogy. In Dirckinck-Holmfeld, L., & Fibiger, B. (Eds.), *Learning in virtual environments* (pp. 31–54). Frederiksberg, Denmark: Samfundslitteratur.

Downes, S. (2005, October). E-learning 2.0. *eLearn Magazine*. Retrieved December 5, 2008, from http://www.elearnmag.org/subpage.cfm?section=articles&article=29-1

Dron, J., & Anderson, T. (2007). Collectives, networks and groups in social software for e-learning. In T. Bastiaens & S. Carliner (Eds.), *Proceedings of World Conference on E-Learning in Corporate, Government, Healthcare, and Higher Education 2007* (pp. 2460–2467). Chesapeake, VA: Association for the Advancement of Computers in Education.

Facer, K., Furlong, J., Furlong, R., & Sutherland, R. (2003). *Screenplay: Children and computing in the home*. London: RoutledgeFalmer. doi:10.4324/9780203380772

Fischer, T., Kretschmer, T., Kugemann, W., & Cullen, J. (2008, October 29–30). *The landscape of Learning 2.0 in Europe: Analysing the Learning 2.0 Database*. Paper presented at the Validation and Policy Options Workshop, Seville, Spain. Retrieved April 30, 2009, from http://is.jrc.ec.europa.eu/pages/documents/FINALPresentationLearning20Database.pdf

Hewling, A. (2006, April 10–12). *PROWE (Personal Repositories Online Wiki Environment)—a first look*. Paper presented at the Fifth International Conference on Networked Learning 2006, Lancaster, UK. Retrieved December 5, 2008, from http://www.networkedlearningconference.org.uk/abstracts/pdfs/05Hewling.pdf

Ito, M., Baumer, S., Bittanti, M., Boyd, D., Cody, R., & Herr, B. … Yardi, S. (2009). *Hanging out, messing around, and geeking out: Kids living and learning with new media*. Cambridge, MA: MIT Press.

Jenkins, H., Purushotma, R., Clinton, K., Weigel, M., & Robison, A. J. (2006). *Confronting the challenges of participatory culture: Media education for the 21st century*. Chicago: MacArthur Foundation. Retrieved August 7, 2009, from http://digitallearning.macfound.org/atf/cf/%7B7E45C7E0-A3E0-4B89-AC9C-E807E1B0AE4E%7D/JENKINS_WHITE_PAPER.PDF

Jones, C. R., Dirckinck-Holmfeld, L., & Lindström, B. (2006). A relational, indirect, meso-level approach to CSCL design in the next decade. *International Journal of Computer-Supported Collaborative Learning, 1*(1), 35–56. doi:10.1007/s11412-006-6841-7

Jones, C. R., Ferreday, D., & Hodgson, V. (2008). Networked learning a relational approach: Weak and strong ties. *Journal of Computer Assisted Learning, 24*(2), 90–102. doi:10.1111/j.1365-2729.2007.00271.x

Jones, C. R., & Ramanau, R. (2009). Collaboration and the net generation: The changing characteristics of first year university students. In C. O'Malley, D. Suthers, P. Reimann, & A. Dimitracopoulou (Eds.), *Proceedings of the Ninth International Conference on Computer Supported Collaborative Learning* (Vol. 1, pp. 237–241). Atlanta, GA: International Society of the Learning Sciences.

Kennedy, G. E., Judd, T. S., Churchward, A., Gray, K., & Krause, K.-L. (2008). First year students' experiences with technology: Are they really digital natives? *Australasian Journal of Educational Technology, 24*(1), 108–122. Retrieved December 5, 2008, from http://www.ascilite.org.au/ajet/ajet24/kennedy.pdf

Kolmos, A., Fink, F. K., & Krogh, L. (Eds.). (2004). *The Aalborg PBL model: Progress, diversity and challenges*. Aalborg, Denmark: Aalborg University Press.

Koschmann, T. (Ed.). (1996). *CSCL: Theory and practice of an emerging paradigm*. Mahwah, NJ: Lawrence Erlbaum.

Kvavik, R. B. (2005). Convenience, communications, and control: How students use technology. In Oblinger, D. G., & Oblinger, J. L. (Eds.), *Educating the Net Generation* (pp. 7.1–7.20). Boulder, CO: EDUCAUSE.

Livingstone, S. (2002). *Young people and new media: Childhood and the changing media environment*. Thousand Oaks, CA: Sage.

Mayfield, A. (2008). *What is social media?* London: iCrossing. Retrieved August 3, 2009, from http://www.icrossing.co.uk/fileadmin/uploads/eBooks/What_is_Social_Media_iCrossing_ebook.pdf

O'Reilly, T. (2005). *What is Web 2.0: Design patterns and business models for the next generation of software*. Retrieved November 7, 2008, from http://www.oreillynet.com/pub/a/oreilly/tim/news/2005/09/30/what-is-web-20.html

Oblinger, D. G., & Oblinger, J. L. (Eds.). (2005a). *Educating the Net Generation*. Boulder, CO: EDUCAUSE.

Oblinger, D. G., & Oblinger, J. L. (2005b). Is it age or IT: First steps toward understanding the Net Generation. In Oblinger, D. G., & Oblinger, J. L. (Eds.), *Educating the Net Generation* (pp. 2.1–2.20). Boulder, CO: EDUCAUSE.

Prensky, M. (2001). Digital natives, digital immigrants. *Horizon, 9*(5), 1–6. doi:10.1108/10748120110424816

Redecker, C. (2009). *Review of Learning 2.0 Practices: Study on the impact of Web 2.0 innovations on education and training in Europe*. Luxembourg: European Commission. Retrieved April 30, 2009, from http://ftp.jrc.es/EURdoc/JRC49108.pdf

Ryberg, T., & Larsen, M. C. (2008). Networked identities: Understanding relationships between strong and weak ties in networked environments. *Journal of Computer Assisted Learning*, *24*(2), 103–115. doi:10.1111/j.1365-2729.2007.00272.x

Salaway, G., Caruso, J. B., & Nelson, M. R. (2008). *The ECAR study of undergraduate students and information technology, 2008*. Boulder, CO: EDUCAUSE Center for Applied Research. Retrieved December 5, 2008, from http://www.educause.edu/ir/library/pdf/ERS0808/RS/ERS0808w.pdf

Selwyn, N. (2008). An investigation of differences in undergraduates' academic use of the Internet. *Active Learning in Higher Education*, *9*(1), 11–22. doi:10.1177/1469787407086744

Siemens, G. (2005). Connectivism: A learning theory for the digital age. *International Journal of Instructional Technology and Distance Learning*, *2*(1), 3–10. Retrieved November 7, 2008, from http://www.itdl.org/Journal/Jan_05/Jan_05.pdf

Sørensen, B. H., Jessen, C., & Olesen, B. R. (Eds.). (2002). *Børn på nettet: Kommunikation og læring (Children on the Internet: Communication and learning)*. Copenhagen: Gads.

Sørensen, B. H., Olesen, B. R., & Audon, L. (2001). *Det hele kører parallelt: De nye medier i børns hverdagsliv (Everything runs in parallel: The new media in children's everyday life)*. Copenhagen: Gads.

Stahl, G. (2006). *Group cognition: Computer support for building collaborative knowledge*. Cambridge, MA: MIT Press.

Wellman, B. (2002). Little boxes, glocalization, and networked individualism. In M. Tanabe, P. van den Besselaar, & T. Ishida (Eds.), *Digital cities II. Computational and sociological approaches. Second Kyoto Workshop on Digital Cities, Kyoto, Japan, October 18–20, 2001. Revised papers: Vol. 2362 Lecture Notes in Computer Science* (pp. 10–25). London: Springer-Verlag.

Wenger, E. (1998). *Communities of practice: Learning, meaning, and identity*. Cambridge, UK: Cambridge University Press.

Wenger, E. (2006). *Learning for a small planet: A research agenda*. Retrieved December 5, 2008, from http://ewenger.com/research/LSPfounding-doc.doc

KEY TERMS AND DEFINITIONS

Digital Natives: A concept initially coined by Marc Prensky to refer to the generation of people born in the 1980s and who are argued to be exceptionally ICT-literate due to their intensive use of and upbringing with the technology. In contrast, older generations who have not grown up with the new technologies are "digital immigrants." The term is similar to and overlaps with concepts such as "Net Generation," "Generation Next," "millennials," and "Generation Y."

Elgg: (http://www.elgg.org/) An open source social networking application, which offers blogging, networking, community creation, RSS feed aggregation, and file sharing features. Elgg was initially intended mainly for educational use as a social networking and e-portfolio creation tool. It has now become a more general social engine or software platform that "empowers individuals, groups and institutions to create their own fully-featured social environment."

Personal Learning Environment (PLE): Typically a combination of web-based systems or applications that help learners take control of and manage their own learning, by providing them with tools for accessing, aggregating, manipulating, and creating digital content to document and share their ongoing learning experiences with others. Some suggest that a PLE should consist of a collection of various "open" Web 2.0 tools selected by the learner as opposed to being systems or environments *per se*, whereas others have developed specialized systems that emphasize personalization and the building of personal e-portfolios (e.g., Elgg and Mahara).

Social Networking Sites: Defined by Boyd and Ellison (2007) as "web-based services that allow individuals to (1) construct a public or semi-public profile within a bounded system, (2) articulate a list of other users with whom they share a connection, and (3) view and traverse their list of connections and those made by others within the system" ("Social network sites: A definition," para. 1).

Virtual Learning Environment (VLE): A software system designed to support teaching and learning in a formal education context. A VLE typically works over the Internet and features a suite of tools to support online teaching and learning (or blended learning), for example discussion forums, chat rooms, content uploading facilities, and in newer systems "Web 2.0" tools such as wikis and blogs. VLEs often incorporate tools for assessment and tracking students' progress. They are sometimes also known as learning management systems (LMSs).

Chapter 17
Activating Assessment for Learning: Are We on the Way with Web 2.0?

Denise Whitelock
The Open University, UK

ABSTRACT

This chapter examines the role Web 2.0 tools can play in promoting the "assessment for learning" agenda. It presents a number of cases of peer, self, and computer assessments that display a range of characteristics proposed by Elliott (2008) for the next generation of assessment tasks. The discussion of the cases reveals a missing characteristic, which is a form of feedback to the students that will take their learning forward—the author calls this "advice for action." It is argued that in order for assessment tasks and tools to become more effective they need to be embedded within a pedagogical framework, which in turn requires a supportive infrastructure as proposed by the 4Ts pyramid. The major components of the pyramid consist of: (1) tool development; (2) staff training; (3) rethinking the assessment tasks; and (4) learning from the assessment tasks.

If we wish to discover the truth about an educational system, we must look into its assessment procedures. (Rowntree, 1987, p. 1)

INTRODUCTION

The current picture of assessment in tertiary education is that there are pockets of change with the advent of e-assessment systems and Web 2.0 tools, and emergence of techniques such as e-portfolios, but the real benefits that have been accrued from the bright shining box of Web 2.0 tools have been in the sphere of learning and teaching. This is because Web 2.0 tools offer new forms of connectivity between barriers as described by Frydenberg in Chapter 7, which facilitate more types of teaching and learning dialogues to take place. This connectivity, with its potential for collaboration, opens the door to what Eijkman, in Chapter 18, describes as a "socially focused and performance-oriented epistemic framework." This means that the focus has more explicitly adopted

DOI: 10.4018/978-1-60566-294-7.ch017

the recommendations found in the social constructivist and situated learning research literature. In other words, Web 2.0 tools facilitate collaboration and offer the potential to move away from the assessment of individual skills to implement a social constructivist view of learning.

However, assessment has remained largely transmission orientated in both conception and in practice (Knight & Yorke, 2003). This is especially true in tertiary education, where the teacher's role is usually to judge student work and to deliver feedback as comments or marks (Shepard, 2000, 2001) rather than to involve students as active participants in the process. The opening section of this chapter addresses the theoretical influences on assessment including the earlier legacy from both cognitive science and constructivist theorists such as Piaget and Bruner, and shows how early web-based assessments were in this vein. The full value of Web 2.0 tools for assessment is still being investigated, and there are few papers published in this area at present, but in parallel with the emergence of the new tools there has been a rethink of assessment and its role in tertiary education. The "assessment for learning" agenda, together with a set of recommendations for "Assessment 2.0" (Elliott, 2008) form the basis for a discussion of a number of technologically supported assessment activities and strategies, however we still have some way to go in order to align Web 2.0 tools with Assessment 2.0. This chapter therefore argues for a new focus of e-assessment that builds upon the Web 2.0 developments but is pedagogically rather than technologically driven. It advocates moving towards an assessment for learning agenda which provides students with advice for action that will assist them on their paths of lifelong learning.

THEORETICAL DRIVERS FOR INFLUENCES ON ASSESSMENT

It is difficult to differentiate or separate assessment from learning, and when we start to investigate the theoretical influences on assessment it is not unreasonable to expect them to be more strongly tied to learning theories than is often found to be the case. This is because developments in assessment have been largely driven by measurement techniques that can account for the validity and reliability of large-scale testing programs, rather than provide students with feedback that will assist them with future learning scenarios. The latter notion is referred to in this chapter as "advice for action." On the other hand, the way in which knowledge creation has been defined and understood has had far-reaching consequences for the way in which education has been delivered (Case, 1996). Consequently, it has affected pedagogical strategies, but often theoretical positions have not been thoroughly worked out at the level of student assessment.

When we examine a constructivist approach to learning we find that knowledge acquisition is asserted as an active, individual process. From the perspective of Piaget (1930) knowledge is developed through the individual continually interacting with and manipulating his or her immediate surroundings. This type of interaction facilitates the construction of a number of mental representations. Induction and the development of a formal rule system can be equated with learning and assessment, and the emphasis of assessment, then, is on testing the acquisition of these types of representations. This paradigm has dominated assessment practices over the years. It is this type of assessment that James (2008) describes as "assessing learning of what is taught" (p. 21). These early ideas do not sit well with the more recent views and ideas about assessment, which have been characterized by Elliott (2008) as "Assessment 2.0," and are discussed later in this chapter.

Further developments within the constructivist paradigm that are of particular interest to the assessment narrative are seen in the work of Bruner (1982), who suggested that performance in assessment tasks will match competence levels depending on the type of help that is available to the student. In fact, he described three different performance levels:

1. the level reached without help;
2. the level reached with help;
3. the scaffolded level found by cooperation.

Bruner's work draws our attention to the level of feedback and support that can be offered to students during formative and summative assessments, and has influenced the development of electronic feedback systems for e-assessment exercises (see Whitelock, 2006).

One of the major problems associated with these approaches is that knowledge is confined to individual learning alone and removed from any sociohistorical context. Crook (1994) also criticizes this theoretical stance because it has little to say about learning *per se* and in particular about cognitive change; one of the goals of assessment is indeed to monitor this type of change. The author of the present chapter concurs with Crook and suggests it has not only told us more about how to represent everyday notions in a computer but has also made more explicit how classification systems develop, and perhaps where they can go wrong.

Another problem is that within this perspective there is a body of knowledge to be learned where there are known stumbling blocks to learners who are assisted to overcome individual difficulties. In turn this has meant that as far as assessment has been concerned students have been asked to present or reproduce a body of knowledge related only to what has been taught, in a cost-effective way (Shavelson, 2007). As one would expect, this approach has been widely criticized. It was Boud and Falchikov (2007) who drew our attention to the problems associated with this type of assessment, in that it limits the process of learning through containing how and what is learned. Gipps (2002) adds her voice to this line of argument by adding that assessment is not divorced from teaching and learning, and that new approaches are required to move the assessment agenda forward. Therefore, what are the main theoretical developments that are available to assist with this new trajectory for assessment?

SOCIAL CONSTRUCTIVISM AND PEER ASSESSMENT

All of the work described above has resulted in a depiction or view of a single learner who has been "abstracting through action" from his or her environment. Learning here has been portrayed as an individual endeavor where the learner's context and culture have been largely ignored. However, in more recent work researchers have realized that when studying learning it must be recognized as a cultural phenomenon that involves a number of social representations, rather than simply investigating autonomous and self-sustained mental representations of individual learners. The main thrust of this latter work has come from the cultural-historical perspective (Cole, 1990; Vygotsky, 1978). Within this sociocultural perspective one of the most important premises is the recognition that individuals shape the cultural setting, which in turn alters and shapes the development of individual minds (Wells & Claxton, 2002). Other schools of thought such as activity theory (Engeström, 1987; Leont'ev, 1947/1981) together with situated cognition (Brown, Collins, & Duguid, 1989; Lave & Wenger, 1991) and the sociocultural studies of Säljö (1987) have influenced our notions of peer interaction and assessment, as well as the role of authenticity in producing engaging assessments that will enhance the students' learning trajectories.

Another important consideration within these theoretical positions has been the key role of tools that are used to mediate action. Within sociocultural theories, how groups of people learn together using a number of tools in different ways and settings becomes more important than the cognitive development of individual learners. This framework provides lenses through which to focus on educational goals (of which assessment is one), dialogue, and pedagogy, which are shaped at different times by different cultures. Dialogue is an important consideration at the social level of these theories, and provides a means to assist learners in discovering how people around them make sense of experience (Mercer & Littleton, 2007). The negotiation of knowledge and understanding is crucial to collaboration and problem solving (Littleton & Häkkinen, 1999; Crook, 1999). Dialogue is also an important feature of the conversational framework presented by Laurillard (2002), where the student and teacher enter into a series of exchanges or interactions (descriptions and re-descriptions) with each other, mediated through educational technology, to achieve understanding of a given domain (see also Luckin et al.'s description of Laurillard's framework, in Chapter 4 of this book).

Sociocultural theories offer powerful descriptions for learning, but the theorists have had little to say about assessment, as such. However, one of the key features of learning in this paradigm is that it is situated within a context (see Chapter 4), to which action is also tied. It therefore seems unreasonable to separate assessment from learning and for it to take place after the learning has taken place (James, 2008). Since learning is no longer seen as an individual endeavor, there is also a case for the learning community to have some say in the assessment process, and so it follows that self, peer, and tutor assessment should be visible within this paradigm. The next section of the chapter describes how the above notions about assessment have developed, and reinforces that there is now strong recognition that assessment should not be separated from the learning context. It culminates in a set of assessment activities known as Assessment 2.0, which have been recommended by Elliott (2008) as the next generation of assessment practices.

ASSESSMENT 2.0 AND WEB 2.0 TOOLS

A sea change in assessment, precipitated by both researchers and practitioners alike, was crystallized by a statement issued by the Assessment Reform Group (ARG), who have rejected the notion of assessment that foregrounds cognitive ability tests that are valued only for their predictive validity (Broadfoot, Daugherty, Gardner, Harlen, James, & Stobart, 2002). The ARG set out to promote better alignment between teaching, learning, and assessment, and have defined the term "assessment for learning" as "the process of seeking and interpreting evidence for use by learners and their teachers to decide where the learners are in their learning, where they need to go and how best to get there" (Broadfoot et al., 2002, p. 2). The 10 principles that they believe underpin assessment for learning are that it:

- is part of effective planning;
- focuses on how pupils learn;
- is central to classroom practice;
- is a key professional skill;
- is sensitive and constructive;
- fosters motivation;
- promotes understanding of goals and criteria;
- helps the learner know how to improve;
- develops the capacity for self (and peer) assessment;
- recognizes all educational achievement.

These principles have been implemented in a number of different ways in a variety of contexts. One key project in this area, known as the Re-Engineering Assessment Practices (REAP) project, was led by David Nicol from the University of Strathclyde. Its aim was to implement and evaluate new models for assessment supported by technology, for large cohorts of first-year students in three Scottish universities. The project team members wanted the students to develop self-regulated learning skills, and so in order to develop the capacity for self-assessment they redesigned activities to involve the learners taking on a more active role in the assessment process. An example of this was the replacement of face-to-face activities with online tasks where students could practice specific skills at their own pace. REAP has defined a set of assessment principles (Nicol & Macfarlane-Dick, 2004; Nicol, 2007), and many of the activities evaluated in this project would be classified as formative assessments. Formative assessment supports and forms part of the ongoing learning cycle, whereas summative assessment is not cyclical and assists with ascertaining the progress made by students at a particular point in time, for example at the end of a unit or course of study.

Among the main advocates of the benefits of formative assessment are Black and Wiliam (2006, 2009); their definition includes peer assessment and emphasizes the role of assessment for learning. It states:

Practice in a classroom is formative to the extent that evidence about student achievement is elicited, interpreted and used by teachers, learners, or their peers, to make decisions about the next steps in instruction that are likely to be better, or better founded, than the decisions they would have taken in the absence of the evidence that was elicited. (Black & Wiliam, 2009, p. 9)

Black and Wiliam recognize the central role feedback plays in formative assessment. The work of Hattie and Temperley (2007) shows the most effective forms of feedback occur when students receive information about the task and how to perform it more effectively. The speed of feedback and its mode of delivery have also been investigated, for example in studies involving the use of free audio recording software tools to provide fast, timely, effective, and easily accessible feedback to learners (see a range of projects funded by the UK Joint Information Systems Committee [JISC], such as ASEL, the Audio Supported Enhanced Learning Project at http://www.aselactive.com/, led by the University of Bradford). Feedback also assists with the fifth of the ARG's 10 principles listed earlier in this section, which states that assessment should be sensitive and constructive. Progress has been made here in parallel with the development of new technological tools and applications. However, there is controversy over the effectiveness of feedback (Wojtas, 1998; Weaver, 2006; Price & O'Donovan, 2008), which can be ignored by students who may only pay attention to the mark or grade awarded to them. These findings suggest that more research is needed about the type and range of comments that are delivered to students (as well as how this is done, and by whom) in order to progress learning. This may be termed "advice for action."

Computer-supported collaborative learning is a powerful research paradigm (Koschmann, 1996, 2001) in which substantial efforts are being made to keep apace with Web 2.0 tool developments, but what about collaborative and peer assessment with Web 2.0 tools? Do they fit more closely this sociocultural view of learning? What form should these assessments take?

Elliott (2008), in his discussion of Assessment 2.0, suggests that in the emerging educational and technological landscape assessment activities should exhibit all of the characteristics in Table 1, although the list is not an exhaustive one. These are not a set of principles and the role of feedback is not overtly specified, nor is how future learning is explicitly supported with this range of activities. Nevertheless, implicit within this list is the recognition that learners are using the new technological tools in powerful and productive ways outside the formal education system (Puttnam, 2007).

Students are personalizing these tools and sharing and negotiating knowledge production. The list of characteristics in Table 1 suggests the adoption of a more personalized assessment agenda that speaks more to andragogy (Knowles, 1984) rather

Table 1. Elliott's (2008, p. 5) characteristics of assessment 2.0 activities

Characteristic	Description
Authentic	Involving real-world knowledge and skills
Personalized	Tailored to the knowledge, skills, and interests of each student
Negotiated	Agreed between the learner and the teacher
Engaging	Involving the personal interests of the students
Recognize existing skills	Willing to accredit the student's existing work
Deep	Assessing deep knowledge—not memorization
Problem oriented	Original tasks requiring genuine problem-solving skills
Collaboratively produced	Produced in partnership with fellow students
Peer and self-assessed	Involving self-reflection and peer review
Tool supported	Encouraging the use of information and communication technology

than pedagogy. This is an argument that is taken even further into the realms of heutagogy (Hase & Kenyon, 2000) in Chapter 4 by Luckin et al., who advocate the concept of learner-generated contexts to assist in making effective use of technology to enable students to manage their own learning. Elliott, however, does not go so far as to "mandate individualised assessment" (p. 5) but stresses more the nature of the evidence that will be produced in future assessment tasks, which may often be distributed across various digital sources such as blogs, wikis, podcasts, etc. and may exist in a range of multimedia formats. Here the focus is on the appropriation of Web 2.0 tools to enhance assessment practice in an authentic manner that, it is suggested, resonates with Luckin et al.'s conceptions of a learner-generated context. We are left with the questions, then, of what assessment is trying to achieve and how we are measuring the learning outcomes.

The cognitive theoretical influences on assessment led to an individualized appraisal of students that is more concerned with checking whether what had been taught could be reproduced, and tests of the nature were considered as a "safeguard for the quality of education" (Havnes & McDowell, 2008, p. 3). However, Knight and Yorke (2003) draw our attention to the fact that there is little evidence to suggest these interventions have improved student learning with the influences of social constructivism. With this recognition there has been a shift towards new forms of assessment (Segers, Dochy, & Cascallar, 2003). These include portfolio learning logs, self and peer assessment, group work, and performance assessment, which can also be formative as well as summative in nature. Here, "formative assessment" refers to any mode of testing that is designed to influence the learning process rather than just measure the final outcomes that contribute to the final grading (i.e., summative testing). The definition of assessment provided by the Quality Assurance Agency for Higher Education (QAA, 2006) in the UK seeks to encompass these new modes of assessment by declaring that assessment is "any process that appraises an individual's knowledge, understanding, abilities or skills" (p. 4).

Hanson's (1993) definition of assessment, which states it is a "representational technique applied by an agency to an individual with the intent of gathering data" (p. 42), fits better with our notions of assessment for learning and the role feedback from assessment can play in influencing learning. This is because the data-gathering exercise (assessment practices) taken as a whole assists teachers in supporting their students' learning but also permits them and employers alike to use them as performance indicators for future occasions. We are then left with the question of how the advent of Web 2.0 tools has contributed to these newer forms of assessment for learning. The remainder of this chapter will examine a range of examples of web-based assessment practice in the light of Elliott's key characteristic of Assessment 2.0, in an effort to understand the part they are playing in contributing to the assessment for learning agenda (Boud, 2000). Unfortunately, there is currently a paucity of examples in the literature that are based purely on a Web 2.0 technology framework, but meanwhile we can evaluate how the new assessment agenda is being addressed and shaped through a range of advances with both Web 1.0 and Web 2.0 social software tools. This is the aim of the next section of the chapter.

NEW FORMS OF ASSESSMENT IN ACTION

The assessment for learning agenda and Elliott's (2008) Assessment 2.0 activities, which fit within this framework, do not discriminate between summative and formative assessments. Yet the summative/formative distinction is a useful one in terms of discussing the following group of web-based assessments that have been selected from the literature. This is because the designers/authors in each case declare the purpose of these assessments in terms of whether they are formative or summative in nature. When the activities or tasks have been designed to formulate a judgment about learning that is reported in terms of grades or scores, and they are underpinned by a set of quality assurance processes, this is known as summative assessment. Four examples of this type of assessment will be discussed first.

Example 1: Authentic Assessment—Open Book, Open Web

Web tools offer the possibility for more authentic assessment to take place online, and although these types of test pre-date Web 2.0 tools, their use has been advocated by researchers such as Herrington and Herrington (1998) and Wiggins (1998). The advantage of using this form of assessment is that candidates' real-life performance skills can be demonstrated in the course of the examination rather than an elicitation of inert knowledge.

A recent research project conducted by Williams and Wong (2009) has drawn on the resources of Web 2.0 tools to investigate the effectiveness of "open book, open web" (OBOW) examinations at a university level. The driver for administering such exams was a desire to adopt a constructivist pedagogy in the design of the exams. Their research took place at U21Global (http://www.u21global.edu.sg/), a solely online graduate school with 4,000 students in 60 centers that has been in operation since 2003. Williams and Wong surveyed all students who had taken traditional summative exams and OBOW final exams. The researchers wanted to test concerns about plagiarism issues, especially that technology exacerbates these problems (McMurtry, 2001), for example by allowing students to share information and exam questions via email (Kleiner & Lord, 1999), and that OBOW exams generally are more susceptible to dishonest practices. In this study the opportunity for cheating in OBOW was ranked lowest by the students (n=54) than any other dimension. The advantages reported included increased flexibility and a format "relevant to business/professional education" (p. 233). Moreover, the intellectual challenge and engaging content of the questions were rated highly by the students. Their survey responses also suggest that there are approximately equal opportunities for cheating with open- and closed-book examinations; it is therefore wiser to choose the option that maximizes student learning, which may well often be the open-book model.

Example 2: Examinations Taken at Home with Self-Diagnosis and Feedback

The next example is from The Open University, UK, where students take their final examination for a short course entitled *Math for Science* in their own home (Whitelock & Raw, 2003). It is a web-based examination that provides immediate feedback and assistance as answers are submitted for each question.

The Math for Science software was built to deduct marks according to the amount of feedback given to a student when he or she answers a question. It was anticipated that the allocation of partial marks for second and third attempts would encourage students to try questions that they might otherwise have skipped due to lack of confidence or knowledge gaps. Specifically, at the simplest level the system was designed to award 100% of the marks for a question to students who answered it correctly on the first attempt, 65% to students who answered correctly after they received a text hint to help them select the correct response, and 35% to those who gave the correct answer after receiving two sets of text hints. Regardless of the correctness or otherwise of the responses and the marks awarded, all students receive a final text message that explains the correct solution to the question before moving on to the next question. This type of feedback is relevant to both student learning and the grading process. It integrates assessment into the teaching and learning feedback loop, and introduces a new level of discourse into the teaching cycle as advocated by Laurillard (2002).

Evaluation of the system has shown that students found it easy to use, and reported learning a lot through the approach, especially when the reasoning for each correct solution was revealed (Whitelock, 2006). They were also pleased to obtain partial credit for their answers. This example illustrates how students can be given "advice for action" not only to assist them in improving their scores but also to help them understand the nature of their misconceptions.

Figure 1. Evidence of food preparation for e-portfolio (Modern Apprenticeship in Hospitality and Catering, West Suffolk College)

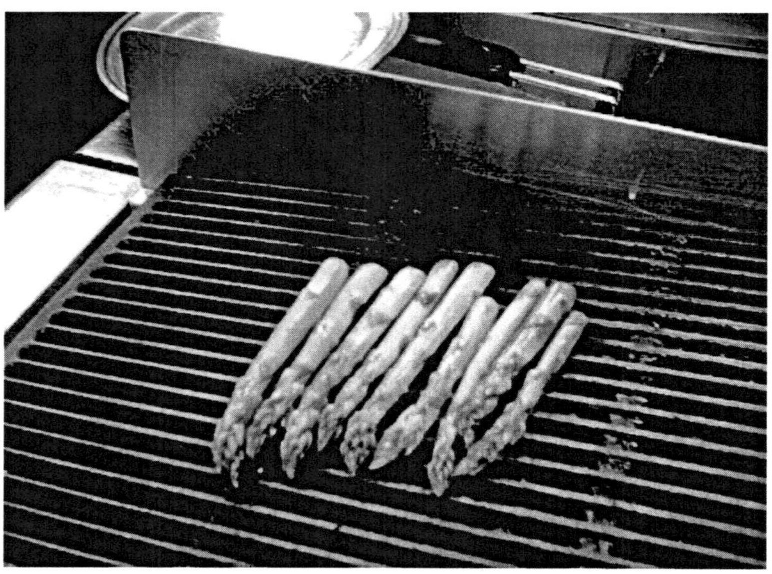

Example 3: E-Portfolios and Mobile Devices

A number of summative examinations in tertiary education institutions not only need to assess a student's knowledge of a given domain, as described in the examples above, but are also required to test a student's performance. These types of assessment are usually found in professional and vocational courses, and often include the construction of a portfolio of evidence of practice. E-portfolios have been developed that can offer a range of features such as log books, case reports, critical event analysis, CVs, individual objectives, and curriculum mapping (see http://www.eportfolios.uk/). An e-portfolio is defined by Sutherland (2007) as "a purposeful aggregation of digital items—ideas, evidence, reflections, feedback etc which 'presents' a selected audience with evidence of a person's learning and/or ability" (para. 2). This was certainly the intention of the tutor who designed the e-portfolio method of assessment for a course for aspiring chefs at West Suffolk College (Whitelock, Ruedel, & Mackenzie, 2006).

The assessment in this case was designed to use primarily photographic material to meet a pedagogical need, that is, to assist students to construct a set of evidence about their practical skills for an e-portfolio. Photographs are "bluetoothed" back to the College via their tutor's laptop, where they are assessed and commented upon. These files are also shared around the class when the relevant underpinning theory is discussed. Figure 1 and Figure 2 show photographic evidence of food preparation and skills required for the *Modern Apprenticeship in Hospitality and Catering* course at West Suffolk College that was captured and saved into a student's e-portfolio.

The course has been able to demonstrate an increase in retention and achievement since using this form of e-assessment. This type of evidence capturing has broken down barriers experienced by students with reading and writing difficulties, and the emphasis on student-generated performance content (Boettcher, 2006) in assessment practice is congruent with the Web 2.0 philosophy and ethos (see Chapter 3).

Figure 2. Evidence of food preparation skill for e-portfolio (Modern Apprenticeship in Hospitality and Catering, West Suffolk College)

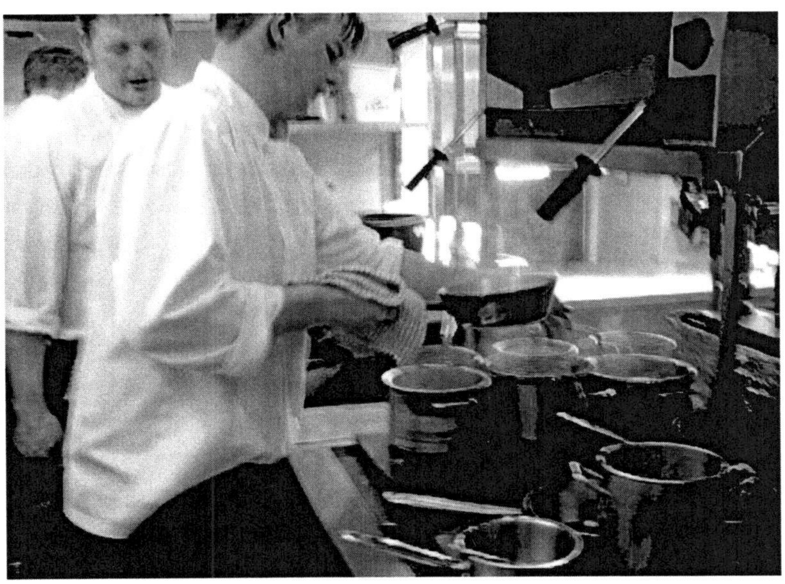

Example 4: Sharing E-Portfolios—The Netfolio Concept

The notion that knowledge and understanding are constituted in and through interaction has considerable currency, and there is a growing body of work that stresses the need to understand the dynamic processes involved in the joint creation of meaning, knowledge, and understanding (Murphy, 2000; Littleton, Miell, & Faulkner, 2004; Miell & Littleton, 2004). The theoretical background here is of social constructivism, which builds upon the notion of interaction with significant others in the learning process. Could these powerful notions be taken one step further with respect to e-portfolios, where students could share and build upon a joint body of evidence and also reflect and revise their own contributions in the process?

The netfolio system (Barbera, 2009) attempts to do just that, by connecting students' e-portfolios into a unique structure in which peer assessment is facilitated simultaneously with individual student assessment. An exploratory study using netfolio was undertaken by Barbera (2009) with 31 students completing a Ph.D. course entitled *Information and the Knowledge Society* at a virtual university that has run all its courses online since 1995. The netfolio is incorporated into the university's virtual learning environment (VLE) and provides feedback to students to improve their final output. This example exploits the participatory, collaborative, and personalization affordances of Web 2.0 to provide students with "advice for learning," as shown by the significant learning gains between the two groups of students.

The students were divided into two groups: one group (Group B) used the netfolio system, while the other (Group A) used a more traditional e-portfolio system. Significant differences were found between the two groups of students. Group B obtained higher grades than Group A. Group B also revised more sections of the work than Group A. This outcome can be explained by the greater visibility of the revision process and the peer assessment function in the netfolio system. This exemplar provides evidence of the role and value of formative peer assessment in improving learning outcomes, a finding also supported by Nicol and Macfarlane-Dick (2006).

Example 5: Peer Assessment and the WebPA Tool

Peer assessment has been used for group work in tertiary education for a number of years before the advent of computerized tools to assist with this activity (Falchikov, 1986; Gatfield, 1999). Traditionally, it has been seen as a way to overcome the difficulties involved with assigning grades in a fair and equitable manner to all members of a team, where one mark for all has been deemed an "unfair" practice. Pond, Coates, and Palermo (2007) have demonstrated that assigning individual marks to team members through peer review also increases the range of marks awarded and avoids the small standard deviation accrued through a single mark for the members of a group.

With the above in mind, an online, peer-moderated marking tool called WebPA (http://webpaproject.lboro.ac.uk/) was developed at Loughborough University that can be used for any type of university group assignment, in any discipline (Loddington, Pond, Wilkinson, & Willmot, 2009). WebPA allows individual tutor customization of the assessment criteria, group size, and number of groups involved in a particular assignment. Students self-assess and peer assess using the given assessment criteria, after which the tutor awards a group mark. The results of staff interviews and a student survey (reported in Loddington et al., 2009) suggest that academics appreciated the time-saving and administrative gains offered by WebPA's automatic calculation of scores, while students rated more highly the pedagogical advantages from using the system. These included more timely feedback that gave them an opportunity to reflect on their work, together with the fact that those who worked hard were rewarded fairly.

To summarize, the above four examples of summative assessment illustrate effective methods of using web technologies to support innovative practices that display a number of Elliott's key characteristics (see Table 2). The use of mobile technologies contributing to the assessment process is also represented within these examples—the chef course, in particular, provides a case study for Pettit and Kukulska-Hulme's (see Chapter 10) investigations into how mobile technologies can be used to cross the borders from informal to formal learning. More importantly, the artifacts collected for the portfolios are also being used in teaching and learning, which contributes to the assessment dialogue cycle. What appears to be missing from Elliott's descriptions, however, is the degree of control given to the student with each type of assessment, that is, time, place, and feedback offered by the assessment process.

THE ASSESSMENT, FEEDBACK, AND LEARNING LOOP

Having examined some recent examples of summative e-assessment practice, let us now turn our attention to formative assessment and what can be achieved in this area with the advent of Web 2.0. We know from the seminal work of Black & Wiliam (2006, 2009) that formative assessment can motivate students and promote learning gains. Formative assessment includes an important feedback element, and can encompass peer assessment as well as self-assessment practices. These strategies assist students in playing a more active role in their own learning (Nicol, 1997), and promote the ability to self-correct (Sadler, 1989). The examples in the first two subsections below illustrate how multiple-choice questions (MCQs)—which have been rather frowned upon as they resonate more with behaviorist rather than constructivist theories and pedagogies—have been used effectively in lecture-theatre settings and group work. This is because MCQs can be used to trigger group discussion that exposes misconceptions and flawed arguments, leading to new joint constructions of knowledge.

Example 6: Instant Surveys or Polls for Assessment

There is now the possibility to undertake instant surveys or polls with a range of tools that are representative of the participatory and collaborative nature of Web 2.0. Electronic voting systems (EVSs), in conjunction with input devices in the form of specialized handsets, or alternatively, mobile devices such as mobile phones and personal digital assistants (PDAs), can be used, during face-to-face lectures, to involve and engage learners in the intellectual discourse. These systems have been applied to a range of subject disciplines such as industrial engineering, management science, electrical engineering, chemistry, applied physics, and psychology (Poulis, Massen, Roberts, & Gilbert, 1998; Draper, Cargill, & Cutts, 2002). The main driver for the use of EVSs in tertiary education has been to encourage active learning and participation by all learners (Simpson & Oliver, 2007), and the potential of these systems depends on the skills of and pedagogical approaches adopted by the instructor. One of the major challenges described by Draper and Brown (2002) is that of creating relevant and engaging questions to ask the students that are pitched at an appropriate level.

More recently, Draper (2009a) has argued for the use of MCQs combined with an EVS to foster deep learning. He calls this approach "catalytic assessment," where he means that the "questions act as initiators either for peer interaction or directly for metacognition which subsequently leads to conceptual learning" (p. 292). His thesis is based

Table 2. Pedagogical drivers and Assessment 2.0 characteristics of summative and formative e-assessment examples discussed in this chapter

Assessment example	Assessment type	Pedagogical driver/rationale	Assessment 2.0 characteristics exhibited
1. Open-book, open-web assessment (Williams & Wong, 2009)	Summative	Change final exam to match constructivist pedagogy and produce an authentic summative e-assessment	• Authentic • Engaging • Recognize existing skills • Deep • Problem oriented • Tool supported
2. Math for Science (Whitelock & Raw, 2003)	Summative	Assist students in self-diagnosing their mathematical skills and performance in order to progress to a second-level science course	• Recognize existing skills • Problem oriented • Self-assessed • Tool supported
3. E-portfolios with mobile devices (Whitelock, Ruedel, & Mackenzie, 2006)	Summative	Use an innovative approach to capture photographic evidence of students' processes (skills) and products in the work environment. Engage and motivate students with reading and writing difficulties, providing them with an alternative method to demonstrate competence.	• Authentic • Problem oriented • Tool supported
4. netfolio (Barbera, 2009)	Summative	Address student concerns about the fairness of group assessment, and encourage reflection and critique	• Authentic • Negotiated • Problem oriented • Collaboratively produced • Peer and self-assessed • Tool supported
5. WebPA (Loddington, Pond, Wilkinson, & Willmot, 2009)	Summative	Increase student confidence in a fair and reliable peer assessment of group work	• Authentic • Engaging • Problem oriented • Collaboratively produced • Peer and self-assessed • Tool supported
6. Electronic voting combined with multiple-choice questions (Draper, 2009a)	Formative	Engage students in active learning, encouraging learning dialogues and collaborative production	• Collaboratively produced • Peer and self-assessed • Tool supported • Deep
7. Mobile computer-supported collaborative learning (Valdivia & Nussbaum, 2009)	Formative	Use a continuous form of e- assessment with mobile devices to support collaborative learning and facilitate self-assessment	• Collaboratively produced • Peer and self-assessed • Tool supported
8. Audio feedback from assessment tasks (Sipple, 2007; Middleton, 2008)	Formative	Provide meaningful feedback that students will refer to in order to improve their learning and performance	• Personalized • Engaging • Tool supported
9. Open Mentor (Whitelock, 2006)	Formative	Implement an electronic marking system for tutors to assist with providing socio-emotive and cognitive feedback to students	• Personalized • Engaging • Recognize existing skills • Deep • Self-assessed • Tool supported

on evidence reported in the literature that six types of MCQ uses are beneficial in this context and can produce substantial learning gains (p. 290):

1. Assertion–reason questions, which can be and have been used with EVS.
2. Taking an MCQ and having the learner generate reasons, for and against each response option, rather than simply ticking one. (This is usually done on paper as a private revision technique.)
3. Confidence-based marking, which is normally delivered by ICT and could be done with EVS with some (but not all) software.
4. Mazur's (1997) method of using brainteasers to prompt peer discussion, which is routinely done using EVS.
5. Having students create MCQs as part of presentations using EVS.
6. Having students create MCQs for use in tests that may be administered either by using EVS or on paper.

Draper does not negate the usual role of formative feedback from MCQs, where questions act as a way to identify student errors and knowledge gaps that can then be diagnosed and remedied, but points the way toward a rethink of MCQs combined with different types of collaborative engagement.

Example 7: Combining PDAs, Group Work, and MCQs

Valdivia and Nussbaum (2009) have also used MCQs to promote collaborative learning and formative assessment. These researchers, while teaching an engineering course, randomly assigned their students into groups of three members, who accessed a set of MCQs from their PDAs. The students discussed their responses to each question and had to reach an agreement before the answer was submitted. The key defining feature (also highlighted by Draper, 2009a) is the design of the questions to reinforce or probe what has already been learned and also move students along the path of building new knowledge.

Valdivia and Nussbaum compared a control group whose members used traditional teaching methods with an experimental group whose members were exposed to 13 mobile computer-supported collaborative learning (m-CSCL) sessions. A comparison of examination results from both groups showed a statistically significant difference, with superior learning gains observed in the students who were exposed to the collaborative learning scenarios with MCQs. Again, it can be seen here that the use of ICT tools in combination with formative assessment strategies is prompting new ways of activating assessment for learning in the Web 2.0 era.

Example 8: Supporting the Feedback Process through Digital Audio

Providing feedback that is powerful and meaningful to students is of concern to tutors, especially when students ignore their comments and only view the mark awarded. Other approaches are being explored and there is a growing interest from tutors in tertiary education in using freely available tools such as Audacity (http://audacity.sourceforge.net/) to provide digital audio feedback to their students. Middleton (2008) defines audio feedback as "formative messages, recorded and distributed as digital audio given to individual students or student groups in response to both ongoing and submitted work, allowing each student to develop their knowledge and the way they learn" (p. 3). He acknowledges that this process can occur between tutors and students as well as between students and their peers.

Distance learning tutors have used audio feedback for many years, and Durbridge (1984) from The Open University found tape-recorded feedback to students effective in clarifying meaning and boosting motivation. However, cassette tapes were difficult to edit; digital audio is an easier medium to manipulate and use. More importantly, the use of digital audio feedback recognizes the role of new online and virtual spaces that can promote learning dialogues. It sits well with offering meaningful and effective student experiences (Rotheram, 2007). Other researchers have found that audio feedback increases students' self-confidence and can result in a change of attitude toward learning (Sipple, 2007). This is a finding mirrored by the work of Ice, Curtis, Phillips, and Wells (2007), who discovered high student satisfaction ratings with the use of audio feedback. This is a technology under the control of the lecturer that does not require complex skills or technical support, and is increasingly being used by tertiary educators in the UK and elsewhere.

Example 9: Open Mentor—Providing Socio-Emotive and Cognitive Feedback

How, though, can tutors become effective broadcasters and deal with the emotional impact of any feedback in whatever medium it is delivered? Designing effective feedback is a challenge for all teaching staff, and finding ways to support them to do this was one of the drivers to develop a web-based tool known as Open Mentor (Whitelock & Watt, 2007). The user interface of this tool is shown in Figure 3.

One of the problems with tutor feedback to students is that a balanced combination of socio-emotive and cognitive support is required, and the feedback needs to be relevant to and appropriate for the assigned grade. Is it possible to capitalize on technology to build training systems for tutors in tertiary education that will support them in generating their feedback to students, and encourage their students to become more reflective learners?

One approach to this question, which can be seen in the work of Whitelock, Watt, Raw, and Moreale (2004), involves building tools to support tutors in the feedback process. Whitelock et al.'s work involved developing an open-source mentoring tool for tutors, known as Open Mentor. This tool analyzes and displays the different types

Figure 3. Open Mentor

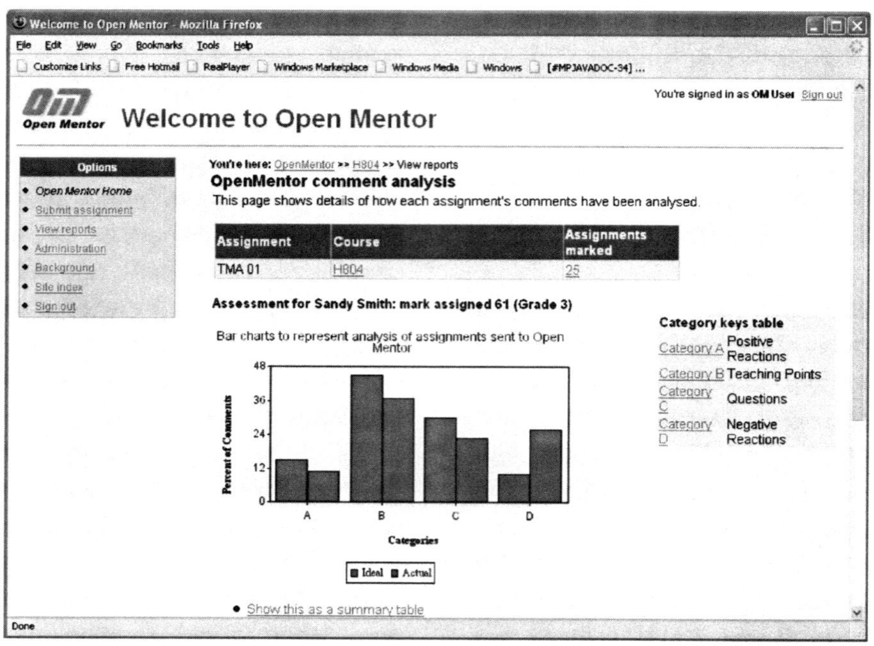

of comments supplied by the tutor as feedback to the student. It then provides reflective comments to the tutor about his or her use of feedback. During the development process it was found that students both expect and receive feedback that is appropriate to the assigned grade. This feedback provides them with the supportive comments they need to feel confident about their level of work. The studies and trials revealed that tutors believed a final mark often speaks for itself, especially in the case of high-achieving students, thus socio-emotive comments of support were not seen as necessary for these students. However, when the students gaining high marks were questioned, they did not always believe that their work was of a high quality even though they had received an excellent mark, because they were not aware of the mean score for the assignment. In other words, they still felt they could be at the bottom of the class even with a high-scoring assignment. Open Mentor therefore guides tutors in providing clearer positive reinforcement for high achievers and prompts tutors to advise all students about how to improve their grades.

Open Mentor works by going through marked assignments, extracting tutor comments and classifying them. Predetermined benchmarks were used to estimate "ideal" distributions of comments for each category, and then display the difference between the actual and the ideal. Although there are "normal" bands of comments of each type, these vary (significantly) depending on the quality of the individual submissions and the number of submissions involved. A large proportion of positive comments in one context may be inappropriate in a second, and coincidental in a third.

To provide an appropriate mentoring framework, Open Mentor is based on Bales' (1950) four main categories of interaction: positive reactions, negative reactions, questions, and answers. These interactional categories illustrate the balance of socio-emotional comments that support the student. It was found that tutors use different types of questions in different ways, both to stimulate reflection and to point out, in a supportive way, that there are problems with parts of an assignment. Open Mentor has been used successfully as a training tool for tutors and prompted reflection and discussion about how to help support students improve their performance in subsequent assignments.

SUMMARY, CONCLUSION, AND RECOMMENDATIONS

Creative and innovative use of ICT tools and technologies has facilitated the adoption of group assessment practices and the provision of timely or instant feedback to students in tertiary education. Tried and tested pedagogical strategies have been enhanced in many of the cases presented in this chapter, and illustrate significant learning gains with the introduction of these technologies. Table 2 summarizes how the practices seen in the four formative assessment examples (in addition to the earlier five examples of summative assessment) are rated with respect to Elliott's Web 2.0 task characteristics. Each of the characteristics is manifested in the nine examples, but negotiated assessment was identified as being exhibited in only one of the examples (netfolio). This could well be because netfolio was used for a doctoral-level course, where the learners have more independence and autonomy.

Evaluations of wikis and blogs for assessment are in their early stages and so have not been included in the cases discussed in this chapter. Nevertheless, the potential role of wikis for self-assessment is implicit in the five-stage wiki activity model proposed by Wheeler in Chapter 9 of this book. Wheeler's findings suggest that wikis can be used to scaffold collaboration and pacing but he does not report that the wiki contributions contributed to the students' overall assessment. Blogging, too, is being used in innovative ways, as seen in Chapter 8. The present chapter has only examined a few cases of innovative Web

2.0 assessments but has illustrated how, even at the summative level, there has been progress on this front. The biggest uptake of social software tools in tertiary education has been with blogs and wikis, however their usage requires further analysis (Kerawalla, Minocha, Kirkup, & Conole, 2009; Wheeler, 2009). These tools have the potential to serve as formative assessment conduits with respect to the educational dialogues that they can promote (Hatzipanagos & Warburton, 2009). Their uses as valuable tools for reflection and self-assessment deserve more thorough and systematic evaluation.

There is general agreement in the assessment field that times are changing and that assessment needs to become embedded in the teaching/learning cycle rather than being used exclusively as a checking device for the awarding institution. E-assessment advocates have tried to address this issue by providing timely and constructive feedback to students through the development of a number of interactive tasks that can be automatically marked. There is also recognition that assessment tasks themselves must change, and this chapter has examined a number of innovative web-based and web-enhanced assessments in light of Elliott's key characteristics of Assessment 2.0 that should contribute to furthering the assessment for learning agenda. One important trait missing from Elliott's list is advice that supports future learning. By this what is meant is that whether a task is assessed by peers, self, or tutors, advice generated from the assessment process should take the students forward to the next stages of their learning journeys.

Peer interaction and assessment often yield advice in terms that are more meaningful for action than that which is provided by the tutor, and this is an area that merits future research. But how can we move from a set of largely summative, "checking" assessment tasks to a framework in which assessment for learning is embedded with the aid of Web 2.0 tools? Luca and Oliver (2002), in their instructional design framework for an online course, advocate learning through authentic and self-regulated activities that are facilitated through (i) instruction, and (ii) reflective tasks. Assessment belongs to the latter set of activities described as reflective tasks, which are supported by self/peer assessment, reflective reports, and discussion board-based dialogue. These reflective tasks could be instantiated in blogs or wikis and therefore lend themselves to Web 2.0 usage; more importantly, however, Luca and Oliver's work illustrates how assessment forms an integral part of the learning process.

Another noteworthy framework has been proposed by Boud and Falchikov (2007). It consists of the following five overlapping phases: (i) identifying self as an active learner; (ii) from known to need—identifying own level of knowledge and the gaps; (iii) practicing testing and judg-

Table 3. Bartlett-Bragg's (2008) pedagogical framework for self-publishing with social software

1. Establishment Learners are actively creating their personalized learning environments with social software, e.g., blogs, wikis, social bookmarking, and aggregation.
2. Interpretation Learners are developing a structure and adapting to their perceived needs.
3. Reflective monologues Learners are publishing to their software platform and establishing their identity, or finding their voice.
4. Reflective dialogues Learners are extending their learning environment by developing social networks.
5. Distributed knowledge artifacts Learners are collaborating with others, distributing their work, and gathering artifacts for review and reflection.

ing; (iv) developing judgment skills over time; and (v) embodying reflexivity and commitment. The attractive feature of this framework is the explicitness of the feedback from peers and tutors to assist the learner in developing a scheme of informed judgment.

A third pedagogical framework, devised by Bartlett-Bragg (2008), emphasizes the use of social software tools such as blogs and wikis as levers for students to receive feedback from beyond the confines of the classroom. Implicit within this notion is that students will increase their locus of assessment through the sharing of their work in a variety of social networks. However, Bartlett-Bragg stresses that this will only occur successfully when social software tools are thoughtfully and properly integrated into students' learning and assessment activities. She has reframed assessment into a five-stage model as illustrated in Table 3.

In Bartlett-Bragg's framework students are self-organizers, and therefore tutors become learning facilitators, exploiting a range of tools and activities in order to assist students in their learning journeys. Tutors also need to guide students in the interpretation phase since the students' perceived needs may not match their learning requirements. At the same time, we know that tutors are experienced and creative guides, but may require assistance and training with the advent of new technological tools. Bartlett-Bragg concedes that there are barriers to the effective implementation of her framework, including those associated with tutors' awareness of the affordances of Web 2.0 tools, organizational constraints, and learners' inhibitions when adopting Web 2.0 tools. It is suggested that the adoption of new assessment frameworks such as those proposed by Bartlett-Bragg (2008), Boud and Falchikov (2007), and Luca and Oliver (2002) necessitates a supportive infrastructure, as set out in the 4Ts pyramid depicted in Figure 4.

The major components of the 4Ts pyramid consist of: (1) tool development; (2) staff training; (3) rethinking the assessment tasks; and (4) learning from the assessment tasks, which include advice for learning. This suite of activities should result in the transfer of learning from assessment tasks and facilitate the implementation of robust pedagogical models that do not just recognize, but also support and enable, the role of assessment for learners and learning. Tool development will continue to take place in the social network arena but adapting these emergent tools for assessment purposes requires further consideration. The production of open source software will make the tools more flexible and easier to adapt to different institutions, disciplines, courses, and sets of individual needs than any commercial, off-the-shelf product.

The provision of feedback that students will actually take note of and that is timely and pertinent to the next phase of their studies warrants more research. The balance of socio-emotive content contained in the feedback cannot be ignored (Draper, 2009b). Assessment practices that leverage feedback such as peer and self-assessment, supported by a range of Web 2.0 tools, start to move us towards what has been described in this chapter as "advice for action."

Figure 4. The 4Ts pyramid to facilitate moving forward with assessment frameworks and Web 2.0 tools

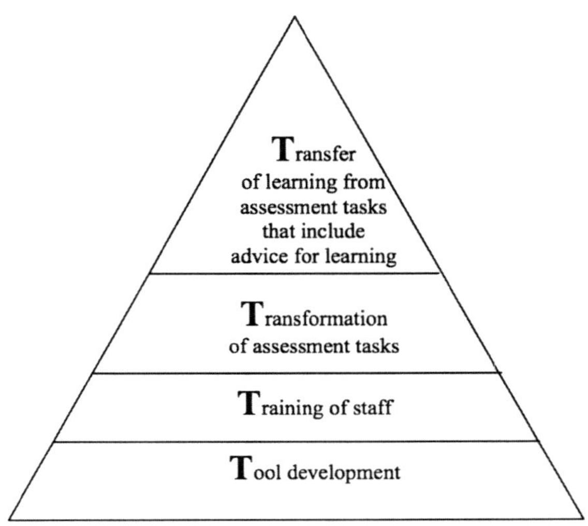

This refers to not just feedback or feed forward, but peer and/or tutor comments that prompt the student to actively change their ideas and ways of organizing their answers and discourse within a given subject domain. Since any feedback that is not fully understood or cannot be acted upon, however pertinent it may be, is likely to be ignored, it will not facilitate learner improvement or confidence. In today's educational climate, with the continued pressure on staff resources, making learning effective, efficient, and engaging is always going to be a challenge—yet it is achievable so long as we manage to maintain our empathy with the learner. Web 2.0 tools and techniques, used in conjunction with appropriate underpinning learning and assessment strategies, can go a long help us achieve this.

ACKNOWLEDGMENT

The author would like to thank all her colleagues at The Open University and Robert Gordon University who have worked on the various projects referred to in this chapter. She is indebted to them for their insightful contributions and good humor.

REFERENCES

Bales, R. F. (1950). A set of categories for the analysis of small group interaction. *American Sociological Review*, *15*(2), 257–263. doi:10.2307/2086790

Barbera, E. (2009). Mutual feedback in e-portfolio assessment: An approach to the netfolio system. *British Journal of Educational Technology*, *40*(2), 342–357. doi:10.1111/j.1467-8535.2007.00803.x

Bartlett-Bragg, A. (2008). Reframing assessment: Using social software to collect and organise learning. In J. Luca & E. Weippl (Eds.), *Proceedings of World Conference on Educational Multimedia, Hypermedia and Telecommunications 2008* (pp. 4020–4024). Chesapeake, VA: Association for the Advancement of Computers in Education.

Black, P., & Wiliam, D. (2006). Developing a theory of formative assessment. In Gardner, J. (Ed.), *Assessment and learning* (pp. 81–100). London: Sage.

Black, P., & Wiliam, D. (2009). Developing a theory of formative assessment. *Educational Assessment, Evaluation and Accountability*, *21*(1), 5–31. doi:10.1007/s11092-008-9068-5

Boettcher, J. V. (2006, February 28). The rise of student performance content. *Campus Technology*. Retrieved November 10, 2009, from http://campustechnology.com/Articles/2006/02/The-Rise-of-Student-Performance-Content.aspx?p=1

Boud, D. (2000). Sustainable assessment: Rethinking assessment for the learning society. *Studies in Continuing Education*, *22*(2), 151–167. doi:10.1080/713695728

Boud, D., & Falchikov, N. (2007). Assessment in the longer term. In Boud, D., & Falchikov, N. (Eds.), *Rethinking assessment in higher education: Learning for the longer term* (pp. 4–13). London: Routledge.

Broadfoot, P., Daugherty, R., Gardner, J., Harlen, W., James, M., & Stobart, G. (2002). *Assessment for learning: 10 principles, Research-based principles to guide classroom practice*. London: Assessment Reform Group. Retrieved October 29, 2009, from http://www.assessment-reform-group.org/CIE3.PDF

Brown, J. S., Collins, A., & Duguid, P. (1989). Situated cognition and the culture of learning. *Educational Researcher*, *18*(1), 32–42.

Bruner, J. S. (1982). The organization of action and the nature of adult–infant transaction. In von Cranach, M., & Harré, R. (Eds.), *The analysis of action* (pp. 313–327). Cambridge, UK: Cambridge University Press.

Case, R. (1996). Changing views of knowledge and their impact on educational research and practice. In Olson, D. R., & Torrance, N. (Eds.), *The handbook of education and human development* (pp. 75–99). Cambridge, MA: Blackwell.

Cole, M. (1990). Cognitive development and formal schooling: The evidence from cross-cultural research. In Moll, L. C. (Ed.), *Vygotsky and education: Instructional implications and applications of sociohistorical psychology* (pp. 89–110). Cambridge, UK: Cambridge University Press.

Crook, C. (1994). *Computers and the collaborative experience of learning*. London: Routledge.

Crook, C. (1999). Computers in the community of classrooms. In Light, P., & Littleton, K. (Eds.), *Learning with computers: Analysing productive interaction* (pp. 102–117). London: Routledge.

Draper, S. W. (2009a). Catalytic assessment: Understanding how MCQs and EVS can foster deep learning. *British Journal of Educational Technology*, *40*(2), 285–293. doi:10.1111/j.1467-8535.2008.00920.x

Draper, S. W. (2009b). What are learners actually regulating when given feedback? *British Journal of Educational Technology*, *40*(2), 306–315. doi:10.1111/j.1467-8535.2008.00930.x

Draper, S. W., & Brown, M. I. (2002). *Use of the PRS (Personal Response System) handsets at Glasgow University*. Retrieved June 22, 2009, from http://www.psy.gla.ac.uk/~steve/ilig/interim.html

Draper, S. W., Cargill, J., & Cutts, Q. (2002) Electronically enhanced classroom interaction. *Australian Journal of Educational Technology*, *18*(1), 13–23. Retrieved August 12, 2008, from http://www.ascilite.org.au/ajet/ajet18/draper.html

Durbridge, N. (1984). Media in course design, No. 9, audio cassettes. In Bates, A. W. (Ed.), *The role of technology in distance education*. Kent, UK: Croom Helm.

Elliott, B. (2008). *Assessment 2.0: Modernising assessment in the age of Web 2.0*. Glasgow: Scottish Qualifications Authority. Retrieved June 22, 2009, from http://www.scribd.com/doc/461041/Assessment-20

Engeström, Y. (1987). *Learning by expanding: An activity-theoretical approach to developmental research*. Helsinki: Orienta-Konsultit Oy.

Falchikov, N. (1986). Product comparisons and process benefits of collaborative peer group and self assessments. *Assessment & Evaluation in Higher Education*, *11*(2), 146–166.

Gatfield, T. (1999). Examining student satisfaction with group projects and peer assessment. *Assessment & Evaluation in Higher Education*, *24*(4), 365–377. doi:10.1080/0260293990240401

Gipps, C. (2002). Sociocultural perspectives on assessment. In Wells, G., & Claxton, G. (Eds.), *Learning for life in the 21st century* (pp. 73–83). Oxford, UK: Blackwell. doi:10.1002/9780470753545.ch6

Hanson, F. A. (1993). *Testing testing: Social consequences of the examined life*. Berkeley, CA: University of California Press.

Hase, S., & Kenyon, C. (2000). From andragogy to heutagogy. *ultiBASE*, *5*(3). Retrieved July 3, 2009, from http://ultibase.rmit.edu.au/Articles/dec00/hase1.pdf

Hattie, J., & Temperley, H. (2007). The power of feedback. *Review of Educational Research*, *77*(1), 81–112. doi:10.3102/003465430298487

Hatzipanagos, S., & Warburton, S. (2009). Feedback as dialogue: Exploring the links between formative assessment and social software in distance learning. *Learning, Media and Technology*, *34*(1), 45–59. doi:10.1080/17439880902759919

Havnes, A., & McDowell, L. (2008). Introduction: Assessment dilemmas in contemporary learning cultures. In Havnes, A., & McDowell, L. (Eds.), *Balancing dilemmas in assessment and learning in contemporary education* (pp. 3–14). New York: Taylor & Francis.

Herrington, J., & Herrington, A. (1998). Authentic assessment and multimedia: How university students respond to a model of authentic assessment. *Higher Education Research & Development*, *17*(3), 305–322. doi:10.1080/0729436980170304

Ice, P., Curtis, R., Phillips, P., & Wells, J. (2007). Using asynchronous audio feedback to enhance teaching presence and students' sense of community. *Journal of Asynchronous Learning Networks*, *11*(2), 3–25.

James, M. (2008). Assessment and learning. In Swaffield, S. (Ed.), *Unlocking assessment: Understanding for reflection and application* (pp. 20–35). London: Routledge.

Kerawalla, L., Minocha, S., Kirkup, G., & Conole, G. (2009). Supporting student blogging in higher education. In Hatzipanagos, S., & Warburton, S. (Eds.), *Handbook of research on social software and developing community ontologies* (pp. 231–247). Hershey, PA: Information Science Reference.

Kleiner, C., & Lord, M. (1999). The cheating game: Cross-national exploration of business students' attitudes, perceptions, and tendencies toward academic dishonesty. *Journal of Education for Business*, *74*(4), 38–42.

Knight, P. T., & Yorke, M. (2003). *Assessment, learning and employability*. Buckingham, UK: Open University Press.

Knowles, M. S. (1984). *Andragogy in action: Applying modern principles in adult learning*. San Francisco: Jossey-Bass.

Koschmann, T. (Ed.). (1996). *CSCL: Theory and practice of an emerging paradigm*. Mahwah, NJ: Lawrence Erlbaum.

Koschmann, T. (2001). Revisiting the paradigms of instructional technology. In G. Kennedy, M. Keppell, C. McNaught, & T. Petrovic (Eds.), *Meeting at the crossroads. Proceedings of the 18th Australasian Society for Computers in Learning in Tertiary Education (ASCILITE) Conference* (pp. 15–22). Melbourne, Australia: Biomedical Multimedia Unit, The University of Melbourne. Retrieved July 3, 2009, from www.ascilite.org.au/conferences/melbourne01/pdf/papers/koschmannt.pdf

Laurillard, D. (2002). *Rethinking university teaching: A conversational framework for the effective use of learning technologies* (2nd ed.). London: RoutledgeFalmer. doi:10.4324/9780203304846

Lave, J., & Wenger, E. (1991). *Situated learning: Legitimate peripheral participation*. Cambridge, UK: Cambridge University Press.

Leont'ev, A. N. (1981). *Problems of the development of mind*. (M. Kopylova, Trans.). Moscow: Progress. (1947).

Littleton, K., & Häkkinen, P. (1999). Learning together: Understanding the processes of computer-based collaborative learning. In Dillenbourg, P. (Ed.), *Collaborative learning: Cognitive and computational approaches* (pp. 20–30). Oxford, UK: Pergamon.

Littleton, K., Miell, D., & Faulkner, D. (Eds.). (2004). *Learning to collaborate, collaborating to learn: Understanding and promoting educationally productive collaborative work*. New York: Nova Science.

Loddington, S., Pond, K., Wilkinson, N., & Willmot, P. (2009). A case study of the development of WebPA: An online peer-moderated marking tool. *British Journal of Educational Technology*, *40*(2), 329–341. doi:10.1111/j.1467-8535.2008.00922.x

Luca, J., & Oliver, R. (2002). Developing an instructional design strategy to support generic skills development. In A. Williamson, C. Gunn, A. Young, & T. Clear (Eds.), *Winds of change in the sea of learning: Charting the course of digital education. Proceedings of the 19th Australasian Society for Computers in Learning in Tertiary Education (ASCILITE) Conference* (pp. 401–411). Auckland, New Zealand: UNITEC Institute of Technology. Retrieved August 12, 2008, from http://www.ascilite.org.au/conferences/auckland02/proceedings/papers/073.pdf

Mazur, E. (1997). *Peer instruction: A user's manual*. London: Prentice Hall.

McMurtry, K. (2001). e-cheating: Combating a 21st century challenge. *T.H.E. Journal*, *29*(4), 36–41.

Mercer, N., & Littleton, K. (2007). *Dialogue and the development of children's thinking: A sociocultural approach*. London: Routledge.

Middleton, A. (2008, June 18–19). *Audio feedback: Timely media interventions*. Paper presented at the Third International Blended Learning Conference, Hertfordshire, UK. Retrieved August 12, 2008, from http://www.herts.ac.uk/fms/documents/teaching-and-learning/blu/conference2008/Andrew-Middleton-2008.pdf

Miell, D., & Littleton, K. (Eds.). (2004). *Creative collaborations*. London: Free Association Books.

Murphy, P. (2000). Gender identifies and the process of negotiation in social interaction. In Joiner, R., Littleton, K., Faulkner, D., & Miell, D. (Eds.), *Rethinking collaborative learning* (pp. 139–160). London: Free Association Books.

Nicol, D. J. (1997). *Research on learning and higher education teaching. UCoSDA Briefing Paper 45*. Sheffield, UK: Universities and Colleges Staff Development Agency.

Nicol, D. J. (2007, May 29–31). *Principles of good assessment and feedback: Theory and practice*. Keynote paper presented at the Re-Engineering Assessment Practices (REAP) International Online Conference. Retrieved August 12, 2008, from http://www.reap.ac.uk/public/Papers/Principles_of_good_assessment_and_feedback.pdf

Nicol, D. J., & Macfarlane-Dick, D. (2006). Formative assessment and self-regulated learning: A model and seven principles of good feedback practice. *Studies in Higher Education*, *32*(2), 199–216. doi:10.1080/03075070600572090

Piaget, J. (1930). *The child's conception of physical causality*. London: Kogan Paul.

Pond, K., Coates, D., & Palermo, O. (2007). Student experiences of peer review marking of team projects. *International Journal of Management Education, 6*(2), 30–43. Retrieved August 12, 2008, from http://www.heacademy.ac.uk/assets/bmaf/documents/publications/IJME/Vol6No2/IJME62Pond.pdf

Poulis, J., Massen, C., Roberts, E., & Gilbert, M. (1998). Physics lecturing with audience paced feedback. *American Journal of Physics*, *66*(5), 439–441. doi:10.1119/1.18883

Price, M., & O'Donovan, B. (2008, August 27–29). *Feedback: All that effort, but what is the effect?* Paper presented at the Fourth Biennial European Association for Research on Learning and Instruction (EARLI)/Northumbria Assessment Conference, Potsdam/Berlin, Germany.

Puttnam, D. (2007, May 8). "In class, I have to power down". *The Guardian*. Retrieved July 4, 2009, from http://education.guardian.co.uk/egweekly/story/0,2074182,00.html

Quality Assurance Agency for Higher Education. (2006). *Code of practice for the assurance of academic quality and standards in higher education. Section 6: Assessment of students* (2nd ed.). Gloucester, UK: QAA. Retrieved July 3, 2009, from http://www.qaa.ac.uk/academicinfrastructure/codeOfPractice/section6/COP_AOS.pdf

Rotheram, B. (2007). Using an MP3 recorder to give feedback on student assignments. *Educational Developments*, *8*(2), 7–11.

Rowntree, D. (1987). *Assessing students: How shall we know them?*London: Kogan Page.

Sadler, D. R. (1989). Formative assessment and the design of instructional systems. *Instructional Science*, *18*(2), 119–144. doi:10.1007/BF00117714

Säljö, R. (1987). The educational construction of learning. In J. T. E. Richardson, M. W. Eysenck, & D. W. Piper (Eds.), *Student learning: Research in education and cognitive psychology* (pp. 101–108). Milton Keynes, UK: Society for Research into Higher Education and Open University Press.

Segers, M., Dochy, F., & Cascallar, E. (Eds.). (2003). *Optimising new modes of assessment: In search of qualities and standards*. Dordrecht, The Netherlands: Kluwer. doi:10.1007/0-306-48125-1

Shavelson, R. J. (2007). Assessing student learning responsibly: From history to an audacious proposal. *Change: The Magazine of Higher Learning*, *39*(1), 26–33. doi:10.3200/CHNG.39.1.26-33

Shepard, L. A. (2000). The role of assessment in a learning culture. *Educational Researcher*, *29*(7), 4–14.

Shepard, L. A. (2001). The role of classroom assessment in teaching and learning. In Richardson, V. (Ed.), *Handbook of research on teaching* (4th ed., pp. 1066–1101). Washington, DC: American Educational Research Association.

Simpson, V., & Oliver, M. (2007). Electronic voting systems for lectures then and now: A comparison of research and practice. *Australasian Journal of Educational Technology*, *23*(2), 187–208. Retrieved July 3, 2009, from http://www.ascilite.org.au/ajet/ajet23/simpson.html

Sipple, S. (2007). Ideas in practice: Developmental writers' attitudes toward audio and written feedback. *Journal of Developmental Education*, *30*(3), 22–31.

Sutherland, S. A. (2007, July 6). A model relating eportfolios to [portfolio] tools? [Electronic mailing list message]. Retrieved July 3, 2009, from https://www.jiscmail.ac.uk/cgi-bin/webadmin?A2=CETIS-PORTFOLIO;%2FPHwFQ;20070706145351%2B0100

Valdivia, R., & Nussbaum, M. (2009). Using multiple choice questions as a pedagogic model for face-to-face CSCL. *Computer Applications in Engineering Education*, *17*(1), 89–99. doi:10.1002/cae.20196

Vygotsky, L. S. (1978). *Mind in society: The development of higher psychological processes* (Cole, M., Trans.). Cambridge, MA: Harvard University Press.

Weaver, M. R. (2006). Do students value feedback? Student perceptions of tutors' written responses. *Assessment & Evaluation in Higher Education*, *31*(3), 379–394. doi:10.1080/02602930500353061

Wells, G., & Claxton, G. (Eds.). (2002). *Learning for life in the 21st century: Sociocultural perspectives on the future of education*. Oxford, UK: Blackwell.

Wheeler, S. (2009). Destructive creativity on the social web: Learning through wikis in higher education. In Hatzipanagos, S., & Warburton, S. (Eds.), *Handbook of research on social software and developing community ontologies* (pp. 497–510). Hershey, PA: Information Science Reference.

Whitelock, D. (2006). Electronic assessment: Marking, monitoring and mediating learning. *International Journal of Learning Technology.*, *2*(2/3), 264–276. doi:10.1504/IJLT.2006.010620

Whitelock, D., & Raw, Y. (2003). Taking an electronic mathematics examination from home: What the students think. In C. P. Constantinou & Z. C. Zacharia (Eds.), *New technologies and their applications in education: Proceedings of the Sixth International Conference on Computer-Based Learning in Science (CBLIS), Volume I* (pp. 701–713). Nicosia, Cyprus: University of Cyprus.

Whitelock, D., Ruedel, C., & Mackenzie, D. (2006). *e-Assessment: Case studies of effective and innovative practice.* Bristol, UK: Joint Information Systems Committee. Retrieved May 30, 2009, from http://kn.open.ac.uk/public/getfile.cfm?documentfileid=12880

Whitelock, D., & Watt, S. (2007). Supporting tutors with their feedback to students. In F. Khandia (Ed.), *Proceedings of the 11th International Computer-Assisted Assessment Conference* (pp. 421–432). Loughborough, UK: Loughborough University.

Whitelock, D., Watt, S., Raw, Y., & Moreale, E. (2004). Analysing tutor feedback to students: First steps towards constructing an electronic monitoring system. *ALT-J Research in Learning Technology*, *11*(3), 31–42.

Wiggins, G. (1998). *Educative assessment.* San Francisco: Jossey-Bass.

Williams, J. B., & Wong, A. (2009). The efficacy of final examinations: A comparative study of closed-book, invigilated exams and open-book, open-web exams. *British Journal of Educational Technology*, *40*(2), 227–236. doi:10.1111/j.1467-8535.2008.00929.x

Wojtas, O. (1998, September). Feedback? No, just give us the answers. *Times Higher Education Supplement*, 7.

KEY TERMS AND DEFINITIONS

4Ts Pyramid: A four-level model representing a suite of activities that should result in the transfer of learning from assessment tasks. These include: (1) tool development; (2) staff training; (3) rethinking the assessment tasks; and (4) learning from the assessment tasks.

Advice for Action: Feedback to students that they will take notice of and use in future learning tasks and assessments.

Assessment for Learning: Represents the goal of achieving a better alignment between teaching, learning, and assessment by acquiring and interpreting evidence that will assist both learners and teachers in determining what has been achieved and how best to move forward in the learning process to attain the desired learning outcomes.

Authentic Assessment: Involves the testing/evaluation of relevant, real-world knowledge and skills.

Formative Assessment: In contrast to summative assessment, refers to any type of assessment or task that provides feedback during the learning process to guide future learning.

Pedagogical Framework: Contains learning and assessment strategies that are well-integrated to achieve a set of given learning outcomes.

Summative Assessment: Assessment that is administered at the end of a learning sequence. It is designed to form a judgment about learning that is often reported in terms of grades or scores and is underpinned by a set of quality assurance processes. See also formative assessment.

Section 3

Web 2.0 and Beyond:

Current Implications and Future Directions for Web-Based Tertiary Teaching and Learning

Chapter 18
Dancing with Postmodernity:
Web 2.0+ as a New Epistemic Learning Space

Henk Eijkman
University of New South Wales at the Australian Defence Force Academy, Australia

ABSTRACT

This chapter addresses a significant theoretical gap in the Web 2.0 (or "Web 2.0+," as it is referred to by the author) literature by analyzing the educational implications of the "seismic shift in epistemology" (Dede, 2008, p. 80) that is occurring. As already identified in Chapter 2, there needs to be a consistency between our own epistemic assumptions and those embedded in Web 2.0. Hence the underlying premise of this chapter is that the adoption of social media in education implies the assumption of a very different epistemology—a distinctly different way of understanding the nature of knowledge and the process of how we come to know. The argument is that this shift toward a radically altered, "postmodernist," epistemic architecture of participation will transform the way in which educators and their students create and manage the production, dissemination, and validation of knowledge. In future, the new "postmodern" Web will increasingly privilege what we may usefully think of as a socially focused and performance-oriented approach to knowledge production. The expected subversion and disruption of our traditional or modernist power-knowledge system, as already evident in the Wikipedia phenomenon, will reframe educational practices and promote a new power-knowledge system, made up of new, social ways in which to construct and control knowledge across the Internet. The chapter concludes by advocating strategies for critical engagement with this new epistemic learning space, and posing a number of critical questions to guide ongoing practice.

DOI: 10.4018/978-1-60566-294-7.ch018

INTRODUCTION: THE SOCIAL WEB AS A NEW SPACE FOR KNOWLEDGE CONSTRUCTION

At its core, this chapter argues that to understand the educational implications of the shift from Web 1.0 to Web 2.0 we have to understand the latter not as a technological but as an epistemological revolution. From that perspective, what sets Web 2.0 apart is that it introduces radical changes in the production, distribution, evaluation, and use of knowledge, to the point that its educational appropriation "involves an apprenticeship in new kinds of knowledge practice" (Beetham, 2007, p. 2). This distinction is set to remain in the foreseeable future, hence from this point forward the term "Web 2.0+" will be used, The plus sign (+) signifies that subsequent iterations will further consolidate and extend this participatory paradigm (Eijkman, in press).

The above implies that, as the chapter will show, the epistemological frameworks of Web 1.0 and Web 2.0+ stand in opposition to each other. Web 2.0+, as a new site of intensified *social* digitization, privileges a social understanding of knowledge and values procedural or performance-oriented knowledge, where the focus is on "knowing how." In contrast, Web 1.0, in common with traditional education, emphasizes a psychological understanding of the nature of knowledge and stresses the individual acquisition of propositional knowledge, which focuses on "knowing what." This drastic shift in the organization and availability of knowledge "opens up many questions about traditional forms of transmission and the organisation of the transmission of knowledge. For example what is taught and learnt, when and how; who is learning and who is teaching and which knowledge is important" (Owen, Grant, Sayers, & Facer, 2006, p. 45).

To illuminate the ways in which Web 2.0+ provides higher education with very different means of creating and evaluating knowledge, the chapter makes explicit the usually implicit assumptions about the nature of knowledge and how it is constructed (Carter & Little, 2007). It illustrates the alignment of both Web 1.0 and traditional education with a modernist epistemic framework, in contrast to Web 2.0+'s more postmodern epistemic stance, with its performance-centered, social understanding of the nature of knowledge. The analysis in the chapter reveals a clear epistemic disconnect between the modernist worlds of Web 1.0 and conventional education practices on the one hand, and the postmodern stance of Web 2.0+ and social constructionist approaches to education on the other. Additionally, given that Web 2.0+ offers users unparalleled access to the ownership and control of knowledge construction, the chapter also identifies the educational impact of a distributed rather than centralized approach to epistemic authority and control, as the knowledge production and justification apparatus is no longer only in the hands of a privileged elite. Consequently, the chapter points out how this new focus on communal participation and control is of such magnitude that it will increasingly disrupt the powerful practices of dominant knowledge institutions to the extent that it may overturn the epistemic base of our current educational power-knowledge system, along with its pedagogic and curricular practices (Foucault, 1980).

A note about the "epistemological": at first glance, a philosophic discussion may seem irrelevant to the practical realities of learning and teaching. However, as will be shown, the epistemic tensions embodied in the postmodern Web are both substantial and significant. Web 2.0+ is above all about engaging educators and learners in very different modes of knowing that demand more mature, open, and transparent forms of authentic, real-world, "non-scholastic social practices" (Lankshear, 2003, p. 177). Web 2.0+'s suite of participatory spaces, which shift learning from being a process of acquiring propositional knowledge to one of acculturation into a community of practice (CoP), pose a fundamental challenge. They are a threat to decontextualized learning, to a psychologistic understanding of knowledge, and to a system in which the authority of knowledge is centralized and vested in educational and professional elites. The heated debates about Wikipedia among educators are indicative of the significance and contested nature of this shift (Eijkman, in press).

In order to guide future development of Web 2.0+ practice away from its digitopian devotees, the chapter advocates a critically reflective approach to this new epistemology and its very different take on the nature of knowledge and the processes of "how we come to know." It argues that despite the challenges this new "digital epistemology" can be the impetus for a thoughtful reshaping of the world of learning, teaching, and research, and for a more inclusive and learning-focused reconfiguration of our current power-knowledge system. Yet its rollout into the educational mainstream also calls for an ability on the part of educators to negotiate among competing worldviews, values, and practices. Consequently, the chapter presents practical strategies focused on the design criteria of coherence, participation, and acculturation, prior to concluding with a set of questions to guide ongoing practice.

Before proceeding, a few points about terms and definitions. First, the combination of limited space and philosophic complexity mean that the picture of the educational implications of Web 2.0+ is, of necessity, painted in broad brush strokes. Second, as noted earlier in this book by Tony Bates (see Chapter 2), readers should not infer from the terms "Web 1.0" and "Web 2.0," and given the Web's perpetual "beta" state, that advances in web technologies represent separate "generations" as if different phases of development somehow consist of disconnected entities on a linear timeline—hence again the reference to the plus sign in "Web 2.0+" (see also Berners-Lee, 2007). Noteworthy also is that a distinction is made between the "modern" and "postmodern" Web, and this is done so rather broadly. For the purposes of the chapter "modern" and its variants refer to the use of digital (Web 1.0) environments that support conventional practices and ways of thinking while "postmodern" refers to Web 2.0+ spaces and their use that take a more deconstructive and open stance. The use of "postmodern" is significant as it is meant to convey a radical rethinking of traditional views and practices that brings a different set of intellectual priorities and theoretical preoccupations to bear (Lather, 1989). Finally, the chapter also refers to "communities" or "networks of practice" and "discourse communities." These terms are used interchangeably to denote the same broad phenomenon, namely a grouping of people who, having a common focus, institutionalize a particular communicative structure (culture, language, and practices), and set of conventions, discourses, power arrangements, institutional hierarchies, vested interests, etc. (Eijkman, 2003; Porter, 1992; Wenger, 1998).

THE SOCIAL WEB AS AN EPISTEMIC MACROSHIFT

As amply described in earlier chapters, such as Chapter 1 (by Dabbagh and Reo) and Chapter 2 (by Bates), among others, Web 2.0 is a rather wide-ranging concept that refers to a broad suite of social networking and mass authoring tools. These tools make it increasingly easy for users to combine or render content in new and novel forms ("mashups"), and do so increasingly in open access content and open source software (Moody, 2006; Burger, 2007; Freedman, 2006). Important for the purposes of the present chapter is that they have two features in common. Their first commonality is that all services and applications are built on a platform of participation (O'Reilly, 2005). Their second common feature is that, at a deeper level, they all exhibit what we may usefully refer to as the social turn in epistemology. All services and platforms, to lesser or greater degrees, are underpinned by a distinctly social understanding of knowledge. All support, in one way or another, a people-centered, participatory paradigm that distributes rather than centralizes epistemic participation *and* authority. The combination of these two features provides higher education with a revolutionary learning environment. It is, above all, the social and participatory nature of the new suite of Internet services and applications that sets them apart from what is now popularly referred to as "Web 1.0." In the new social Web, "collaboration, contribution and community are the order of the day and there is a sense in which some think that a new 'social fabric' is being constructed before our eyes" (Anderson, 2007, p. 4). As is made plain throughout this book, educators increasingly recognize that in one way or another the postmodern Web's rich participation-driven suite of social networking and mass authoring tools redefine the way we use the Internet for learning, teaching, and research (e.g., Lankshear, 2003; Downes, 2006; Alexander, 2006; Hinchcliffe, 2006; Selwyn, 2008; Crook, 2008; Eijkman, 2008). The social Web's more mature architecture of participation and its social-performative epistemology irrevocably change the way people now engage with one another and with online content in the quest for knowledge.

The literature associates the postmodern Web with two core features of pivotal importance from an educational-philosophic standpoint, namely an architecture of participation supporting communal collaboration (see for instance Chapter 7), and a socially focused and performance-oriented epistemic framework. In terms of its architecture of participation and communal collaboration, and as stressed by Brown and Duguid (2002), by foregrounding people and connectivity rather than information "Web 2.0 is about a scaling up of participation that creates new possibilities for sharing and network effects" (Crook, 2008, p. 8). There is here a real focus on *users as generators as well as consumers* of multimedia forms of communication. In practice, the repositioning of users as "first class entities" means, for example, that static, read-only "pages" are replaced by dynamic blogs and wikis that feature the capacity for interaction and social writing (Cormode & Krishnamurthy, 2008). Internet users now have the flexibility to find, organize, share, and create information in *locally* meaningful ways but with *global* accessibility (Boyd, 2005).

Web 2.0+ also features a socially focused and performance-oriented epistemic framework. By way of introductory explanation, as this is explained in more detail below, the underpinning epistemic framework of the postmodern Web foregrounds two key elements, the social and the performative. There is a distinct emphasis on the social nature of knowledge and a privileging of procedural knowledge that is focused on a preference for "knowing how" (rather than propositional, "knowing what" knowledge). The postmodern digital episteme, borrowing from Lyotard (1979/1984), is said to be oriented toward a performance epistemology so called because the knowing that counts is "knowing as ... an ability to perform" (Lankshear, 2003, p. 183). The emerging epistemic picture of the postmodern Web reveals it is more comfortable with a social epistemology, a distinctly sociological view in which knowledge is not a reflection of empirical reality but is always mediated by and situated in discourse communities. Although a detailed discussion is out of scope, such a social constructionist position is quite different from the much-feted social constructivist stance (see for instance Eijkman, 2003; Hruby, 2001). In any case, as the curators of "digital assets" are also therefore increasingly communal rather than institutional, user ownership and control over knowledge production are greatly strengthened, allowing users to generate content with decreasing reference to geographic, cultural, institutional, and disciplinary boundaries and constraints (Schiltz, Truyen, & Coppens, 2007).

The participatory architecture on which the Web is now based has made it a much more sociable and egalitarian people-centered space. We can begin to see how postmodern web practices, being less amenable to domination by technophiles as well as professional and educational elites, undermine or disrupt our current power-knowledge system. The technical and conceptual architecture of the postmodern Web and its subsequent iterations (such as "Web 3.0"—see Chapter 20) has irrevocably shifted the emphasis away from the modernist Web's primary role as a hierarchic, top-down information repository and its associated "information fetishism" (Brown & Duguid, 2002). Gone, therefore, is the largely read-only information page metaphor and the focus on one-way flows of expert-validated information, in which the authority of knowledge was safely vested in academia.

While not underestimating the continued need for critical appraisal of these changes as advocated by Keen (2007) and many others, when taken together, the essentially distinctive feature of all of Web 2.0+'s applications and services is their emphasis on sociability, on more open and transparent participation in the communal production, sharing, and ownership of knowledge. The postmodern Web's much richer connective matrix makes it a very different place to what it was before. Arguably, this epistemic shift is of such magnitude that it will generate internal tensions in our current elitist power-knowledge system and its pedagogic and curricular practices, to a point where the stresses will precipitate either its stagnation or the breakthrough of a new, more participatory power-knowledge system (Eijkman, 2008; Hinchcliffe, 2006).

It should also become increasingly clear that this shift in web-based social practices, while driven by technology, is not reducible to it. The truly important transformation is epistemological, not merely technological, for it is the former rather than the latter that drives the pressure for change in our current power-knowledge system. What we are facing is a fundamental transformation in the way Internet users, in their everyday lives, can easily shape not just content but also the way content is organized (Hinchcliffe, 2006). Central to the *sound* educational use of the postmodern Web is how we, as educators, will respond to it at the level of epistemology.

WEB 2.0+: POWER AND KNOWLEDGE

The differences between Web 1.0 and Web 2.0+ are such that they invite a cultural shift in our epistemological framework, that is, in our understanding of the nature of knowledge and its authority—and particularly so when applied to formal education. Lankshear (2003) stresses that these new web-based technologies challenge our epistemological assumptions about what constitutes knowledge and knowing in the digital age. To begin with, Web 2.0+ shifts the emphasis from the individual to the collective, which in turn changes how "knowers" are constituted in relationship to other "knowers" as well as "the relative significance of, and balance among, different modes of knowing" (Lankshear, 2003, p. 177).

The point here is that Web 2.0+ reflects a powerful social drive for a shift from control to participation (Goodwin, 1999). Whereas the focus of the modernist Web was on the consumption of expert-validated knowledge, the participatory operating principle of the postmodern Web blurs the distinction between the production and consumption of knowledge, and hence that between producers and consumers and the control they have over knowledge. The participatory turn also positions participants differently vis-à-vis a vastly expanded, less hierarchically situated, and more culturally diverse range of "others." Furthermore, the extensive increase in the power of users in terms of control and ownership of knowledge has two immediate effects on the ways in which knowledge is constructed. It is far less constrained by cultural, institutional, or disciplinary boundaries, and because of its grassroots, bottom-up approach it is much more open to alternative viewpoints and perspectives that challenge or even subvert our hegemonic power-knowledge systems (Foucault, 1980; Ugoretz, 2006).

Though a detailed discussion is out of scope, suffice to say that for Foucault (1975/1977) the goals of power and those of knowledge are interdependent: "there is no power relation without the correlative constitution of a field of knowledge, nor any knowledge that does not presuppose and constitute at the same time power relations" (p. 27). Hence our prevailing knowledge system, with its rules, procedures, and limits, is inextricably linked to issues of power. The postmodern Web poses a deep-seated challenge to our "industrial model" power-knowledge system. It defies many of its accepted rules and regularities. It overthrows some of its limits and exclusions. It opens up the "conditions of possibility" by extending the range of what is possible and legitimate to "write," and how and where one can "write." It questions accepted norms about what counts as reason, argument, and evidence (note the simultaneous rise in concern about plagiarism), and what constitutes valid and valuable knowledge (Foucault, 1969/1972). The once solid boundaries around the ownership of epistemic authority have, to borrow from Marx, "melt[ed] into air" (quoted by Berman, 1982, p. 23). Nowhere is this epistemic tension more visible than in Wikipedia, the iconic symbol of this clash of educational civilizations, that Web 2.0+ phenomenon students love and academics love to hate (Eijkman, in press).

Wikipedia and the Epistemic Paradigm War

Wikipedia, as one of Web 2.0+'s best-known services, is a pertinent example of the postmodern episteme at work. It is in effect the public face of the struggle between old- and new-paradigm thinking about the nature of knowledge and the location of its authority.

While some academics are less concerned about Wikipedia and even see value in a more open and user-driven approach to knowledge creation and ownership, many are overwhelmingly suspicious and reject it outright as a source of trustworthy knowledge. At the epistemic level many educators see the Wikipedia phenomenon as a call to arms, to defend the cause of certainty, objectivity, universal "Truth," and academia's authority against the forces of intellectual darkness. In a nutshell, what they see as postmodern relativism (See Eijkman, in press; Keen, 2007; Ugoretz, 2006; Garfinkel, 2008; Child, 2007). At one level, what is at stake in the battle over Wikipedia is the *current* reluctance or willingness of many academics to engage with user-driven and communally curated knowledges in which they cease to have sole power over knowledge production and its justification. Wikipedia showcases how the process of and control over knowledge creation has become much more open, transparent, and egalitarian. Web 2.0+ offers educational networks of practice a novel and open, borderless world. Wikipedia is a symbol of a communal power-sharing approach to the authority of knowledge. At a deeper, structural and systemic level and for better and/or worse, Wikipedia is the iconic disruptor of the long-accepted rules and regularities that make up our power-knowledge system. Wikipedia contests its established limits and exclusions, its current "conditions of possibility" and customary norms about what counts as valid and valuable knowledge (Eijkman, in press).

Given the largely unknown effects of these new approaches, and that wikis are also one of the most iconic platforms of the postmodern Web and increasingly used by educators, w*hat is at stake here is the manner in which the postmodern epistemic framework of these and other Web 2.0+ platforms will be appropriated by educators*. For instance, to what extent will the imposition of modernist epistemic conventions about knowledge and learning work against the grain when applied to Web 2.0+ and its architecture of participatory knowledge construction, distributed control, and acculturation?

Let us now cast our gaze upon the future epistemic framework of the postmodern Web, and see how its unruly elements will increasingly disrupt our current power-knowledge system and its curricular and pedagogic practices. At the same time our gaze must confront the reality that this new, intensified socio-digital power-knowledge system will in turn also institutionalize its own type of educational power-knowledge system, the impact of which is not yet verifiable in this early stage of development, and given the choices educators have at their disposal.

THE NATURE OF THE POSTMODERN EPISTEMIC FRAMEWORK

It is important to locate Web 2.0+ technologies within the wider sociological and epistemological landscape. From this worldview, the postmodern Web's architecture of participation and communal collaboration are sustained by a socially focused and performance-oriented epistemic framework. Two core elements drive this epistemic framework, a distinctly social or sociological theory of knowledge and an epistemological focus on procedural knowledge concerned with "performativity" (Lyotard, 1979/1984). Both stand in opposition to the conventional epistemology dominant in modernist education and Web 1.0 practices, which privilege an individualist or psychologist theory of knowledge and have a focus on propositional knowledge.

A Social Epistemology

Web 2.0+, by providing new forms, arenas, and resources for the social construction of knowledge and easy, extensive, access to a vast range of networks of practice, enables the collaborative and egalitarian construction, exchange, and publishing of knowledge (Crook, 2008; Freedman, 2006). From this perspective, the knowing subject is not the individual but the discourse community to which he or she belongs. Knowledge is understood as being socially constructed and knowing is an inherently social rather than individual process. Hence the reference point for knowledge is neither internal (the individual mind) nor external (the empirical world) but social, namely the discourse community (Wenger, 1998; Gergen, 1999; Eijkman, 2003). From this empirically non-foundational epistemic vantage point, learning is understood as something that occurs "primarily *outside* the head, between participants in social relationship" (Eijkman, 2003, p. 145, emphasis in original). This sociological or social epistemological stance and its egalitarian or democratic impulse will progressively begin to disrupt the dominant, modernist psychologistic (individualistic) view of knowledge and learning, and the associated web-based practices.

In other words, the discourse communities to which we belong always mediate everything we perceive and come to know, so that "the 'reality' that we impute to the 'worlds' we inhabit is a [socially] constructed one" (Bruner, 2003, p. 169). As such, knowledge is, succinctly put, what a discourse community believes at a point in time, or what beliefs it "institutionalizes" in its culture and in its prevalent power-knowledge system. This makes knowledge a *sociocultural* artifact, a product of historically situated interchanges among members of particular discourse community at a particular instance. It follows from this that our knowledge of the world is always partial and situated, with no one interpretation being superior to another. Knowledge and truth are epistemically (though not morally) relative and therefore not universally valid or true. This perspective is thus inherently open to multiple knowledge claims, and is naturally compatible with a world in which the authority of knowledge is distributed, and in which knowledge claims are always subject to negotiation (Rorty, 1979, 1989; Toulmin, 1990; Gee, 1999; Gergen, 1999; Eijkman, 2003; Eijkman & Clarke 2007).

As the social is always the beginning and endpoint of all learning, gaining knowledge is always a social project, even if it is undertaken individually. For example, even the fictional character Robinson Crusoe, although he was alone, saw, interpreted, and acted upon "his" island not as a culturally abstracted individual, but as a member of his (albeit geographically distant) discourse community (Gergen, 1999). This is what sets the social constructionist position apart from constructivism, in that it is a *social theory of learning*, whereas constructivism is a *theory of social learning* (Wenger, 1998). Succinctly put, "these technologies represent a paradigm shift with specific and multiple impacts on the nature of knowledge in society, and therefore on the nature of learning" (Beetham & Sharpe, 2007, p. 1). One impact of the shift in epistemic emphasis from the individual to the collective is that it changes the constitution of "knowers" and what it means "to know" (Lankshear, 2003).

A Performance Epistemology

Lyotard (1979/1984) proposed that the two closely intertwined impulses of post-industrialism and postmodernism, which are now clearly evident in the deeper incursions of Web 2.0+'s social digitization into everyday life, irrevocably change the status of knowledge. He argued that the post-industrial intensification and entrenchment of new technologies and the postmodernist demise of belief in modernist grand narratives shifted the emphasis from propositional to procedural or performance-focused knowledge. Accordingly, under current postmodern conditions of intensified digitization, knowledge has become a commodity governed by the principle of performativity, defined as "the endless optimization" of performance (Lyotard, 1993, p. 25). In the postmodern Web, therefore, knowledge is not so much concerned with "truth" as with "high performativity," with knowledge that enhances the ability to perform efficiently (Lyotard, 1979/1984). Modernist epistemology, education, scientific research, and their associated practices within Web 1.0 foreground text-based propositional knowledge (knowing what). However, the kind of knowing involved in Web 2.0+'s social practices is, as Lankshear (2003, p. 183) asserts, "very different from this ... much of the knowing that is involved in the new spaces might better be understood in terms of a performance epistemology—knowing as an ability to perform." This has immense consequences for the two key tasks to which knowledge is put, namely learning and research, and how we do so within the diverse postmodern spaces of Web 2.0+.

FACING THE FUTURE: WEB 2.0+ AND DANCING THE POSTMODERN TANGO

The upshot is that as Web 2.0+ becomes an integral element in online learning, its new performance-focused epistemology will increasingly pose a challenge to those educational, scientific, and web-based practices that are still firmly embedded in a conventional modernist epistemology. While the exact implications for Web 2.0+-based educational practices are still unclear, since these have yet to fully enter the educational mainstream, what is becoming more and more apparent is that the impact of this digital epistemology will be considerable (Lankshear, 2003).

Despite the constructivist push, a modernist Cartesian epistemology still underpins much of the educational world of Web 1.0. From this modernist, psychologistic perspective (which incidentally encompasses activity theory, and even social constructivism), knowledge, in the final analysis, always resides in and belongs to individuals. The acquisition of knowledge is understood as a product of individual mental functioning, even if some see the individual as being, to various degrees, socially situated (Jonassen, 1991; Wertsch, 1998). In this model, knowledge is acquired through cognitive skills, and its authority continues to lie with academics who ultimately own and control the learning process (Hruby, 2001; Rorty, 1979; Gergen, 1999). Because knowledge formation occurs primarily *inside* the heads of individuals, the individual knower remains the ultimate epistemological unit of analysis (Eijkman, 2003). Moreover, and recognizing successful constructivist opposition, this modernist perspective, as still reflected in Laurillard's (2002) work, makes it easier for formal learning environments to expose students to abstract, second-order knowledges by presenting them with teacher-mediated descriptions of the world rather than encouraging them to engage in direct experience of the world.

As attested to by learning management systems (LMSs) all over the globe, crammed with lecture notes, readings, and PowerPoint presentations, this modernist educational episteme easily finds a home in the equally modernist-inclined spaces of Web 1.0, with its top-down, read-only information-page approach to discipline-based, validated knowledge. On the other hand, the postmodern episteme embedded in Web 2.0+ offers quite different pathways to learning and research. The postmodern Web, especially when pressed into service for educational purposes, represents a window of opportunity to address long-standing issues in learning and teaching. Yet at the same time these issues pose a systemic challenge to conventional epistemology, and to those education, research, and web-based practices that remain largely committed to it.

Critically progressive educators recognize that while Web 2.0+ and its postmodern episteme open up new educational vistas, they also pose new challenges of their own (see for example Aldrich, 2006; Beniger, 1989; Boyd, 2008; Goldberg, 2000; Keen, 2007; Welch, 2008). The central question about deploying Web 2.0+ in formal education is how to *critically* appropriate the postmodern Web and its social-performative epistemology for learning. There may be various methods to appropriate Web 2.0+ for educational purposes, and in such a way that its epistemic framework aligns with that of a similar, social constructionist, epistemological point of departure. Two possible strategies are suggested below.

First, as evident in the underlying theme of this chapter, as a first move it would be useful to replace an emphasis on the technological with a systemic focus on the epistemological. This makes it clear that we are invited to engage with knowledge in new ways, and that this invitation has an "RSVP" attached to it. In other words, we are asked for a response to this reframing of knowledge, of knowers, of the processes of coming to know, and of what knowing is valued (Siemens, 2008).

A second strategy to assist in critically appropriating Web 2.0+ involves considering our potential and/or intended use of Web 2.0+ tools, techniques, and applications, and the impact vis-à-vis our desired learning outcomes along three fundamental design criteria: the degree of epistemic coherence, the scale of participation, and the extent to which learning focuses on acculturation. To guide us in selecting the most appropriate Web 2.0+ tools and deciding how to deploy them we can ask, in relation to the specific context and desired learning aims and outcomes, "What levels of epistemic coherence, participation, and acculturation would be most appropriate?" As shown in Figure 1 each criterion offers a continuum of choices rather than a forced dichotomous, "either/or" situation. This enables educators to select their desired position on each criterion and identify consequences, consider the impact of trade-offs, anticipate potential issues, modify strategies, and identify research issues.

The Degree of Epistemic Coherence

Whereas to date our knowledge structure has been largely text based, the new social Web makes possible the multimodal structuring of knowledge by multiple communities or networks (Heim, 1999; Weinberger, 2006). The epistemic

Figure 1. Continua of choices for engaging with the new epistemic space to design and implement Web 2.0+-based e-learning

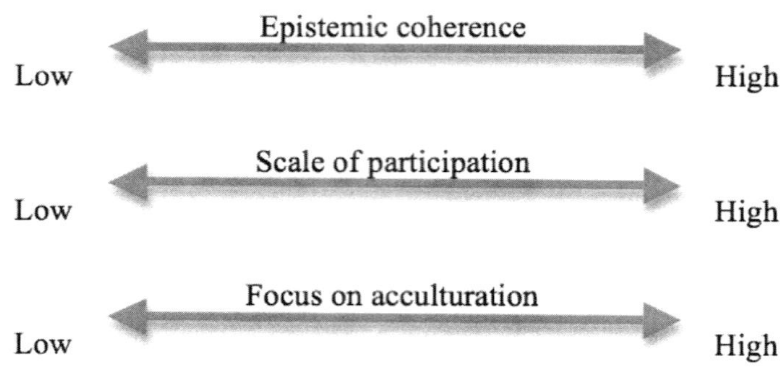

stance of the postmodern Web is such that "the creation, circulation, valuation and use of knowledge have changed" (Beetham, 2007, p. 2). This calls for a critical evaluation of both the old and new epistemes, taking into account their advantages and disadvantages, and a rethink and reframing of their related pedagogic, curricular, and research practices. While there appears to be a great deal of disjuncture between the modern and postmodern worlds of both higher education and the Web, there may also be valuable pedagogic and curricular trade-offs to be made, with the possibility of hybrid epistemic positionings. Evaluating epistemic alignment necessitates a cost-benefit analysis: specifically, what are the potential benefits of epistemic alignment between the planned educational or research activity and the social-performative epistemology of Web 2.0+, what are the possible costs of lower levels of alignment or even misalignment, and how do we resolve this issue of alignment to optimize learning?

The essence is that Web 2.0+, as Beetham (2007, p. 2) points out, is not just about "offering learners the technologies they are likely to use in the knowledge economy [but] … involves *an apprenticeship in new kinds of knowledge practice*" (emphasis added). It is therefore important that we, as educators, also enter into and make this apprenticeship explicit, first to ourselves, and then to our students. The question is about alignment—broadly put, it is about how we and our students can engage productively in such an epistemic apprenticeship.

A case in point may be seen in academic dishonesty or plagiarism. For example, is there a possible connection between the alleged explosion of, and concern about, plagiarism and the immersion of students in an intensified and increasingly intrusive digital environment with a very different epistemic stance? Are there some fundamental contradictions when students are, on the one hand, subject to a traditional educational process, while on the other hand simultaneously immersed in the epistemic world of Web 2.0+? Could it be that part of the plagiarism problem is that educators and students have disparate epistemic understandings and expectations about knowledge, its construction, and its ownership? Is there an epistemic mismatch between the postmodern digital epistemologies that students encounter on the Web and the traditional epistemic practices and expectations of academia? What are the differences in the epistemic framing of students and educators in a postmodern web environment, and how might these differences contribute to epistemic dissonance? Overall, when discussing plagiarism there is value in explicitly exploring the issues at a deeper epistemic level, so as to ascertain perceptions about the ownership of knowledge and its academic and professional "control" mechanisms, let alone what constitutes reliable knowledge and the importance of "truth." It is the tendency in traditional educational practices to position students as passive consumers of academically acceptable practices, policies, and procedures on knowledge production that may increasingly be out of step with students' web-based experiences and activities. Dialogue with students at the level of epistemology may well have something to offer here.

At a broader, more generic level, questions about the design of learning activities that make use of Web 2.0+ platforms might include the following:

- To what extent is the planned activity or program of activities a high-stakes, high-risk endeavor, and how should this influence the level of engagement with Web 2.0+ platforms, especially if students and/or educators are unfamiliar with the epistemic implications?
- How conventional are the educational and epistemic worldviews of the institution, teaching staff, and students? What scaffolding is needed to promote a smooth transition toward the effective educational use of the postmodern Web?
- How important, in a specific pedagogic-curricular context, is propositional knowledge, compared to procedural-performance knowledge? How can specific Web 2.0+ applications and/or services best support the acquisition of such knowledges?
- What balance will work best here, and given this expected balance, how do the Web 2.0+ tools to be used support or work against this chosen epistemic position?
- If there is an epistemic mismatch between the digital environment and legitimate educational expectations, what are the potential effects, and how can they be dealt with?
- Is an explicit awareness of any epistemic differences helpful in itself? For example, is it useful for students and educators to have an understanding about how they are framed both vis-à-vis one another on the Web and vis-à-vis web content and the knowledge construction process? Will an acknowledgment of degrees of alignment or misalignment make it possible to proactively incorporate useful allowances or ameliorative strategies?

From this perspective both the modernist and postmodernist positions have to be reviewed for their relevance, strengths, and limitations (cf. Castells, 1996, Gee, Hull, & Lankshear, 1996). If the rather hasty dismissal of Wikipedia by many academics is any indication, those wedded to a conventional epistemology may find such an epistemic review, let alone possible reframing, quite challenging (Eijkman, in press).

As noted in Chapter 2, the point is that if educators really want to capitalize on Web 2.0+'s affordances they need to begin to seriously consider the epistemological implications and how to achieve a critical alignment between their epistemological stance and that of the social Web. In the final analysis, when appropriated for educational purposes, it is not the digital technology but the epistemic worldview of educators that will determine how students, educators, and other "knowers" are framed and conceptualized, and how effectively the technology will be deployed for learning and research. One way of putting this issue firmly on the table, so to speak, is to encourage educators—and students—to expand current discussions about Wikipedia. As a hot topic it is ideally placed to provide a platform for further exploring issues around the different perceptions of knowledge, authority, and control, and illuminating how Web 2.0+ differs markedly from conventional academic practices in terms of the way it frames participants in educational endeavors.

The Scale of Participation

Central to the postmodern Web is the shift from control to participation, and consequently the problematic "passionate drive to keep the Internet as free of authority and control as possible" (Lankshear, 2003, p. 175). Issues around control and authority are, however, central to education as we know it, while the democratization of knowledge sits at the core of the postmodern Web. This places educational values and concerns about what constitutes useful/valid knowledge and how it should be generated and used in direct opposition to Web 2.0+'s democratic ideals. The deep tensions inherent in the participation–control continuum pose the most profound challenge to higher education and its authority over knowledge, and will therefore need to be the focal point for deliberation, critical analysis, and research.

At any rate, the postmodern Web's preference for the optimization of participation in content construction and subsequent role as a disruptive epistemology are clearly visible in its focus on open access, people centeredness, the dissolution of boundaries between consumption and production of content, and the distribution of ownership and control. In short, there is a dramatic change in knowledge production practices as Web 2.0+ applications and services tend toward pushing or drawing students and educators into more collaborative methods of learning and inquiry that, even when not explicit, implicitly remove layers of control (Thompson, 2007; Crook, 2008). As explained in more detail in the next subsection, this tension between conventional education's need for control and the Web's focus on broader participation poses a major barrier to the open rather than institutionally-closed uptake of Web 2.0+ platforms at the level of their epistemology. This is exemplified by Huijser's (2008, p. 48) observation that "[t]he main threat of using SNSs [social networking sites] in an educational context arises from a perceived lack of control over the educational space, because of the public nature of such sites, contrasting sharply with more traditional closed environments such as learning management systems" (see also Chapter 14 in this book by Huijser and Sankey).

The democratization of knowledge, while having important positive aspects for learning, also attracts critical debate. Many educators are concerned about the perceived danger of the "cult of the amateur" (Keen, 2007) and its threat to scholarly authority. Traditional education is inherently opposed to the democratizing tendencies of the postmodern Web—and not all of it unreasonably so. We may be best able to avoid any unproductive polarization by drawing on the work of Basil Bernstein (1996) and approaching the matter as being about a fundamental disagreement regarding the degree to which learning environments ought to be either strongly or weakly framed and classified. To elaborate, according to Bernstein (1996; see also Eijkman, 2003) conventional learning operates within a strongly "classified" and strongly "framed" education system. Disciplines have strongly classified, that is, strictly defined knowledge boundaries, and the learning and teaching processes and their associated discourses are also tightly defined or framed. In contrast, and courtesy of its open knowledge-creation processes, the postmodern Web's participatory framework has a distinct preference for weak classification of content (having minimal or no boundaries) and weak framing (Eijkman, 2003). The traditional educational paradigm, with its strongly classified curricular structuring and strongly framed learning processes, appears distinctly anti-participatory compared to the model seen in Web 2.0+.

The tensions inherent in the "strong-versus-weak" framing and classification approaches are, for instance, clearly evident in the traditional reluctance to involve students in any stage of the curriculum/learning design process other than evaluation. Moreover, this is an issue of increased importance in the context of educational planning for Web 2.0+ and its participatory framework. In other words, the ethos of the social Web also calls for the inclusion of students in educational design and planning, to elicit information about their everyday experiences of Web 2.0+ and their expectations of using Web 2.0+ for formal educational purposes (Lohnes & Kinzer, 2007; Eijkman & Herrmann, 2009; see also Chapter 3). Educators need to pay more attention to promoting student participation in planning for the use of social media premised on a participatory ethic (Selwyn, 2007).

In essence, determining the optimum scale of participation in educational Web 2.0+ environments calls for a rethink about how the social Web positions educators and students differently in knowledge-creation processes, and how they can best participate together in planning, learning, and inquiry within and using these environments. The issue about the scale of participation within a program of study relates to the extent to which educators are willing to empower students as co-producers rather than mere consumers of knowledge, and conversely, the readiness of students to engage more actively in this process. On this basis, any perceived threat to scholastic authority

> *only materialises if we stay locked in a binary framework of "educator versus student." The concept of co-creation by contrast allows us to think about the educational context as a space where educators and students are both implicated in a community of co-creators. This applies especially to Web 2.0 technologies as both students and teachers potentially bring different skills to the table, and are thus joined in a collaborative learning journey (Huijser, 2008, p. 49).*

The key question here is this: to what extent are we, as educators, ready for the challenge to (thoughtfully) step out of our "authoritative" comfort zone without compromising the value and validity of the knowledges our students will produce? Put another way, to what degree can we promote a participatory mindset, balancing this with our need and desire to remain masters within our walled-in, cloistered courtyards?

It seems inevitable that Web 2.0+'s architecture of participation will involve various degrees of curricular and pedagogic deinstitutionalization. In other words, Web 2.0+-based learning activities and initiatives are likely to be less contained or restrained by institutional boundaries and restrictions such as the established roles of students, educators, and the WWW—the "Wide Wild World" (Eijkman & Clarke, 2007)—in the knowledge production process, reinforced by the longstanding focus on closed institutional intranets and LMSs. Presently, instead of seeing this as a window of opportunity for constructive change, there is a general tendency for both institutions and educators to be wary of the pressure for greater student participation and autonomy; they are interpreting the new practices and affordances rather negatively as constituting a serious slippage in their capacity to control and manage the educational experience (Bernstein, 1996; Crook, 2008; Eijkman, 2004; Huijser, 2008).

Resistance to the participatory turn in Web 2.0+ is likely to result in an educationally-disruptive digital disconnect and legitimacy crisis (Kenway & Bullen, 2005; Levin & Arafeh, 2002). Students familiar with Web 2.0+ applications and services are likely to increasingly question the authoritarian appropriation of democratic and participatory Web 2.0+ practices in formal educational settings, if not now, certainly more so in the future. This scenario is especially likely if their educational use of Web 2.0+ bears little or no resemblance to their everyday experiences, in which they are positioned as co-owners and co-producers of knowledge.

In considering the optimum scale of participation for a learning context, educators may ask:

- What degree of participation would best suit the planned program of study? What level of participation would motivate students to learn most effectively? To what extent can students participate as co-producers of a curriculum? How can their voices be heard and represented in the planning process? How can participation be best negotiated before, during, and after the planning and implementation phases?
- To what degree can we frame students as co-producers of knowledge? What are the advantages of doing so? What are the personal, professional, and/or institutional enablers and inhibitors to this end?
- What support structures and mechanisms are useful for both educators and students in promoting participation and helping them become accustomed to their new roles as co-producers?
- To what extent can participation in the educational experience match the inherent participatory expectations of Web 2.0+? To what extent can formal learning activities tap into the open access provided by the Wide Wild World of the Web, rather than enclosing students and learning within the confines of an LMS?

Learning as Acculturation

Web 2.0+ enables access to authentic, real-world practices and communities on an unprecedented scale. The default epistemic position of the postmodern Web is to reframe participants as actively-contributing, cosmopolitan members of global networks of practice (Wenger, 1998; Eijkman, 2003). From this viewpoint, the focus of learning is not on content *per se* but on acculturation. For students, as newcomers to a CoP, learning is about becoming progressively familiar with the culture, discourse, knowledge, worldviews, dispositions, and practices of the community they are joining. This entails placing students on the most productive trajectories of participation to enable them to progress from "novices" to fully competent "insiders" of their respective community (Wenger, 1998; Eijkman, 2003, 2004). It is arguable that all our learning, regardless of if it is formal or informal, and whether it is undertaken individually or collectively, from childhood on, is about acculturation into the knowledge system and practices of one or more communities or networks of practice (Gee, 1999). Accordingly, in the postmodern Web,

The model of e-learning as being a type of content, produced by publishers, organized and structured into courses, and consumed by students, is turned on its head. Insofar as there is content, it is used rather than read—and is, in any case, more likely to be produced by students than courseware authors. And insofar as there is structure, it is more likely to resemble a language or a conversation rather than a book or a manual (Downes, 2006, emphasis added).

In comparison to conventional learning and its emphasis on propositional knowledge, learning as acculturation favors a performative epistemology, as promoted in Web 2.0+. Therefore, acculturation is most effective when students are permitted to embark on trajectories of legitimate peripheral participation in practice-focused, first-order or experiential knowledge development, in which efforts concentrate on direct and authentic experiences of the world rather than institutionally mediated abstract descriptions of it (Lave & Wenger, 1991; Wenger, 1998; Eijkman, 2003).

Hence both learning as acculturation and Web 2.0+ facilitate participatory pathways in which learning morphs from *learning about* to *learning to be* productive members of CoPs (Wenger, 1998). Web 2.0+'s preference for a performance epistemology shifts the attention away from the conventional emphasis on propositional knowledge (knowing what) toward procedural knowledge (knowing how), where knowing "as an ability to perform" is central. This immediately moves the focus to mature forms of authentic, non-scholastic social practices, and thereby invites substantive changes in curriculum and pedagogy (Lankshear, 2003).

The crux here is to consider where we, as educators, are willing to position our understanding of learning on this continuum, and how that position will frame our curricular and pedagogic orientation as content or acculturation centered. Questions we may profitably ask include the following:

- To what extent does the relevant discipline or profession favor propositional knowledge (content) or procedural knowledge (acculturation) in its dominant curricular and pedagogic practices?
- How do these conventional curricular and pedagogic preferences align with the acculturative-performative emphasis of Web 2.0+?
- What are the perceived advantages of shifting toward a more acculturative stance for student learning? What challenges does it pose for the educator, institution, and discipline? What challenges does it pose for students?
- What strategies are likely to support an effective transition to a more weakly classified and weakly framed Web 2.0+ learning environment?

One effective approach to giving students a real sense of acculturation-over-time is to take up and extend Matthew Allen's proposal to shift the emphasis of online engagement from participation in short-term, semester-based units to immersion and active involvement in long-term, program-based communities of practice. As Allen (1999) noted over a decade ago,

> *the really important step forward that universities can take is to begin fostering communities that are less specifically connected to units and are, instead, about issues, subjects, disciplines or professions. ... Student membership of these communities should become integral to their course completion; where necessary, whole components of the course should become (instead of "study") knowledge-based community participation. (p. 9)*

We can enhance the impact value of such a move in at least two ways. First, we can provide these online communities with a Web 2.0+ environment that optimizes both local and global interaction and participation. This connects students at least in some ways to their institutional as well as wider, global networks of practice. Second, and with a focus on retaining alumni within the institutional community, it is worth considering the establishment of post-institutional Web 2.0+-based communities through which graduates can enjoy continued access to their institutional, program-based community and selected institutional benefits, rather than "cutting them off" upon program completion as has usually been the case.

And so we can view acculturation in tertiary education and the postmodern Web through both a short and long-term lens. At a unit-of-study level we can take steps to attempt to strike an appropriate balance between supplied content and acculturation. At a program level we can begin to rethink the provision of online communities by enabling students to maintain personal awareness of their acculturation through the ability to capture and track their achievements as they progress on their trajectories of participation throughout—and perhaps even beyond—their programs of study. The aim of such a long-term Web 2.0+ presence is to connect students more consistently to the culture, language, concepts, expectations, and practices of their real-world discourse communities (Bizzell, 1992), and to do so continuously rather than in an ad hoc fashion, in ways that allow them, their educators, and the institution to ascertain and celebrate progress.

NOT A CONCLUSION, BUT A BEGINNING: TOWARD A SYSTEMIC POSTMODERN WORLDVIEW

It is clear that Web 2.0+ provides curriculum and pedagogy with a very different epistemic space. The highly participatory tools, technologies, and practices that enable multiple ways of seeing and knowing undermine the power and gatekeeping role of academia. Traditional knowledge structures and approaches, including the ability of an elite few to decide what constitutes trustworthy knowledge, are denaturalized as epistemic processes and epistemic authority are opened up and made much more transparent. The very different understanding about the nature of knowledge as a social rather than individual phenomenon, in its production, assessment, and validation, has far-reaching theoretical and practical consequences for learning, teaching, and research.

Moving toward full integration of the social Web into the domain of higher education will be a challenging process requiring the resolution of major tensions and deep-seated dilemmas. As Chowcat, Phillips, Popham, and Jones (2008) highlight, much of this will be about identifying drivers, inhibitors, and disruptors:

we will refine our understanding of the trends and, especially, the emerging disruptions through dialogue with the expert community and by engaging in other activities. Activities will include "sandpit" events (where small groups can engage in-depth with specific technologies to evaluate their educational potential), commissioning a small number of action research projects, and identifying exemplar projects to form the basis of case studies. (p. 6)

For example, participation can, in different circumstances and in different ways, be as much a driver as a disruptor and inhibitor of good practice. Action research projects can be useful here as a way forward in providing for evidence-based practice. Take the tensions inherent in the popularly conceived participation–control dichotomy—again, although there is not the scope here to explore this topic in the depth it deserves, linked to these different directions regarding the centralized or democratic authority of knowledge are extremely important considerations. It is crucial these are fully and critically explored in ways that transcend mindless conservatism on one side and unquestioning digitopian enthusiasm on another, and that go beyond reductionist thinking that places these two perspectives in an unproductive "either/or" dichotomy.

In addition, given the variable exposure of learners and educators to the relatively new social media applications and services, there exist opportunities for a collaborative and strategic approach to the implementation of Web 2.0+ spaces for learning in higher education. Planning and design will benefit, at the immediate educational level, from consultation with students and other stakeholders. It is clear, as well, that given the systemic nature of the change inherent in Web 2.0+, institutions stand to benefit greatly from a systemic rather than piecemeal approach to implementation. Educational leaders and administrators should, for example, consider systematizing the introduction of Web 2.0+ by commissioning dedicated strategic and operational plans. Also, in view of the fact that social inequities will undoubtedly continue to prevail, it will be especially valuable in this context to research and assess not just the digital but also the epistemic divides, and to do so with critical intent to ensure that *all* social groups will benefit from any transformation of our current power-knowledge system (Eijkman, 2003).

In conclusion, and drawing on the work of Beetham (2007, p. 5), it is suggested that from a minimalist perspective researchers and practitioners at least consider the following questions with regard to the expanded use of the social Web for learning:

- What are the *critical choices* we as educators make, not just with respect to our educational use of social media but in relation to its underpinning epistemological assumptions and worldview?
- What *practices, habits, and patterns* of use emerge from these epistemic choices? What impact do different patterns of use have on curriculum, pedagogy, student learning, and research?
- What are the *critical moments* in the changing relationships that educators, researchers, and students experience when learning, teaching, or researching with Web 2.0+ social media?
- How can we define *effective learning and research* in epistemically different Web 2.0+ environments? What skills, strategies, aptitudes, and approaches are most effective and useful in such environments?
- How can participants best *integrate and personalize* their formal and informal learning strategies, their online and offline social networks, and their academic and peer-created knowledges?
- What changes need to occur in *institutional policies and technological practices* in order to integrate the social Web effectively into the educational mainstream?

All in all, we find ourselves in an exploratory phase of working with the postmodern Web, and this, to use Boorstin's (1980) metaphor, gives us a "fertile verge;" a broad liminal "betwixt and between" space within which we can act and research—and do so simultaneously, as action researchers—if we want to (Chowcat et al., 2008). We will find ourselves ever more in an educational frontier region where two different epistemic paradigms will increasingly meet and mingle, and in which we can acculturate ourselves, our students, and our institutions into new, groundbreaking epistemic practices.

REFERENCES

Aldrich, C. (2006, November 20). Second Life is not a teaching tool [Web log post]. *The Learning Circuits Blog*. Retrieved October 12, 2008, from http://learningcircuits.blogspot.com/2006/11/second-life-is-not-teaching-tool.html

Alexander, B. (2006). Web 2.0: A new wave of innovation for teaching and learning? *EDUCAUSE Review*, *41*(2), 32–44.

Allen, M. (1999, March). *Don't be a troll! Using the Internet for successful higher education*. Paper presented at Higher Education '99, Sydney.

Anderson, P. (2007). *What is Web 2.0? Ideas, technologies and implications for education*. Bristol, UK: Joint Information Systems Committee. Retrieved November 28, 2008, from http://www.jisc.ac.uk/media/documents/techwatch/tsw0701b.pdf

Beetham, H. (2007). *Learners' experiences of e-learning. A briefing for the PVC Network: e-learning Special Interest Group*. Bristol, UK: Joint Information Systems Committee. Retrieved September 6, 2008, from http://www.jisc.ac.uk/media/documents/programmes/elearningpedagogy/pspvcelearningsigbriefingpaperfinal.pdf

Beetham, H., & Sharpe, R. (Eds.). (2007). *Rethinking pedagogy for a digital age: Designing and delivering e-learning*. London: Routledge.

Beniger, J. R. (1989). *The control revolution: Technological and economic origins of the information society*. Cambridge, MA: Harvard University Press.

Berman, M. (1982). *All that is solid melts into air: The experience of modernity*. New York: Simon & Schuster.

Berners-Lee, T. (2007, March 27). Giant Global Graph [Web log post]. *timbl's blog*. Retrieved May 23, 2008, from http://dig.csail.mit.edu/breadcrumbs/node/215

Bernstein, B. (1996). *Pedagogy, symbolic control and identity: Theory, research, critique*. London: Taylor & Francis.

Bizzell, P. (1992). *Academic discourse and critical consciousness*. Pittsburgh, PA: University of Pittsburgh Press.

Boorstin, D. J. (1980). *The fertile verge: Creativity in the United States. An address given at the Carnegie Symposium on Creativity, the Inaugural Meeting of the Library of Congress Council of Scholars, November 19–20, 1980*. Washington, DC: Library of Congress.

Boyd, D. (2005). Why Web 2.0 matters: Preparing for glocalization [Web log post]. *apophenia*. Retrieved March 17, 2008, from http://www.zephoria.org/thoughts/archives/2005/09/05/why_web20_matte.html

Boyd, D. (2008). None of this is real. In Karaganis, J. (Ed.), *Structures of participation in digital culture* (pp. 132–157). New York: Social Science Research Council.

Brown, J. S., & Duguid, P. (2002). *The social life of information*. Boston: Harvard Business School Press.

Bruner, J. (2003). The narrative construction of reality. In Mateas, M., & Sengers, P. (Eds.), *Narrative intelligence* (pp. 41–62). Amsterdam: John Benjamins.

Burger, T. N. (2007, January 22). Libraries facilitate open access to information with open source software. *Linux.com*. Retrieved August 29, 2008, from http://www.linux.com/articles/59491

Carter, S. M., & Little, M. (2007). Justifying knowledge, justifying method, taking action: Epistemologies, methodologies, and methods in qualitative research. *Qualitative Health Research, 17*(10), 1316–1328. doi:10.1177/1049732307306927

Castells, M. (1996). *The rise of the network society*. Oxford, UK: Blackwell.

Child, M. L. (2007, February 26). Professors split on wiki debate. *The Harvard Crimson*. Retrieved November 6, 2008, from http://www.thecrimson.com/article.aspx?ref=517305

Chowcat, I., Phillips, B., Popham, J., & Jones, I. (2008, July) *Harnessing technology: Preliminary identification of trends affecting the use of technology for learning*. Coventry, UK: Becta. Retrieved January 19, 2009, from http://emerging-technologies.becta.org.uk/upload-dir/downloads/page_documents/partners/ht_trends_july08.pdf

Cormode, G., & Krishnamurthy, B. (2008). Key differences between Web 1.0 and Web 2.0. *First Monday, 13*(6). Retrieved January 19, 2009, from http://www.uic.edu/htbin/cgiwrap/bin/ojs/index.php/fm/article/viewArticle/2125/1972

Crook, C. (2008). *Web 2.0 technologies for learning: The current landscape—opportunities, challenges and tensions*. Coventry, UK: Becta. Retrieved January 10, 2009, from http://research.becta.org.uk/upload-dir/downloads/page_documents/research/web2_technologies_learning.pdf

Dede, C. (2008). A seismic shift in epistemology. *EDUCAUSE Review, 43*(3), 80–81. Retrieved January 9, 2009, from http://www.educause.edu/ir/library/pdf/ERM0837.pdf

Downes, S. (2006, October 16). *Learning networks and connective knowledge*. Retrieved January 9, 2009, from http://it.coe.uga.edu/itforum/paper92/paper92.html

Eijkman, H. (2003). *Online learning as curricular justice? A critical framework for higher education*. Unpublished Ph.D. dissertation, University of Canberra, Canberra, Australia.

Eijkman, H. (2004, November 26–28). *Contingency, curriculum and solidarity: A social constructionist response to the academic divide in Australian higher education*. Paper presented at the 33rd Annual Philosophy of Education Society of Australasia Conference. Melbourne, Australia.

Eijkman, H. (2008). Web 2.0 as a non-foundational network-centric learning space. *Campus-Wide Information Systems*, *25*(2), 93–104. doi:10.1108/10650740810866567

Eijkman, H. (in press). How academics view Wikipedia: Web 2.0+ and the change in academic power-knowledge arrangements. *Campus-Wide Information Systems*.

Eijkman, H., & Clarke, B. (2007). Towards a participatory learning and assessment culture in higher education: Leveraging aocial rechnologies to reframe our curricular practices. In K. Fernstrom (Ed.), *Readings in technology in education: Proceedings of the International Conference on Information Communication Technologies in Education*. Abbostsford, BC: University of the Fraser Valley.

Eijkman, H., & Herrmann, A. (2009, March 25–27) *Beyond stereotyping: Understanding student readiness for network centric learning*. Paper presented at the Defence Academies and Colleges eLearning Conference, Stellenbosch, South Africa.

Foucault, M. (1972). *The archaeology of knowledge*. (A. M. Sheridan-Smith, Trans.). London: Tavistock. (1969).

Foucault, M. (1977). *Discipline and punish: The birth of the prison*. (A. M. Sheridan-Smith, Trans.). Harmondsworth, UK: Penguin. (1975).

Foucault, M. (1980). *Power/knowledge: Selected interviews and other writings, 1972–77* (Gordeon, C., Ed.). Brighton, UK: Harvester.

Freedman, T. (Ed.). (2006). *Coming of age: An introduction to the new World Wide Web*. Ilford, UK: Terry Freedman. Retrieved November 25, 2008, from http://fullmeasure.co.uk/Coming_of_age_v1-2.pdf

Garfinkel, S. L. (2008, November/December). Wikipedia and the meaning of truth: Why the online encyclopedia's epistemology should worry those who care about traditional notions of accuracy. *Technology Review*, 84–86.

Gee, J. P. (1999). *Language, learning, and latecomers: Discourses in education*. Unpublished manuscript.

Gee, J. P., Hull, G., & Lankshear, C. (1996). *The new work order: Behind the language of the new capitalism*. Sydney: Allen & Unwin.

Gergen, K. J. (1999). *An invitation to social construction*. London: Sage.

Goldberg, K. (2000). *The robot in the garden: Telerobotics and telepistemology in the age of the Internet*. Cambridge, MA: MIT Press.

Goodwin, B. C. (1999). From control to participation via a science of qualities. *ReVision*, *21*(4), 26–35.

Heim, M. (1999). *Transmogrification*. Retrieved February 7, 2009, from http://www.mheim.com/files/transmog.pdf

Hinchcliffe, D. (2006, September 4). All we got was Web 1.0, when Tim Berners-Lee actually gave us Web 2.0 [Web log post]. *Dion Hinchcliffe's Web 2.0 Blog*. Retrieved October 8, 2009, from http://web2.socialcomputingjournal.com/all_we_got_was_web_10_when_tim_bernerslee_actually_gave_us_w.htm

Hruby, G. G. (2001). Sociological, postmodern, and new realism perspectives in social constructionism: Implications for literacy research. *Reading Research Quarterly*, *36*(1), 48–62. doi:10.1598/RRQ.36.1.3

Huijser, H. J. (2008). Exploring the educational potential of social networking sites: The fine line between exploiting opportunities and unwelcome imposition. *Studies in Learning, Evaluation, Innovation and Development, 5*(3), 45–54. Retrieved September 15, 2008, from http://sleid.cqu.edu.au/include/getdoc.php?id=708&article=199&mode=pdf

Jonassen, D. H. (1991). Evaluating constructivistic learning. *Educational Technology*, *31*(9), 28–33.

Keen, A. (2007). *The cult of the amateur: How today's Internet is killing our culture*. New York: Doubleday.

Kenway, J., & Bullen, E. (2005). Globalizing the young in the age of desire: Some educational policy issues. In Apple, M. W., Kenway, J., & Singh, M. (Eds.), *Globalizing education: Policies, pedagogies, & politics* (pp. 31–43). New York: Peter Lang.

Lankshear, C. (2003). The challenge of digital epistemologies. *Education Communication and Information*, *3*(2), 167–186. doi:10.1080/14636310303144

Lather, P. (1989, August 25–27). *Deconstructing/deconstructive inquiry: Issues in feminist research methodologies*. Paper presented at the New Zealand Women's Studies Association Conference, Christchurch, New Zealand.

Laurillard, D. (2002). *Rethinking university teaching: A conversational framework for the effective use of learning technologies* (2nd ed.). London: RoutledgeFalmer. doi:10.4324/9780203304846

Lave, J., & Wenger, E. (1991). *Situated learning: Legitimate peripheral participation*. New York: Cambridge University Press.

Levin, D., & Arafeh, S. (2002). *The digital disconnect: The widening gap between Internet-savvy students and their schools*. Washington, DC: Pew Internet & American Life Project. Retrieved October 28, 2009, from http://www.pewinternet.org/~/media//Files/Reports/2002/PIP_Schools_Internet_Report.pdf.pdf

Lohnes, S., & Kinzer, C. (2007). Questioning assumptions about students' expectations for technology in college classrooms. *Innovate: Journal of Online Education, 3*(5). Retrieved January 12, 2009, from, http://www.innovateonline.info/index.php?view=article&id=431

Lyotard, J.-F. (1984). *The postmodern condition: A report on knowledge*. (G. Bennington & B. Massumi, Trans.). Minneapolis, MN: University of Minnesota Press. (1979).

Lyotard, J.-F. (1993). A svelte appendix to the postmodern question. In *Political writings* (pp. 25–29). (Readings, B., & Geiman, K. P., Trans.). Minneapolis, MN: University of Minnesota Press.

Moody, G. (2006, February 22). Parallel universes: Open access and open source. *LWN.net*. Retrieved May 17, 2008, from http://lwn.net/Articles/172781/

O'Reilly, T. (2005). *What is Web 2.0: Design patterns and business models for the next generation of software*. Retrieved May 17, 2008, from http://www.oreillynet.com/pub/a/oreilly/tim/news/2005/09/30/what-is-web-20.html

Owen, M., Grant, L., Sayers, S., & Facer, K. (2006). *Social software and learning*. Bristol, UK: Futurelab. Retrieved January 12, 2009, from http://www.futurelab.org.uk/resources/documents/opening_education/Social_Software_report.pdf

Porter, J. (1992). *Audience and rhetoric: An archaeological composition of the discourse community*. Upper Saddle River, NJ: Prentice Hall.

Rorty, R. (1979). *Philosophy and the mirror of nature*. Princeton, NJ: Princeton University Press.

Rorty, R. (1989). *Contingency, irony, and solidarity*. Cambridge, UK: Cambridge University Press.

Schiltz, M., Truyen, F., & Coppens, H. (2007). Cutting the trees of knowledge: Social software, information architecture and their epistemic consequences. *Thesis Eleven, 89*(1), 94–114.

Selwyn, N. (2007, October 16–17). *Web 2.0 applications as alternative environments for informal learning—a critical review*. Paper presented at the CERI-KERIS International Expert Meeting on ICT and Educational Performance, Cheju Island, South Korea. Retrieved March 2, 2008, from http://www.oecd.org/dataoecd/32/3/39458556.pdf

Selwyn, N. (Ed.). (2008). *Education 2.0? Designing the web for teaching and learning*. London: Teaching and Learning Research Programme, Institute of Education, University of London. Retrieved January 12, 2009, from http://www.tlrp.org/tel/files/2008/11/tel_comm_final.pdf

Siemens, G. (2008, May 21). A seismic shift in epistemology [Web log post]. *elearnspace*. Retrieved January, 9, 2009, from http://www.elearnspace.org/blog/2008/05/21/a-seismic-shift-in-epistemology/

Thompson, J. (2007). Is Education 1.0 ready for Web 2.0 students? *Innovate: Journal of Online Education, 3*(4). Retrieved February 11, 2008, from http://www.innovateonline.info/index.php?view=article&id=393

Toulmin, S. E. (1990). *Cosmopolis: The hidden agenda of modernity*. New York: Free Press.

Ugoretz, J. (2006, June 9). Three stars and a chili pepper: Social software, folksonomy, and user reviews in the college context. *Academic Commons*. Retrieved January 12, 2009, from http://www.academiccommons.org/commons/essay/Ugoretz-social-software-folksonomy

Weinberger, D. (2006). *The new shape of knowledge: From trees to piles of leaves* [Webcast]. Retrieved January 16, 2009, from http://webcast.oii.ox.ac.uk/?view=Webcast&ID=20051130_109

Welch, D. J. (2008) Virtual worlds: Moving beyond today. *EDUCAUSE Review, 43*(5), 12–13. Retrieved January 16, 2009, from http://www.educause.edu/ir/library/pdf/ERM0858.pdf

Wenger, E. (1998). *Communities of practice: Learning, meaning, and identity*. Cambridge, MA: Cambridge University Press.

Wertsch, J. V. (1998). *Mind as action*. New York: Oxford University Press.

KEY TERMS AND DEFINITIONS

Acculturation: An approach to learning in which the focus is not content *per se* but on framing students as newcomers to a community of practice (CoP) and setting them on effective trajectories of participation to enable them to become fully familiar with the culture, discourse, knowledge, worldviews, dispositions, and practices of that community.

Discourse Community: This term is used interchangeably with "communities of practice" and "networks of practice" to refer to the same broad phenomenon, namely, an assemblage of people who, having a common focus, institutionalize a particular communicative structure (culture, language, and practices), conventions, power arrangements, institutional hierarchies, and vested interests.

Epistemology: The field of study concerned with the nature, origin/sources, and validity of knowledge.

Social Epistemology: Also known as "social constructionism" or "non-foundational epistemology." Refers to a distinctly sociological rather than a psychological or empirical understanding of knowledge and ways of knowing. Its central tenet is that the interests, values, and power-knowledge arrangements of the social (or discourse) communities to which we belong shape our conceptions of reality and its social formation.

Modernism: For the purposes of this chapter, "modernism" and its variants are used as a shorthand term to refer to ideas and practices associated with Industrial Age scientific thinking and conventional educational practices predominantly informed by psychological theories of learning.

Postmodernism: For the purpose of this chapter, the term "postmodern" is used to describe ideas and practices that adopt a more deconstructive and open stance toward modernist certainties. Postmodernism stresses the fragmentary and fragile nature of social reality and therefore rejects grand narratives, objective accounts of reality, and notions of universal truths and progress. Its use here conveys a radical questioning of traditional educational certainties, views, and practices in line with a very different set of intellectual priorities and theoretical preoccupations.

Web 2.0+: Web 2.0 is a generic term popularly used to describe a broad suite of web-based applications and services that, designed on ideals of participation, enable individuals anywhere to easily form rich and decentralized social networks based on common interests and to collaboratively create, distribute, share and recreate content from multiple sources, leveraging their collective intelligence or "wisdom of crowds." In this chapter, the term "Web 2.0+" is used; the plus sign (+) implies that the Web will continue to evolve with future iterations that will further consolidate and extend this participatory paradigm (see also Eijkman, in press).

Chapter 19
Web 2.0 and Professional Development of Academic Staff

Belinda Tynan
University of New England, Australia

Cameron Barnes
University of New England, Australia

ABSTRACT

This chapter argues that the latest wave of Web 2.0 technologies has the potential to transform online learning. To realize this potential, universities must rethink the way in which they develop academic skills in online teaching. The current emphasis on training academics to teach online using learning material and learning management systems has yielded mixed results. Too much of the focus has been on "top-down" models of change. Web 2.0 technologies favor "bottom-up" approaches to staff development, approaches that leverage the power, ease of use, and flexibility of Web 2.0 technologies. These have a better chance to produce the constructivist, student-centered online learning that is now widely regarded as the ideal. The authors use fictional accounts in order to capture some of the issues involved.

INTRODUCTION

This chapter examines the implications of Web 2.0 technologies for academic staff development. It argues that the cheapness, ease of use, and speed with which Web 2.0 tools can be deployed empowers academics as well as students. These new technologies provide university teaching staff with alternatives to "shovelware" (Morrison & Anglin, 2006) approaches to online learning. Web 2.0 technologies call for new models of staff development and training—approaches that suit decentralized, collaborative learning within academic communities of practice. As in a previous discussion (Barnes & Tynan, 2007), the authors of the present chapter draw upon fictional accounts and characters in order to capture some of the issues involved.

THE CONCEPT OF WEB 2.0

Web 2.0 has received tremendous attention since 2005. As the origins and history of the Web 2.0

DOI: 10.4018/978-1-60566-294-7.ch019

concept have been discussed in other chapters, there is no need to repeat this material here. Following O'Reilly (2005), Anderson asserts that Web 2.0 "has, at its heart, a set of at least six powerful ideas" (2007, p. 2). These are:

- Individual production and user-generated content;
- Harnessing the power of the crowd;
- Data on an epic scale;
- Architecture of participation;
- Network effects;
- Openness.

As will be discussed later in this chapter, these ideas are crucial for universities. They provide an alternative to current approaches to online learning that depend on "one-size-fits-all" models.

LIVING AND TEACHING IN A CONNECTED WORLD

Today, we live in a connected world. Nothing demonstrates this more forcefully than the increasing flood of mobile phones. There are over 3.3 billion mobile phone subscriptions worldwide ("Mobile phone users reach 3.3bn," 2008). This is almost three times the number of fixed landline phones (1.3 billion). More than 2 billion people send or receive SMS messages, and at an astonishing rate—for example, the Gartner group predicted that over 2.3 trillion SMS messages would be sent in 2008 (Gartner, Inc., 2007). In addition, over 825 million mobile phone subscribers across the globe use their mobiles to connect to the Internet (Ahonen, 2008). Accessing online content—movies, video clips, music, and podcasts—has driven an explosive demand in mobile devices. According to market research company iSuppli, 163 million MP3 players and other personal media devices were sold worldwide in 2007 (cellular-news, 2007).

Along with the increase in the number of mobile devices, there has been a rapid growth in personal computer (PC) ownership. In countries such as Australia and the United States, PC ownership is reaching saturation point. According to Ahonen (2008), at some time in 2008, the number of PCs on desktops around the world would exceed the 1 billion mark. Partly as a result of the growing ubiquity of PCs, the global total of Internet users has reached a staggering 1.4 billion (Miniwatts Marketing Group, 2008). Although ownership is concentrated in the developed world, falling unit costs and cheaper telecommunications are expected to result in an explosion in third-world computer ownership over the next few decades.

Even more remarkable than the spread of modern communications has been the rapid growth of Web 2.0 applications. MySpace (http://www.myspace.com/), one of the two largest social networking sites on the Web, is an example of social computing on an unprecedented scale. In early 2008, the number of active users on MySpace allegedly was in excess of 110 million. The MySpace community reads billions of pages every day—as many as 4.5 billion MySpace pages over a single 24-hour period in January 2008, for instance. More than 300,000 new users join MySpace daily. Every day, 8 million new images are added and 60,000 fresh videos are uploaded to the site (Owyang, 2008).

Despite this activity, MySpace is not alone. Archrival Facebook (http://www.facebook.com/) advertised that it had 60 million active users and 6 million active user groups in early 2008 (Owyang, 2008). MySpace and Facebook are only part of the picture. There is also a very long tail. Outside the U.S., other social networking sites claim significant market shares. These challengers include Badoo, Orkut, Friendster, Bahu, Hi5, Faceparty, and Habbo, to name but a few. Collectively, the second- and third-tier Web 2.0 platforms add up to a significant online presence.

Blogs are another area in which growth seems to have been breathtaking. The Technorati (http://www.technorati.com/) site tracks traffic at 112.8 million blogs (and counts 250 million pieces of tagged social media). In April 2007, the creation of new blogs was running at 120,000 new blogs a day. At this point, there were 1.5 million blog posts each day: 17 every second (Sifry, 2007). Today's figures are almost certainly much higher. For most of 2007, the number of blogs was doubling every six months.

There is an element of "hype" in many of these statistics. The owners of sites such as MySpace and Facebook have every reason to include inactive accounts in their totals. It has been observed that "only a fraction of registered users ever go back. And only a fraction of them use the site on any kind of regular basis" (Glaser, 2007, "The rise of MySpace and Facebook," para. 3). If site owners exaggerate the size of their user base, this makes the raw statistics even more impressive. Every day, Facebook users view over 3 billion images on the site, and upload an additional 14 million new ones (Beaver, 2007; Owyang, 2008). YouTube's figures indicate that in December 2007 alone, 77.6 million viewers in the U.S. watched 3.2 billion online videos (41.6 videos per viewer), almost a third of the 10 billion online videos watched by Americans in the same month (comScore, 2008).

Web 2.0 technologies such as wikis, RSS syndication, and tag-based folksonomies have resulted in a fundamental shift in the way the Web is used. For most of its short history, the Web worked on a delivery model—content creators were a small minority. The majority of users were passive consumers of content. Like the printing press, radio, or television before it, the Web seemed significant primarily in that it represented a cheaper and faster way of disseminating content. With Web 2.0, the Web has moved to another model: one that could theoretically support universal or near-universal participation. In a Web 2.0 world, all users can simultaneously be content creators, even if in practice it is doubtful that all would wish to do so (Anderson, 2007).

Tools allowing online social networking and user-generated content have existed for more than two decades. Long before blogs and wikis, there were email lists, Usenet newsgroups, Internet chat, and bulletin boards. The WELL, possibly the oldest online community still in existence, was created as long ago as 1985. The first virtual worlds were text based and have a history stretching far back into the distant past of the Internet. The earliest game worlds were developed in the 1970s. (See Chapter 1 in this book for a more detailed discussion of the history and evolution of social software.)

The older generation of technologies never achieved the popularity of successful Web 2.0 applications. In 1993 there were 45,000 bulletin board systems (BBSs) in the United States. The total number of BBS subscribers was only 12 million. Even The WELL had no more than 6,600 members. Usenet had a mere 2 million subscribers (Sproll & Faraj, 1993).

What happened? The difference is the latest tools are free, almost ridiculously easy to use, and designed with flexibility and interoperability in mind (Kamel Boulos, Maramba, & Wheeler, 2006; Parker & Chao, 2007). If they are not quite yet "transparent technologies" (as is the case with the fixed line telephone or the ballpoint pen), they are not far from this point. If this characterization seems extreme, consider the change from the command-line interfaces of the 1980s to today's widget-driven Web 2.0 world. Any blogger capable of cutting and pasting a few lines of code can install one of hundreds of "widgets" (small, portable applications) within minutes. Widgets have been used to customize blogs, wikis, personal spaces, and other web pages, providing services (such as news feeds), games, new products, and tools, including online chat (Stroud, 2008).

Although academics are among the most "wired" people in the world in terms of their access to the Internet (Allport, 2001), they are less "wired" than many of their students in the popular sense of the term. With few exceptions, teaching staff and the latest cohort of undergraduates live in different technological worlds (Barnes & Tynan, 2007; see also Chapter 16). Academic staff speak of "keeping up." Occasionally, they wonder aloud whether it is worth the effort to engage with current trends. For many students, the question simply does not arise. They have already made the leap.

Terence Littleton, a lecturer in 18th-century literature and fan of the Rolling Stones, slid behind the wheel and slipped a bootleg CD into the player. Sixties rock filled the sedan as he drove towards the motorway. In the distance, the glass and brick towers of the University flamed with the rising sun. He didn't like Mondays. This Monday was no exception. His first appointment was with an educational developer from the Learning Center. Not his idea. The hints from his Department Head had been gentle at first. When Terence hadn't responded, pointed reference was made to the promotions round. Well, he had outlasted deconstruction, so he'd probably survive constructivism. Hmm, that was good. He'd save that one...

ISSUES, CONTROVERSIES, PROBLEMS

No university in Australia is without a learning management system (LMS) or virtual learning environment (VLE) of some kind. These systems are widely regarded by university decision-makers as the preferred solution to the task of taking universities from traditional forms of teaching to the web-based environment. For a number of years, most universities have favored commercial solutions. The most popular have been established products such as WebCT and Blackboard. However, open source solutions (including Sakai and Moodle) are now emerging as alternatives to proprietary software. The growing impact of Web 2.0 technologies has also led to changes in the feature set of proprietary and open source solutions alike. Tools such as wikis and blogs now supplement more familiar tools like discussion boards/forums and chat applications.

The question arises as to how successful the LMS-based approach has been. The Web has long been hyped as the "magic bullet" that will finally result in the realization of social constructivist approaches to university teaching (Chickering & Ehrmann, 1996; Conole, 2004; Holt & Challis, 2007). The literature provides numerous "war stories" about engagement and change processes (Goodyear & Jones, 2003; Weaver, Spratt, & Nair, 2008). There are also tales of transformative experiences in which individual academics energetically grasp the potential of new forms of teaching (Hannon, 2008).

For all this debate, and despite the funding that has been pumped into the development of web-based learning systems, the results have frequently been disappointing in constructivist terms (Pratt, 2005; Salmon, 2005; Jones & Muldoon, 2007). Critics have described many LMS-based course materials as "shovelware" (Morrison & Anglin, 2006). Reporting on a study of the relations between educational developers and their clients at an unnamed Australian university, Hannon (2008) refers to the common themes arising from his research, which

were related to the low uptake of online learning among teaching staff: the time required to train in the learning management system and to set up an online course, poor pedagogy associated with online teaching, and the limitations with the functionality of online learning systems. (p. 23)

These problems are not confined to a single Australian university, and are perhaps generalizable to many institutions elsewhere in the developed world (Heaton-Shrestha, Edirisingha, Burke, & Linsey, 2005; Pratt, 2005; Salmon, 2005; Benson & Palaskas, 2006; Wise & Quealy, 2006; Jones & Muldoon, 2007).

Susan Hill, the educational developer, was friendlier than Terence had expected. He was not, however, inclined to give an inch. She asked him about his teaching approach. Terence replied that he felt the same way about teaching as his students did about learning. They disliked the latter almost as much as he detested the former. When Susan raised the issue of new technologies, Terence bristled. These, he said, meant endless emails, long hours wasted wrestling with technology, and no time to do the things that mattered. If only she knew how many times he'd answered the same emails on Tristram Shandy ... As this point, Susan broke in. How would he like to reduce the number of emails he received?

By and large, the new pedagogies remain marginal to the way most universities actually work. The installation of an institutional LMS tends not to transform institutional pedagogies, although counter examples exist (Steel & Hudson, 2001; Heaton-Shrestha et al., 2005). As Kirkup and Kirkwood (2005) observe, "teaching staff appropriate those technologies which they can incorporate into their teaching activity most easily, that offer affordances for what they already do, rather than those which radically change teaching and learning practices" (p. 188). Jamieson (2004) asserts that part of the reason for this conservatism is the extent to which teaching modes in higher education are shaped by convention. University teachers have "traditionally progressed from the experience of learning in the classroom to teaching in the classroom" (p. 22).

An important issue is the manner in which institutional imperatives have driven professional development. Primary responsibility for professional development usually falls onto small, centralized units within universities (Bird, 2004; Holt & Challis, 2007; Weaver et al., 2008; O'Connell, Benson, & Samarawickrema, 2006). The mission of such units is often defined by their institutional strategic plans. Academic development activities are therefore often target driven. Organizational pressures, such as the need to meet project timelines, trump pedagogic considerations (Wozniak, Scott, & Atkinson, 2005; Coates, James, & Baldwin, 2005). One example is the extent to which professional development activities are often structured around the release of a new LMS. Another is the immense amount of effort expended on exemplar online courses, which all too often later wither away in the absence of continued support (Hannon, 2008). As a result, there is a wide discrepancy between best practice in online teaching and what is actually achieved across institutions, according to Hannon. Not surprisingly, he warns of "incongruencies in educational development practice" (p. 27).

Academic staff use online environments in a variety of ways, many of which are only weakly underpinned by sound and effective pedagogical and instructional goals (Heaton-Shrestha et al., 2005; Jones & Muldoon, 2007). As Ryan (1998) pointed out over a decade ago:

Clicking icons no more of itself stimulates learning than entering a library. Learning depends on the motivation of students and the nature of materials they engage with. Many current online materials are simply static pages with a few hypertext links and a constrained pathway through the text. (p. 18, emphasis in original)

The situation has hardly changed in 10 years. In many universities, the move to online learning has largely consisted of putting existing unit materials on the Web. Converting course notes into Adobe Acrobat (PDF) format or HTML has become a goal in itself. Such an approach is firmly behaviorist. Constructivist goals have been lost in the drive to reduce costs or to achieve ill-considered institutional goalposts. In a recent case study, Weaver et al. (2008) observe that:

if the way in which the majority of WebCT sites are perceived by students ... is any indication, this objective is not being achieved. Students demand more than a repository dump—they want and need active and enthusiastic engagement from their teachers. Our results indicate that, due to a perceived lack of institutional support and adequate resourcing, many staff are forced to adopt a teacher centred approach in their online teaching. (p. 39)

As Conole (2004) warns, if we see a LMS simply as a content repository, we are missing the point. Teacher-centered practices not only continue, but are actually encouraged as support for well-designed print materials drops off in the rush to go online (McLoughlin & Visser 2003; Oliver, 2003; Oliver, 2005).

In Web 2.0 terms, recent trends appear startlingly old fashioned. University managements insist that academic staff create their online learning materials using tools (like proprietary learning material systems) that are already obsolete. Institutions persist in constructing silos at the very moment that silos have gone out of fashion. And for what benefit? Existing methods of web-based teaching are unlikely to suit users who already enjoy total freedom over how they engage with others online. For what purpose do we invest in discussion boards and online chat rooms, when the latest generation of students has already moved on? With these points in mind, it is probably time to consider the concept of Web 2.0 and what it might mean for academic teaching and staff development.

Before Terence could reply, Susan took out two lapel microphones. She slipped one onto her coat. The other she attached to Terence's battered tweed jacket. Out came her wireless laptop. After a second or two, she began firing questions. In spite of himself, Terence found himself answering them. She had done her homework, and the questions were the ones that students typically asked. A dozen answers later, Susan detached the microphone and motioned Terence to do the same. As he fumbled with his lapel, Susan steered the cursor expertly over her screen. A few clicks later, she announced that the audio file had been loaded into the electronic reserve for his unit. It was now available for any student who wanted to listen.

ENGAGING WITH STUDENTS

In addition, universities need to start listening to their students. Sharpe, Benfield, Lessner, and DeCicco (2005) have noted the general scarcity of studies that foreground the user experience. In particular, when conducting their research, they were disappointed by the absence of published studies in which the learner's voice is central. Recent work by Creanor, Trinder, Gowan, and Howells (2006) and Conole, de Laat, Dillon, and Darby (2006) go some way in part to address this. But it is surprising that it has taken so long for the learner experience to reach center stage. This point is all the more crucial if universities are to come to terms with the world of Web 2.0 technologies, which the latest generation of undergraduates have made particularly their own.

Terence didn't believe her. However, when he went to his unit reserve, the file was there. As it played, he had to agree, it would do. Much better than many of his bootlegs of ancient Stones concerts! Susan decided on a little flattery: He spoke well, she pointed out. She was sure that his students would enjoy being able to download audio files of his lectures. They could listen and relisten until they understood. She could show him how to record his next lecture. Was he aware of the audio series on English novelists from South Africa? She seemed to remember that there was one on Laurence Sterne. A Canadian university had one on Tristram Shandy, and another institution from New Zealand had a lecture on comic writing from the 18th century. If he liked, they could add links to each of these external resources to his unit reserve this morning.

MOVING TOWARD WEB 2.0

As mentioned earlier, Anderson (2007) identified six main ideas that feature prominently within Web 2.0. These are individual production and user-generated content, harnessing the power of the crowd, data on an epic scale, architecture of participation, network effects, and openness. Anderson's six main ideas provide us with clear guidance as to how we might move forward.

Individual Production and User-Generated Content

The proprietary learning material systems that are now employed in most universities have largely served their purpose. In a Web 2.0 world, it is anachronistic to expect that academic staff need to be able write HTML (or depend on the services of those who have this skill) in order to create online learning materials. The latest generation of website creation tools such as Google Page Creator (http://pages.google.com/), SynthaSite (http://www.synthasite.com/), and Jimdo (http://www.jimdo.com/) show that it is possible to build systems that allow anyone to create attractive, functional web pages in minutes. The task for universities is either to duplicate these systems at an institutional level, or to steer their academic staff towards free tools (such as SynthaSite) that allow their users to create pages and download them to local servers for secure hosting.

There is also a need to steer academic staff towards the range of Web 2.0 tools that can simplify the task of producing new forms of teaching materials. Sites such as SlideShare (http://www.slideshare.net/) simplify the sharing of lecture slides and audio, while others like Gcast (http://www.gcast.com/) make it possible for individuals to create podcasts without the intervention of sound technicians, or even without the use of computer. With Gcast, for example, users can simply phone in their podcasts. Embedding the Gcast player in a web page is just a matter of copying and pasting a few lines of HTML.

No less important is the potential of such sites for more active, student-centered approaches to learning. There is a growing body of research literature that clearly demonstrates that active engagement in online learning environments is effective and highly desired by students (Creanor et al., 2006; Weaver et al., 2008). Ramsden (2003) has long discussed and promoted student-cantered approaches to learning. Even delivering traditional lectures as digital audio opens up a range of new strategies for stimulating learning. We have known for considerable time that audio can enhance motivation and engagement (Durbridge, 1984). Learner control has a huge role to play and is consistent with the intentions behind Web 2.0 technologies (Dron, 2007). Students can replay such lectures as many times as they like, and when and where they choose. If they are uncertain at any point, they can pause and rerun the recording. There is good evidence that students benefit from such podcast lectures (Tynan & Colbran, 2006; Lee & Chan, 2007). More importantly, access to tools such as Gcast means that students can edit recordings, add their comments, and send the remixed materials on to other students. The ease of use inherent in Web 2.0 tools means that academic staff can explore forms of teaching that would be inconceivable even a few years ago. This clearly stands in stark contrast with current approaches, in which teaching staff and students alike are forced to master unfriendly, proprietary interfaces before online learning can begin.

Terence was almost convinced. Then he remembered the last time he had attempted to add some materials to the University's LMS. "That's all very well," he heard himself say, "but that means knowing how to write in that web gobbledygook. I can't." Susan was ready for this. "But, you don't," came the reply. Susan explained what he could do using the right tools. He could post his PowerPoints using SlideShare. SlideShare would also allow him to produce a Sharecast, which combined an audio file with a PowerPoint presentation. If he liked, he could use Gcast to create podcasts, and YouTube or Google Video to post video clips. He could collect links to full-text journal articles using delicious or any one of a number of similar social bookmarking applications. She could send him the URLs. These tools would create web addresses that he could just copy and paste into the unit reserve. What's more, if he uploaded his lectures, millions of people around the world could listen to him. He could explain to them exactly why Tristram Shandy was such a great novel. In the process, he could refer people to the book he published a while back, and to his articles (she understood that he had written quite a few!). In fact, she could show him how to gather all his articles together in electronic form and make them available from a single page. Terence was not quite certain. It also seemed so dazzlingly easy. "Show me," he said.

The Power of the Crowd

Anderson's second idea is equally critical. Web 2.0 technologies and techniques such as social bookmarking, tagging, and folksonomies have changed the way knowledge is sought out, organized, and evaluated. Tools such as delicious not only make it easier for academic staff to provide students with the digital equivalent of a list of readings, they also open up new avenues for students to build and share their own collections of citations, references, and full-text materials. These technologies hold out the promise of truly collaborative forms of learning.

Data on an Epic Scale

Anderson's third big idea relates to data on an epic scale. Wikipedia (http://en.wikipedia.org/) provides the perfect illustration of this point. In December 2007, a notice on the Wikipedia site proclaimed that the online encyclopedia included 9.25 million articles in 253 languages, totaling 1.74 billion words. It is almost certainly the largest single encyclopedia created in modern times. For certain tasks, Wikipedia has become the first choice for finding information. Even academic librarians have begun to rely upon it as a ready reference tool. The most astonishing thing about Wikipedia is its open nature: there are no subscription fees and it has been written entirely by a worldwide network of volunteers. In the majority of cases, anyone who is prepared to register as a contributor can write and edit articles.

Experiments have already been undertaken at universities around the world with the use of Wikipedia as a teaching tool. From the University of Tartu in Estonia to the University of Virginia in the USA, students are typically asked to improve existing Wikipedia articles or write new ones. An example is the successful experiment conducted at the University of East Anglia in 2007. Master's students in an international politics program were asked to edit and write Wikipedia articles on Middle Eastern affairs (Birke, 2007). Even more ambitious was a project at the University of New South Wales, Australia, in which students were set the task of filling in gaps and correcting errors in around 150 Wikipedia articles in immunology and related topics (Moses, 2007). The result is a virtuous circle, in which students learn firsthand how knowledge is created, develop research skills, and improve the quality of Wikipedia at the same time. The prospect of truly utopian projects in the collective creation of reference materials and even textbooks is astounding.

Architecture of Participation

Anderson's fourth idea refers to the architecture of participation. Anderson describes one aspect of this idea in the following terms:

the architecture of participation occurs when, through normal use of an application or service, the service itself gets better. To the user, this appears to be a side effect of using the service, but in fact, the system has been designed to take the user interactions and utilise them to improve itself ... (2007, p. 19).

Wikipedia provides an example of this principle, but it can also be applied to university teaching. The latest generation of Web 2.0 tools offers academics the opportunity to hand over part of the responsibility for building teaching materials to their students. Tagging, social bookmarking, and other collaboration and sharing technologies mean that students can contribute to the creation of electronic reserves, readings lists, and assignment guides.

Network Effects

The second-to-last big idea relates to network effects. Anderson explains the network effect thus:

The Network Effect is a general economic term used to describe the increase in value to the existing users of a service in which there is some form of interaction with others, as more and more people start to use it. (2007, p. 20)

The implications for university teaching in a Web 2.0 world are clear. In most LMS systems, social tools are limited to the course or unit level. They operate to facilitate communication among individuals enrolled in the same subject. Why not open up these tools to permit social interactivity between students across the institution? Anderson further argues that

Educationalists should bear this in mind when reviewing new or proposed Web 2.0 services and their potential role in educational settings. As one lecturer recently found out, it is easier to join with the herd and discuss this week's coursework online within Facebook (a popular social networking site) than to try and get the students to move across to the institutional VLE. (2007, p. 21)

Anderson may be wrong here—it is far from clear that most students would relish the intrusion of academics into their social spaces (see Chapters 3 and 15 in this book).

Openness

Hannon (2008) notes that earlier "innovative approaches to learning technologies were constrained by a technology centred repertoire which framed a nexus between learning technologies and institutional strategy" (p. 27). Institutional strategies are important; however, we need to disconnect such strategies from a reliance on proprietary systems and specific platforms. Such approaches are at variance with Web 2.0 principles, which represent the new rules of the game.

WHO IS MANAGING THE LEARNING?

At present, the answer to the above question is ambiguous. Universities have built learning materials systems, but (in practice) no one is in control. At the level of the individual unit or course, academics are using LMSs in many different ways. Some of these are excellent, but, as discussed earlier, others tend merely to reproduce traditional, behaviorist forms of university teaching.

Perhaps the time has come to transfer management of the learning to academics and students, to take it out of the hands of the LMS managers or administrators. In truth, they probably will not miss what they never had. The growing range of Web 2.0 tools mean that most universities can probably well do without the expensive, "one-size-fits-all" proprietary systems that have been the focus of so much effort and expenditure. This is not tantamount to saying that universities should leave everything to individual initiative—they still need to provide an infrastructure for web-based teaching, but this infrastructure can be cut down, more open, and more flexible.

Most importantly of all, universities need to leverage the speed and user friendliness of Web 2.0 tools. Past experience has shown that one of the greatest disincentives to the uptake and use of LMS systems by academics has been the adverse impact on staff workloads (Heaton-Shrestha et al., 2005). It would be nice to think that the new technologies would sell themselves, but this is perhaps too optimistic. Facilitating a switch to Web 2.0-based teaching and learning involves a major change management exercise. It means undoing many of the mistakes of the past. The first place to start is for professional development units to begin to acquaint themselves with the new technologies, and the possibilities and pitfalls they present. Before they can assist others, they need to assist themselves.

If university managers want improvements in online teaching, they must be prepared to pay for it. This means greater investment in pedagogy rather than technology *per se*. As Kim and Bonk (2006) have found, teachers of online environments feel that "monetary support for and pedagogical competency of online instructors would most significantly affect the success of their online programs" (p. 25). Kim and Bonk also found that:

pedagogical skill was deemed more important than technological skill for effective online teaching. With regard to the needs for pedagogical competency of online instructors, a majority of the respondents expected that online instructors would typically have received some sort of training in online teaching either internally or externally by the year 2010. (p. 25)

One of the most important incentives for academics to make greater use of online learning is the example of their peers. More attention needs to be given to the support of "innovators" and "early adopters" at the level of the school or department. Such individuals need to be formally acknowledged by their institutions, and rewarded in tangible ways for their contributions. These might take the form of awards, time relief, promotion, or additional support. The crucial point is that idealism and enthusiasm can carry innovators only so far.

Moreover, universities need to move away from centralized approaches to staff development. At some institutions, such as Kingston University in the UK, "technology champions" have been useful. These are specialist staff seconded to the Faculties and tasked with providing informal support to academics (Heaton-Shrestha et al., 2005). "Grassroots" rather than "top-down" approaches to change management are what are required.

Students are another group that requires a hearing. We must continue to investigate how learners engage with technologies. This task, as discussed earlier, is well overdue (Conole & Creanor, 2007). The question of how learners actually engage with learning and with their teachers and peers in web-based environments has yet to be fully explored.

Back in her office elsewhere in the Faculty, Susan put on a cup of tea. Terence had been nowhere as difficult as she had feared, despite the Head's warnings. If he became a champion of new technologies in his Department, he could make a difference. His experience as a Rolling Stones bootlegger made him something of an audio technician. This would help in so many ways. She'd been lucky that a friend had mentioned his hobby on the weekend. But, would his enthusiasm stick? Could he be persuaded to adopt more active learning approaches? She could regard today's encounter as a small victory, but would it last? The electric kettle began to bubble, signaling its impatience. Well, one down ...

CONCLUSION

The focus in this chapter has been on the implications of Web 2.0 technologies for capacity building in academic development. There is much evidence that academic staff are not engaging adequately with new technologies for teaching and learning. Their professional development needs are being neglected. Furthermore, current programs and initiatives are failing to sufficiently address the issue of academic workloads. It is time to change direction. The advent of Web 2.0 provides academic staff with a new generation of easy-to-use, swift, and powerful tools. Unlooked for, and unasked for, they may well be exactly what academics need. The task for university decision makers and staff development units is to see that these tools get into academic hands, along with appropriate types and levels of training, development, and support.

REFERENCES

Ahonen, T. T. (2008). When there is a mobile phone for half the planet: Understanding the biggest technology [Web log post]. *Communities Dominate Brands*. Retrieved February 12, 2008, from http://communities-dominate.blogs.com/brands/2008/01/when-there-is-a.html

Allport, C. (2001). Educating and organizing globally: Perspectives on the Internet and higher education. *Australian Universities Review, 44*(1/2), 21–27.

Anderson, P. (2007). *What is Web 2.0? Ideas, technologies and implications for education*. Bristol, UK: Joint Information Systems Committee. Retrieved February 12, 2008, from http://www.jisc.ac.uk/media/documents/techwatch/tsw0701b.pdf

Barnes, C., & Tynan, B. (2007). The adventures of Miranda in the brave new world: Learning in a Web 2.0 millennium. *ALT-J Research in Learning Technology*, *15*(3), 189–200.

Beaver, D. (2007). Facebook photos infrastructure [Web log post]. *The Facebook Blog*. Retrieved February 19, 2008, from http://blog.facebook.com/blog.php?post=2406207130

Benson, R., & Palaskas, T. (2006). Introducing a new learning management system: An institutional case study. *Australasian Journal of Educational Technology, 22*(4), 548–567. Retrieved February 19, 2008, from http://www.ascilite.org.au/ajet/ajet22/benson.html

Bird, J. (2004). Professional navel gazing: Flexible learning professionals into the future. In R. Atkinson, C. McBeath, D. Jonas-Dwyer, & R. Phillips (Eds.), *Beyond the comfort zone: Proceedings of the 21st Australasian Society for Computers in Learning in Tertiary Education (ASCILITE) Conference* (pp. 123–133). Perth, Australia: The University of Western Australia. Retrieved February 12, 2008, from http://www.ascilite.org.au/conferences/perth04/procs/bird.html

Birke, S. (2007, March 19). Off to wik we go. *The Times*, 2. cellular-news. (2007, October 31). *New applications boost small/medium display market*. Retrieved February 12, 2008, from http://www.cellular-news.com/story/27086.php

Chickering, A. W., & Ehrmann, S. C. (1996). Implementing the seven principles: Technology as lever. *AAHE Bulletin, 49*(2), 3–6. Retrieved June 22, 2008, from http://www.tltgroup.org/programs/seven.html

Coates, H., James, R., & Baldwin, G. (2005). A critical examination of the effects of learning management systems on university teaching and learning. *Tertiary Education and Management, 11*(1), 19–36.

comScore. (2008, February 8). *U.S. Internet users viewed 10 billion videos online in record-breaking month of December, according to comScore video matrix*. Retrieved February 22, 2008, from http://www.comscore.com/press/release.asp?press=2051

Conole, G. (2004). E-learning: The hype and the reality. *Journal of Interactive Media in Education*. Retrieved February 22, 2008, from http://www-jime.open.ac.uk/2004/12/conole-2004-12.pdf

Conole, G., & Creanor, L. (2007). *In their own words: Exploring the learner's perspective on e-learning*. Bristol, UK: Joint Information Systems Committee. Retrieved December 6, 2008, from http://www.jisc.ac.uk/media/documents/programmes/elearningpedagogy/iowfinal.pdf

Conole, G., de Laat, M., Dillon, T., & Darby, J. (2006). *JISC LXP: Student experiences of technologies. Final report.* Bristol, UK: Joint Information Systems Committee. Retrieved July 17, 2008, from http://www.jisc.ac.uk/media/documents/programmes/elearningpedagogy/lxp-projectfinalreportdec06.pdf

Creanor, L., Trinder, K., Gowan, D., & Howells, C. (2006). *LEX: The Learner Experience of e-Learning—Final project report*. Bristol, UK: Joint Information Systems Committee. Retrieved February 22, 2008, from http://www.jisc.ac.uk/uploaded_documents/LEX%20Final%20Report_August06.pdf

Dron, J. (2007). *Control and constraint in e-learning: Choosing when to choose*. Hershey, PA: Information Science Reference.

Durbridge, N. (1984). Media in course design, No. 9, audio cassettes. In Bates, A. W. (Ed.), *The role of technology in distance education*. Kent, UK: Croom Helm.

Gartner, Inc. (2007, December 17). *Gartner says mobile messages to surpass 2 trillion messages in major markets in 2008*. Retrieved February 12, 2008, from http://www.gartner.com/it/page.jsp?id=565124

Glaser, M. (2007, August 29). Your guide to social networking online. *Media Shift*. Retrieved June 16, 2008, from http://www.pbs.org/mediashift/2007/08/your-guide-to-social-networking-online241.html

Goodyear, P., & Jones, C. (2003). Implicit theories of learning and change: Their role in the development of e-learning environments in higher education. In Naidu, S. (Ed.), *Learning and teaching with technology: Principles and practice* (pp. 29–42). London: Routledge.

Hannon, J. (2008). Doing staff development: Practices, dilemmas and technologies. *Australasian Journal of Educational Technology, 24*(1), 15–29. Retrieved July 17, 2008, from http://www.ascilite.org.au/ajet/ajet24/hannon.pdf

Heaton-Shrestha, C., Edirisingha, P., Burke, L., & Linsey, T. (2005). Introducing a VLE into campus-based undergraduate teaching: Staff perspectives on its impact on teaching. *International Journal of Educational Research, 43*(6), 370–386. doi:10.1016/j.ijer.2006.07.001

Holt, D., & Challis, D. (2007). From policy to practice: One university's experience of implementing strategic change through wholly online teaching and learning. *Australasian Journal of Educational Technology, 23*(1), 110–131. Retrieved July 17, 2008, from http://www.ascilite.org.au/ajet/ajet23/holt.html

Jamieson, P. (2004). The university as workplace: Preparing lecturers to teach in online environments. *Quarterly Review of Distance Education, 5*(1), 21–27.

Jones, D., & Muldoon, N. (2007). The teleological reason why ICTs limit choice for university learners and learning. In R. Atkinson & C. McBeath (Eds.), *ICT: Providing choices for learners and learning. Proceedings of the 24th Australasian Society for Computers in Learning in Tertiary Education (ASCILITE) Conference* (pp. 450–459). Singapore: Nanyang Technological University. Retrieved June 22, 2008, from http://www.ascilite.org.au/conferences/singapore07/procs/jones-d.pdf

Kamel Boulos, M. N., Maramba, I., & Wheeler, S. (2006). Wikis, blogs and podcasts: A new generation of web-based tools for virtual collaborative clinical practice and education. *BMC Medical Education, 6*(41). Retrieved June 22, 2008, from http://www.biomedcentral.com/1472-6920/6/41

Kim, K. J., & Bonk, C. J. (2006). The future of online teaching and learning in higher education: The survey says.... *EDUCAUSE Quarterly, 29*(4), 22–30. Retrieved June 22, 2008, from http://www.educause.edu/ir/library/pdf/EQM0644.pdf

Kirkup, G., & Kirkwood, A. (2005). Information and communications technologies (ICT) in higher education teaching—a tale of gradualism rather than revolution. *Learning, Media and Technology, 30*(2), 185–199. doi:10.1080/17439880500093810

Lee, M. J. W., & Chan, A. (2007). Reducing the effects of isolation and promoting inclusivity for distance learners through podcasting. *Turkish Online Journal of Distance Education, 8*(1), 85–104. Retrieved February 22, 2008, from http://tojde.anadolu.edu.tr/tojde25/pdf/article_7.pdf

McLoughlin, C., & Visser, T. (2003). Quality e-learning: Are there universal indicators? In C. McLoughlin, P. LeCornu, & W. Jackson (Eds.), *Sustaining quality learning environments: Proceedings of the 16th Open and Distance Learning Association of Australia (ODLAA) Biennial Conference*. Canberra, Australia: Canberra Institute of Technology.

Miniwatts Marketing Group. (2008, July 1). *World Internet usage*. Retrieved July 17, 2008, from http://www.internetworldstats.com/stats.htm

Mobile phone users reach 3.3bn. (2008, May 27). *The Australian*. Retrieved July 17, 2008, from http://www.theaustralian.com.au/australian-it/mobile-phone-users-reach-33bn/story-e6fr-galx-1111116448670

Morrison, G., & Anglin, G. J. (2006). An instructional design approach for effective shovelware: Modifying materials for distance education. *Quarterly Review of Distance Education, 7*(1), 63–74.

Moses, A. (2007, October 31). Wikipedia project is a class act. *The Sydney Morning Herald*. Retrieved February 12, 2008, from http://www.smh.com.au/news/web/wikipedia-project-is-a-class-act/2007/10/31/1193618940842.html

O'Connell, M., Benson, R., & Samarawickrema, G. (2006). Professional development for professional developers: Who's learning about e-learning from whom? In L. Markauskaite, P. Goodyear, & P. Reimann (Eds.), *Who's learning? Whose technology? Proceedings of the 23rd Australasian Society for Computers in Learning in Tertiary Education (ASCILITE) Conference* (pp. 599–602). Sydney: University of Sydney. Retrieved February 12, 2008, from http://www.ascilite.org.au/conferences/sydney06/proceeding/pdf_papers/p169.pdf

O'Reilly, T. (2005). *What is Web 2.0: Design patterns and business models for the next generation of software*. Retrieved February 12, 2008, from http://www.oreillynet.com/pub/a/oreilly/tim/news/2005/09/30/what-is-web-20.html

Oliver, R. (2003). Exploring benchmarks and standards for assuring quality online teaching and learning in higher education. In C. McLoughlin, P. LeCornu, & W. Jackson (Eds.), *Sustaining quality learning environments: Proceedings of the 16th Open and Distance Learning Association of Australia (ODLAA) Biennial Conference*. Canberra, Australia: Canberra Institute of Technology.

Oliver, R. (2005). Quality assurance and e-learning: Blue skies and pragmatism. *ALT-J Research in Learning Technology, 13*(3), 173–187.

Owyang, J. (2008, January 9). Social network stats: Facebook, MySpace, Reunion (Jan, 2008) [Web log post]. *Web Strategy by Jeremiah Owyang*. Retrieved February 12, 2008, from http://www.web-strategist.com/blog/2008/01/09/social-network-stats-facebook-myspace-reunion-jan-2008/

Parker, K. R., & Chao, J. T. (2007). Wiki as a teaching tool. *Interdisciplinary Journal of Knowledge and Learning Objects, 3*, 57–72. Retrieved February 15, 2008, from http://www.ijklo.org/Volume3/IJKLOv3p057-072Parker284.pdf

Pratt, J. (2005). The fashionable adoption of online learning technologies in Australian universities. *Journal of the Australian and New Zealand Academy of Management, 11*(1), 57–73.

Ramsden, P. (2003). *Learning to teach in higher education* (2nd ed.). London: Routledge.

Ryan, Y. (1998). Time and tide: Teaching and learning online. *Australian Universities Review, 41*(1), 14–19. Retrieved August 5, 2009, from http://www.aur.org.au/archive/41-01/aur_41-01.pdf

Salmon, G. (2005). Flying not flapping: A strategic framework for e-learning and pedagogical innovation in higher education institutions. *ALT-J Research in Learning Technology, 13*(3), 201–218.

Sharpe, R., Benfield, G., Lessner, E., & DeCicco, E. (2005). *Final report: Scoping study for the pedagogy strand of the JISC e-learning programme*. Bristol, UK: Joint Information Systems Committee. Retrieved July 17, 2008, from http://www.jisc.ac.uk/uploaded_documents/scoping%20study%20final%20report%20v4.1.doc

Sifry, D. (2007, April 5). The state of the live web, April 2007 [Web log post]. *Sifry's Alerts*. Retrieved February 12, 2008, from http://www.sifry.com/alerts/archives/000493.html

Sproll, L., & Faraj, S. (1993). Atheism, sex, and databases: The net as a social technology. In Kiesler, S. (Ed.), *Culture of the Internet* (pp. 35–51). Mahwah, NJ: Lawrence Erlbaum.

Steel, J., & Hudson, A. (2001). Educational technology in learning and teaching: The perceptions and experiences of teaching staff. *Innovations in Education and Teaching International, 38*(2), 103–111. doi:10.1080/13558000010030158

Stroud, R. (2008). Social networking: An age-neutral commodity—Social networking becomes a mature web application. *Journal of Direct, Data and Digital Marketing Practice, 9*(3), 278–292. Retrieved August 5, 2009, from http://www.palgrave-journals.com/dddmp/journal/v9/n3/pdf/4350099a.pdf

Tynan, B., & Colbran, S. (2006). Podcasting, student learning and expectations. In L. Markauskaite, P. Goodyear, & P. Reimann (Eds.), *Who's learning? Whose technology? Proceedings of the 23rd Australasian Society for Computers in Learning in Tertiary Education (ASCILITE) Conference* (pp. 825–832). Sydney: University of Sydney. Retrieved January 12, 2008, from http://www.ascilite.org.au/conferences/sydney06/proceeding/pdf_papers/p132.pdf

Weaver, D., Spratt, C., & Nair, C. S. (2008). Academic and student use of a learning management system: Implications for quality. *Australasian Journal of Educational Technology, 24*(1), 30–41. Retrieved February 19, 2008, from http://www.ascilite.org.au/ajet/ajet24/weaver.pdf

Wise, L., & Quealy, J. (2006). At the limits of social constructivism: Moving beyond LMS to re-integrate scholarship. In L. Markauskaite, P. Goodyear, & P. Reimann (Eds.), *Who's learning? Whose technology? Proceedings of the 23rd Australasian Society for Computers in Learning in Tertiary Education (ASCILITE) Conference* (pp. 899–907). Sydney: University of Sydney. Retrieved February 20, 2008, from http://www.ascilite.org.au/conferences/sydney06/proceeding/pdf_papers/p158.pdf

Wozniak, H., Scott, K., & Atkinson, S. (2005). The balancing act: Managing emerging issues of elearning projects at the University of Sydney. In H. Goss (Ed), *Balance, fidelity, mobility: Maintaining the momentum? Proceedings of the 22nd Australasian Society for Computers in Learning in Tertiary Education (ASCILITE) Conference* (pp. 735–745). Brisbane, Australia: Queensland University of Technology. Retrieved February 20, 2008, from http://www.ascilite.org.au/conferences/brisbane05/blogs/proceedings/86_Wozniak.pdf

KEY TERMS AND DEFINITIONS

Learning Management System (LMS): An application that automates many of the administrative processes involved in online teaching. Close synonyms include "course management system" (CMS), "managed learning environment" (MLE), and "virtual learning environment" (VLE).

Short Message Service (SMS): The technology used to send and receive short, text-based messages on mobile phones. Also commonly known as "text messaging."

Social Constructivist: This is the branch of educational theory that focuses on the social contexts of learning. Following Lev Vygotsky (1896–1934), social constructivists see knowledge as mutually constructed.

Social Networking Sites: These are websites designed to support an online community of users with similar interests. Well-known examples include MySpace and Facebook, although there are many others that exist.

Web 2.0: A term that refers to the latest thinking on how software developers and end-users should best make use of the Web. Web 2.0 ideas depend on the central concept of the "Internet as a platform." Although there is occasional disagreement, the term is properly pronounced "web two point oh."

Web 2.0 Technologies: When used by educational researchers and practitioners this term refers to applications such as blogs, wikis, podcasting, and social networking, which permit the creation and remixing of user-generated content. The same term is also used by technical writers to refer to specific toolsets (such as AJAX and CCS) that are used to create Web 2.0 sites.

Widget: A small code snippet that can be installed into an HTML (web) page by any non-coding page owner to provide some specialized functionality. Widgets are typically free to the end-user and perform one or more simple tasks.

Chapter 20
When the Future Finally Arrives:
Web 2.0 Becomes Web 3.0

Matt Crosslin
The University of Texas at Arlington, USA

ABSTRACT

This chapter examines how the World Wide Web could possibly change over the next 10 years into a concept increasingly being referred to as "Web 3.0," and how these changes might affect education. It examines how Web 3.0 concepts such as cloud computing, the Semantic Web, and the three-dimensional (3-D) Web are currently being explored and realized. A possible future online learning scenario is also described and analyzed to help visualize these possibilities for education. The author hopes that providing an understanding of and insight into how the Internet and related technologies may continue to develop and evolve in the next several years will help educators be better prepared for the future of online learning.

INTRODUCTION

As technology grows and changes, some people like to sit back and see where the ride takes them. Others prefer to keep an eye on where the ride is going—they have learned from the past that if one fails to keep an eye on the future, he or she could end up with a broken Betamax player and a stack of video tapes that no longer play on anyone's machine. In education, knowing what the future holds is especially critical when dealing with technology. Educators are no longer dealing with making technology decisions for themselves; they now have to make decisions for entire classes or even entire departments or schools. Knowing what is coming around the bend in technology could make the difference between creating a cutting-edge classroom or an odd collection of useless gadgets in the corner of a bland, normal classroom.

"Web 2.0" is one of the many technology buzz-words that has gained the attention of the academic world recently. Many educators are beginning to grasp the concept of Web 2.0—but what comes

DOI: 10.4018/978-1-60566-294-7.ch020

after that? If Web 2.0 is here, what will Web 3.0 look like? Will it be a revamped attempt to create a three-dimensional (3-D) Web, or something entirely different? What will all of this mean for educators who are still trying to implement Web 2.0 tools and concepts in their classes?

Web 2.0 and its pedagogical implications have been examined thoroughly in other chapters in this book. This chapter will only touch on the basics of Web 2.0 that are pertinent to the discussion of the future of the World Wide Web beyond Web 2.0. The chapter will address the following objectives:

1. Examine how Web 2.0 will pave the way for Web 3.0;
2. Define what the term "Web 3.0" is currently understood to mean;
3. Examine the benefits and pitfalls this may have for education;
4. Predict how Web 3.0 will interact with the 3-D Web in the classroom of the future.

BACKGROUND

To some, the term "Web 2.0" implies a new version of the World Wide Web—one that is perhaps better than "Web 1.0." This implication might lead some educators to wonder if they are falling behind in technological knowledge, especially since there was never an announcement made about how to access this new version of the Web. Fortunately, this is not the case.

Web 2.0 does imply something new, but this new factor has more to do with how web design is approached instead of a new version of the Internet itself. O'Reilly Media recognized the confusion that some people have over this issue and decided to give the term a precise—although somewhat lengthy and complex—definition in 2005. Tim O'Reilly (2005) listed seven features or characteristics that define Web 2.0:

- The World Wide Web as platform (instead of a computer desktop);
- Utilizing collective intelligence (allowing users to contribute);
- Web services driven by databases (mainly SQL based);
- No more software release cycles (more frequent updates);
- Use of lightweight programs and languages (such as RSS or PHP);
- Applications that work on multiple devices (computers, cellphones [mobile phones], etc.);
- Lightweight user interfaces (based on AJAX) for richer experiences.

Some of these features are still developing and evolving; therefore, Web 2.0 has yet to be completely realized (Alexander, 2006). Full realization of Web 2.0, however, is probably only a matter of time and effort.

As O'Reilly (2005) points out, none of the above features use or require new types of programs or programming languages. The databases that web services are driven by, such as MySQL, have existed for years. So have the open source languages, such as PHP, that are used to end software release cycles. AJAX (which stands for Asynchronous JavaScript and XML) is also nothing new. All of the technological terms used by O'Reilly in the list above are the underlying architecture that allows the real point of Web 2.0 to shine: website users can collaboratively contribute to the site while online—in contrast with working on something alone offline before uploading it. Many have used the phrase "read/write Web" to quickly and concisely describe the nature of Web 2.0 (in contrast to "read-only Web," which describes Web 1.0).

With more classes offered online every year, and still more face-to-face classes integrating the Internet into daily lessons, educators are beginning to wonder if Web 2.0 will affect their classroom experience. Two areas in which the influences and effects of Web 2.0 might be felt are in online tool availability and course design. As examined in other chapters, Web 2.0 tools can be used for a variety of teaching and learning purposes in tertiary education. As tools change and expand, instructional designers will have a larger range of options for educational technologies and, therefore, course design will also be affected. One of the positive side benefits of the Web 2.0 movement is that many companies are offering their services for free. For example, several websites provide web browser-based, Microsoft Office-like services at no cost. Blogs, wikis, photo editing, video recording, podcasts, and many other tools can all be found online for low or no cost. Because of this, certain tools that were once out of reach for some educators are now being offered online, sometimes even in multiple versions or "flavors." As these tools are offered through lightweight interfaces built on existing technologies, many older computers can take advantage of the latest Web 2.0 sites.

As web users become accustomed to collaborating and contributing, will some instructors see a greater desire among students to work in groups and even contribute to the course content itself? Some feel that students will lose interest in technology once it is used in education (Anderson, 2007). Course design will need to reflect this collaborative mindset in order to keep students engaged in the learning process.

FROM WEB 2.0 TO WEB 3.0

Most people probably will look at the term "Web 2.0" and wonder, "Will there be a Web 3.0?" The answer to that question is, "Most likely." Discussion about Web 3.0 is ongoing, with many still divided on what it will entail. Web 2.0-based information resources such as Wikipedia and the blogosphere, and online technology news forums, are probably the best sources for tracking the ongoing discussion as it unfolds. The term "Web 3.0" can apply to many different (though sometimes overlapping) concepts, including the Semantic Web, the 3-D Web, and the "read/ write/execute" Web. All of these possibilities rely on Web 2.0 first being fully realized; despite the fact that this is not yet the case, work is currently progressing on all Web 3.0 concepts.

Cloud Computing and the Semantic Web

As noted earlier, Web 2.0 is commonly seen as the "read/write" Web. Users do not just read websites—they actively contribute content. Some sites, such as Facebook, are taking the concept of user-contributed content to the next level by giving users the ability to add their own generated code to the website (using an Application Programming Interface or API). This concept is sometimes called the "read/write/execute" Web or "cloud computing" (because computer functions happen somewhere off in the Internet "cloud" instead of locally on a desktop). As computing power increases, this may give website users the means to safely alter the code of a website itself based on personal preferences. In education, companies could begin granting website users the ability to submit user-created interfaces for specific programs targeted at specific disciplines. For example, in health education, an instructor might develop custom scenarios where students examine the effects of different lifestyle choices on the human body. Instead of being limited to prewritten conditions defined by the website, educators may use a set of open source APIs to build scenarios that reflect actual conditions in their students' communities. Adventurous teachers may even some day have the ability to allow students to modify online courses as a class project. Using the previous example, students could begin writing their own APIs to create scenarios for other students to solve. This would give students the chance to use higher-order thinking skills, as well as construct knowledge for others to learn through collaboration. The challenge for websites seeking to offer services like this for education is that they will need to incorporate APIs and other resources that are powerful enough to be useful at the same time that they are easy to learn and use.

According to Anderson (2007), the Semantic Web is basically a newer way of looking at organizing and searching the Internet. The Semantic Web will aim to aggregate Internet data and transform it into machine-searchable information, thus making future web searches incredibly accurate. No longer will the end-user have to scroll through pages and pages of unrelated (and often questionable) content to find exactly what he or she needs. Even more intriguing than this is the concept that sites on the Semantic Web will be able to start reproducing functions that mirror human intelligence (Anderson, 2007). For example, websites currently are unable to distinguish between a nut that is eaten and a nut that is used with a bolt. Searching for something about a specific nut and bolt combination will yield results that contain information about all types of nuts. The web user still has to filter through all of these results to find what her or she is looking for. Once these results are tagged and rated, web searches will become more accurate. The benefit of accurate web searching has enormous implications for education. Web searches could actually become part of a classroom discussion—not just something that has to be done after the discussion is over, due to the fact that the time taken to filter results may be prohibitive.

The 3-D Web

Another possibility for Web 3.0 might be a 3-D version of the Internet built on 3-D graphics. This is a possibility that is being promoted by the Web3D Consortium (http://www.web3d.org/). A 3-D World Wide Web might eventually look something like Second Life (SL at http://www.secondlife.com/) or some other immersive online virtual environment, with website designers creating 3-D virtual spaces instead of two-dimensional (2-D) pages. Another possibility might be a new 3-D interface for surfing the current Web.

Currently, 3-D environments such as SL must be run in a separate program installed on the desktop that connects to content online. If the Web 2.0 goal of "Internet as a platform" and the Web 3.0 goal of "read/write/execute" Web are fully realized, virtual environments might possibly run natively inside of a web browser at some point. Eventually, the current information Web and various virtual environments may merge to become one integrated world. Some software development companies are creating SL clients that have integrated web browsers inside of them. Clicking on an object in SL with an embedded web link will bring up a transparent web browser next to the user's SL avatar (3-D virtual representation of a person). Depending on the future direction of the Internet, this could be what surfing the Web could become. Surfers will have a virtual avatar that explores 3-D islands and cities online, and then displays more information about various organizations, companies, schools, and individuals by bringing up a website within the virtual world.

Two factors currently hinder this from being viable for educational purposes: space on virtual worlds can be costly and difficult to create, and there are several different virtual worlds to choose from that are unable to interact and interoperate with one another. Why buy space in one world that may not work with the one that most of your students are on? Why even try to propose buying something that is out of your budget in the first place? Questions like this could possibly convince some to not even consider using a virtual world in teaching and learning. Fortunately, solutions are being worked on for these issues (see the Virtual World Interoperability wiki site at http://vwinterop.wikidot.com/). In October 2007, representatives from 23 companies and organizations met to work on a set of standards that would grant members from one online world the ability to enter other worlds with the same account. If this agreement can be reached, picking an online virtual world in which to create a virtual space will become analogous to choosing a hosting company with which to host a website.

What about the difficulty of creating an online virtual space? This activity does have a steep learning curve, but so did HTML when it was first introduced. Many tools have been created through the years that help even the worst technophobes create their own sites in minutes. For years now, web hosting companies have offered free templates for users that sign up for their services. People began learning code for themselves. Eventually, all of this will happen for 3-D virtual worlds as well.

Of course, many universities and colleges prefer to host websites on their own servers. These institutions are also likely to favor hosting their own virtual spaces, versus outsourcing to a third party (i.e., paying for hosting on some corporately controlled server). This is understandable due to the fact that some institutions may have policies in place to provide security and simplified authentication for all online university applications. Also, virtual worlds hosted on external servers can be unpredictable. Anyone that has tried to present information about SL on Wednesday morning has found out the hard way that this period of time is scheduled maintenance time, during which SL is closed! Hosting their own virtual worlds would give institutions control over many issues like this. Some open source virtual world programs already exist, and some companies like SL are working on releasing their code as open source in the future. Once again, the learning curve on hosting a virtual world is steep, but can also be learned just like any other computer code.

Benefits of Web 3.0 for Education

The importance of online 3-D interactions can be thought about in light of two crucial educational factors: social presence and immediacy. Social presence is an awareness of other people (students, teachers, etc.) in a course and the involvement of those people in the communication process (Xu, 2005). Lev Vygotsky, as well as several other learning theorists, assert that social interaction is an important factor in the learning process. Several studies have examined the importance of social presence in learning (Tu & McIsaac, 2002). The challenge for online learning is that many of the factors that lead to social presence, such as facial expressions and eye contact, cannot be experienced online. Some day, virtual avatars will be able to replicate many of these missing factors (Derene, 2008). Web 3.0 sites focused on communication and educational tagging could also one day contribute functions that increase social presence by adding new levels of interaction through a web browser (instead of outside of a web browser in a separate application).

In general, immediacy refers to the perceived (as opposed to actual) distance between people who are communicating (Woods & Baker, 2004). Some researchers have found that teachers who can decrease perceived distance in classrooms will see an increase in learning (Swan, 2002). Once again, personal avatars may possibly help increase some of the factors that also increase immediacy. Also, cloud computing and the Semantic Web could someday contribute sites that increase communication between class participants, thereby increasing immediacy.

The obvious benefit of virtual worlds for online education is the realism of 3-D design—although immersing students into complex, engaging tasks is also very important (Herrington, Reeves, & Oliver, 2007). This realism is not quite photorealistic, or even up to the same level as video gaming, but advances are made every year in graphics technology. One benefit of this realism is its effect on communication. Current online communication is often limited to lines of text or an audio or video conference. Video conferencing is constantly improving, however it can still sometimes be expensive or low quality, and the interaction with objects on screen is limited. In virtual worlds, people communicate through 3-D representations of themselves (avatars) that they can customize. Avatars come complete with facial expressions and realistic movements that can interact with other objects on screen. Some environments, such as SL, already have voice communication features built in. Spatial audio technology gives an illusion of direction and depth in communication, while users speak into a microphone as they would in a normal conversation.

This realism can also help with online activities. Historical re-enactments, object design, role playing, and field trips can all go beyond mere discussion and static, 2-D photographs. For example, instead of just talking about Morocco and looking at images of the country on websites, students could actually visit a 3-D recreation of key Moroccan landmarks in SL. Students in architecture classes could construct and share interactive 3-D models of their ideas instead of just drawing them. History students studying about Hell's Kitchen (a neighborhood of Manhattan in New York City, once the bastion of poor Irish Americans and part of the New York underworld) can enter into a virtual re-enactment in SL straight from the 1980s. Other examples of sites of interest for educators in SL can be found in the quick-start tour guide at edumuve.com (2009). Realistic virtual environments could even possibly give rise to a greater level of simulation-based learning, mainly because real people could be behind the simulation rather than a set of preprogrammed computer responses. The current direction of 3-D virtual environments indicates that these simulations could also be user designed—not dictated by a software company board. This could greatly expand the meaning of the "anywhere" part of "anywhere, anytime" learning.

To some degree, not all of these ideas are just speculation. Some groups and organizations are already beginning to experiment with online learning inside of 3-D virtual environments. For example, the Sloodle project (http://www.sloodle.org/) is exploring how to integrate the Moodle course management system with the SL online virtual environment. SL has its own open source scripting language, the Linden Scripting Language, which grants SL objects permission to connect to the World Wide Web. Moodle is also written in open source web languages. Since connecting one open source language to another is fairly straightforward, the Sloodle project was born. Some of the accomplishments that the Sloodle project has already achieved include creating a password-protected 3-D learning "room," designing new ways to communicate using chats and calendars in a 3-D environment, and even scripting a "quiz chair" that feeds questions to a user's avatar, moving up or down based on the correctness of the answers. The open nature of Web 2.0 and its architecture of participation as manifested in Moodle have helped the Sloodle project move forward in a manner that would not have worked as easily with other learning management systems.

As stated earlier, the main benefit of the Semantic Web will be accurate and intelligent searches on the Web. But what about cloud computing? Using an API sounds interesting, but is that really just something for an information technology (IT) class? Cloud computing could possibly benefit any educational discipline by opening the door for more active learning online. APIs can be designed to be used by people with no programming experience. Students will no longer just sit back and read content online, maybe commenting or replying to a few things here and there. They will be able to contribute to the lesson by creating programs and plugins of their own.

3-D Hardware

The development of the 3-D Web could also possibly be driven by the development of 3-D hardware to enhance the online experience. Video games and online virtual worlds are already designed in 3-D, so those environments will be ready for the new devices as soon as they are manufactured.

Holographic (3-D) monitors already exist, but tend to be large, expensive machines with small screens. Recent breakthroughs in technology have led experts to speculate that someday, companies will be making affordable, full-screen holographic monitors with screen sizes that rival today's large screen giants—ready for home and educational uses (Greene, 2007).

Just as there are already holographic monitors, 3-D scanners and printers already exist. Of course, these are also large and expensive. As with holographic monitors, advances are being made every year to bring down their sizes and prices. The basic idea behind a 3-D scanner is that an object is placed on a scanner bed, scanned by lasers, and virtually recreated inside a computer graphics program (Wayner, 2007). This image can then be manipulated and sent anywhere in the world. A 3-D printer then takes this scan and recreates (sometimes even in full color) the object out of some type of plastic substance (Simkins, 2008).

3-D scanners and printers will someday make incredible tools for education. Any object that is needed in a virtual world could be scanned in at the touch of a button. This would make creating an online space much easier. Students can work on an idea for an object—say, a new idea for a toothbrush design—in a virtual environment, and then "print" the design and test it out. 3-D printers would also make replacing supplies extremely fast and convenient. If a student breaks the last protractor in mathematics class, all the teacher has to do is to download the relevant template and print out a new one. The possibilities are endless.

User interaction within virtual environments is also being improved every day. Digital cameras are being designed that track movements of hands and other objects (Tabuchi, 2007). Users may no longer have to use a mouse or joystick to control virtual avatars—they will just move around in front of a screen and their avatar will follow or mimic their moves and facial expressions. Software already exists that can map the movement of a person's head to a graphic character. This will take interaction within virtual worlds to an all-new level of realism.

FUTURE TRENDS

Predicting the future is a tricky business. Many inventions have been predicted through the years that have never come to fruition, while some inventions like the Internet have taken off in directions that no one could have ever predicted. The popularity of the science fiction genre in general would suggest that many people are still intrigued and curious, thinking and dreaming about possible futures.

The Internet as it is currently known may still go in other directions that no one can currently predict. The recent popularity of personal smartphones has opened up a whole new world in the form of a true mobile Internet experience. Will the Internet migrate to bigger, holographic screens, or to smaller, pocket-sized mobile devices? Will consumers come to prefer portability over realism? If the Web 2.0 goal of "applications that work on multiple devices" becomes a reality, there may be no clear global preference on these issues. Students may be able to choose to visit a virtual world on a large screen at home, and on their pocket-sized mobile device while on the move.

Taking in to account all of the previously discussed changes to the Internet, what could online learning look like 10 years into the future? First of all, let us assume that all ideas previously discussed become fully realized as expected, and that they are designed to work and interact with one another. With this assumption, a fairly impressive vision of the future of learning comes into view. Take the following scenario, for example (which only uses technology that currently exists or that is currently being developed).

An Example of Online Learning 10 Years in the Future

Morning arrives for our online learner as she stumbles out of bed to the sound of her handheld computer's notification ringtone. Picking up her handheld, she sees a list of due dates for some of her courses, and two missed text messages. One of the messages is a question from one of her group members in her engineering class. It seems that one of her partners has run into a snag with their project. This would probably be a good day to see how the project is progressing, so she sends a quick audio message out to all members to suggest some times on their shared calendar that they can meet that day in their institution's virtual world.

She walks across the room to her personal media center. Since television signals and Internet are both delivered to one large, wide-screen, high-definition, holographic, 3-D, multi-touch-screen monitor, most people just have one center in their house for communication and entertainment purposes. Price breakthroughs have also brought the cost of these media centers down to the level of today's laptops. Our online learner takes her center off of standby, and the screen jumps to life as her center connects to the Internet. As it connects, she looks around at the unusual virtual world on her screen, her brain still a little foggy on just where she left her avatar. She sees a few people walking around in medieval clothes and turns her head to the right slightly. The view on her screen reacts to her head movement and the view shifts to the right. She notices the Globe Theater standing off in the distance. Ah, yes! She was attending a virtual re-enactment of a Shakespeare play here last night for her English class. She wonders if she remembered to save any of the recordings she made. With a flick of her wrist, a list of files on her hard drive flashes on to the screen in front of her. With a few waves of her index finger, she quickly finds her files from *A midsummer night's dream*. She captured some great clips, so her project is sure to be a success.

A flashing note at the side of the screen indicates that one of her group members has responded to her message about a meeting. She decides to wait until all of the responses have come in before bringing up her calendar. Another note pops up to let her know that her professor will be starting his class in about one minute, so she decides it is time to get ready for class.

Pointing at the inventory button on screen, she pulls up her premade avatar selection. No time to go for a custom look today. Since she is going to do some course work, she decides to use a realistic avatar. Her sleek, stylish dragon-like alter ego will have to wait for social time. Her computer takes the most recent image that she tagged of herself in her online picture storage area and creates a realistic virtual persona using automated 3-D image creation software. She then chooses the clothes that she wants her avatar to wear from a selection of photographs that are tagged as "school casual," and those appear on her virtual representation. The cameras that are embedded in her media center follow the movements of her hands, lips, arms, and eyes to make her avatar mimic the exact same movements. She puts on her microphone (for voice chat) as a final preparation for class.

Time to teleport her avatar to sculpture class. She says the word *"favorites"* out loud, and a list of online bookmarks appears, floating between her and the virtual world behind it. She searches through the list and sees that the instructor had sent the entire class an updated meeting location this morning and her bookmark had already updated itself. A notice from her online calendar floats in front of her field of view, reminding her that it is her turn to have progress on her art project critiqued in sculpture class. Panic sets in for a brief moment as she asks herself, "What project?" She then notices that she had left herself a note stating that she had worked on her sculpture last week; it has been ready to critique for a few days. Her notice also serves up the sculpture project design file (her blueprint for creating the real object), so with a flick of her wrist she sends it to the corner of her screen to keep it handy for later. As she finally teleports to class, a security alert flashes on the screen and reminds her that she needs to swipe her student card to gain access to the virtual room. She pulls out her student ID, touches it to the screen and the scene in front of her changes. The Globe Theater slow fades to darkness and her virtual art class fades quickly in to view.

The instructor begins a few moments after our online learner arrives and tells her that it is now time to critique the progress of her project. She touches the file at the corner of her screen and drags it to the display table in the center of the virtual classroom. After confirming that she wants to share this object with others, the file image floating in front of her fades away and her sculpture project design manifests itself on the virtual table for all to see. She then takes the actual project and places it on her 3-D scanner. A laser scans down her project, and an exact virtual replica appears in the classroom. The students in her class gather around the artwork and begin giving feedback on how well her work is progressing when compared to the design file next to it. Her design file is also connected to a collection of videos that she made of herself creating the sculpture. Her instructor notices these and watches a few clips to see how she is using standard techniques in the project.

Feedback begins streaming in from students. Most just comment through the in-world audio, knowing that feedback sessions are recorded for future reference. Some look around the Internet and send her links to images and other files online that may give her some ideas. All of the feedback is stored in an online folder, tagged to match this project. The learner has rated some users as "most trusted," so their critiques float to the top of the list in her folder. She will probably read all her feedback, but knows that these classmates best understand what she is trying to accomplish with her project. She has also sorted her classmates by those that actually seem to be paying attention and those that just say something to ensure a decent "participation" grade from the instructor. No other classmates can see these tags, but they are all aware that they all do this for one another. Those that read the syllabus carefully know that the instructor can also see these tags, and will actually use them when determining participation grades.

One student notices a few similarities between our learner's sculpture and van Gogh's painting style. The instructor suggests that students look for some information on van Gogh to see which of his pieces could have influenced the sculpture. Our learner pulls up an information browser that floats virtually before her on the screen and tells the browser *"search: van Gogh; filter: academic."* She chooses to use her academic search filter so that online results will be filtered by what other students and teachers have deemed to have "academic relevance." All of her results are excellent resources on van Gogh. She decides that she really likes the first three results. She scans through the links and finds two images that she thinks influenced her sculpture the most. She then tags these images and, with a flick of her wrist, sends those links and tags to her classmates. As other links and tags come in from other students, they start to see a pattern emerging: most students (including our learner) seem to think that the sculpture being critiqued was influenced by van Gogh's *The starry night*. One student also found a link to a 3-D representation of this painting in Second Life. This virtual representation received high ratings from other art teachers on a virtual world ratings site. Since SL is part of the open virtual worlds agreement, the instructor suggests that they teleport their avatars there for about five minutes or so to take a look and provide additional input.

Within a few seconds, the entire class has teleported to the location of the van Gogh simulation in SL. The simulation turns out to not just be a 3-D model to look at, but an entire section of an SL island dedicated to recreating *The starry night* in life-sized accuracy. The simulation gives visitors a sense of actually being inside of a van Gogh painting. There are a few comments and messages tagged on different areas of the island. The visibility of these can be turned on or off by each user, but most students know by now to leave them visible when on virtual field trips—the instructor always takes some of them and uses them as examples. The instructor chooses a few tags that are labeled as "academic" in nature and discusses the ways that van Gogh has influenced painters through the years. He compliments our learner on achieving a nice use of influence in her sculpture, without becoming too derivative.

Following several minutes spent discussing and reading comments from other visitors, the instructor teleports the entire class to an online virtual Earth simulation to see a historical view of the Saint Rémy de Provence of south France, where van Gogh painted *The starry night*. Students switch from contemporary view to the particular historical view highlighted by the instructor (larger cities and popular areas of Earth can have as many as 100 historical views) to immerse themselves in van Gogh's world for a minute. They sift through some comments and tags left by previous visitors, and add a few comments. After a few moments, a shared alarm from the class group calendar flashes in front of everyone—time to critique the next project. The instructor waves his hand at a "back to class" script he installed in his course, and the classroom quickly fades back into view.

As our learner settles in to observe and comment on the next sculpture, she notices that three classmates have sent her private feedback. She is anxious to read these, but knows that the instructor is tracking all of his students' movements in class to make sure they are staying on task. Pulling up those comments at this moment would cause that action to be noted in her personal class log, as would reading the three new video messages she had received, or checking to see what deals her online auction tracker had found for her. She and a few other students did not believe at first that this instructor was serious about checking the logs—until they got their first participation grade. No more multi-tasking in this class! (She will save that for her English class, in which there is no participation grade …)

At the end of class, the instructor goes over a few last-minute details, and then the entire room vanishes, leaving students standing in an open virtual field in the temporary class area of their institution's virtual world. No matter where class begins or ends up going, the instructor seems to get the classroom back to this spot every time. The popularity of virtual classes outgrew the institution's server capacity, so no one class has a permanently assigned space anymore. Instructors are assigned a temporary spot on the virtual class field and a time to meet. They are also given a movable classroom template that can actually be used in any online virtual world. Our learner's online class sometimes randomly meets in worlds other than the one her institution runs in.

In five minutes another class will probably appear on the spot where she is standing, so our learner decides to move to the commons area. She finally gets a chance to catch up on messages. She decides to put her avatar to sleep and access her messages from her handheld device while sitting in her favorite real-world couch. Several messages about her engineering class have come in while she was in the sculpture class. Her virtual learning environment calendar has also highlighted the times that all group members are available. Since our learner is the group leader, it is her responsibility to pick a time and reserve an online virtual meeting spot. With a few touches of her screen, she has the whole meeting planned.

Our learner has about an hour until the synchronous group meeting for her engineering class will commence. The first thing she takes care of is looking through the private messages she received during her critique session. She is hoping for some deeper feedback on her work—maybe something that someone was afraid to bring up in class. Some of her classmates are still very reluctant to share with the class due to the possible risk of saying something wrong. She pulls up her messages on her handheld (because her handheld is wireless and "syncs" instantly with her media center). She ends up becoming pretty frustrated with the messages received. They are just all fluffy, filler messages that say "cool work" and contain other useless feedback. She realizes that these messages are from students hoping to get more participation points from the instructor. She decides to tag these messages for the instructor as feedback for her project. That way, the instructor will read them and the students that sent them will not receive any points for wasting her time.

Our learner decides that it is time to put aside study and relax for a while by seeing if her favorite webcast has released another episode. No such luck, but the site that tracks her web videos for her has picked up on the fact that she searched for van Gogh recently, and lets her know about a new van Gogh documentary that recently aired on the History Channel. She decides to watch the video, and uses her handheld as a remote control to play the documentary on her media center screen. Her sleeping avatar fades out of view and the video leaps to 3-D life in front of her. As the video plays, our learner stops it every so often to read viewer comment tags on certain scenes. One tag, in particular, gives her an idea for her sculpture. Having detected that this video has the same tags as her art project, the media center is keeping her project ideas folder floating at the right-hand side of the screen. Our learner touches the tags and slides her finger in an upward, right-hand motion. This sends a copy of the tags flying in to her ideas folder. Next, she uses the index finger of both hands to create a highlighted section of the video and throws that into to her ideas folder. A warning pops up in front of her field of view that states the video she just saved is copyrighted, will only display for her, and cannot be transferred to anybody else. The video will also delete itself in three days. She is given the option to purchase permanent rights to the image, but she declines and accepts the trial educational license. She will just have to remember to look at it again before it erases itself from her folder. She also smiles to herself, wondering how boring television was before it was connected to the Internet, or even before touch screens were added.

The documentary ends about 15 minutes before her meeting is scheduled to start. She decides it would be a good idea to review the progress on her group project prior to the meeting. For her engineering class, she and her classmates have been working on a better cover for the web interface glove they use in class. The current one has not been updated in a couple of years, so it is a little bulky for some of the current applications. Her media center notices that she is looking at her notes for her engineering class, and pulls up a list of new tags related to her group project. Her group members seem to have recently been surfing the information Web for ideas. She has received about a dozen new images and two new video notes. These notes seem to contain some good ideas, so she makes her own video notes and enables her avatar. The address link for her virtual meeting is already in her avatar's field of view, so with a touch of the screen she teleports to the preset meeting location.

Within a few seconds, all group members are present and chatting about upcoming assignments. Their avatars gather around a virtual table, and a working 3-D virtual model of the glove interface design appears before them. Their instructor has invited several engineering experts into the class to provide critique and feedback on projects as they develop. The students' project has several tags attached to it, so apparently the outside reviewers have visited since the last meeting a few days ago. Information on these tags is sometimes rather direct and blunt, but ultimately very helpful.

The group spends at least half an hour pouring over the suggestions. Some are accepted and some are tweaked a little before they are added to the model. After all of the required tweaks are made, the group decides that it is time to test their glove cover out in real life. Each group member sends a copy of the model to his or her own 3-D printer. In a matter of minutes, a plastic model has been molded out of plastic dust inside each of their printing devices. All of the group members snap their new covers on to their engineering gloves and direct their avatars to leave the virtual meeting spot to test out the design. To save time, group members have previously agreed that all real-life testing would be asynchronous.

Our learner roams through several virtual worlds, testing out different tasks at random—all of them involving some feature of the glove interface. She records several notes to herself and her group. She also sees that several other notes have been added by her fellow group members. At this point, she decides to leave the organization and tagging of feedback notes until later, since it is now time to head off to work. She switches the clothes on her avatar to a set from her album marked "professional," and teleports her avatar to her virtual workplace.

Analysis of the Future Example

Predicting the future can be entertaining, but the big question behind all of this needs to be, "How can/does this improve education?" The learner in this scenario was able to collaborate with other learners synchronously and asynchronously. She was able to construct meaning from previous experiences and share it with others. She was also able to integrate her learning, including the various designs and theories, with real-life experiences. From a pedagogical perspective, all of this is already possible in online teaching and learning today. Therefore, improvements in technology should not necessarily be seen as brand-new or revolutionary educational innovations, but rather as refinements or improvements building upon what is already being accomplished by teachers, learners, and institutions across the globe.

Also, as seen in the scenario, if the instructor does not place careful and thoughtfully considered limits on interaction, students may be tempted to "use the system" to manipulate grades or avoid attending to the learning tasks and objectives at hand. Greater levels of socialization among students could also possibly create opportunities for them to lose focus, thus instructors may need to create guidelines to direct socialization in a manner that keeps students on task and on track. (Other chapters in this book provide in-depth coverage of the problems and pitfalls of Web 2.0 and social software in education.)

CONCLUSION

As fascinating as predicting the future can be, it is imperative to realize that all of these ideas are speculative, at best. This chapter has attempted to look at some technologies that are currently in development to see how they might come together to improve and enhance online experiences overall, and online educational experiences specifically. All of the technologies previously discussed will need to be researched to see if there are actual educational benefits in their usage beyond their "ghee-whiz" or "coolness" factors.

Some of the emerging technologies explored in this chapter might take off in directions that are impossible to foresee. Some of them may never result in viable educational solutions at all—unless forward-thinking educational researchers and practitioners push them in that direction. This is precisely why educators need to keep a close eye on new technologies as they develop: without their voice in the development process, these future ideas will be driven solely by the entertainment (e.g., gaming) or business industries and their respective interests, and the outcomes may be rendered unusable or of limited use for educational purposes and settings.

REFERENCES

Alexander, B. (2006). Web 2.0: A new wave of innovation for teaching and learning? *EDUCAUSE Review, 41*(2), 33–44. Retrieved June 5, 2008, from http://www.educause.edu/ir/library/pdf/ERM0621.pdf

Anderson, P. (2007). *What is Web 2.0? Ideas, technologies and implications for education*. Bristol, UK: Joint Information Systems Committee. Retrieved June 30, 2008, from http://www.jisc.ac.uk/media/documents/techwatch/tsw0701b.pdf

Derene, G. (2008, March 21). Motion capture ready to bring next-gen avatars to gaming, movies, medicine, the military and more (with video!). *Popular Mechanics*. Retrieved July 1, 2008, from http://www.popularmechanics.com/technology/industry/4264771.html?series=6

edumuve.com. (2008). *Sites of interest to educators in Second Life*. Retrieved July 1, 2008, from http://edumuve.com/tour/

Greene, K. (2007, April 24). Practical holographic video, *Technology Review*. Retrieved July 1, 2008 from http://www.technologyreview.com/read_article.aspx?id=18572.

Herrington, J., Reeves, T. C., & Oliver, R. (2007). Immersive learning technologies: Realism and online authentic learning. *Journal of Computing in Higher Education*, *19*(1), 65–84. doi:10.1007/BF03033421

O'Reilly, T. (2005). *What is Web 2.0: Design patterns and business models for the next generation of software*. Retrieved January 10, 2008, from http://www.oreillynet.com/pub/a/oreilly/tim/news/2005/09/30/what-is-web-20.html

Simkins, M. (2008, March 15). 3-D printing a goo goo, *TechLearning*. Retrieved July 1, 2008, from http://www.techlearning.com/showArticle.php?articleID=196605073

Swan, K. (2002). Immediacy, social presence, and asynchronous discussion. In Bourne, J., & Moore, J. C. (Eds.), *Elements of quality online education* (*Vol. 3*, pp. 157–172). Needham, MA: Sloan Consortium.

Tabuchi, H. (2007, November 21). Making "Second Life" more like real life. *MSNBC*. Retrieved July 1, 2008, from http://www.msnbc.msn.com/id/21917042/

Tu, C.-H., & McIsaac, M. (2002). The relationship of social presence and interaction in online classes. *American Journal of Distance Education*, *16*(3), 131–150. doi:10.1207/S15389286AJDE1603_2

Wayner, P. (2007, April 5). Beaming up 3-D objects on a budget. *New York Times*. Retrieved July 1, 2008, from http://www.nytimes.com/2007/04/05/business/05scan.html?ex=1336190400&en=0344a82aae2a277b&ei=5124&partner=permalink&exprod=permalink

Woods, R., & Baker, J. (2004). Interaction and immediacy in online learning. *International Review of Research in Open and Distance Learning, 5*(2). Retrieved July 7, 2008, from http://www.irrodl.org/index.php/irrodl/article/view/186/268

Xu, Y. (2005). Creating social presence in online environment. In B. Hoffman (Ed.), *Encyclopedia of educational technology*. San Diego, CA: San Diego State University. Retrieved January 11, 2008, from http://coe.sdsu.edu/eet/articles/creatsp/start.htm

KEY TERMS AND DEFINITIONS

Avatar: Three-dimensional (3-D) self-created representation of a computer user used within an online virtual world or environment.

Cloud Computing: An Internet-based concept where the development and use of computer programs occurs over Internet connections rather than on a local desktop.

Immediacy: The perceived distance between people that are communicating.

Online Virtual Environment: An Internet-based simulation area intended to be used for interaction among users separated by distance.

Semantic Web: An extension of the World Wide Web where the semantics of information and services posted on the Web are clearly defined, resulting in the possibility of the servers and software on the Web understanding the requests of users more clearly.

Social Presence: An awareness of other people in a course and the involvement of these people in the communication process.

Web 2.0: A term that describes the evolving nature of web programming and design in a manner that emphasizes dynamic collaboration, contribution, and sharing over static information presentation.

Chapter 21
Stepping over the Edge: The Implications of New Technologies for Education

Gráinne Conole
The Open University, UK

ABSTRACT

This chapter considers the impact of Web 2.0 technologies on education and, in particular, how these new technologies are changing learning and teaching practices. It considers their fundamental characteristics and looks at the implications for learners, teachers, and institutions. It argues that the impact on practice can be both positive and negative, and that as a consequence, educational institutions need to develop new policies and strategies. The chapter concludes with two approaches to making sense of and harnessing these new technologies. The first is an example of applying Web 2.0 approaches to facilitating greater dialogue and sharing of learning and teaching ideas, through a social networking site for design. The second argues for greater use of metaphors and other forms of meaning making as a mechanism for understanding Web 2.0 technologies in an educational context.

INTRODUCTION

There is now a growing body of empirical evidence on the impact of Web 2.0 technologies on education—see, for example, the European Union (EU) study on "Learning 2.0" (Redecker, 2009; Redecker, Ala-Mutka, Bacigalupo, Ferrari, & Punie, 2009), the Becta research project examining use of Web 2.0 in schools in the UK (Crook & Harrison, 2008), the U.S. National Science Foundation's task force on cyberlearning (NSF, 2008), the most recent *Horizon* reports on future technological trends (New Media Consortium, 2008, 2009, 2010), and the Organisation for Economic Co-operation and Development's investigation into "new millennium learners" (Pedró, 2006), in addition to the various other chapters in this book. The central message across these reports and reviews is encapsulated in the following quote from a white paper on new media literacies by Jenkins, Purushotma, Clinton, Weigel, and Robison (2006):

DOI: 10.4018/978-1-60566-294-7.ch021

According to a recent study from the Pew Internet & American Life project (Lenhardt & Madden, 2005), more than one-half of all teens have created media content, and roughly one third of teens who use the Internet have shared content they produced. In many cases, these teens are actively involved in what we are calling participatory cultures ... A growing body of scholarship suggests potential benefits of these forms of participatory culture, including opportunities for peer-to-peer learning, a changed attitude toward intellectual property, the diversification of cultural expression, the development of skills valued in the modern workplace, and a more empowered conception of citizenship.

The new skills for this, according to Jenkins et al., include play, performance, simulation, appropriation, multitasking, distributed cognition, collective intelligence, judgment, transmedia navigation, networking, and negotiation. The list seems to encapsulate a lot of the potential of what Web 2.0 technologies can offer in an educational context. However, fostering these new skills suggests a need for radical transformation of the educational curriculum.

This chapter reflects on how Web 2.0 technologies are being used in education. The central focus is a critique of the impact of new technologies on education, which raises a number of key questions: What new digital literacy skills are needed? What does it mean to be a teacher or learner in this new environment? What are the implications for organizational structures and processes? What new learning spaces need to be developed to harness the potential of new technologies? The title "Stepping over the edge" is used to indicate that we are poised on the threshold of major change in education. A taxonomy of tools is used as a basis for critiquing the characteristics of Web 2.0 technologies and the associated positive and negative impacts on practice. The chapter then looks at the implications for learners (how they learn and how they are supported in their learning), teachers (how they design and assess learning), and educational institutions (in terms of the learning spaces—real and virtual—they provide for learners). Two examples of approaches to harnessing Web 2.0 technologies are then presented: (i) a description of a social networking site for discussing and sharing learning and teaching ideas; and (ii) a discussion of the types of meaning making and metaphors that might be used to better understand and represent the digital environment. The chapter concludes by considering the impact of Web 2.0 technologies on education and the potential implications for the future.

THE EVOLUTION OF TECHNOLOGIES

With a historic lens, it is evident that there are key step changes in terms of technological development that have acted as catalytic triggers in education. Cook, White, Sharples, Davis, and Sclater (2007) use Bush's (1945) seminal article "As we may think" as a starting point. In the article, Bush described the first system with hypertext capability that was in essence the forerunner of the Internet developed decades later. Following the timeline forward, there are other obvious triggers: the rise of the personal computer (PC) (and individual computer ownership); the Internet (providing access to increasing quantities of digital information and new forms of electronic communication); the uptake of institutional learning management systems (LMSs) / virtual learning environments (VLEs); mobile technologies; and, in recent years, the introduction of social networking and Web 2.0 tools (Downes, 2005; Alexander, 2006; Anderson, 2007).

Pea considers technological developments and their impact on practice in five stages (Pea, 2008; NSF, 2008, p. 11), focusing in particular on how progressive waves of technology have changed the "ether" of mediation. The first phase is "cultural mediation" (i.e., standard human communication in face-to-face settings, primarily through speech). The second phase is "symbol mediation" (i.e., through more abstract symbolic representations such as letters—alphabets and written text—and numbers—and associated mathematical language and notation). The third phase is "communication mediation" (i.e., first-wave communication technologies such as the phone, radio, and television). The fourth phase is "network mediation" (the emergence of networks and the Internet). Finally, the fifth, current phase, is described by Pea as "cyberinfrastructure mediation" (i.e., cloud computing, ubiquitous access and constant contact, smart technologies, and sensor networks). These phases emphasize the development of technologies, as well as the co-evolution of tools and users. Pea argues that as a result of these changes, how we learn has evolved substantially as well, echoing similar arguments emerging from empirical studies of the "Net Generation" (see the subsection "Implications for learners" under the "Implications" section later in this chapter, as well as Chapter 16 of this book). With respect to thinking about this in terms of designing for learning, in her presentations Diana Laurillard often quotes Wolpert (2003):

It is only with causal beliefs that technologies become possible and it was technology—the ability to physically interact with the environment—that made life easier ... The adaptive evolutionary advantage in making tools was enormous. (p. 1714)

We may argue about the subtleties of which technologies to foreground, nonetheless for each new technological development there is an associated set of ripples of change in terms of the impact on individual practices and roles, and the structure of organizations. For example, word processors signaled the demise of the traditional secretarial role, and email changed the way in which we communicate within organizations (Conole, White, & Oliver, 2007). These changes in practice work both at an individual level and at the level of organizational culture. The rise of new integrated learning environments to support students required institutions to take stock of their information technology structures and the nature of the associated support provision required for these new systems. Just when institutions were beginning to get "comfortable" with LMS/VLEs in place, Web 2.0 technologies emerged, raising fundamental issues about the balance of institutionally supported systems versus loosely coupled systems. Web 2.0 technologies challenge not only the type of technical support that institutions might provide, but also the way in which learning might be designed, delivered, and supported.

WEB 2.0 TECHNOLOGIES: FUNCTIONALITY AND IMPACT ON PRACTICE

A taxonomy developed by the author (Conole, 2006) classified tools according to how they were being used. The focus was not on the most technologically advanced, but rather on the tools that had the most radical impact on learning and teaching. Not surprisingly, word processing, email, and the Internet emerged as the tools that had made the most significant differences, changing the way people create and distribute information, altering organizational structures and associated roles with some roles disappearing and new professions emerging, and arguably even altering the very nature and worth of knowledge itself.

Table 1 lists these functional characteristics, and contrasts the original pre-2005 tools described in the aforementioned taxonomy with current Web 2.0 tools. This time divide is somewhat arbitrary, but is meant mainly as an indicative marker to signal the emergence of Web 2.0 tools. Some of the tools listed in the final column of Table 1 were around pre-2005, however their impact on practice only started to occur to any significant extent post-2005. The intention here is not to be comprehensive, but rather to provide illustrative

Table 1. Changing toolsets against functionality

Function	Tools pre-2005	Web 2.0 tools and beyond
Text and data manipulation	Word, spreadsheets, databases	Google Docs and Spreadsheets
Presentation and dissemination	PowerPoint, PDF, the HTML-based information Web	SlideShare, Flickr, YouTube, AJAX technologies, Flash animations
Data analysis	Quantitative tools (e.g., SPSS), qualitative tools (e.g., NVivo)	Tools to manipulate multimedia, enable annotation of data, and perform collaborative data analysis
Information seeking and handling	Search engines and portals	Google + Wikipedia, RSS feeds
Information storage and management	Bibliographic tools (e.g., EndNote), e-journals, repositories	Social bookmarking, blogs, wikis
Personal management	Online diary tools, to-do lists	Online shared calendar services and to-do lists ("remember the milk")
Project management	Project manager	Collaborative working environments specifically designed to support project work (e.g., SharePoint)
Communication	Email, discussion forums, chat	Audio and video conferencing (e.g., Skype, Elluminate), blogging, podcasts, microblogging (e.g., Twitter)
Visualization and brainstorming	Image manipulation tools (e.g., Photoshop), mind-mapping tools	Gliffy, sense making tools (e.g., Compendium, Cohere)
Guidance and support	Wizards, toolkits	Pedagogical planners, specialized networks and online communities, social networking sites (e.g., MySpace, Facebook, LinkedIn), immersive 3-D virtual worlds (e.g., Second Life)
Evaluation and assessment	E-assessment tools, LMS/VLEs	Shift toward personal learning environments; use of aggregators like Google, Pageflakes, and Netvibes

tools for each functional characteristic, and to consider what, if any, fundamental shifts and differences the new technologies create.

What is most noticeable in trying to map current tools to this taxonomy is that the functional classifications that were adequate to describe tools up to 2005 are inadequate to describe Web 2.0 tools. In particular, they do not reflect the core characteristics of Web 2.0 approaches (such as user-generated content, networked communities, interactivity, participation, sharing, and remixing)—practices captured in phrases such as "the wisdom of the crowds" (Surowiecki, 2004) and "the architecture of participation" (O'Reilly, 2004). Also, it is significant that many of the post-2005 tools are available as free, online services. Classification against individual functionality breaks down with Web 2.0 technologies, because they are multifaceted in nature, that is, they can be used for a range of functions, not just one specific purpose. Another feature of Web 2.0 technologies is that information can be easily transmitted between tools and services—functionality created in one tool can be embedded or made available in another. For example, the "embed" function enables SlideShare presentations or YouTube videos to be incorporated into blogs and run *in situ* in that environment. This enables users to create their own personal environments, and to consume information at locations and in formats they choose/control. The emphasis on the social and collaborative characteristics of these new tools is very prominent, as is the shift from desktop tools to web services—emphasizing the assumption that there is near-ubiquitous access to the Internet.

What can be seen with this snapshot is further evidence of the co-evolution of tools and users depicted in Pea's (2008) five stages of development, discussed earlier. Some tools remain as core elements, but aspects of their functionality change. For example, word processing is a fundamental activity as a means of manipulating existing text or creating new text. But the introduction of online tools such as Google Docs now combines some of the best features of word processors with the collaborative power of wikis, providing new ways in which people can construct knowledge. Sharing PowerPoint slides on Slideshare means that a greater audience has access to presentations, and adding audio or video to these enhances their value and potentially their uptake by others. Blogs and wikis also change the way in which we create knowledge. Blogs can be used for reflective purposes, but also can serve as personal digital repositories; they function simultaneously as personal tools and dissemination channels. Wikis enable group collaboration and co-construction of ideas. Kerawalla, Minocha, Kirkup, and Conole (2008, 2009) undertook a detailed study of students' use of blogs and identified a range of uses, tailored to individual needs. Similar patterns of appropriation and personalization occur with other tools, so each individual will have his or her own set of tools, adapted to his or her own particular needs and interests. Other tools hint at new practices and ways of doing things—such as three-dimensional (3-D) immersive virtual worlds like Second Life or new tools for visualizing and representing knowledge and creating connections and meaning, such as Compendium (Okada & Buckingham Shum, 2006) and Cohere (Buckingham Shum, 2008). The boundaries of individuals and communities blur through the interconnected nature of social networks and the blogosphere, with information being simultaneously transmitted through multiple channels to different communities and audiences.

WEB 2.0 TECHNOLOGIES IN EDUCATION

Having given a general outline of new technologies and how they can be used, this section provides an overview of their use in an educational context. The aim is not to be comprehensive; more detailed case studies and examples are provided elsewhere in this book, as well as the references provided at the very beginning of this chapter. Instead, the aim is to give a snapshot of how these technologies are being used, before moving on to consider the implications of this for learners, teachers, and educational institutions.

In a comprehensive review conducted as part of a study on "Learning 2.0" commissioned by the Institute for Prospective Technological Studies (IPTS) of the European Commission's Joint Research Centre (JRC), Redecker (2009) identified over 200 illustrative case studies of the use of Web 2.0 technologies in learning and teaching. The report developed a framework, iLANDS (innovative lands for learning), which helped conceptualize and structure the findings of the review, illustrating the ways that social computing tools are being used in education. The case studies spanned the educational spectrum from K-12 through tertiary education and into informal contexts, and covered a range of different disciplinary domains. From the cases reviewed, 16 were chosen for more in-depth analysis, focusing in particular on cases that demonstrated innovative use of technologies and those that exemplified accessibility and inclusion issues. Table 2 lists some illustrative examples.

What these examples show is the variety of ways in which the tools are being used to foster new forms of dialogue and collaboration, co-construction of knowledge, and reflection. They demonstrate how the tools are being used to satisfy different discipline needs, foster specific types of learning approaches, and address various educational challenges such as diversity, accessibility, and cultural issues.

Table 2. Examples of the use of Web 2.0 technologies in education

Project	Link
MELT (Metadata Ecology for Learning and Teaching) http://info.melt-project.eu/	Concerned with improving the quality of metadata for educational resources
Open Living Labs http://www.openlivinglabs.eu/	A European network of "living labs"
LeMill (Learning Mill) http://www.lemill.net/	A web community for finding, authoring, and sharing learning resources
Notschool http://www.notschool.net/	An online alternative to traditional schooling for disaffected children
Schome (Not School—Not Home—Schome) http://www.schome.ac.uk/	Use of virtual worlds with gifted and talented children
Welker's Wikinomics http://welkerswikinomics.wetpaint.com/	A wiki-based resource for Economics
MOSEP (More Self-Esteem with my E-Portfolio) http://www.mosep.org/	Use of e-portfolios in a range of different contexts

THE CHARACTERISTICS OF THE NEW TECHNOLOGIES AND IMPACT ON PRACTICE

Reviewing the use of Web 2.0 tools in different educational contexts, such as the examples given in the last section, provides a perspective on some of the inherent differences between these and earlier tools. Table 3 synthesizes some of the characteristics that define these new technologies and outlines their impact on practice (both positive and negative). Each of the areas of change is then covered in greater detail in the subsections that follow.

Free Resources

The Internet has enabled access to a vast amount of information, and with the advent of the open educational resources (OER) movement (Brown & Adler, 2008), access to free resources. However, finding *appropriate* resources and knowing how to use them is a specialized skill; many learners, despite being competent technology users, lack the appropriate academic literacy skills to appropriate these free resources for their learning (Lankshear & Knobel, 2007). McAndrew (2006) considered Web 2.0 characteristics and compared them against the way in which OERs are developed and used,

Table 3. Characteristics of new technologies and associated impact on practice

Change	Positive impact	Negative impact
Free resources	Specialized niche use	Inappropriate academic literacy skills
Ubiquitous access	Technology as a core tool for learning	Narrower but deeper digital divide
Multiple communication and distribution channels	Increased opportunity for peer and tutor dialogue. Information repurposed to meet different needs	Fragmentation of voice. No centralized repository of knowledge
Free tools and services	Access and personalization	Lack of institutional control
Media-rich representations	New forms of sense making	Lack of new forms of digital literacy
User-generated content and social profiling	Variety and acknowledging individual contributions. Knowledge sharing and community building	Quality assurance issues. Inappropriate descriptions and use of personal information for other purposes

with specific reference to the context of The Open University's OpenLearn (http://openlearn.open.ac.uk/) website. For example, he argues that such sites align well with the long-tail phenomenon by providing access to specialist subjects. Similarly, the social tools and features associated with the site enable users to contribute ideas and adapt content, providing an example of user-generated content—a key aspect of Web 2.0—and the broader notion of users adding value within a Web 2.0 context.

Ubiquitous Access

Web 2.0 practices rely on scale: user-generated content, the wisdom of the crowds, and collective knowledge building. Such scale requires easy access, and in this respect, in the developed world at least, we are approaching a state of near-ubiquitous access, with wireless Internet (e.g., Wi-Fi) almost universally available. The percentage of those online is approaching 100% in most developing countries, however the digital divide is still evident—narrower but deeper (Warschauer, 2003).

Multiple Communication and Distribution Channels

The variety of communicative channels and multiple distribution mechanisms for retrieving and aggregating information means that there are a multitude of opportunities for finding resources and communicating with peers and experts. However, this has also led to a "fragmentation of voice"—there is no longer one definitive source of knowledge, no one "expert." Learners need to develop strategies for finding and validating appropriate resources. Learners and teachers have a range of digital tools to use to communicate (email, chat, blogs, audio and video conferences, social networking sites, etc.); there is no single communicative channel. This multiplicity can be confusing and disorientating for those involved.

Free Tools and Services

The availability of free tools means that students can appropriate and personalize these for their individual learning needs. However, there is a tension between these tools and those under institutional control. If students are able to use free email tools, wikis, blogs, etc., what is the function of an institutional LMS? What, if any, tools and services should institutions be providing? (Dalsgaard, 2006; see also Chapter 14 in this book)

Media-Rich Representation

The richness of the new media opens up the possibility for new forms of representation, providing new opportunities in terms of sense making (Okada, Buckingham Shum, & Sherborne, 2008). However, this raises issues in terms of whether teachers and students have the appropriate digital literacy skills to utilize these representations (Brown, 2006).

User-Generated Content and Social Profiling

The user participation and social practices of Web 2.0 technologies clearly provide immense opportunities in terms of fostering collaboration for co-construction and sharing of knowledge, but raise a number of issues about quality, copyright, and privacy.

IMPLICATIONS

This section looks at some of the implications of the new technologies and the shifting patterns of use—for learners, teachers, and educational institutions. It focuses on the impact on different stakeholders within the educational system, and argues that the boundaries between roles is blurring as users adopt multiple and complex identities in the digital environment.

Implications for Learners

Students are changing in terms of how they interact with technologies and use them to support their learning. This is the overarching finding from a growing body of empirical research that looks at how students are using technologies (Conole, de Laat, Dillon, & Darby, 2008; Conole, 2008; Salaway, Caruso, & Nelson, 2007; Kennedy et al., 2006; Baird & Mercedes, 2006). This includes the research outputs of a learner experience program funded by JISC in the UK (see JISC, 2010a, 2010b for information and links to the various outputs), surveys of the use of technologies carried out in the United States, Australia, and Hong Kong, as well as a wider body of research exploring the notion of the "Net Generation." A note of caution needs to be struck, however, as this evidence is primarily from a western perspective, and the experiences of those in developing countries are likely to be fundamentally different. (Indeed, studies indicate that rather than following the regular trajectory of technological developments adopted by western countries, some developing countries "leap frog" the use of technologies, skipping a technology generation—a good example of this is the way in which mobile technologies are being used in Africa. An edited volume containing an international comparison of e-learning policy and developments supplies a valuable snapshot of the issues faced by different countries [Carr-Chellman, 2005], and a more recent handbook provides useful case studies of research and development activities in e-learning from around the globe [Andrews & Haythornthwaite, 2007].)

Nevertheless with the abovementioned caveat the evidence does point to significant changes in how students are appropriating technologies for learning, which are likely to be mirrored more broadly in time. The empirical data is compelling. Students see technologies as core tools for learning, PC and laptop ownership is high, broadband connectivity in the home the norm. They complement PC/laptop ownership with a range of mobile devices—phones and MP3 players being the most common. They use a variety of tools and resources to support their learning, appropriating these tools to their own personal preferred styles of communication and ways of learning. The Internet is their primary information resource—particularly through Google and Wikipedia, but also through suggestions from peer networks. Uptake of social networking tools is rising rapidly, from participation in social networks like MySpace and Facebook, to user-generation of content via blogs, wikis, and media sharing sites such as YouTube and Flickr. Just as some technologies are on the rise, others are in decline: TV and email are being replaced by online, on-demand video and social networking tools such as Skype and Twitter.

Kennedy, Judd, Churchward, Gray, and Krause (2008) provide a good summary of current perspectives in this area, and Michael Wesch encapsulates many aspects of today's students through his engaging YouTube videos—*Web 2.0... The machine is us/ing us* (Wesch, 2007b) and *A vision of students today* (Wesch, 2007a)—as well as through his own use of technologies in his classroom to teach digital ethnography (see, for example, Wesch, 2008). Some researchers argue that the way in which these students learn is different—that they are used to small, bite-sized chunks of information, multimodal and multifaceted representation; that they learn through experiential interaction, rather than through guided, step-by-step instruction. However, others argue that despite the fact that they have grown up immersed in these technologies, they lack the skills necessary to harness these for academic purposes. For example, they may know how to navigate the Internet to find information, but may not have the ability to critically evaluate resources and assess their academic value (see Chapter 16).

Implications for Teachers and Support Staff

In contrast to students, the change in teachers is less radical (Ertmer, 2005). While it is true that an increasing number of teachers are using technologies to support both their teaching and research, use of new technologies is far from ubiquitous, and in many instances is still in the realms of the innovators and early adopters. Some are engaging in the blogosphere and participating in communities of interest through social networking tools like Facebook or Elgg, however overall these spaces are still dominated by those with an interest in the technologies themselves, rather than mainstream academics. This is despite fairly significant investment in promoting innovations in the use of technologies in a number of countries.

Nonetheless, staff roles are changing as a consequence of the increasing impact of technologies. Teachers have to juggle a complex range of duties associated with teaching, research, and administration. The boundaries in terms of roles are no longer clear. Professional development in understanding and using technologies is more important than ever, but many institutions struggle to provide adequate and targeted support; this is further exacerbated by the fact that teachers lack the time and incentive to explore new technologies and have competing calls on their time, most notably a general drive to focus on research.

The teacher–student nexus is also under threat. In an information-rich, Web 2.0 world where the focus is on user-generated content, peer dialogue, and co-construction of knowledge, the notion of teacher as "expert" and student as "receiver" makes little sense. Therefore, there is a disjuncture between student use of the technologies and academic use, with students increasingly developing their own sophisticated personal learning environment of tools and resources to support their learning, while teachers grapple to keep up with the latest technological fad. To label it simply as a generational effect is too simplistic. More fundamental is the cultural context within which teachers work; research is still privileged over teaching, and so for many, investing the time to experiment with new technologies and apply them to their practice is a low priority. In addition, use of social tools by their nature has a peer dimension—that is, the value of use is multiplied if other peers with similar interests are using them as well; students are in peer networks, but the same cannot be said for academics. Currently, the majority of teachers are not connected in this way, and hence the potential benefits of such networks are not apparent to them. Participation in the blogosphere or via microblogging services such as Twitter, or immersion in 3-D virtual worlds, only have true value if others are contributing, and if what they are saying is of interest to you as an individual, that is, if it adds value to your practice. Academics currently struggle to see the practical benefits of these tools, being overwhelmed by the sheer quantity and potential possibilities, and intimidated by the fact that incorporation of these new approaches will require a fundamental change in their role as "teacher," along with an associated loss of authority.

Similarly, those with a support role in institutions—educational developers, technical staff, librarians, and those in strategy/policy positions—are not engaging with these new technologies to the same extent as students. Those who are enthusiastic about using technologies face a frustrating battle trying to convince their colleagues of the importance and impact of these new technologies, finding themselves contending against outdated arguments and concepts about technologies, which relate to the way things used to be and have little or nothing to do with the reality of today's digital environment. Providing the right kind of professional development to enable staff to understand and use new technologies is a major issue. What kind of support is needed? Who should do it? Who will provide ongoing support and advice? Educational developers, librarians, and learning technologists all provide aspects of this, but it is unclear what the right balance should be, and different institutions adopt different approaches. More importantly, the constantly changing support structures within institutions and reassignment of responsibility for professional development to different stakeholders in the system suggest that neither policymakers nor users are happy with the services received—workshops only skim the surface of the possibilities of how new tools can be used; advice and guidance and examples tend to be generic and never specific enough to meet an individual's needs at the time he or she requires them. How can teachers and support staff keep up with the latest in research and development in a field that is moving very fast, and where technologies are continuing to develop? Furthermore, a key characteristic of these new technologies is "learning by doing"—users need to be immersed in and "play with" the affordances that these new digital environments offer, and hence over time get a sense of how they can change practice.

(Refer to Chapter 19 in this book for more coverage of the implications of Web 2.0 for academic staff, with an emphasis on their professional development needs.)

Implications for Institutions

The rise of Web 2.0 has served to illustrate that most educational institutions are working with inappropriate and outmoded legacy systems and environments, which are fundamentally at odds with the new approaches, and any attempt to incorporate new tools into the existing mix of technologies is like opening a hornet's nest of associated problems and issues (Sheehan, 2008). There is a tension between institutionally provided systems (such as email and LMS/VLEs) and freely available web services. This is problematic from a number of perspectives (Sclater, 2008). Firstly, many institutional tools are made available to the students only for the duration of their studies. This is a particular issue for tools such as blogs and e-portfolios, which are designed to act as long-term repositories of information; students may be reluctant to commit to inputting information into an institutional system if they cannot then access it after their course has finished. Secondly, institutions tend to set very low limits on the amount of space associated with email accounts; in contrast, free services such as Google Mail (Gmail) offer unlimited space. Thirdly, many students are already using existing tools with which they are familiar and satisfied, and may not want to switch to institutional ones. Fourthly, institutional tools are often inferior in terms of richness and functionality.

However, Sclater goes on to argue that not providing *any* institutional services is not necessarily the solution. Institutions have, on the whole, developed robust support packages for the technologies they provide—including backup facilities, quick responses to malfunctions, and a range of support and help. Student-facing tools, such as LMS/VLEs, are integrated with key institutional systems such as student records, the library, and finance systems. There is usually a consistency in terms of the interface and corporate brand, and compliance with accessibility guidelines. In addition, LMS/VLEs have valuable tracking facilities, which enable teachers to monitor student activities and identify emergent patterns of use.

Just as roles are under threat, so too are organizational structures, and potentially the longer-term viability of educational institutions. The traditional structure of tertiary education institutions, in particular—into academic departments and a range of support services (finance, human resources, student services, information and support services, etc.) was designed long before the invention of the Web. As technologies have become increasingly mission critical in the last 15 years, institutions have had to engage in a continual cycle of reorganization to accommodate the impact technologies have had on their organizational processes. By and large, however, these reorganizations have tended to be piecemeal, for example involving a local review of information services or an educational development unit, rather than entailing a more holistic review of all the interconnected components of the system. Arguably, the potential impact of technologies is now so profound that more radical, systemic change is needed. If we were designing a new university from scratch, harnessing the affordances of new technologies, what would it look like? (Walton, Weller, & Conole, 2009). The information flow through the system is radically different in a digital world, and hence there is a need for reconceptualization of the best processes to support this. New ways of communicating and working together, distributing experience between real and virtual spaces, require a different way of using the physical environment—tiered lecture theatres designed for one-to-many broadcasting are immensely out of sync with these new patterns of working. The suggestion that we need radical change also infers that piecemeal, bottom-up interventions are inadequate; instead, it is likely that top-level strategy and policy are needed to ensure that the change is indeed systemic. Such strategic change will require vision and an in-depth understanding of the new media, and it is debatable as to whether most senior managers have the appropriate skills to accomplish this.

As businesses have migrated online, new business models have emerged, and it seems self-evident that the same will need to occur in education. In a world in which content and services are free, what are students actually paying for? Are there existing models that could be adapted—eBay or Amazon.com for education? Or, do we need new models tailored to the specific needs of the education system?

MAKING SENSE OF THE COMPLEXITY

So far, the chapter has provided an overview of the characteristics of new technologies and considered their impact on learners, teachers, and educational institutions. The central message is that Web 2.0 technologies are beginning to have an increasingly important influence in education, and this trend is likely to continue. The chapter has also demonstrated that there are associated issues with this increased use, and a set of unintended consequences (as illustrated in Table 2). Many learners and teachers lack the necessary new digital literacy skills to maximize their potential—for students, in terms of utilizing new technologies to support their learning; for teachers, in terms of designing educational activities using new technologies. There is little evidence at the moment of leadership at the institutional level in terms of Web 2.0-informed strategies and policies to provide appropriate digital spaces and learning environments to facilitate learning and teaching.

This section will introduce two approaches that might be helpful in terms of harnessing new technologies for learners, teachers, and institutions. The first is an example of a social networking site for finding, sharing, and discussing learning and teaching ideas. Primarily designed for teachers and support staff, this resource could equally well be used by students as a space to aggregate their learning resources, and to share and discuss them with other students. The second addresses the complexity that new technologies bring, and suggests how notions of metaphors (and other methods of meaning making) might be used to provide different lenses on the digital landscape, and to help users navigate through this space.

These examples address specific issues in an educational context. Firstly, how can we design pedagogically effective learning activities for our students that are relevant for their needs and context, and that harness the affordances of the new technologies? Secondly, how can we navigate the complex digital landscape and make sense of the space; how can we represent it and use different metaphors to describe different aspects of the activities occurring?

Example One: New Design, New Pedagogy

A fundamental feature of the new technologies is that it is no longer possible for any one individual to be an expert; teachers cannot be expected to be up to date with all the latest tools and their potential uses. The very nature of Web 2.0 is about collective wisdom—can we leverage this to provide teachers with the relevant, just-in-time support they need?

The Open University Learning Design Initiative (OULDI at http://ouldi.open.ac.uk/) has developed a suite of tools and resources to help teachers exploit new technologies for learning (Conole, 2009). These include conceptual tools, an online social networking tool called Cloudworks, and a tool for visualizing designs called CompendiumLD. Conole and Culver (2010) provide a description of the vision behind the development of Cloudworks and the first phases of design and evaluation of the site. Cloudworks adopts a Web 2.0-based philosophy, and is intended to be an evolving, dynamic community of tools, resources, and users associated with learning design. The site is based on the notion of social objects, which Engeström (2005) defines as follows:

the term "social networking" makes little sense if we leave out the objects that mediate the ties between people. Think about the object as the reason why people affiliate with each specific other and not just anyone ... The fallacy is to think that social networks are just made up of people. They're not; social networks consist of people who are connected by a shared object. (para. 3, emphasis in original)

Cloudworks is built on the premise that there is a network of social objects associated with learning design: tools, resources, approaches to design, and people. The site is designed to facilitate connections between these objects.

Figure 1 shows the home page for the Cloudworks site. Cloudworks aims to: (i) apply the best of Web 2.0 in an appropriate way to an educational context; and (ii) build on existing practice, while providing an environment that enables teachers to adopt more of a social networking approach to their practice. The core social object in Cloudworks is a "cloud." This can be anything to do with learning and teaching, and could include:

- a short description of some aspect of a teacher's practice;
- a more detailed design plan (a lesson plan, a case study, or some form of visual representation of the design);
- a resource for use in a particular teaching context, such as a learning object or open educational resources;
- a design template or a pedagogical schema (i.e., a specific structured approach to thinking about design);
- a link to a site providing information on a specific tool and how it can be used;
- a description of a design or pedagogical tool;
- a request for advice on a particular teaching problem;
- a link to a paper or research project describing a particular pedagogical intervention or approach.

Each cloud is "social" in that others can comment on it, and an evolving dialogue associated with the cloud can be generated. Anyone can browse the site, but to add clouds or comment on existing clouds, users have to register with the site. Each user has an associated profile, and any social objects users put in are automatically assigned to them, adding value to their profiles.

Clouds can be aggregated into "cloudscapes." A cloudscape can be created around a particular shared interest, event, or activity. For example, cloudscapes can be associated with conferences

Figure 1. The Cloudworks home page

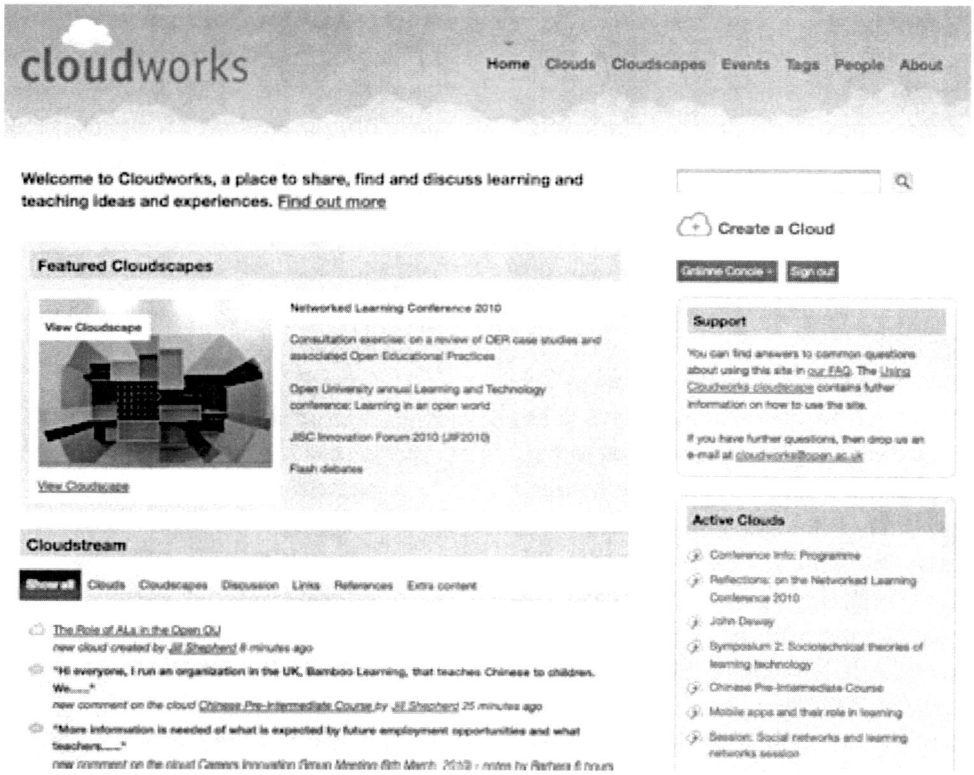

or workshops, with research projects or institutions. Cloudscapes can also be set up to aggregate and discuss clouds associated with a particular pedagogical approach, or as a space to discuss the use of a particular tool. Individuals can choose to "follow" cloudscapes and/or people; all of the social objects they are following are automatically added to their dynamic "cloudstream." Thus in a sense, Cloudworks is a combination of a Web 2.0 repository, blog, and microblog. Other functionality includes user-generated tagging, RSS feeds for different levels of the site, activity streams, user recommendations (such as voting and favorites), and connection to other sites (via links and embedding). Current technical developments include the creation of different language versions of the site, the building of an API (application programming interface) to connect with other social networking sites, and the release of an open source version.

Example Two: Navigating the Digital Space—New Metaphors for Meaning Making

A key theme of this chapter has been the complexity of the digital space. There is a need for new approaches to help navigate through the digital environment, and also to help make sense of it and the impact it is having on our lives. Simplistic descriptions of the digital environment replicating physical spaces are no longer appropriate; it is necessary to take a more holistic view and describe technologies and users together, emphasizing the connections between them. The second example focuses on how metaphors and other mechanisms for meaning making might be applied to describe technologies and how they are being used.

Metaphors are powerful ways of meaning making—how we use metaphors influences the way we think about the world around us. In their book, *Metaphors we live by*, Lakoff and Johnson (1980) suggest that metaphors not only make our thoughts more vivid and interesting, but also structure our perceptions and understanding:

We have found, on the contrary, that metaphor is pervasive in everyday life, not just in language but in thought and action. Our ordinary conceptual system, in terms of which we both think and act, is fundamentally metaphorical in nature. (p. 3)

This section will begin by considering some of the limitations of the ways in which technologies have been described to date, before suggesting some alternative approaches that emphasize the holistic, interconnected relationship between tools and users.

With the advent of the Web and the introduction of the concept of hyperlinks and connections between web pages, the notion of the digital space quickly took hold. In an educational context "virtual universities" were created, replicating real campus spaces with virtual cafés, libraries, and lecture halls. Interestingly, virtual 3-D worlds use similar ideas with the creation of islands and the replication of the physical world through virtual objects. The Windows operating system also uses a spatial metaphor, "the desktop," as a means of describing the tools and functions of the system. Windows replicates ideas of files and folders, and objects on a desk. However, the way in which we now use computers is radically different to what it was previously. Information no longer needs to be "filed" in one place—it can have multiple locations and multiple connections, and searching makes hierarchical filing redundant (Weinberger, 2007). As the patterns of use of the Internet have developed, and as tools have emerged with new functionalities resulting in changes of use and practice, simple spatial descriptions have become inadequate as a means of describing what is happening.

In addition to a spatial description, it is necessary to consider the temporal, functional, and connected properties of the digital environment. It has become evident that as in the real world, virtual space also has a temporal dimension—things happen over different timeframes, and for some activities within the virtual space it is important to be able to represent this temporal dimension. Functionality is another important facet we need to take account of. What are the different things tools can do? What are the inputs and outputs associated with different tools in use? What is the information flow through the digital space? Finally, the Web 2.0 philosophy emphasizes the social dimensions of the Web, hence means of representing connectivity are also needed. These four aspects of the digital space are described in Table 4.

Derntl, Parrish, and Botturi (2010), in describing design representations, argue that

A universal language or documentation system that will suit all these needs is likely impossible, just as no language can be taken as the medium of humankind, be it English or Esperanto, for

Table 4. Descriptions of the digital space

Focus	Aspects of the digital space this emphasizes
Spatial	Made up of objects that are connected in a typology of hyperlinks
Temporal	Evolving over time, with events happening over different timeframes
Functional	Represented as the different functions of the tools; tools acting on "data" in the system leading to transformation in some way
Connected	A connected network of different types of objects (tools, resources, people) interacting

capturing all forms of cultural expression that exist. (p. 188, emphasis in original)

With this as a given, is it possible to better articulate what different representations of the digital space are for? Moreover, are there new metaphors and forms of meaning making we should be applying to articulate new properties and patterns of use that arise as tools and users co-evolve?

Morgan's (1986) work on organizational metaphors provides a useful illustration of how notions of metaphors might be adapted and applied to understand the use of technologies. Conole, White, and Oliver (2007) provide a discussion of Morgan's metaphors in an e-learning context, focusing on five metaphors: organizations as machines (emphasizing the structural aspects of organizations), brains (adopting an information processing systems perspective), organisms (where the organization is seen as a living ecosystem), cultures (the organization is made up of mini-cultures with different customs and values), and political systems (highlighting the relationship between different interests, conflicts, and power dynamics).

Comparing these with the foci outlined in Table 4, the spatial, temporal, and functional dimensions are evident if we view the digital environment as a machine or brain. However, what is potentially very powerful is application of Morgan's notions of organism, culture, and political system. These ideas have much to offer in terms of better describing the connected nature of the Internet. In fact, the organisms metaphor is already being applied to some extent with reference to technology—researchers talk of "ecosystems" and "learning ecologies" as a means of describing the interaction of users and technologies (see, for example, Brown, 1999 and Siemens, 2003, as well as Chapter 1 in this book). Engeström (2007) also uses a biological metaphor through considering the notion of mycorrhizae as one method of understanding complex modern working practices—nodal, interconnected, mainly unseen, and distributed. Siemens (2005, 2006) proposes the notion of connectivism, maintaining that the metaphor of a network better describes the modern learning environment than the more traditional learning theories. In connectivism, learning is the process of establishing links between nodes to form a network. (See Chapters 2, 3, and 7 in this book for more on connectivism.)

These metaphors are beginning to give us new insights into the digital environment, and ways of describing what is happening. There is a need to continue to explore different metaphorical approaches. The application of the cultural metaphor could be helpful in terms of understanding different communities and their practices and values. Similarly, the political metaphor could help us to articulate power dynamics within a system and conflicts—one example of this is the tensions between institutional systems and loosely coupled free tools described earlier. Given the behind-the-scenes power dynamics that are evolving, what are the implications for practice, for instance, in the financial relationship that has been forged between Google and Wikipedia (e.g., see Rogers, 2006), altering the way information is rendered to the user? Likewise, what are the implications of restrictions in access to the Internet as a result of clampdowns in fundamentalist regimes?

In addition to metaphors, new ideas for meaning making and visualization have emerged in recent years, which can be used to make sense of the connections between the social objects in the digital space and to help users navigate through the digital environment (see, for example, Buckingham Shum & Okada, 2008 for a description of knowledge cartography for open sense-making communities). Mindmaps and visual argumentation tools are increasingly used within education, both by students and teachers. In the OULDI work, an argumentation tool, Compendium (http://compendium.open.ac.uk/), has been adapted as a tool for helping teachers to visualize learning designs (Conole, Brasher, Cross, Weller, Clark,

Figure 2. Visual design representations in CompendiumLD

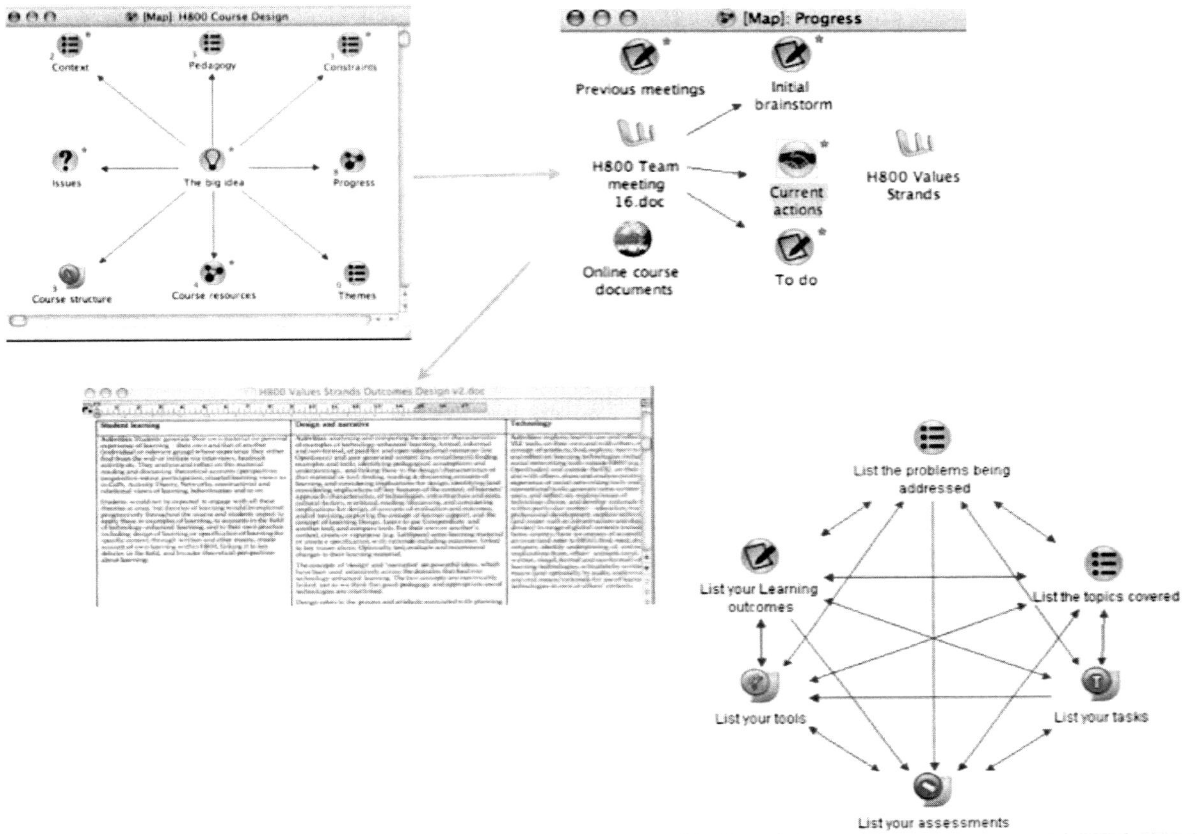

& Culver, 2008). The result is CompendiumLD (http://compendiumld.open.ac.uk/).

Figure 2 shows some of the different visual representations that can be created in CompendiumLD. The Learning Activity Management System (LAMS at http://www.lamsfoundation.org/) tool also provides a visual representation, focusing on the sequences of tasks within a learning activity. LAMS can be used not only as a design tool, but also as a runtime environment for the students. Cohere (http://cohere.open.ac.uk/) is a web-based tool in which ideas can be networked together in terms of their relationships and meaning.

These and other tools are beginning to enable us to embed more meaning in the objects and connections within the digital space. The tools can also be used to navigate through the digital space, providing particular narrative paths of meaning to address different goals or interests. In terms of education, these narrative trails could potentially be created either by the teacher or the student. In the case of the former, designs are produced by the teacher and then used as narrative trails to guide students' learning paths; in the latter case, the student actively employs these tools to construct meaning.

CONCLUSION AND IMPLICATIONS FOR THE FUTURE

Despite the hype and rhetoric, Web 2.0, and more specifically (E-)Learning 2.0, are still relatively new phenomena that have not yet penetrated mainstream education. Nevertheless, the affordances of Web 2.0 technologies and analysis of how they are beginning to be adopted in educational contexts suggest they could have a profound impact in the near future. Additionally, there are a number of potential side effects of the increased use of Web 2.0 that we need to be aware of, particularly in relation to vulnerable communities. Negative social practices like cyberbullying and online grooming are already beginning to emerge. There are also issues in terms of the "openness" of social networking, such as the ways in which disclosing personal data on sites like Facebook might then be appropriated for other purposes (see Grimmelmann, 2009 for an analysis of privacy issues associated with social networking sites). There are also issues in terms of equity of access, as well as the digital literacy skills needed to make sense of these new digital spaces and use them effectively for academic and learning purposes.

This chapter has considered the characteristics of new technologies and their impact on both organizations and individuals within an educational context. It has provided some alternative suggestions for new ways in which we can make sense of this complex landscape. This can be done through specialized tools to guide understanding, as well as through the use of different kinds of representations of the space, and metaphors to help meaning making. The chapter has argued that there are significant implications for teachers and their roles. Currently, the majority of teachers lack any personal direct experience of Web 2.0-based social software, and there are no institutional incentives for them to try out and experiment with these tools. At the institutional level, there is little evidence of a corporate understanding of these tools as well, coupled with a lack of vision for how social computing can be used. Policies on the use of Web 2.0 technologies are generally inadequate, and there is a paucity of appropriate training and support to promote greater usage of these tools.

What is evident is that uncertainty and change are the norm. It is clear that we are now working in an environment of constant flux, where the future is unpredictable and where changes appear to be ever more rapid and fundamentally radical in terms of their implications. No one individual can be an expert in all the tools and the potential ways in which they can be used. The approach needs to shift to harnessing the networked aspects of new technologies, so that individuals foster their own set of meaningful connections to support their practice, whether this be teachers seeking connections to support them in developing and delivering their teaching, or learners in search of connections to support and evidence their learning.

It has been argued in this chapter that we need to be mindful that tools do not exist in isolation, and that tools and users co-evolve. As technologies become more and more a fundamental part of our working practice, we evolve in the use of the tools and appropriate them to meet our needs, yet at the same time our own practices are evolving and being influenced/altered by the affordances of the tools and what they enable us to do.

As claimed at the start of the chapter, the implications of these new technologies for education are profound. Unintended consequences of use will arise, misuse and abuses of the system will occur, and the digital divide is still present (Warschauer, 2003)—it may be narrower, but it is getting deeper, and those not engaging with technologies or without access are getting left further and further behind. We need to be mindful that the egalitarian, liberal view of new technologies is a myth; power dynamics remain, niches develop and evolve. Applications of metaphorical notions of ecology, culture, and politics can help us better understand and deal with these complexities.

The chapter has suggested that a range of new skills is needed—for learners, teachers, support staff, and senior policymakers. They need skills to enable them to navigate through and make sense of the digital space; to cope with change and the exponential development of new tools; to deal with new notions of space, time, and boundaries; and to operate in a multifaceted and fast-moving environment. Educators have to accept that it is impossible to keep up with the rate of change, so strategies must be developed to empower individual learners to create and customize their own personal digital environments. These personal environments could consist of supporting tools and networks, selected by the student, to facilitate access to and use of relevant information for his or her needs. The new skills that are required apply across the range of stakeholders involved in education, from students to senior managers, not just a selective minority. Harnessing the potential of the technologies to provide better and more engaging learning opportunities and experiences for students should remain the ultimate goal. The challenges may be daunting, but the possibilities are truly exciting.

REFERENCES

Alexander, B. (2006). Web 2.0: A new wave of innovation for teaching and learning? *EDUCAUSE Review, 41*(2), 32–44. Retrieved December 21, 2008, from http://www.educause.edu/ir/library/pdf/erm0621.pdf

Anderson, P. (2007). *What is Web 2.0? Ideas, technologies and implications for education.* Bristol, UK: Joint Information Systems Committee. Retrieved December 21, 2008, from from http://www.jisc.ac.uk/media/documents/techwatch/tsw0701b.pdf

Andrews, R., & Haythornthwaite, C. (Eds.). (2007). *The SAGE handbook of e-learning research.* London: Sage.

Baird, D. E., & Mercedes, A. (2006). Neomillennial user experience design strategies: Utilizing social networking media to support "always on" learning styles. *Journal of Educational Technology Systems, 34*(1), 5–32. doi:10.2190/6WMW-47L0-M81Q-12G1

Brown, J. S. (1999, March 20–23). Learning, working, and playing in the digital age. Address delivered at the AAHE 1999 Conference on Higher Education, Washington, DC. Retrieved December 21, 2008, from http://www.ntlf.com/html/sf/jsbrown.pdf

Brown, J. S. (2006). New learning environments for the 21st century: Exploring the edge. *Change: The Magazine of Higher Learning, 38*(5), 18–24. doi:10.3200/CHNG.38.5.18-24

Brown, J. S., & Adler, R. P. (2008). Minds on fire: Open education, the long tail, and Learning 2.0. *EDUCAUSE Review, 43*(1), 16–32. Retrieved December 21, 2008, from http://net.educause.edu/ir/library/pdf/ERM0811.pdf

Buckingham Shum, S. (2008). Cohere: Towards Web 2.0 argumentation. In P. Besnard, S. Doutre, & A. Hunter (Eds.), *Proceedings of the 2008 Conference on Computational Models of Argument* (pp. 97–108). Amsterdam: IOS Press.

Buckingham Shum, S., & Okada, A. (2008). Knowledge cartography for open sensemaking communities. *Journal of Interactive Media in Education.* Retrieved December 21, 2008, from http://jime.open.ac.uk/2008/10/jime-2008-10.pdf

Bush, V. (1945). As we may think. *Atlantic Monthly, 176*(1), 101–108.

Carr-Chellman, A. A. (Ed.). (2005). *Global perspectives on e-learning: Rhetoric and reality.* Thousand Oaks, CA: Sage.

Conole, G. (2006). What impact are technologies having and how are they changing practice? In McNay, I. (Ed.), *Beyond mass higher education: Building on experience* (pp. 81–95). Maidenhead, UK: Society for Research into Higher Education and Open University Press.

Conole, G. (2008). Listening to the learner voice: The ever-changing landscape of technology use for language students. *ReCALL, 20*(2), 124–140. doi:10.1017/S0958344008000220

Conole, G. (2009). Capturing practice and scaffolding learning design. In Tait, A., Vidal, M., Bernath, U., & Szucs, A. (Eds.), *Distance and e-learning in transition: Learning innovation, technology and social challenges* (pp. 579–593). London and Hoboken, NJ: International Society for Technology in Education and John Wiley & Sons.

Conole, G., Brasher, A., Cross, S., Weller, M., Clark, P., & Culver, J. (2008). Visualising learning design to foster and support good practice and creativity. *Educational Media International*, *45*(3), 177–194. doi:10.1080/09523980802284168

Conole, G., & Culver, J. (2010). The design of Cloudworks: Applying social networking practice to foster the exchange of learning and teaching ideas and designs. *Computers & Education*, *54*(3), 679–692. doi:10.1016/j.compedu.2009.09.013

Conole, G., de Laat, M., Dillon, T., & Darby, J. (2008). "Disruptive technologies", "pedagogical innovation": What's new? Findings from an in-depth study of students' use and perception of technology. *Computers & Education*, *50*(2), 511–524. doi:10.1016/j.compedu.2007.09.009

Conole, G., White, S., & Oliver, M. (2007). The impact of e-learning on organisational roles and structures. In Conole, G., & Oliver, M. (Eds.), *Contemporary perspectives in e-learning research: Themes, methods and impact on practice* (pp. 69–81). London: RoutledgeFalmer.

Cook, J., White, S., Sharples, M., Davis, H., & Sclater, N. (2007). The design of learning technologies. In Conole, G., & Oliver, M. (Eds.), *Contemporary perspectives in e-learning research: Themes, methods and impact on practice* (pp. 55–68). London: RoutledgeFalmer.

Crook, C., & Harrison, C. (2008). *Web 2.0 technologies for learning at Key Stages 3 and 4: Summary report*. Coventry, UK: Becta. Retrieved June 8, 2010, from http://research.becta.org.uk/upload-dir/downloads/page_documents/research/web2_ks34_summary.pdf

Dalsgaard, C. (2006). Social software: E-learning beyond learning management systems. *European Journal of Open, Distance and E-Learning*, *9*(2). Retrieved December 21, 2008, from http://www.eurodl.org/materials/contrib/2006/Christian_Dalsgaard.htm

Derntl, M., Parrish, P., & Botturi, L. (2010). Beauty and precision: Weaving complex educational technology projects with visual instructional design languages. *International Journal on E-Learning*, *9*(2), 185–202.

Downes, S. (2005, October). E-learning 2.0. *eLearn Magazine*. Retrieved December 21, 2008, from http://www.elearnmag.org/subpage.cfm?section=articles&article=29-1

Engeström, J. (2005, April 13). Why some social network services work and others don't—Or: the case for object-centered sociality [Web log post]. *Zengestrom.com*. Retrieved December 21, 2008, from http://www.zengestrom.com/blog/2005/04/why_some_social.html

Engeström, Y. (2007). From communities of practice to mycorrhizae. In Hughes, J., Jewson, N., & Unwin, L. (Eds.), *Communities of practice: Critical perspectives* (pp. 41–54). London: Routledge. doi:10.4324/NOE0415364737.ch4

Ertmer, P. A. (2005). Teacher pedagogical beliefs: The final frontier in our quest for technology integration? *Educational Technology Research and Development*, *53*(4), 25–39. doi:10.1007/BF02504683

Grimmelmann, J. (2009). Saving Facebook. *Iowa Law Review*, *94*(4), 1137–1206.

Jenkins, H., Purushotma, R., Clinton, K., Weigel, M., & Robison, A. J. (2006). *Confronting the challenges of participatory culture: Media education for the 21st century*. Chicago: MacArthur Foundation. Retrieved December 21, 2008, from http://digitallearning.macfound.org/atf/cf/%7B7E45C7E0-A3E0-4B89-AC9C-E807E1B0AE4E%7D/JENKINS_WHITE_PAPER.PDF

Joint Information Systems Committee. (2010a). *Learner experiences of e-learning: Phase 1*. Retrieved June 8, 2010, from http://www.jisc.ac.uk/whatwedo/programmes/elearningpedagogy/learneroutcomes.aspx

Joint Information Systems Committee. (2010b). *Learner experiences of e-learning: Phase 2*. Retrieved June 8, 2010, from http://www.jisc.ac.uk/whatwedo/programmes/elearningpedagogy/learnerexperience.aspx

Kennedy, G., Krause, K.-L., Gray, K., Bennett, S., Maton, K., Dalgarno, B., & Bishop, A. (2006). Questioning the Net Generation: A collaborative project in Australian higher education. In L. Markauskaite, P. Goodyear, & P. Reimann (Eds.), *Who's learning? Whose technology? Proceedings of the 23rd Australasian Society for Computers in Learning in Tertiary Education (ASCILITE) Conference* (pp. 413–417). Sydney: University of Sydney. Retrieved December 21, 2008, from http://www.ascilite.org.au/conferences/sydney06/proceeding/pdf_papers/p160.pdf

Kennedy, G. E., Judd, T. S., Churchward, A., Gray, K., & Krause, K.-L. (2008). First year students' experiences with technology: Are they really digital natives? *Australasian Journal of Educational Technology, 24*(1), 108–122. Retrieved December 21, 2008, from http://www.ascilite.org.au/ajet/ajet24/kennedy.pdf

Kerawalla, L., Minocha, S., Kirkup, G., & Conole, G. (2008). Characterising the different blogging behaviours of students on an online distance learning course. *Learning, Media and Technology, 33*(1), 21–33. doi:10.1080/17439880701868838

Kerawalla, L., Minocha, S., Kirkup, G., & Conole, G. (2009). An empirically grounded framework to guide blogging in higher education. *Journal of Computer Assisted Learning, 25*(1), 31–42. doi:10.1111/j.1365-2729.2008.00286.x

Lakoff, G., & Johnson, M. (1980). *Metaphors we live by*. Chicago: University of Chicago Press.

Lankshear, C., & Knobel, M. (2007). Researching new literacies: Web 2.0 practices and insider perspectives. *E-learning, 4*(3), 224–240. doi:10.2304/elea.2007.4.3.224

McAndrew, P. (2006, October 26–27). *Motivations for OpenLearn: The Open University's open content initiative*. Paper presented at the OECD experts meeting on open educational resources, Barcelona. Retrieved December 21, 2008, from http://kn.open.ac.uk/public/getfile.cfm?documentfileid=10026

Morgan, G. (1986). *Images of organization*. Newbury Park, CA: Sage.

National Science Foundation. (2008). Fostering learning in a networked world: the cyberlearning opportunity and challenge. *A 21st century agenda for the National Science Foundation* (Report of the NSF task force on cyberlearning). Retrieved December 21, 2008, from http://www.nsf.gov/pubs/2008/nsf08204/nsf08204.pdf

New Media Consortium. (2008). *The Horizon Report: 2008 edition*. Austin, TX: NMC. Retrieved June 8, 2010, from http://www.nmc.org/pdf/2008-Horizon-Report.pdf

New Media Consortium. (2009). *The Horizon Report: 2009 edition*. Austin, TX: NMC. Retrieved June 8, 2010, from http://www.nmc.org/pdf/2009-Horizon-Report.pdf

New Media Consortium. (2010). *The Horizon Report: 2010 edition*. Austin, TX: NMC. Retrieved June 8, 2010, from http://www.nmc.org/pdf/2010-Horizon-Report.pdf

O'Reilly, T. (2004). *The architecture of participation*. Retrieved December 21, 2008, from http://www.oreillynet.com/pub/a/oreilly/tim/articles/architecture_of_participation.html

O'Reilly, T. (2005). *What is Web 2.0: Design patterns and business models for the next generation of software*. Retrieved December 21, 2008, from http://www.oreillynet.com/pub/a/oreilly/tim/news/2005/09/30/what-is-web-20.html

Okada, A., & Buckingham Shum, S. (2006, September 3–6). *Knowledge mapping with Compendium in academic research and online education*. Paper presented at the 22nd International Council for Open and Distance Education (ICDE) World Conference, Rio de Janeiro.

Okada, A., Buckingham Shum, S., & Sherborne, T. (Eds.). (2008). *Knowledge cartography: Software tools and mapping techniques*. London: Springer-Verlag.

Pea, R. (2008, November 6). *Fostering learning in the networked world*. Keynote presentation delivered at Becta's Research Conference 2008: Exploring technology-enabled change in education, Sheffield, UK. Retrieved December 21, 2008, from http://events.becta.org.uk/download.cfm?resID=38800&download_url=http://events.becta.org.uk/content_files/corporate/resources/events/2008/november/pea_fostering_learning.pdf

Pedró, F. (2006). *The new millennium learners: Challenging our views on ICT and learning*. Retrieved December 21, 2008, from http://www.oecd.org/dataoecd/1/1/38358359.pdf

Redecker, C. (2009). *Review of Learning 2.0 practices: Learning 2.0, the impact of Web 2.0 innovations on education and training in Europe*. Saville, Spain: Institute for Perspective Technological Studies.

Redecker, C., Ala-Mutka, K., Bacigalupo, M., Ferrari, A., & Punie, Y. (2009). *Learning 2.0: The impact of Web 2.0 innovations on education and training in Europe*. Saville, Spain: Institute for Perspective Technological Studies.

Rogers, G. (2006, March 8). Google Reference, a Wikipedia partnership? [Web log post]. *Googling Google*. Retrieved December 21, 2008, from http://www.zdnet.com/blog/google/google-reference-a-wikipedia-partnership/124

Salaway, G., Caruso, J. B., & Nelson, M. R. (2007). *The ECAR study of undergraduate students and information technology, 2007*. Boulder, CO: EDUCAUSE Center for Applied Research. Retrieved December 21, 2008, from http://www.educause.edu/ir/library/pdf/ers0706/rs/ERS0706w.pdf

Sclater, N. (2008). *Large-scale open source e-learning systems at the Open University UK*. Boulder, CO: EDUCAUSE Center for Applied Research. Retrieved December 21, 2008, from http://www.educause.edu/ir/library/pdf/ERB0812.pdf

Sheehan, M. C. (2008). *Higher education IT and cyberinfrastructure: Integrating technologies for scholarship*. Boulder, CO: EDUCAUSE Center for Applied Research. Retrieved December 21, 2008, from http://www.educause.edu/ir/library/pdf/ers0803/rs/ERS0803w.pdf

Siemens, G. (2003). *Learning ecology, communities, and networks: Extending the classroom*. Retrieved Decemeber 21, 2008, from http://www.elearnspace.org/Articles/learning_communities.htm

Siemens, G. (2005). Connectivism: A learning theory for the digital age. *International Journal of Instructional Technology and Distance Learning, 2*(1), 3–10. Retrieved Decemeber 21, 2008, from http://www.itdl.org/Journal/Jan_05/Jan_05.pdf

Siemens, G. (2006). *Knowing knowledge*. Vancouver, BC: Lulu.

Surowiecki, J. (2004). *The wisdom of crowds: Why the many are smarter than the few and how collective wisdom shapes business, economies, societies, and nations*. New York: Doubleday.

Walton, A., Weller, M., & Conole, G. (2009). SocialLearn—widening participation and sustainability of higher education. In Tait, A., Vidal, M., Bernath, U., & Szucs, A. (Eds.), *Distance and e-learning in transition: Learning innovation, technology and social challenges* (pp. 691–699). London and Hoboken, NJ: International Society for Technology in Education and John Wiley & Sons.

Warschauer, M. (2003). *Technology and social inclusion: Rethinking the digital divide*. Cambridge, MA: MIT Press.

Weinberger, D. (2007). *Everything is miscellaneous: The power of the new digital disorder*. New York: Times.

Wesch, M. (2007a, October 12). *A vision of students today* [Video file]. Retrieved June 8, 2010, from http://www.youtube.com/watch?v=dGCJ46vyR9o

Wesch, M. (2007b, March 8). *Web 2.0... The machine is us/ing us* [Video file]. Retrieved June 8, 2010, from http://www.youtube.com/watch?v=6gmP4nk0EOE

Wesch, M. (2008, June 17). *A portal to media literacy*. Guest lecture delivered at the University of Manitoba, Winnipeg, MB. Retrieved June 8, 2010, from http://umanitoba.ca/ist/production/streaming/podcast_wesch.html

Wolpert, L. (2003). Causal belief and the origin of technology. *Philosophical Transactions of the Royal Society A: Mathematical, Physical & Engineering Sciences, 361*(1809), 1709–1719.

KEY TERMS AND DEFINITIONS

Web 2.0: A term coined by O'Reilly (2005). It refers to the collective technologies associated with the Web, emphasizing the user-focused, collaborative aspects of the affordances of these technologies. It stands in contrast with the first phase of web technologies ("Web 1.0"), which were essentially information focused.

Affordances: Refers to the perceived and actual properties of a thing, primarily those functional properties that determine just how the thing could possibly be used. It originates from work on Gibson in the 1970s and has been used in relation to technological affordances in the last decade or so.

Learner Voice: A term that has come into use in recent years to describe research that is exploring the student's perspective, concerns, and right to be heard in educational design and decision making. In particular, it has been appropriated to refer to students' use and experience of learning technologies.

Metaphors: Ways to describe or make sense of things. A metaphor is a figure of speech used to help others understand something.

Meaning Making / Sense Making: The ability to make sense or meaning of a complex situation.

Learning Management System / Virtual Learning Environment (LMS/VLE): Overarching online learning and teaching systems that have become increasingly important in educational institutions in the last decade. The systems include a set of tools to support the delivery of online education, which provide facilities for communication (e.g., chat, forums), reflection and collaboration (e.g., blogs, wikis), and assessment (e.g., drop boxes for assignments, e-portfolios for aggregating learning evidence). VLE/LMSs include commercial products such as Blackboard as well as open source systems such as Moodle.

Compilation of References

Abbitt, J. T. (2007). Exploring the educational possibilites for a user-driven social content system in an undergraduate course. [from http://jolt.merlot.org/documents/abbitt.pdf]. *Journal of Online Learning and Teaching*, *3*(4), 437–447. Retrieved November 4, 2008.

Ahonen, T. T. (2008). When there is a mobile phone for half the planet: Understanding the biggest technology [Web log post]. *Communities Dominate Brands*. Retrieved February 12, 2008, from http://communities-dominate.blogs.com/brands/2008/01/when-there-is-a.html

Alberta Provincial Government. (2008). *Alberta access planning framework*. Edmonton, AB: Alberta Advanced Education and Technology.

Albrechtsen, H., Andersen, H. H. K., Bødker, S., & Pejtersen, A. M. (2001). *Affordances in activity theory and cognitive systems engineering*. Roskilde, Denmark: Risø National Laboratory.

Aldrich, C. (2006, November 20). Second Life is not a teaching tool [Web log post]. *The Learning Circuits Blog*. Retrieved October 12, 2008, from http://learningcircuits.blogspot.com/2006/11/second-life-is-not-teaching-tool.html

Alexander, S. (2001). E-learning developments and experiences. *Education + Training*, *43*(4/5), 240–248. doi:10.1108/00400910110399247

Alexander, B. (2004). Going nomadic: Mobile learning in higher education. *EDUCAUSE Review*, *39*(5), 28–35. Retrieved December 6, 2008, from http://www.educause.edu/ir/library/pdf/ERM0451.pdf

Alexander, B. (2006). Web 2.0: A new wave of innovation for teaching and learning? *EDUCAUSE Review*, *41*(2), 32–44. Retrieved December 21, 2008, from http://www.educause.edu/ir/library/pdf/erm0621.pdf

Alexander, B. (2008). Social networking in higher education. In Katz, R. N. (Ed.), *The tower and the cloud: Higher education in the age of cloud computing* (pp. 197–201). Boulder, CO: EDUCAUSE.

Allan, S. (2006). *Online news: Journalism and the Internet*. Maidenhaid, UK: Open University Press.

Allen, C. (2004, October 13). Tracing the evolution of social software [Web log post]. *Life With Alacrity*. Retrieved February 12, 2006, from http://www.lifewithalacrity.com/2004/10/tracing_the_evo.html

Allen, E. I., & Seaman, J. (2006). *Making the grade: Online education in the United States, 2006*. Needham, MA: Sloan Consortium.

Allen, E. I., & Seaman, J. (2008). *Staying the course: Online education in the United States, 2008*. Needham, MA: Sloan Consortium.

Allen, M. (1999, March). *Don't be a troll! Using the Internet for successful higher education*. Paper presented at Higher Education '99, Sydney.

Allport, C. (2001). Educating and organizing globally: Perspectives on the Internet and higher education. *Australian Universities Review*, *44*(1/2), 21–27.

Anderson, J. (2006). *The e-mature learner*. Retrieved November 29, 2008, from http://tre.ngfl.gov.uk/uploads/materials/24875/The_emature_learner_John_Anderson.doc

Anderson, P. (2007). *What is Web 2.0? Ideas, technologies and implications for education*. Bristol, UK: Joint Information Systems Committee. Retrieved January 8,

2009, from http://www.jisc.ac.uk/media/documents/techwatch/tsw0701b.pdf

Anderson, T. (2004). Toward a theory of online learning. In Anderson, T., & Elloumi, F. (Eds.), *Theory and practice of online learning* (pp. 33–60). Athabasca, AB: Athabasca University.

Anderson, T. (2007a, April 30). On groups, networks and collectives [Web log post]. *Virtual Canuck*. Retrieved July 2, 2007, from http://terrya.edublogs.org/2007/04/30/on-groups-networks-and-collectives/

Anderson, T. (2007b, June 25–29). *Social Learning 2.0*. Keynote paper presented at World Conference on Educational Multimedia, Hypermedia, and Telecommunications 2007, Vancouver, BC. Retrieved June 27, 2007, from http://www.slideshare.net/terrya/educational-social-software-edmedia-2007/

Anderson, T. (Ed.). (2008). *The theory and practice of online learning* (2nd ed.). Athabasca, AB: Athabasca University Press. Retrieved April 29, 2010, from http://www.aupress.ca/books/120146/ebook/99Z_Anderson_2008-Theory_and_Practice_of_Online_Learning.pdf

Andreasen, L. B. (2006). Weblogs as forums for discussion—an alternative to the computer conference as a standard in online learning? In Buhl, M., Holm Sørensen, B., & Meyer, B. (Eds.), *Media and ICT—learning potentials* (pp. 71–88). Copenhagen: Danish University of Education Press.

Andrews, R., & Haythornthwaite, C. (Eds.). (2007). *The SAGE handbook of e-learning research*. London: Sage.

Apple. (2008). *MobileMe*. Retrieved November 20, 2008, from http://www.apple.com/mobileme/

Apple. (2008). *Podcasting Frequently Asked Questions (FAQ)*. Retrieved October 29, 2008, from http://support.apple.com/kb/HT1597

Arenas, E. (2008). Personal learning environments: Implications and challenges. In D. Orr, P. A. Danaher, G. Danaher, & R. E. Harreveld (Eds.), *Lifelong learning: Reflecting on successes and framing futures. Keynote and refereed papers from the Fifth International Lifelong Learning Conference* (pp. 54–59). Rockhampton, Australia: Central Queensland University Press.

Argyris, C. (1999). *On organizational learning* (2nd ed.). Oxford, UK: Blackwell.

Arias, E. G., Eden, H., Fischer, G., Gorman, A., & Scharff, E. (2000). Transcending the individual human mind—creating shared understanding through collaborative design. *ACM Transactions on Computer-Human Interaction*, *7*(1), 84–113. doi:10.1145/344949.345015

Armstrong, T. (1994). *Multiple intelligences in the classroom*. Alexandria, VA: Association for Supervision and Curriculum Development.

Astin, A. (1985). *Achieving educational excellence: A critical assessment of priorities and practices in higher education*. San Francisco: Jossey-Bass.

Atkinson, R. (2006). Podcasting: Do you really need to know? *HERDSA News*, *28*(2), 20–22.

Attwell, G. (2007). Personal learning environments: The future of e-learning? *eLearning Papers*, *2*(1). Retrieved December 11, 2007, from www.elearningeuropa.info/files/media/media11561.pdf

Augar, N., Raitman, R., & Zhou, W. (2004). Teaching and learning online with wikis. In R. Atkinson, C. McBeath, D. Jonas-Dwyer, & R. Phillips (Eds.), *Beyond the comfort zone: Proceedings of the 21st Australasian Society for Computers in Learning in Tertiary Education (ASCILITE) Conference* (pp. 95–104). Perth, Australia: The University of Western Australia. Retrieved February 10, 2008, from http://www.ascilite.org.au/conferences/perth04/procs/augar.html

Augoustinos, M., & Walker, I. (1996). *Social cognition*. London: Sage.

Australian Flexible Learning Framework. (2007). *"PUT THE HARD WORD ON 'EM" campaign report*. Brisbane, Australia: AFLF. Retrieved December 15, 2007, from http://pre2009.flexiblelearning.net.au/flx/webdav/shared/NCP/HARD_WORD.pdf

Avery, S., Brooks, R., Brown, J., Dorsey, P., & O'Connor, M. (2001). Personal knowledge management: Framework for integration and partnerships. In P. Smith (Ed.), *Proceedings of the Association of Small Computer Users in Education (ASCUE) Conference* (pp. 29–39). Myrtle Beach, SC: ASCUE.

Aviram, R., & Talmi, D. (2004). *The impact of ICT on education: The three opposed paradigms, the lacking discourse*. Retrieved November 1, 2008, from http://www.elearningeuropa.info/extras/pdf/ict_impact.pdf

Baer, J. (2007, December 19). "Digital natives" under attack! (as a metaphor) [Web log post]. *Digital Natives Blog*. Retrieved December 3, 2008, from http://blogs.law.harvard.edu/digitalnatives/2007/12/19/digital-natives-under-attack-as-a-metaphor/

Baggetun, R., & Wasson, B. (2006). Self-regulated learning and open writing. *European Journal of Education, 41*(3/4), 452–473.

Baird, D. E., & Mercedes, A. (2006). Neomillennial user experience design strategies: Utilizing social networking media to support "always on" learning styles. *Journal of Educational Technology Systems, 34*(1), 5–32. doi:10.2190/6WMW-47L0-M81Q-12G1

Baker, J. R., & Moore, S. M. (2008). Blogging as a social tool: A psychological examination of the effects of blogging. *Cyberpsychology & Behavior, 11*(6), 747–749. doi:10.1089/cpb.2008.0053

Bales, R. F. (1950). A set of categories for the analysis of small group interaction. *American Sociological Review, 15*(2), 257–263. doi:10.2307/2086790

Barab, S. A., & Roth, W.-M. (2006). Intentionally-bound systems and curricular-based ecosystems: An ecological perspective on knowing. *Educational Researcher, 35*(5), 3–13. doi:10.3102/0013189X035005003

Barbera, E. (2009). Mutual feedback in e-portfolio assessment: An approach to the netfolio system. *British Journal of Educational Technology, 40*(2), 342–357. doi:10.1111/j.1467-8535.2007.00803.x

Barnes, C., & Tynan, B. (2007). The adventures of Miranda in the brave new world: Learning in a Web 2.0 millennium. *ALT-J Research in Learning Technology, 15*(3), 189–200.

Barnes, J. M. (1995, April 18–22). *Embodiment, hermeneutic, alterity, and background relations on the Internet*. Paper presented at the Annual Meeting of the American Educational Research Association, San Francisco.

Barnes, K., Marateo, R., & Ferris, S. (2007). Teaching and learning with the Net Generation. *Innovate: Journal of Online Education, 3*(4). Retrieved December 4, 2008, from http://www.innovateonline.info/index.php?view=article&id=382

Barnwal, R. (2007, January 21). Web 2.0 is all about understanding the economic value of social interaction. *AlooTechie*. Retrieved July 20, 2008, from http://www.alootechie.com/news/1977.asp

Barrett, H. C., & Garrett, N. (2009). Online personal learning environments: Structuring electronic portfolios for lifelong and life-wide learning. *Horizon, 17*(2), 142–152. doi:10.1108/10748120910965511

Barsky, E., & Purdon, M. (2006). Introducing Web 2.0: Social networking and social bookmarking for health librarians. *Journal of the Canadian Health Libraries Association, 27*(3), 65–67. Retrieved March 29, 2008, from http://article.pubs.nrc-cnrc.gc.ca/RPAS/RPViewDoc?_handler_=HandleInitialGet&calyLang=eng&journal=jchla&volume=27&articleFile=c06-024.pdf

Barth, S. (2005, October 1). Personal toolkit: A framework for personal knowledge management tools. *KMWorld*. Retrieved November 1, 2008, from http://www.kmworld.com/Authors/AuthorDetails.aspx?AuthorID=508

Bartlett-Bragg, A. (2008). Reframing assessment: Using social software to collect and organise learning. In J. Luca & E. Weippl (Eds.), *Proceedings of World Conference on Educational Multimedia, Hypermedia and Telecommunications 2008* (pp. 4020–4024). Chesapeake, VA: Association for the Advancement of Computers in Education.

Bates, A. W. (1981). Radio: The forgotten medium? Studies in the use of radio programming and audio-cassettes in Open University courses. In *Papers on broadcasting, No. 185*. Milton Keynes, UK: Institute of Educational Technology, The Open University.

Bates, A. W., & Poole, G. (2003). *Effective teaching with technology in higher education: Foundations for success*. San Francisco: Jossey-Bass.

Bates, A. W. (2000). *Managing technological change: Strategies for college and university leaders*. San Francisco: Jossey-Bass.

Batson, T. (2008, January 16). A new social context for information. *Campus Technology*. Retrieved January 18, 2009, from http://campustechnology.com/

articles/2008/01/a-new-social-context-for-information.aspx

Beaver, D. (2007). Facebook photos infrastructure [Web log post]. *The Facebook Blog*. Retrieved February 19, 2008, from http://blog.facebook.com/blog.php?post=2406207130

Beetham, H. (2007). *Learners' experiences of e-learning. A briefing for the PVC Network: e-learning Special Interest Group*. Bristol, UK: Joint Information Systems Committee. Retrieved September 6, 2008, from http://www.jisc.ac.uk/media/documents/programmes/elearningpedagogy/pspvcelearningsigbriefingpaperfinal.pdf

Beetham, H., & Sharpe, R. (Eds.). (2007). *Rethinking pedagogy for a digital age: Designing and delivering e-learning*. London: Routledge.

Beldarrain, Y. (2006). Distance education trends: Integrating new technologies to foster student interaction and collaboration. *Distance Education*, *27*(2), 139–153. doi:10.1080/01587910600789498

Beniger, J. R. (1989). *The control revolution: Technological and economic origins of the information society*. Cambridge, MA: Harvard University Press.

Benkler, Y. (2008, November/December). The university in the networked economy and society: Challenges and opportunities. *EDUCAUSE Review, 43*(6), 59–60. Retrieved January 8, 2009, from http://www.educause.edu/ir/library/pdf/ERM0866.pdf

Bennett, S., Maton, K., & Kervin, L. (2008). The 'digital natives' debate: A critical review of the evidence. *British Journal of Educational Technology*, *39*(5), 775–786. doi:10.1111/j.1467-8535.2007.00793.x

Benson, A. D., & Whitworth, A. (2007). Technology at the planning table: Activity theory, negotiation and course management systems. *Journal of Organisational Transformation and Social Change*, *4*(1), 75–92. doi:10.1386/jots.4.1.75_1

Benson, R., & Palaskas, T. (2006). Introducing a new learning management system: An institutional case study. *Australasian Journal of Educational Technology, 22*(4), 548–567. Retrieved February 19, 2008, from http://www.ascilite.org.au/ajet/ajet22/benson.html

Benzie, R. (2007, May 3). Facebook banned for Ontario staffers. *The Star*. Retrieved July 21, 2007, from http://www.thestar.com/News/article/210014

Bereiter, C. (2002). *Education and mind in the knowledge age*. Mahwah, NJ: Lawrence Erlbaum.

Berg, J., Berquam, L., & Christoph, K. (2007). Social networking technologies: A "poke" for campus services. *EDUCAUSE Review, 42*(2), 32–44. Retrieved February 3, 2008, from http://educause.edu/ir/library/pdf/erm0721.pdf

Berman, M. (1982). *All that is solid melts into air: The experience of modernity*. New York: Simon & Schuster.

Berners-Lee, T. (2000). *Weaving the Web*. New York: HarperCollins.

Berners-Lee, T. (2007, March 27). Giant Global Graph [Web log post]. *timbl's blog*. Retrieved May 23, 2008, from http://dig.csail.mit.edu/breadcrumbs/node/215

Berners-Lee, T., Hendler, J., & Lassila, O. (2001). The Semantic Web. *Scientific American*, *284*(5), 29–37. doi:10.1038/scientificamerican0501-34

Bernstein, B. (1996). *Pedagogy, symbolic control and identity: Theory, research, critique*. London: Taylor & Francis.

Beshears, F. M. (2005, October 4). Viewpoint: The economic case for creative commons textbooks. *Campus Technology*. Retrieved March 10, 2007, from http://campustechnology.com/articles/40535/

Bird, J. (2004). Professional navel gazing: Flexible learning professionals into the future. In R. Atkinson, C. McBeath, D. Jonas-Dwyer, & R. Phillips (Eds.), *Beyond the comfort zone: Proceedings of the 21st Australasian Society for Computers in Learning in Tertiary Education (ASCILITE) Conference* (pp. 123–133). Perth, Australia: The University of Western Australia. Retrieved February 12, 2008, from http://www.ascilite.org.au/conferences/perth04/procs/bird.html

Birke, S. (2007, March 19). Off to wik we go. *The Times*, 2. cellular-news. (2007, October 31). *New applications boost small/medium display market*. Retrieved February 12, 2008, from http://www.cellular-news.com/story/27086.php

Bizzell, P. (1992). *Academic discourse and critical consciousness*. Pittsburgh, PA: University of Pittsburgh Press.

Black, P., & Wiliam, D. (2006). Developing a theory of formative assessment. In Gardner, J. (Ed.), *Assessment and learning* (pp. 81–100). London: Sage.

Blaug, R. (2000). Outbreaks of democracy. In L. Panitch & C. Leys (Eds.), *Socialist Register 2000: Necessary and unnecessary utopias* (pp. 145–160). Pontypool, UK: Merlin. Retrieved November 29, 2008, from http://socialistregister.com/index.php/srv/article/view/5739/2634

Blaug, R. (2007). Cognition in a hierarchy. *Contemporary Political Theory*, *6*(1), 24–44. doi:10.1057/palgrave.cpt.9300276

Bleed, R. (2001). A hybrid campus for the new millennium. *EDUCAUSE Review*, *36*(1), 17–24. Retrieved January 20, 2008, from http://net.educause.edu/ir/library/pdf/erm0110.pdf

Blogs move student learning beyond the classroom: An interview with Alex Halavais. (2004, December). *Online Classroom*, 4, 8.

Blood, R. (2000, September 7). Weblogs: A history and perspective. *Rebecca's Pocket*. Retrieved April 29, 2010, from http://www.rebeccablood.net/essays/weblog_history.html

Boettcher, J. V. (2006, February 28). The rise of student performance content. *Campus Technology*. Retrieved November 10, 2009, from http://campustechnology.com/Articles/2006/02/The-Rise-of-Student-Performance-Content.aspx?p=1

Boorstin, D. J. (1980). *The fertile verge: Creativity in the United States. An address given at the Carnegie Symposium on Creativity, the Inaugural Meeting of the Library of Congress Council of Scholars, November 19–20, 1980.* Washington, DC: Library of Congress.

Boud, D., & Sampson, J. (1996). *Learning contracts: A practical guide*. London: RoutledgeFalmer.

Boud, D. (2000). Sustainable assessment: Rethinking assessment for the learning society. *Studies in Continuing Education*, *22*(2), 151–167. doi:10.1080/713695728

Boud, D., & Falchikov, N. (2007). Assessment in the longer term. In Boud, D., & Falchikov, N. (Eds.), *Rethinking assessment in higher education: Learning for the longer term* (pp. 4–13). London: Routledge.

Boud, D., & Lee, A. (2005). Peer learning as pedagogic discourse for research education. *Studies in Higher Education*, *30*(5), 501–516. doi:10.1080/03075070500249138m

Boyd, D. (2008). Why youth (heart) social network sites: The role of networked publics in teenage social life. In Buckingham, D. (Ed.), *Youth, identity, and digital media* (pp. 119–142). Cambridge, MA: MIT Press.

Boyd, D. (2007). The significance of social software. In Burg, T. N., & Schmidt, J. (Eds.), *BlogTalks reloaded: social software research & cases* (pp. 15–30). Norderstedt, Germany: Books on Demand.

Boyd, D. (2008). None of this is real. In Karaganis, J. (Ed.), *Structures of participation in digital culture* (pp. 132–157). New York: Social Science Research Council.

Boyd, D. (2005). Why Web 2.0 matters: Preparing for glocalization [Web log post]. *apophenia*. Retrieved March 17, 2008, from http://www.zephoria.org/thoughts/archives/2005/09/05/why_web20_matte.html

Boyd, D. (2008, January 16). The Economist debate on social "networking" [Web log post]. *Futurelab*. Retrieved March 3, 2009, from http://blog.futurelab.net/2008/01/the_economist_debate_on_social.html

Boyd, D. M. (2004). Friendster and publicly articulated social networking. In E. Dykstra-Erickson & M. Tscheligi (Eds.), *Proceedings of the SIGCHI Conference on Human Factors in Computing Systems* (pp. 1279–1282). New York: Association for Computing Machinery.

Boyd, D. M., & Ellison, N. B. (2007). Social network sites: Definition, history, and scholarship. *Journal of Computer-Mediated Communication, 13*(1). Retrieved October 11, 2008, from http://jcmc.indiana.edu/vol13/issue1/boyd.ellison.html

Brabazon, T. (2002). Point, click and graduate: Student motivation in the information age. In *Digital hemlock: Internet education and the poisoning of teaching* (pp. 128–152). Sydney: University of New South Wales Press.

Braun, V., & Clarke, V. (2006). Using thematic analysis in psychology. *Qualitative Research in Psychology*, *3*(2), 77–101. doi:10.1191/1478088706qp063oa

Broadfoot, P., Daugherty, R., Gardner, J., Harlen, W., James, M., & Stobart, G. (2002). *Assessment for learning: 10 principles, Research-based principles to guide classroom practice*. London: Assessment Reform Group. Retrieved October 29, 2009, from http://www.assessment-reform-group.org/CIE3.PDF

Brown, J. S., & Adler, R. P. (2008). Open education, the long tail, and Learning 2.0. *EDUCAUSE Review*, *43*(1), 18–32.

Brown, J. S., Collins, A., & Duguid, P. (1989). Situated cognition and the culture of learning. *Educational Researcher*, *18*(1), 32–42.

Brown, J. S., & Duguid, P. (2002). *The social life of information*. Boston: Harvard Business School Press.

Brown, J. S. (2006). New learning environments for the 21st century: Exploring the edge. *Change: The Magazine of Higher Learning*, *38*(5), 18–24. doi:10.3200/CHNG.38.5.18-24

Brown, J. S. (1999, March 20–23). Learning, working, and playing in the digital age. Address delivered at the AAHE 1999 Conference on Higher Education, Washington, DC. Retrieved December 21, 2008, from http://www.ntlf.com/html/sf/jsbrown.pdf

Brown, J. S., & Adler, R. P. (2008). Minds on fire: Open education, the long tail, and Learning 2.0. *EDUCAUSE Review, 43*(1), 16–32. Retrieved December 21, 2008, from http://net.educause.edu/ir/library/pdf/ERM0811.pdf

Brown, T. H. (2005). Beyond constructivism: Exploring future learning paradigms. *Education Today, 2005*(2). Retrieved January 11, 2006, from http://www.bucks.edu/IDlab/Beyond_constructivism.pdf

Brownstein, E., & Klein, R. (2006). Blogs: Application in science education. *Journal of College Science Teaching*, *35*(6), 18–22.

Bruner, J. (2003). The narrative construction of reality. In Mateas, M., & Sengers, P. (Eds.), *Narrative intelligence* (pp. 41–62). Amsterdam: John Benjamins.

Bruner, J. S. (1982). The organization of action and the nature of adult–infant transaction. In von Cranach, M., & Harré, R. (Eds.), *The analysis of action* (pp. 313–327). Cambridge, UK: Cambridge University Press.

Bruns, A. (2005). *Gatewatching: Collaborative online news production*. New York: Peter Lang.

Bruns, A. (2008). *Blogs, Wikipedia, Second Life, and beyond: From production to produsage*. New York: Peter Lang.

Bruns, A., & Humphreys, S. (2005). Wikis in teaching and assessment: the M/Cyclopedia project. In D. Riehle (Ed.), *Proceedings of the 2005 International Symposium on Wikis* (pp. 25–32). New York: Association for Computing Machinery. Retrieved June 6, 2008, from http://www.wikisym.org/ws2005/proceedings/paper-03.pdf

Bruns, A., & Humphreys, S. (2007). Building collaborative capacities in learners: The M/cyclopedia project revisited. In A. Désilets & R. Biddle (Eds.), *Proceedings of the 2007 International Symposium on Wikis* (pp. 1–10). New York: Association for Computing Machinery. Retrieved November 4, 2008, from http://www.wikisym.org/ws2007/_publish/Bruns_WikiSym2007_MCyclopedia.pdf

Bruns, A., & Jacobs, J. (Eds.). (2006). *Uses of blogs*. New York: Peter Lang. Chowcat, I., Phillips, B., Popham, J., & Jones, I. (2008, July) *Harnessing technology: Preliminary identification of trends affecting the use of technology for learning*. Coventry, UK: Becta. Retrieved February 12, 2009, from http://emergingtechnologies.becta.org.uk/upload-dir/downloads/page_documents/partners/ht_trends_july08.pdf

Bryant, L. (2007). Emerging trends in social software for education. In *Emerging technologies for learning* (Vol. 2, pp. 9–18). Coventry, UK: Becta. Retrieved October 28, 2008, from http://partners.becta.org.uk/upload-dir/downloads/page_documents/research/emerging_technologies07_chapter1.pdf

Bryant, T. (2006). Social software in academia. *EDUCAUSE Quarterly, 29*(2), 61–64. Retrieved March 14, 2008, from http://net.educause.edu/ir/library/pdf/eqm0627.pdf

Buckingham, D. (2007). Digital media literacies: Rethinking media education in the age of the Internet. *Research in Comparative and International Education*, *2*(1), 43–55. doi:10.2304/rcie.2007.2.1.43

Buckingham, D. (2006). Defining digital literacy. *The Nordic Journal of Digital Literacy*, *1*(4), 263–276.

Buckingham Shum, S. (2008). Cohere: Towards Web 2.0 argumentation. In P. Besnard, S. Doutre, & A. Hunter (Eds.), *Proceedings of the 2008 Conference on Computational Models of Argument* (pp. 97–108). Amsterdam: IOS Press.

Buckingham Shum, S., & Okada, A. (2008). Knowledge cartography for open sensemaking communities. *Journal of Interactive Media in Education*. Retrieved December 21, 2008, from http://jime.open.ac.uk/2008/10/jime-2008-10.pdf

Bulik, B. S. (2008). Does your company need a chief blogger? *Advertising Age*, *79*(15), 24.

Bumgardner, J. (2006). *Building tag clouds in Perl and PHP*. Cambridge, MA: O'Reilly.

Burger, T. N. (2007, January 22). Libraries facilitate open access to information with open source software. *Linux.com*. Retrieved August 29, 2008, from http://www.linux.com/articles/59491

Burgess, J. (2006). Blogging to learn, learning to blog. In Bruns, A., & Jacobs, J. (Eds.), *Uses of blogs* (pp. 105–114). New York: Peter Lang.

Burgos, D., Tattersall, C., & Koper, R. (2007). Re-purposing existing generic games and simulations for e-learning. *Computers in Human Behavior*, *23*(6), 2656–2667. doi:10.1016/j.chb.2006.08.002

Bush, V. (1945). As we may think. *Atlantic Monthly*, *176*(1), 101–108.

Butler, C. K. (2006). Blogging their way through academe. *U.S. News & World Report*, *140*(13), 48–51.

Butterfield, S. (2003, March 24). An article complaining about 'social software' and a rebuttal from Ross Mayfield [Web log post]. *Syllogue*. Retrieved February 10, 2006, from http://www.sylloge.com/personal/2003_03_01_s.html#91273866

Byron, M. (2005). Teaching with Tiki. *Teaching Philosophy*, *28*(2), 108–113.

Calvani, A. (2005). *Reti, comunità e conoscenza: Costruire e gestire dinamiche collaborative (Networks, community and knowledge: Building and managing dynamic collaboration)*. Trento, Italy: Erickson.

Cameron, M., & Fox, J. (2007, September 4–6). *Whose e-learning is it anyway? A case study exploring the boundaries between social networks and VLE courses*. Paper presented at the 14th Association for Learning Technology Conference, Nottingham, UK.

Campbell, G. (2007). *Jon Udell's interviews with innovators*. Retrieved December 20, 2007, from http://itc.conversationsnetwork.org/shows/detail3451.html

Candy, P. (1991). *Self-direction for lifelong learning*. San Francisco: Jossey-Bass.

Candy, P. (2002). *Information literacy and lifelong learning* [White paper]. Prague, The Czech Republic: UNESCO.

Carmichael, J. (2005, November 3). A new deal for fireside chats? *Teachers College Record*. Retrieved December 29, 2008, from http://www.tcrecord.org/Content.asp?ContentId=12231

Carr, W., & Kemmis, S. (1986). *Becoming critical: Knowing through action research*. Geelong, Australia: Deakin University Press.

Carr-Chellman, A. A. (Ed.). (2005). *Global perspectives on e-learning: Rhetoric and reality*. Thousand Oaks, CA: Sage.

Carrick Institute for Learning and Teaching in Higher Education. (2007). *Places & spaces for learning seminars*. (Draft report). Retrieved November 13, 2009, from http://www.altc.edu.au/system/files/resources/Consolidated%20Report%20P%20%20S%20Seminars%20without%20slides%20ref%20v%200%205%20_5_.pdf

Carroll, D. (2008). Dorion Carroll: Technorati. In Jones, B. L. (Ed.), *Web 2.0 heroes: Interviews with 20 Web 2.0 influencers* (pp. 55–78). Indianapolis, IN: Wiley.

Carter, S. M., & Little, M. (2007). Justifying knowledge, justifying method, taking action: Epistemologies, methodologies, and methods in qualitative research. *Qualitative Health Research*, *17*(10), 1316–1328. doi:10.1177/1049732307306927

Case, R. (1996). Changing views of knowledge and their impact on educational research and practice. In Olson, D. R., & Torrance, N. (Eds.), *The handbook of education and human development* (pp. 75–99). Cambridge, MA: Blackwell.

Caspersz, D., Skene, J., & Wu, M. T. W. (2006). Managing cultural diversity in student teams: A proposed conceptual framework. In A. Bunker & I. Vardi (Eds.), *Critical visions: Thinking, learning and researching in Higher Education. Proceedings of the 29th Higher Education Research and Development Society of Australasia (HERDSA) Annual Conference* (pp. 73–80). Milperra, Australia: HERDSA. Retrieved December 13, 2007, from http://www.herdsa.org.au/wp-content/uploads/conference/2006/Caspersz.PDF

Castells, M. (2001). *The Internet galaxy: Reflections on the Internet, business, and society*. New York: Oxford University Press.

Castells, M. (1996). *The rise of the network society*. Oxford, UK: Blackwell.

Centre for Information Behaviour and the Evaluation of Research. (2008). *Information behaviour of the researcher of the future*. London: CIBER, University College London. Retrieved December 6, 2008, from http://www.bl.uk/news/pdf/googlegen.pdf

Chalmers, M. (2004). A historical view of context. *Computer Supported Cooperative Work, 13*(3/4), 223–247. doi:10.1007/s10606-004-2802-8

Chan, A., & Lee, M. J. W. (2005). An MP3 a day keeps the worries away: Exploring the use of podcasting to address preconceptions and alleviate pre-class anxiety amongst undergraduate information technology students. In D. H. R. Spennemann & L. Burr (Eds.), *Good practice in practice: Proceedings of the Student Experience Conference* (pp. 58–70). Wagga Wagga, Australia: Charles Sturt University. Retrieved November 30, 2005, from http://www.csu.edu.au/division/studserv/sec/papers/chan.pdf

Chan, A., & McLoughlin, C. (2007). Choice, communication and learner autonomy: The development of social competence skills using podcasting technologies. In R. Atkinson & C. McBeath (Eds.), *ICT: Providing choices for learners and learning. Proceedings of the 24th Australasian Society for Computers in Learning in Tertiary Education (ASCILITE) Conference* (pp. 132–134). Singapore: Nanyang Technological University. Retrieved April 23, 2008, from http://www.ascilite.org.au/conferences/singapore07/procs/chan-poster.pdf

Chan, A., Frydenberg, M., & Lee, M. J. W. (2007). Facilitating cross-cultural learning through collaborative skypecasting. In J. J. Ekstrom (Ed.), *Proceedings of the 2007 ACM Information Technology Education Conference* (pp. 59–66). New York: Association for Computing Machinery.

Chang, Y.-F., & Schallert, D. L. (2005). The design for a collaborative system of English as foreign language composition writing of senior high school students in Taiwan. In P. Goodyear, D. Sampson, D. J.-T. Yang, Kinshuk, T. Okamoto, R. Hartley, & N.-S. Chen (Eds.), *Proceedings of the Fifth IEEE International Conference on Advanced Learning Technologies* (pp. 774–775). Los Alamitos, CA: IEEE Computer Society.

Chemero, A. (2003). An outline of a theory of affordances. *Ecological Psychology, 15*(2), 181–195. doi:10.1207/S15326969ECO1502_5

Chickering, A., & Gamson, Z. (1987). Seven principles for good practice in undergraduate education. *AAHE Bulletin, 39*(7), 3–7.

Chickering, A. W., & Ehrmann, S. C. (1996). Implementing the seven principles: Technology as lever. *AAHE Bulletin, 49*(2), 3–6. Retrieved June 22, 2008, from http://www.tltgroup.org/programs/seven.html

Child, M. L. (2007, February 26). Professors split on wiki debate. *The Harvard Crimson*. Retrieved November 6, 2008, from http://www.thecrimson.com/article.aspx?ref=517305

Chowcat, I., Phillips, B., Popham, J., & Jones, I. (2008, July) *Harnessing technology: Preliminary identification of trends affecting the use of technology for learning*. Coventry, UK: Becta. Retrieved January 19, 2009, from http://emergingtechnologies.becta.org.uk/upload-dir/downloads/page_documents/partners/ht_trends_july08.pdf

Chu, M., & Meulemans, Y. N. (2008). The problems and potential of MySpace and Facebook usage in academic libraries. *Internet Reference Services Quarterly, 13*(1), 69–85. doi:10.1300/J136v13n01_04

Churchill, D., & Hedberg, J. (2008). Learning object design considerations for small-screen handheld devices. *Computers & Education, 50*(3), 881–893. doi:10.1016/j.compedu.2006.09.004

Cigognini, M. E., Mangione, G. R., & Pettenati, M. C. (2007a). E-learning design nell'apprendimento (in) formale (E-learning design for (in)formal learning). *TD: Tecnologie Didattiche, 41*, 16–22. Retrieved November 1, 2008, from http://www.tdmagazine.itd.cnr.it/PDF41/4_Cigognini_Mangione_Pettenati_TD41.pdf

Cigognini, M. E., Mangione, G. R., & Pettenati, M. C. (2007b, September 5–6). *Favouring a critical, creative and ethical use of the network resources through Web 2.0 applications*. Paper presented at the Towards a Social Science of Web 2.0 Conference, York, UK. Retrieved October 24, 2007, from http://www.york.ac.uk/res/siru/web2.0/cigognini.htm

Cigognini, M. E., Pettenati, M. C., & Paoletti, G. (2008). Personal knowledge management skills model for expert lifelong learners: A validation method. In J. M. Nunes & M. A. McPherson (Eds.), *Proceedings of the IADIS International Conference e-Learning 2008* (pp. 215–222). Lisbon: International Association for Development of the Information Society.

Cigognini, M. E., Pettenati, M. C., Paoletti, G., & Edirisingha, P. (2008, June 11–14). *Guiding learners to become knowledgeable Learners 2.0*. Paper presented at the European Distance and E-learning Network (EDEN) 2008 Annual Conference, Lisbon, Portugal.

Clark, W., Logan, K., Luckin, R., Mee, A., & Oliver, M. (2009). Beyond Web 2.0: Mapping the technology landscapes of young learners. *Journal of Computer Assisted Learning, 25*(1), 56–69. doi:10.1111/j.1365-2729.2008.00305.x

Clark, D., & Walsh, S. (2004). *iPod-learning*. Brighton, UK: Epic Group.

Clarke, D. (2003, April 21–25). *Practice, role and position: Whole class patterns of participation*. Paper presented at the Annual Meeting of the American Educational Research Association, Chicago.

Clausen, S. K., & Jacobsen, M. K. (2008). *Læringspotentialer i social software* (Learning potential in social software). Unpublished Master's thesis, Aalborg University, Aalborg, Denmark.

Cluett, L., & Skene, J. (2007). A new(er) dimension to online learning communities: Using web tools to engage students. In R. Atkinson & C. McBeath (Eds.), *Student engagement: Proceedings of the 16th Annual Teaching Learning Forum*. Perth, Australia: The University of Western Australia. Retrieved April 23, 2008, from http://lsn.curtin.edu.au/tlf/tlf2007/refereed/cluett.html

Cluett, L., Skene, J., & Hogan, J. (2007). *The NODE summary report: Findings of a 2006–07 survey into UWA students' experiences with, access to and expectations of ICT*. Perth, Australia: Univesity of Western Australia. Retrieved April 23, 2008, from http://www.student-services.uwa.edu.au/ss/learning/networking_smarter/llrs_projects/publications?f=249629

Coates, H., James, R., & Baldwin, G. (2005). A critical examination of the effects of learning management systems on university teaching and learning. *Tertiary Education and Management, 11*(1), 19–36.

Cochrane, T. (2008). Mobile Web 2.0: The new frontier. In R. Atkinson & C. McBeath (Eds.), *Hello! Where are you in the landscape of educational technology? Proceedings of the 25th Australasian Society for Computers in Learning in Tertiary Education (ASCILITE) Conference* (pp. 177–186). Melbourne, Australia: Deakin University. Retrieved December 3, 2008, from http://www.ascilite.org.au/conferences/melbourne08/procs/cochrane.pdf

Cole, M. (1990). Cognitive development and formal schooling: The evidence from cross-cultural research. In Moll, L. C. (Ed.), *Vygotsky and education: Instructional implications and applications of sociohistorical psychology* (pp. 89–110). Cambridge, UK: Cambridge University Press.

Collis, B., & Moonen, J. (2008). Web 2.0 tools and processes in higher education: Quality perspectives. *Educational Media International, 45*(2), 93–106. doi:10.1080/09523980802107179

Commission of the European Communities. (2000). *A memorandum on lifelong learning*. Commission staff working paper. Brussels: European Commission. Retrieved November 1, 2008, from http://www.bologna-berlin2003.de/pdf/MemorandumEng.pdf

Commission of the European Communities. (2007). *e-Skills for the 21st century: Fostering competitiveness, growth and jobs*. Communication from the Commission to the Council, the European Parliament, the European Economic and Social Committee and the Committee of the Regions. Brussels: European Commission. Retrieved November 1, 2008, from http://ec.europa.eu/enterprise/sectors/ict/files/comm_pdf_com_2007_0496_f_en_acte_en.pdf

Community College Survey of Student Engagement. (2007). *Committing to student engagement: Reflections on CCSSE's first five years. 2007 findings*. Austin, TX: Community College Leadership Program, The University of Texas at Austin. Retrieved December 6, 2008, from http://www.ccsse.org/publications/2007NatlRpt-final.pdf

comScore. (2007). *Social networking goes global*. Retrieved March 3, 2009, from http://www.comscore.com/Press_Events/Press_Releases/2007/07/Social_Networking_Goes_Global

comScore. (2008, February 8). *U.S. Internet users viewed 10 billion videos online in record-breaking month of December, according to comScore video matrix*. Retrieved February 22, 2008, from http://www.comscore.com/press/release.asp?press=2051

Conference Board of Canada. (1991). *Employability skill profile: The critical skills required of the Canadian workforce*. Ottawa, ON: Conference Board of Canada.

Conference Board of Canada. (2008). *Canada's "missing" trade with Asia*. Ottawa, ON: Conference Board of Canada.

Conole, G., & Dyke, M. (2004). What are the affordances of information and communication technologies? *ALT-J Research in Learning Technology*, *12*(2), 113–124.

Conole, G. (2008). Listening to the learner voice: The ever-changing landscape of technology use for language students. *ReCALL*, *20*(2), 124–140. doi:10.1017/S0958344008000220

Conole, G., Brasher, A., Cross, S., Weller, M., Clark, P., & Culver, J. (2008). Visualising learning design to foster and support good practice and creativity. *Educational Media International*, *45*(3), 177–194. doi:10.1080/09523980802284168

Conole, G., & Culver, J. (2010). The design of Cloudworks: Applying social networking practice to foster the exchange of learning and teaching ideas and designs. *Computers & Education*, *54*(3), 679–692. doi:10.1016/j.compedu.2009.09.013

Conole, G., de Laat, M., Dillon, T., & Darby, J. (2008). "Disruptive technologies", "pedagogical innovation": What's new? Findings from an in-depth study of students' use and perception of technology. *Computers & Education*, *50*(2), 511–524. doi:10.1016/j.compedu.2007.09.009

Conole, G., White, S., & Oliver, M. (2007). The impact of e-learning on organisational roles and structures. In Conole, G., & Oliver, M. (Eds.), *Contemporary perspectives in e-learning research: Themes, methods and impact on practice* (pp. 69–81). London: RoutledgeFalmer.

Conole, G. (2006). What impact are technologies having and how are they changing practice? In McNay, I. (Ed.), *Beyond mass higher education: Building on experience* (pp. 81–95). Maidenhead, UK: Society for Research into Higher Education and Open University Press.

Conole, G. (2009). Capturing practice and scaffolding learning design. In Tait, A., Vidal, M., Bernath, U., & Szucs, A. (Eds.), *Distance and e-learning in transition: Learning innovation, technology and social challenges* (pp. 579–593). London and Hoboken, NJ: International Society for Technology in Education and John Wiley & Sons.

Conole, G. (2004). E-learning: The hype and the reality. *Journal of Interactive Media in Education*. Retrieved February 22, 2008, from http://www-jime.open.ac.uk/2004/12/conole-2004-12.pdf

Conole, G., & Creanor, L. (2007). *In their own words: Exploring the learner's perspective on e-learning*. Bristol, UK: Joint Information Systems Committee. Retrieved December 6, 2008, from http://www.jisc.ac.uk/media/documents/programmes/elearningpedagogy/iowfinal.pdf

Conole, G., de Laat, M., Dillon, T., & Darby, J. (2006). *JISC LXP: Student experiences of technologies. Final report*. Bristol, UK: Joint Information Systems Committee. Retrieved September 23, 2008, from http://www.jisc.ac.uk/media/documents/programmes/elearningpedagogy/lxpprojectfinalreportdec06.pdf

Converso, J. A., Schaffer, S. P., & Guerra, I. J. (1999). *Distributed learning environment: Major functions, implementation, and continuous improvement*. Tallahassee, FL: Learning Systems Institute, Florida State University.

Cook, J., White, S., Sharples, M., Davis, H., & Sclater, N. (2007). The design of learning technologies. In Conole,

G., & Oliver, M. (Eds.), *Contemporary perspectives in e-learning research: Themes, methods and impact on practice* (pp. 55–68). London: RoutledgeFalmer.

Copley, J. (2007). Audio and video podcasts of lectures for campus-based students: Production and evaluation of student use. *Innovations in Education and Teaching International, 44*(4), 387–399. doi:10.1080/14703290701602805

Cormier, D. (2008). Rhizomatic education: Community as curriculum. *Innovate: Journal of Online Education, 4*(5). Retrieved July 2, 2008, from http://www.innovateonline.info/index.php?view=article&id=550

Cormode, G., & Krishnamurthy, B. (2008). Key differences between Web 1.0 and Web 2.0. *First Monday, 13*(6). Retrieved April 30, 2009, from http://www.uic.edu/htbin/cgiwrap/bin/ojs/index.php/fm/article/viewArticle/2125/1972

Creanor, L., Trinder, K., Gowan, D., & Howells, C. (2006). *LEX: The Learner Experience of e-Learning—Final project report*. Bristol, UK: Joint Information Systems Committee. Retrieved December 3, 2008, from http://www.jisc.ac.uk/uploaded_documents/LEX%20Final%20Report_August06.pdf

Creswell, J. W. (2002). *Educational research: Planning, conducting, and evaluating quantitative and qualitative research*. Upper Saddle River, NJ: Pearson Education.

Cronje, J. (2006). Real learning in virtual environments. In Martin, A., & Madigan, D. (Eds.), *Digital literacies for learning* (pp. 34–41). London: Facet.

Cronon, W. (1998). "Only Connect ... " The goals of a liberal education. *The American Scholar, 67*(4), 73–80.

Crook, C. (1994). *Computers and the collaborative experience of learning*. London: Routledge.

Crook, C. (1999). Computers in the community of classrooms. In Light, P., & Littleton, K. (Eds.), *Learning with computers: Analysing productive interaction* (pp. 102–117). London: Routledge.

Crook, C. (2008). *Web 2.0 technologies for learning: The current landscape—opportunities, challenges and tensions*. Coventry, UK: Becta. Retrieved January 10, 2009, from http://research.becta.org.uk/upload-dir/downloads/page_documents/research/web2_technologies_learning.pdf

Crook, C., & Harrison, C. (2008). *Web 2.0 technologies for learning at Key Stages 3 and 4: Summary report*. Coventry, UK: Becta. Retrieved June 8, 2010, from http://research.becta.org.uk/upload-dir/downloads/page_documents/research/web2_ks34_summary.pdf

Crowe, C., & Tonkin, J. (2006). Fifteen megabytes of fame blogging, learning and assessment. *Synergy*, 24. Retrieved December 20, 2006, from http://www.itl.usyd.edu.au/synergy/article.cfm?articleID=287

Cubric, J. (2007). Wiki-based process framework for blended learning. In A. Désilets & R. Biddle (Eds.), *Proceedings of the 2007 International Symposium on Wikis* (pp. 11–24). New York: Association for Computing Machinery. Retrieved November 4, 2008, from http://www.wikisym.org/ws2007/_publish/Cubric_WikiSym2007_BlendedLearningFramework.pdf

Cunningham, W., & Leuf, B. (2001). *The wiki way: Quick collaboration on the Web*. New York: Addison-Wesley.

Curry, A. (2004). *iPodder—A brief history*. Retrieved April 23, 2005, from http://www.ipodder.org/history

Dabbagh, N. (2002). Evolution of authoring tools. *Educational Technology, 42*(4), 24–32.

Dabbagh, N. (2004). Distance learning: Emerging pedagogical issues and learning designs. *Quarterly Review of Distance Education, 5*(1), 37–49.

Dabbagh, N., & Bannan-Ritland, B. (2005). *Online learning: Concepts, strategies, and application*. Upper Saddle River, NJ: Prentice Hall.

Dabbagh, N., & Benson, A. (2007). Technology, globalization, and distance education: Pedagogical models and constructs. In Levy, J., Thompson, J., & Hayden, M. (Eds.), *Handbook of Research in International Education* (pp. 188–198). Thousand Oaks, CA: Sage.

Dalsgaard, C. (2006). Social software: E-learning beyond learning management systems. *European Journal of Open, Distance and E-Learning, 9*(2). Retrieved April 29, 2010, from http://www.eurodl.org/materials/contrib/2006/Christian_Dalsgaard.htm

Dalsgaard, C., & Mathiasen, H. (2008). Self-organized learning environments and university students' use of social software: A systems theoretical perspective. *International Journal of Instructional Technology and*

Distance Learning, 5(2), 3–15. Retrieved April 29, 2010, from http://itdl.org/Journal/Feb_08/Feb_08.pdf

Daniels, H. (2001). *Vygotsky and pedagogy*. London: RoutledgeFalmer.

Darbyshire, P., & Burgess, S. (2006). Strategies for dealing with plagiarism and the Web in higher education. *Journal of Business Systems, Governance and Ethics, 1*(4), 27–39. Retrieved April 2, 2007, from http://www.jbsge.vu.edu.au/issues/vol01no4/Darbyshire-Burgess.pdf

Davi, A., Frydenberg, M., & Gulati, G. J. (2007). Blogging across the disciplines: Integrating technology to enhance liberal learning. *Journal of Online Learning and Teaching, 3*(3), 222–233. Retrieved November 4, 2008, from http://jolt.merlot.org/vol3no3/frydenberg.pdf

Davis, A. (2009, January 3). Friended by Mom and Dad on Facebook. *ABC News*. Retrieved February 14, 2009, from http://abcnews.go.com/OnCampus/story?id=6555853&page=1

Davis, M. (2008). *Semantic wave 2008 report: Industry roadmap to Web 3.0 & multibillion dollar market opportunities. Executive Summary.* Washington, DC: Project 10X.

Davydov, V. (1995). The influence of L. S. Vygotsky on education theory, research, and practice. (S. T. Kerr, Trans.). *Educational Researcher, 24*(3), 12–21.

de Byl, P., & Taylor, J. (2007). A Web 2.0/Web3D hybrid platform for engaging students in e-learning environments. *Turkish Online Journal of Distance Education, 8*(3), 108–127. Retrieved December 5, 2008, from http://tojde.anadolu.edu.tr/tojde27/pdf/article_7.pdf

de Certeau, M. (1984). The practice of everyday life. (S. Rendall, Trans.) Berkeley, CA: University of California Press. (1980)

De Fazio, T. (2002). *Studying part-time without stress*. Crows Nest, Australia: Allen & Unwin.

de Guerrero, M. C. M., & Villamil, O. S. (2000). Activating the ZPD: Mutual scaffolding in L2 peer revision. *Modern Language Journal, 84*(1), 51–68. doi:10.1111/0026-7902.00052

Debenham, M. (2007, February). Epistolary interviews on-line: a novel addition to the researcher's palette. *JISC TechDis*. Retrieved April 29, 2010, from http://www.techdis.ac.uk/index.php?p=3_7_31_1

Dede, C. (1996). Emerging technologies and distributed learning. *American Journal of Distance Education, 10*(2), 4–36. doi:10.1080/08923649609526919

Dede, C. (2008). A seismic shift in epistemology. *EDUCAUSE Review, 43*(3), 80–81. Retrieved January 9, 2009, from http://www.educause.edu/ir/library/pdf/ERM0837.pdf

Deleting Online Predators Act of 2006, H. R. 5319, 109th Cong. (2006).

Derene, G. (2008, March 21). Motion capture ready to bring next-gen avatars to gaming, movies, medicine, the military and more (with video!). *Popular Mechanics*. Retrieved July 1, 2008, from http://www.popularmechanics.com/technology/industry/4264771.html?series=6

Derntl, M., Parrish, P., & Botturi, L. (2010). Beauty and precision: Weaving complex educational technology projects with visual instructional design languages. *International Journal on E-Learning, 9*(2), 185–202.

Desharnais, R. A., & Limson, M. (2007). Designing and implementing virtual courseware to promote inquiry-based learning. *Journal of Online Learning and Teaching, 3*(1), 30–39. Retrieved October 11, 2007, from http://jolt.merlot.org/vol3no1/desharnais.pdf

Developing the pedagogy andragogy heutagogy continuum. (2008). Retrieved November 29, 2008, from http://learnergeneratedcontexts.pbworks.com/PAH

Dey, A. K. (2001). Understanding and using context. *Personal and Ubiquitous Computing, 5*(1), 4–7. doi:10.1007/s007790170019

DiCamilla, F., & Antón, M. (1997). Repetition in the collaborative discourse of L2 learners: A Vygotskian perspective. *Canadian Modern Language Review, 53*(4), 609–633.

Dick, W., & Carey, L. (1996). *The systematic design of instruction* (4th ed.). New York: HarperCollins.

Dickey, M. D. (2004). The impact of web-logs (blogs) on student perceptions of isolation and alienation in a web-based distance-learning environment. *Open Learning, 19*(3), 279–291. doi:10.1080/0268051042000280138

Dirckinck-Holmfeld, L. (2002). Designing virtual learning environments based on problem oriented project pedagogy. In Dirckinck-Holmfeld, L., & Fibiger, B. (Eds.), *Learning in virtual environments* (pp. 31–54). Frederiksberg, Denmark: Samfundslitteratur.

Dixon, C., & Greeson, M. (2006). *Recasting the concept of podcasting (Part I)*. Retrieved September 20, 2006, from http://news.digitaltrends.com/talkback109.html

Donath, J., & Boyd, D. (2004). Public displays of connection. *BT Technology Journal, 22*(4), 71–82. doi:10.1023/B:BTTJ.0000047585.06264.cc

Donato, R. (1994). Collective scaffolding on second language learning. In Lantolf, J., & Appel, G. (Eds.), *Vygotskian approaches to second language research* (pp. 33–56). Westport, CT: Ablex.

Dorsey, P. A. (2001). *Personal knowledge management: educational framework for global business*. Retrieved February 18, 2007, from http://www.millikin.edu/pkm/pkm_istanbul.html

Dourish, P. (2004). What we talk about when we talk about context. *Personal and Ubiquitous Computing, 8*(1), 19–30. doi:10.1007/s00779-003-0253-8

Downes, S. (2004). Educational blogging. *EDUCAUSE Review, 39*(5), 14–26. Retrieved January 21, 2007, from http://net.educause.edu/ir/library/pdf/ERM0450.pdf

Downes, S. (2005, October). E-learning 2.0. *eLearn Magazine*. Retrieved December 21, 2008, from http://www.elearnmag.org/subpage.cfm?section=articles&article=29-1

Downes, S. (2006). *Learning networks and connective knowledge*. Retrieved March 12, 2008, from http://it.coe.uga.edu/itforum/paper92/paper92.html

Downes, S. (2006). *Understanding learning networks*. Keynote presentation delivered at the Fourth EDEN Research Workshop, Castelldelfels, Spain. Retrieved December 6, 2008, from http://www.downes.ca/files/spain.ppt

Downes, S. (2006, June 5). *The students own education*. Presentation delivered at the Vice Chancellor's Forum: Towards a Global Online University, The Open University, Milton Keynes, UK.

Downes, S. (2007). Learning networks in practice. In *Emerging technologies for learning* (Vol. 2, pp. 19–27). Coventry, UK: Becta. Retrieved October 28, 2008, from http://partners.becta.org.uk/upload-dir/downloads/page_documents/research/emerging_technologies07_chapter2.pdf

Draper, S. W. (2009a). Catalytic assessment: Understanding how MCQs and EVS can foster deep learning. *British Journal of Educational Technology, 40*(2), 285–293. doi:10.1111/j.1467-8535.2008.00920.x

Draper, S. W. (2009b). What are learners actually regulating when given feedback? *British Journal of Educational Technology, 40*(2), 306–315. doi:10.1111/j.1467-8535.2008.00930.x

Draper, S. W., & Brown, M. I. (2002). *Use of the PRS (Personal Response System) handsets at Glasgow University*. Retrieved June 22, 2009, from http://www.psy.gla.ac.uk/~steve/ilig/interim.html

Draper, S. W., Cargill, J., & Cutts, Q. (2002) Electronically enhanced classroom interaction. *Australian Journal of Educational Technology, 18*(1), 13–23. Retrieved August 12, 2008, from http://www.ascilite.org.au/ajet/ajet18/draper.html

Dreyfus, H. L. (2001). *On the Internet*. London: Routledge.

Dron, J. (2007). *Control and constraint in e-learning: Choosing when to choose*. Hershey, PA: Information Science Publishing.

Dron, J., & Anderson, T. (2007). Collectives, networks and groups in social software for e-learning. In T. Bastiaens & S. Carliner (Eds.), *Proceedings of World Conference on E-Learning in Corporate, Government, Healthcare, and Higher Education 2007* (pp. 2460–2467). Chesapeake, VA: Association for the Advancement of Computers in Education.

Dron, J., & Bhattacharya, M. (2007). Lost in the Web 2.0 jungle. In J. M. Spector, D. G. Sampson, T. Okamoto, Kinshuk, S. A. Cerri, M. Ueno, & A. Kashihara (Eds.), *Proceedings of the Seventh International Conference on Advanced Learning Technologies* (pp. 895–896). Los Alamitos, CA: IEEE Computer Society.

Dror, I. E. (2008). Technology enhanced learning: The good, the bad, and the ugly. *Pragmatics & Cognition, 16*(2), 215–223. doi:10.1075/p&c.16.2.02dro

Drucker, P. (1969). *The age of discontinuity: Guidelines to our changing society*. New York: Harper & Row.

Du, H. S., & Wagner, C. (2007). Leaning with weblogs: Enhancing cognitive and social knowledge construction. *IEEE Transactions on Professional Communication, 15*(1), 1–16. doi:10.1109/TPC.2006.890848

du Boulay, B., Coultas, J., & Luckin, R. (2007). *How compelling is the evidence for the effectiveness of e-Learning in the post-16 sector? A review of the literature in higher education, the health sector and work-based learning and a post-review stakeholder consultation*. Bath, UK: Eduserv. Retrieved November 29, 2008, from http://www.reveel.sussex.ac.uk/files/Version4.2.pdf

Duffy, T., & Cunningham, D. (1996). Constructivism: Implications for the design and delivery of instruction. In Jonassen, D. H. (Ed.), *Handbook of Research for Educational Communications and Technology*. New York: Simon & Schuster Macmillan.

Durbridge, N. (1984). Media in course design, No. 9, audio cassettes. In Bates, A. W. (Ed.), *The role of technology in distance education*. Kent, UK: Croom Helm.

Dziuban, C., Moskal, P., & Hartman, J. (2003). Higher education, blended learning and the generations: Knowledge is power—no more. In Bourne, J., & Moore, J. C. (Eds.), *Elements of quality online education: Engaging communities* (pp. 85–100). Needham, MA: The Sloan Consortium.

Earth System Research Laboratory. (2008). *Outreach at ERSL*. Retrieved December 20, 2008, from http://www.esrl.noaa.gov/outreach/index.html

Ebersbach, A., Glaser, M., & Heigl, R. (2006). *Wiki: Web collaboration*. Berlin: Springer-Verlag.

Ede, L., & Lunsford, A. (1990). *Singular texts / plural authors*. Carbondale, IL: Southern Illinois University Press.

Edirisingha, P., & Salmon, G. (2007). *Pedagogical models for podcasts in higher education*. Retrieved May 27, 2008, from http://hdl.handle.net/2381/405

Edirisingha, P., Rizzi, C., Nie, M., & Rothwell, L. (2007). Podcasting to provide teaching and learning support for an undergraduate module on English language and communication. *Turkish Online Journal of Distance Education, 8*(3), 87–107. Retrieved December 14, 2007, from http://tojde.anadolu.edu.tr/tojde27/pdf/article_6.pdf

Edirisingha, P., Salmon, G., & Fothergill, J. (2006, June 15). *Enriching a blended learning environment with podcasts and e-tivities: A case study*. Paper presented at the First International Blended Learning Conference: Promoting dialogue in innovation and practice, Hatfield, UK.

Edirisingha, P., Salmon, G., & Fothergill, J. (2007). Profcasting—a pilot study and guidelines for integrating podcasts in a blended learning environment. In U. Bernath & A. Sangrà (Eds.), *Research on competence development in online distance education and e-learning: Selected papers from the 4th EDEN Research Workshop in Castelldefels/Spain, October 25–28, 2006* (pp. 127–137). Oldenberg, Germany: BIS-Verlag der Carl von Ossietzky Universität Oldenburg.

Edson, J. (2007, June 25). Curriculum 2.0: User-driven education. *The Huffington Post*. Retrieved December 10, 2007, from http://www.huffingtonpost.com/jonathan-edson/curriculum-20-userdri_b_53690.html

EDUCASE Learning Initiative. (2006). *Learner-centered concepts*. Retrieved November 1, 2008, from http://www.educause.edu/content.asp?page_id=940&bhcp=1

EDUCAUSE Learning Initiative. (2005). *7 things you should know about wikis*. Retrieved October 28, 2009, from http://www.educause.edu/ir/library/pdf/ELI7004.pdf

EDUCAUSE Learning Initiative. (2006). *7 things you should know about Facebook*. Retrieved January 28, 2009, from http://net.educause.edu/ir/library/pdf/ELI7017.pdf

edumuve.com. (2008). *Sites of interest to educators in Second Life*. Retrieved July 1, 2008, from http://edumuve.com/tour/

Efimova, L., & Fiedler, S. (2004). Learning webs: Learning in weblog networks. In P. Kommers, P. Isaias, & J. M. Nunes (Eds.), *Proceedings of the IADIS International Conference Web Based Communities 2004* (pp. 490–494). Lisbon: International Association for Development of the Information Society.

Eijkman, H. (2008). Web 2.0 as a non-foundational network-centric learning space. *Campus-Wide Information Systems, 25*(2), 93–104. doi:10.1108/10650740810866567

Eijkman, H. (in press). How academics view Wikipedia: Web 2.0+ and the change in academic power-knowledge arrangements. *Campus-Wide Information Systems*.

Eijkman, H. (2003). *Online learning as curricular justice? A critical framework for higher education*. Unpublished Ph.D. dissertation, University of Canberra, Canberra, Australia.

Eijkman, H. (2004, November 26–28). *Contingency, curriculum and solidarity: A social constructionist response to the academic divide in Australian higher education*. Paper presented at the 33rd Annual Philosophy of Education Society of Australasia Conference. Melbourne, Australia.

Eijkman, H., & Clarke, B. (2007). Towards a participatory learning and assessment culture in higher education: Leveraging aocial rechnologies to reframe our curricular practices. In K. Fernstrom (Ed.), *Readings in technology in education: Proceedings of the International Conference on Information Communication Technologies in Education*. Abbostsford, BC: University of the Fraser Valley.

Eijkman, H., & Herrmann, A. (2009, March 25–27) *Beyond stereotyping: Understanding student readiness for network centric learning*. Paper presented at the Defence Academies and Colleges eLearning Conference, Stellenbosch, South Africa.

Eisenstadt, M. (2007). Does Elearning have to be so awful? (Time to mashup or shutup). In J. M. Spector, D. G. Sampson, T. Okamoto, Kinshuk, S. A. Cerri, M. Ueno, & A. Kashihara (Eds.), *Proceedings of the Seventh International Conference on Advanced Learning Technologies* (pp. 6–10). Los Alamitos, CA: IEEE Computer Society.

Eldon, E. (2007, September 10). Facebook to take over Stanford classroom [Web log post]. *VentureBeat*. Retrieved November 4, 2008, from http://venturebeat.com/2007/09/10/facebook-to-take-over-stanford-classroom/

E-learning—the virtual classroom. (2005, October 27). In *M/cyclopedia of new media*. Retrieved January 8, 2009, from http://wiki.media-culture.org.au/index.php/E-Learning_-_The_Virtual_Classroom

Elgort, I. (2007). Using wikis as a learning tool in higher education. In R. Atkinson & C. McBeath (Eds.), *ICT: Providing choices for learners and learning. Proceedings of the 24th Australasian Society for Computers in Learning in Tertiary Education (ASCILITE) Conference* (pp. 233–238). Singapore: Nanyang Technological University. Retrieved May 3, 2008, from http://www.ascilite.org.au/conferences/singapore07/procs/elgort.pdf

Elgort, I., Smith, A. G., & Toland, J. (2008). Is wiki an effective platform for group work? *Australian Journal of Educational Technology, 24*(2), 189–210. Retrieved June 5, 2008, from http://www.ascilite.org.au/ajet/ajet24/elgort.pdf

Elliott, B. (2008). *Assessment 2.0: Modernising assessment in the age of Web 2.0*. Glasgow: Scottish Qualifications Authority. Retrieved June 22, 2009, from http://www.scribd.com/doc/461041/Assessment-20

Ellison, N. (2007, December 5–7). *Facebook use on campus: A social capital perspective on social network sites*. Presentation delivered at the EDUCAUSE Center for Applied Research Symposium, Boca Raton, FL. Retrieved February 14, 2009, from http://www.educause.edu/ir/library/pdf/ECR0713.pdf

Elola, I. (2005). *The complexity of revision in an intermediate-level Spanish language classroom and the creation of a foreign language revision model*. Unpublished Ph.D. dissertation, The University of Iowa, Iowa City, IA.

Engeström, Y. (1987). *Learning by expanding: An activity-theoretical approach to developmental research*. Helsinki: Orienta-Konsultit Oy.

Engeström, Y. (1999). Innovative learning in work teams: Analyzing cycles of knowledge creation in practice. In Engeström, Y., Miettinen, R., & Punamäki, R.-L. (Eds.), *Perspectives on Activity Theory* (pp. 377–404). Cambridge, UK: Cambridge University Press.

Engeström, Y. (2007). From communities of practice to mycorrhizae. In Hughes, J., Jewson, N., & Unwin, L. (Eds.), *Communities of practice: Critical perspectives* (pp. 41–54). London: Routledge. doi:10.4324/NOE0415364737.ch4

Engeström, J. (2005a, June 10–11). *Object-centered sociality*. Paper presented at Reboot 7, Copenhagen.

Retrieved July 23, 2008, from http://aula.org/people/jyri/presentations/reboot7-jyri.pdf

Engeström, J. (2005b, April 13). Why some social network services work and others don't—Or: the case for object-centered sociality [Web log post]. *Zengestrom.com*. Retrieved July 23, 2008, from http://www.zengestrom.com/blog/2005/04/why_some_social.html

Entwistle, N., & Tait, H. (1990). Approaches to learning, evaluations of teaching, and preferences for contrasting academic environments. *Higher Education, 19*(2), 169–194. doi:10.1007/BF00137106

Ertmer, P. A. (2005). Teacher pedagogical beliefs: The final frontier in our quest for technology integration? *Educational Technology Research and Development, 53*(4), 25–39. doi:10.1007/BF02504683

Eshet-Alkalai, Y. (2004). Digital literacy: A conceptual framework for survival skills in the digital era. *Journal of Educational Multimedia and Hypermedia, 13*(1), 93–106.

Essex, C. (2006). Podcasting: A new medium for distance learning. In M. R. Simonson & M. Crawford (Eds.), *Proceedings of the 2006 Association for Educational Communications and Technology (AECT) International Convention* (pp. 136–139). North Miami Beach, FL: Nova Southeastern University.

European Centre for the Development of Vocational Training. (2008). *European e-Skills 2008 Conference: Implementing a long-term e-skills strategy in Europe*. Retrieved November 1, 2008, from http://eskills.cedefop.europa.eu/conference2008/

European Union. (2006). Recommendation of the European Parliament and of the Council of 18 December 2006 on key competences for lifelong learning (2006/962/EC). *Official Journal of the European Union, 49*(L 394), 10–18. Retrieved November 1, 2008, from http://eur-lex.europa.eu/LexUriServ/LexUriServ.do?uri=OJ:L:2006:394:0010:0018:EN:PDF

Eustace, K. (2003). Educational value of e-learning in conventional and complementary computing education. In S. Mann & A. Williamson (Eds.), *Proceedings of the 16th Annual Conference of the National Advisory Committee on Computing Qualifications* (pp. 53–62). Hamilton, New Zealand: NACCQ.

Evans, C. (2008). The effectiveness of m-learning in the form of podcast revision lectures in higher education. *Computers & Education, 50*(2), 491–498. doi:10.1016/j.compedu.2007.09.016

Facebook. (2009). In *Wikipedia, the free encyclopedia*. Retrieved April 11, 2009, from http://en.wikipedia.org/wiki/Facebook

Facebook. (2009). *Statistics*. Retrieved April 13, 2009, from http://www.facebook.com/press/info.php?statistics

Facer, K., Furlong, J., Furlong, R., & Sutherland, R. (2003). *Screenplay: Children and computing in the home*. London: RoutledgeFalmer. doi:10.4324/9780203380772

Falchikov, N. (1986). Product comparisons and process benefits of collaborative peer group and self assessments. *Assessment & Evaluation in Higher Education, 11*(2), 146–166.

Farabaugh, R. (2007). "The isle is full of noises": Using wiki software to establish a discourse community in a Shakespeare classroom. *Language Awareness, 16*(1), 41–56. doi:10.2167/la428.0

Farabaugh, P., Farabaugh, R., & Freeland, S. (2005, November 7). *Using wikis in teaching and learning*. Workshop delivered as part of the University of Maryland Baltimore Country Teaching, Learning and Technology Brown Bag workshop series, Baltimore, MD. Retrieved June 5, 2008, from http://www.umbc.edu/studio/videos/qtdetail?ID=380

Farmer, J. (2006). Blogging to basics: How blogs are bringing online education back from the brink. In Bruns, A., & Jacobs, J. (Eds.), *Uses of blogs* (pp. 91–103). New York: Peter Lang.

Feenberg, A. (1998). *Questioning technology*. London: Routledge.

Feenberg, A. (2002). *Transforming technology: A critical theory revisited* (2nd ed.). Oxford, UK: Oxford University Press.

Feldstein, M. (2006). In defense of walled gardens [Web log post]. *e-Literate*. Retrieved December 11, 2008, from http://mfeldstein.com/in_defense_of_walled_gardens/

Felix, U. (2005). E-learning pedagogy in the third millennium: The need for combining social and cognitive constructivist approaches. *ReCALL, 17*(1), 85–100. doi:10.1017/S0958344005000716

Ferguson, R., Clough, G., & Hosein, A. (2007). Postgraduate blogs: Beyond the ordinary research journal. In S. Wheeler & N. Whitton (Eds.), *Beyond control: Learning technology for the social network generation. Research Proceedings of the 14th Association for Learning Technology Conference* (pp. 179–188). Oxford, UK: ALT.

Fiedler, S. (2004). Personal webpublishing as a reflective conversational tool for self-organized learning. In Burg, T. N. (Ed.), *BlogTalks* (pp. 190–216). Wien, Austria: Libri.

Fiedler, S., & Pata, K. (2009). Distributed learning environments and social software: In search for a framework of design. In Hatzipanagos, S., & Warburton, S. (Eds.), *Handbook of research on social software and developing community ontologies* (pp. 151–164). Hershey, PA: Information Science Reference. doi:10.4018/978-1-60566-208-4.ch011

Fiedler, S., & Kieslinger, B. (2006). Adapting to changing landscapes in education. In T. Hug, M. Lindner, & P. A. Bruck (Eds.), *Micromedia & E-learning 2.0: Gaining the big picture. Proceedings of Microlearning Conference 2006* (pp. 78–89). Innsbruck, Austria: Innsbruck University Press.

Fink, L. (2005, September 16). Making textbooks worthwhile. *Chronicle of Higher Education*. Retrieved March 10, 2007, from http://chronicle.com/weekly/v52/i04/04b01201.htm

Firdyiwek, Y. (1999). Web-based courseware tools: Where is the pedagogy? *Educational Technology, 39*(1), 29–34.

Fischer, G. (2001, August 11–14). *Communities of interest: Learning through the interaction of multiple knowledge systems*. Paper presented at the 24th Information Systems Research Seminar in Scandinavia, Bergen, Norway. Retrieved July 21, 2007, from http://l3d.cs.colorado.edu/~gerhard/papers/iris24.pdf

Fischer, T., Kretschmer, T., Kugemann, W., & Cullen, J. (2008, October 29–30). *The landscape of Learning 2.0 in Europe: Analysing the Learning 2.0 Database*. Paper presented at the Validation and Policy Options Workshop, Seville, Spain. Retrieved April 30, 2009, from http://is.jrc.ec.europa.eu/pages/documents/FINALPresentationLearning20Database.pdf

Forte, A., & Bruckman, A. (2006). From Wikipedia to the classroom: Exploring online publication and learning. In S. A. Barab, K. E. Hay, & D. T. Hickey (Eds.), *Proceedings of the Seventh International Conference on Learning Sciences* (pp. 182–188). Atlanta, GA: International Society of the Learning Sciences.

Foucault, M. (1980). *Power/knowledge: Selected interviews and other writings, 1972–77* (Gordeon, C., Ed.). Brighton, UK: Harvester.

Foucault, M. (1972). *The archaeology of knowledge*. (A. M. Sheridan-Smith, Trans.). London: Tavistock. (1969).

Foucault, M. (1977). *Discipline and punish: The birth of the prison*. (A. M. Sheridan-Smith, Trans.). Harmondsworth, UK: Penguin. (1975).

Frand, J. L. (2000). The information-age mindset: Changes in students and implications for higher education. *EDUCAUSE Review, 35*(5), 14–24.

Frand, J., & Hixon, C. (1999). *Personal knowledge management: Who, what, why, when, where, how?* Retrieved November 1, 2008, from http://www.anderson.ucla.edu/faculty/jason.frand/researcher/speeches/PKM.htm

Franklin, T., & van Harmelen, M. (2007). *Web 2.0 for learning and teaching in higher education*. London: The Observatory of Borderless Higher Education. Retrieved April 28, 2008, from http://www.obhe.ac.uk/resources-new/pdf/651.Pdf

Freedman, T. (Ed.). (2006). *Coming of age: An introduction to the new World Wide Web*. Ilford, UK: Terry Freedman. Retrieved November 25, 2008, from http://fullmeasure.co.uk/Coming_of_age_v1-2.pdf

Friedman, T. L. (2007). *The world is flat: A brief history of the twenty-first century* (3rd ed.). New York: Picador.

Frielick, S. (2004). Beyond constructivism: An ecological approach to e-learning. In R. Atkinson, C. McBeath, D. Jonas-Dwyer, & R. Phillips (Eds.), *Beyond the comfort zone: Proceedings of the 21st Australasian Society for Computers in Learning in Tertiary Education (ASCILITE) Conference* (pp. 328–332). Perth, Australia: The University of Western Australia. Retrieved from http://www.ascilite.org.au/conferences/perth04/procs/pdf/frielick.pdf

Friesen, N., & Hopkins, J. (2008). Wikiversity; or education meets the free culture movement: An ethnographic investigation. *First Monday, 13*(10). Retrieved October 16, 2008, from http://www.uic.edu/htbin/cgiwrap/bin/ojs/index.php/fm/rt/printerFriendly/2234/2031

Frosch, D. (2007, May 15). Pentagon blocks 13 web sites from military computers. *The New York Times*. Retrieved July 21, 2007, from http://www.nytimes.com/2007/05/15/washington/15block.html

Fry, R. (2005a). *Get organised.* New York: Thomson Delmar Learning.

Fry, R. (2005b). *How to study*. New York: Thomson Delmar Learning.

Frydenberg, M. (2006). Principles and pedagogy: The two P's of podcasting in the information technology classroom. In D. Colton, W. J. Tastle, M. Hensel, & A. A. Abdullat (Eds.), *Proceedings of ISECON 2006* (§3354). Chicago, IL: Association of Information Technology Professionals. Retrieved November 27, 2006, from http://isedj.org/isecon/2006/3354/ISECON.2006.Frydenberg.pdf

Frydenberg, M. (2008a). Wikis as a tool for collaborative course management. *Journal of Online Learning and Teaching, 4*(2), 169–181. Retrieved November 4, 2008, from http://jolt.merlot.org/vol4no2/frydenberg0608.pdf

Frydenberg, M. (2008b). Slickr: A multi-tiered web development capstone project using databases, web services, and AJAX. *Information Systems Education Journal, 6*(37). Retrieved November 4, 2008, from http://isedj.org/6/37/ISEDJ.6(37).Frydenberg.pdf

Fuchs-Kittowski, F., & Kohler, J. (2006). Wiki communities in the context of work processes. In D. Riehle (Ed.), *Proceedings of the 2005 International Symposium on Wikis* (pp. 33–39). New York: Association for Computing Machinery. Retrieved June 6, 2008, from http://www.wikisym.org/ws2005/proceedings/paper-04.pdf

Gachuhi, D., & Matiru, B. (1987). Active learning. In *Distance Education—By Design Symposium '87 Papers* (pp. 1–21). Barrhead, AB: Alberta Correspondence School.

Galusha, J. M. (1997). *Barriers to learning in distance education.* Retrieved June 19, 2008, from http://www.infrastruction.com/barriers.htm

Ganley, B. (2004, October 11). Images, words and students finding their way [Web log post]. *Bgblogging.* Retrieved November 19, 2009, from http://bgblogging.com/2004/10/11/images-words-and-students-finding-their-way/

Gardner, H. (1983). *Frames of mind: The theory of multiple intelligences.* New York: Basic.

Gardner, H. (1993). *Multiple intelligences: The theory in practice.* New York: Basic.

Gardner, H. (2000). *Intelligence reframed: Multiple intelligences for the 21st century.* New York: Basic.

Garfinkel, S. L. (2008, November/December). Wikipedia and the meaning of truth: Why the online encyclopedia's epistemology should worry those who care about traditional notions of accuracy. *Technology Review*, 84–86.

Garnett, F., & Ecclesfield, N. (2008). Colloquium; Developing an organisational architecture of participation. *British Journal of Educational Technology, 39*(3), 468–474. doi:10.1111/j.1467-8535.2008.00839.x

Garrison, D. R., & Kanuka, H. (2004). Blended learning: Uncovering its transformative potential in higher education. *The Internet and Higher Education, 7*(2), 95–105. doi:10.1016/j.iheduc.2004.02.001

Garrison, D. R. (2007). Online community of inquiry review: Social, cognitive and teaching presence issues. *Journal of Asynchronous Learning Networks, 11*(1), 61–72.

Garrison, D. R., & Anderson, T. (2003). Community of inquiry. In *E-learning in the 21st century: A framework for research and practice* (pp. 22–31). London: RoutledgeFalmer. doi:10.4324/9780203166093

Gartner, Inc. (2007, December 17). *Gartner says mobile messages to surpass 2 trillion messages in major markets in 2008.* Retrieved February 12, 2008, from http://www.gartner.com/it/page.jsp?id=565124

Gatfield, T. (1999). Examining student satisfaction with group projects and peer assessment. *Assessment & Evaluation in Higher Education, 24*(4), 365–377. doi:10.1080/0260293990240401

Gaver, W. W. (1996). Situating Action II: Affordances for interaction: The social is material for design. *Ecological Psychology, 8*(2), 111–129. doi:10.1207/s15326969eco0802_2

Gee, J. P. (2003). *What video games have to teach us about learning and literacy*. New York: Palmgrave.

Gee, J. P., Hull, G., & Lankshear, C. (1996). *The new work order: Behind the language of the new capitalism*. Sydney: Allen & Unwin.

Gee, J. P. (1999). *Language, learning, and latecomers: Discourses in education*. Unpublished manuscript.

Geith, C. (2008). Teaching and learning unleashed with Web 2.0 and open educational resources. In Katz, R. N. (Ed.), *The tower and the cloud: Higher education in the age of cloud computing* (pp. 219–226). Boulder, CO: EDUCAUSE.

Georgia College & State University. (2005). *The iPod at GC&SU: A pocketful of learning*. Retrieved March 2, 2006, from http://ipod.gcsu.edu

Gergen, K. J. (1999). *An invitation to social construction*. London: Sage.

Gibson, J. J. (1979). *The ecological approach to visual perception*. Boston: Houghton Mifflin.

Gibson, J. J. (1977). The theory of affordances. In Shaw, R., & Bransford, J. (Eds.), *Perceiving, acting, and knowing: Toward an ecological psychology* (pp. 67–82). Hillsdale, NJ: Lawrence Erlbaum.

Gipps, C. (2002). Sociocultural perspectives on assessment. In Wells, G., & Claxton, G. (Eds.), *Learning for life in the 21st century* (pp. 73–83). Oxford, UK: Blackwell. doi:10.1002/9780470753545.ch6

Giridharadas, A. (2010, April 18). In many parts of the world, a cellphone is sufficient. *The New York Times/ The Observer*.

Glaser, M. (2007, August 29). Your guide to social networking online. *Media Shift*. Retrieved June 16, 2008, from http://www.pbs.org/mediashift/2007/08/your-guide-to-social-networking-online241.html

Godwin-Jones, R. (2003). Blogs and wikis: Environments for on-line collaboration. *Language Learning & Technology, 7*(2), 12–16. Retrieved January 10, 2008, from http://llt.msu.edu/vol7num2/pdf/emerging.pdf

Goldberg, K. (2000). *The robot in the garden: Telerobotics and telepistemology in the age of the Internet*. Cambridge, MA: MIT Press.

Golder, S. A., Wilkinson, D., & Huberman, B. A. (2007, June). Rhythms of social interaction: Messaging within a massive online network. In C. Steinfield, B. Pentland, M. Ackerman, & N. Contractor (Eds.), *Proceedings of Third International Conference on Communities and Technologies* (pp. 41–66). London: Springer.

Golding, W. (1954). *The lord of the flies*. London: Faber & Faber.

Gonella, L., & Pantò, E. (2008). Didactic architectures and organization models: A process of mutual adaptation. *eLearning Papers, 9*. Retrieved July 20, 2008, from http://www.elearningeuropa.info/files/media/media15973.pdf

Goodman, E., & Moed, A. (2006, November 4–8). *Community in mashups: The case of personal geodata*. Paper presented at the 20th ACM Conference on Computer Supported Cooperative Work, Banff, AB. Retrieved March 19, 2008, from http://mashworks.net/images/5/59/Goodman_Moed_2006.pdf

Goodwin, B. C. (1999). From control to participation via a science of qualities. *ReVision, 21*(4), 26–35.

Goodyear, P. (2006). Technology and the articulation of vocational and academic interests: Reflections on time, space and e-learning. *Studies in Continuing Education, 28*(2), 83–98. doi:10.1080/01580370600750973

Goodyear, P., & Jones, C. (2003). Implicit theories of learning and change: Their role in the development of e-learning environments in higher education. In Naidu, S. (Ed.), *Learning and teaching with technology: Principles and practice* (pp. 29–42). London: Routledge.

Gould, C., & Brown, D. (2003). *Constructivism and practice*. Lanham, MD: Rowman & Littlefield.

Graves, W. H. (2005). Improving institutional performance through IT-enabled innovation. *EDUCAUSE Review, 40*(6), 78–99. Retrieved February 14, 2009, from http://www.educause.edu/ir/library/pdf/ERM0564.pdf

Gray, K., Thompson, C., Clerehan, R., Sheard, J., & Hamilton, M. (2008). Web 2.0 authorship: Issues of referencing and citation for academic integrity. *The Internet and Higher Education, 11*(2), 112–118. doi:10.1016/j.iheduc.2008.03.001

Green, H., & Hannon, C. (2007). *Their space: Education for a digital generation*. London: Demos. Retrieved December 2, 2007, from http://www.demos.co.uk/files/Their%20space%20-%20web.pdf

Green, H., Facer, K., Rudd, T., Dillon, P., & Humphreys, P. (2005). *Personalisation and digital technologies*. Bristol, UK: Futurelab. Retrieved October 23, 2007, from http://www.futurelab.org.uk/resources/documents/opening_education/Personalisation_report.pdf

Green, K. C. (2007). *The 2007 National Survey of Information Technology in U.S. Higher Education*. Encino, CA: The Campus Computing Project. Retrieved December 6, 2008, from http://www.campuscomputing.net/sites/www.campuscomputing.net/files/2007-CCP_0.pdf

Greene, K. (2007, April 24). Practical holographic video, *Technology Review*. Retrieved July 1, 2008 from http://www.technologyreview.com/read_article.aspx?id=18572.

Greenfield, A. (2006). *Everyware: The dawning age of ubiquitous computing*. Berkeley, CA: New Riders.

Greeno, J. G. (1994). Gibson's affordances. *Psychological Review, 101*(2), 236–342. doi:10.1037/0033-295X.101.2.336

Grey, D. (2006, June 21). *Looking at personal knowledge management*. Retrieved November 1, 2008, from http://kmwiki.wikispaces.com/PKM

Grimmelmann, J. (2009). Saving Facebook. *Iowa Law Review, 94*(4), 1137–1206.

Gross, R., & Acquisti, A. (2005). Information revelation and privacy in online social networks. In S. De Capitani di Vimercati & R. Dingledine (Eds.), *Proceedings of the 2005 ACM workshop on Privacy in the Electronic Society* (pp. 71–80). New York: Association for Computing Machinery.

Grudin, J. (2001). Desituating action: Digital representation of context. *Human-Computer Interaction, 16*(2/3), 269–286. doi:10.1207/S15327051HCI16234_10

Guess, A. (2007, August 20). In Second Life, there's no fallout. *Inside Higher Ed*. Retrieved from http://insidehighered.com/news/2007/08/20/secondlife

Gunawardena, C., Lowe, C., & Anderson, T. (1997). Analysis of a global online debate and the development of an interaction analysis model for examining social building of knowledge in computer conferencing. *Journal of Educational Computing Research, 17*(4), 397–431.

Gunter, B. (2009). Blogging—private becomes public and public becomes personalized. *Aslib Proceedings: New Information Perspectives, 61*(2), 120–126.

Gurak, L. J., & Antonijevic, S. (2008). The psychology of blogging: You, me, and everyone in between. *The American Behavioral Scientist, 52*(1), 60–68. doi:10.1177/0002764208321341

Hamburg, I., Engert, S., & Anke, P. (2008). Communities of practice and Web 2.0 to support learning in SMEs. In O. Cernian (Ed.), *Proceedings of the Sixth Romanian Educational Network (RoEduNet) International Conference* (pp. 152–155). Craiova, Romania: Faculty of Automation, Computers and Electronics, University of Craiova.

Hannon, J. (2008). Doing staff development: Practices, dilemmas and technologies. *Australasian Journal of Educational Technology, 24*(1), 15–29. Retrieved July 17, 2008, from http://www.ascilite.org.au/ajet/ajet24/hannon.pdf

Hanson, F. A. (1993). *Testing testing: Social consequences of the examined life*. Berkeley, CA: University of California Press.

Hargis, J., & Wilcox, S. M. (2008). Ubiquitous, free, and efficient online collaboration tools for teaching and learning. *Turkish Online Journal of Distance Education, 9*(4), 9–17. Retrieved December 5, 2008, from http://tojde.anadolu.edu.tr/tojde32/pdf/notes_for_editor_1.pdf

Hartman, J., Moskal, P., & Dziuban, C. (2005). Preparing the academy of today for the learner of tomorrow. In Oblinger, D. G., & Oblinger, J. L. (Eds.), *Educating the Net Generation* (pp. 6.1–6.15). Boulder, CO: EDUCAUSE.

Hase, S., & Kenyon, C. (2000). From Andragogy to Heutagogy. *ultiBASE, 5*(3). Retrieved July 12, 2008, from http://ultibase.rmit.edu.au/Articles/dec00/hase1.pdf

Hattie, J., & Temperley, H. (2007). The power of feedback. *Review of Educational Research, 77*(1), 81–112. doi:10.3102/003465430298487

Hatzipanagos, S., & Warburton, S. (2009). Feedback as dialogue: Exploring the links between formative assessment and social software in distance learning. *Learning, Media and Technology, 34*(1), 45–59. doi:10.1080/17439880902759919

Haughey, M. (2007, May 14). Some community tips for 2007: Seven tips on how to run a successful community [Web log post]. *Fortuitious*. Retrieved December 10, 2007, from http://fortuito.us/2007/05/some_community_tips_for_2007

Havenstein, H. (2007, November 14). Forget Generations X and Y: Here comes Generation V. *Computerworld*. Retrieved February 22, 2008, from http://www.computerworld.com/s/article/9046879/Forget_Generations_X_and_Y_Here_comes_Generation_V

Havnes, A., & McDowell, L. (2008). Introduction: Assessment dilemmas in contemporary learning cultures. In Havnes, A., & McDowell, L. (Eds.), *Balancing dilemmas in assessment and learning in contemporary education* (pp. 3–14). New York: Taylor & Francis.

Haythornthwaite, C. (2005). Social networks and Internet connectivity effects. *Information Communication and Society, 8*(2), 125–147. doi:10.1080/13691180500146185

Heaton-Shrestha, C., Edirisingha, P., Burke, L., & Linsey, T. (2005). Introducing a VLE into campus-based undergraduate teaching: Staff perspectives on its impact on teaching. *International Journal of Educational Research, 43*(6), 370–386. doi:10.1016/j.ijer.2006.07.001

Heeren, E. S. (2007). *Exploring the new literacies: Instruction and assessment practices of middle school master teachers of Internet literacy*. Unpublished Ed.D. dissertation, The University of Memphis, Memphis, TN.

Heim, M. (1999). *Transmogrification*. Retrieved February 7, 2009, from http://www.mheim.com/files/transmog.pdf

Helms, D. (2007a). *Drug use and abuse*. Retrieved November 2, 2007, from http://druguseandabuse.ning.com/

Helms, D. (2007b). *Group project*. Retrieved November 2, 2007, from http://www.msjc.edu/hs/hs123_group_project.html

Henri, F., Charlier, B., & Limpens, F. (2008). Understanding PLE as an essential component of the learning process. In J. Luca & E. Weippl (Eds.), *Proceedings of World Conference on Educational Multimedia, Hypermedia and Telecommunications 2008* (pp. 3766–3770). Chesapeake, VA: Association for the Advancement of Computers in Education.

Henshaw, R. G. (2008). A singular vision for a disparate future: Technology adoption patterns in higher learning through 2035. *Innovate: Journal of Online Education, 4*(6). Retrieved June 24, 2008, from http://www.innovate.info/index.php?view=article&id=533

Heppell, S. (2006, June 5). *It's a new millennium, it's a new century*. Presentation delivered at the Vice Chancellor's Forum: Towards a Global Online University, The Open University, Milton Keynes, UK.

Herrington, J., & Kervin, L. (2007). Authentic learning supported by technology: Ten suggestions and cases of integration in classrooms. *Educational Media International, 44*(3), 219–236. doi:10.1080/09523980701491666

Herrington, J., & Herrington, A. (1998). Authentic assessment and multimedia: How university students respond to a model of authentic assessment. *Higher Education Research & Development, 17*(3), 305–322. doi:10.1080/0729436980170304

Herrington, J., Reeves, T. C., & Oliver, R. (2007). Immersive learning technologies: Realism and online authentic learning. *Journal of Computing in Higher Education, 19*(1), 65–84. doi:10.1007/BF03033421

Hewitt, A., & Forte, A. (2006, November 4–8). *Crossing boundaries: Identity management and student/faculty relationships on the Facebook*. Paper presented at the 2006 20th Anniversary Conference on Computer Supported Cooperative Work, Banff, AB.

Hewling, A. (2006, April 10–12). *PROWE (Personal Repositories Online Wiki Environment)—a first look*. Paper presented at the Fifth International Conference on Networked Learning 2006, Lancaster, UK. Retrieved December 5, 2008, from http://www.networkedlearning-conference.org.uk/abstracts/pdfs/05Hewling.pdf

Hicks, T. (2006). Expanding the conversation: A commentary toward revision of Swenson, Rozema, Young, McGrail, and Whitin. *Contemporary Issues in Technology and Teacher Education, 6*(1), 46–55. Retrieved November 4, 2008, from http://www.editlib.org/f/21862

Higher Education Opportunity Act of 2008, Pub. L. No. 110-315, 122 Stat. 3078 (2008).

Hilton, J. (2006). The future for higher education: Sunrise or perfect storm? *EDUCAUSE Review, 41*(2), 58–71. Retrieved November 1, 2008, from http://net.educause.edu/ir/library/pdf/erm0623.pdf

Hiltz, S. R. (1986). The virtual classroom: Using computer-mediated communication for university teaching. *The Journal of Communication, 36*(2), 95–104. doi:10.1111/j.1460-2466.1986.tb01427.x

Hiltz, S. R., & Turoff, M. (1978). *The network nation: Human communication via computer*. Reading, MA: Addison-Wesley.

Hinchcliffe, D. (2006, September 4). All we got was Web 1.0, when Tim Berners-Lee actually gave us Web 2.0 [Web log post]. *Dion Hinchcliffe's Web 2.0 Blog*. Retrieved October 8, 2009, from http://web2.socialcomputingjournal.com/all_we_got_was_web_10_when_tim_bernerslee_actually_gave_us_w.htm

Hirvela, A. (1999). Collaborative writing: Instruction and communities of readers and writers. *TESOL Journal, 8*(2), 7–12.

Hoare, S. (2007, November 5). Students tell universities: Get out of MySpace! *The Guardian*. Retrieved February 21, 2009, from http://www.guardian.co.uk/education/2007/nov/05/link.students

Hodgkinson-Williams, C., Slay, H., & Siebörger, I. (2008). Developing communities of practice within and outside higher education institutions. *British Journal of Educational Technology, 39*(3), 433–442. doi:10.1111/j.1467-8535.2008.00841.x

Holt, D., & Challis, D. (2007). From policy to practice: One university's experience of implementing strategic change through wholly online teaching and learning. *Australasian Journal of Educational Technology, 23*(1), 110–131. Retrieved July 17, 2008, from http://www.ascilite.org.au/ajet/ajet23/holt.html

Homik, M., & Melis, E. (2006). Using blogs for learning logs. In *Proceedings of the Fourth International ePortfolio Conference*. Champlost, France: European Institute for E-Learning. Retrieved April 29, 2010, from http://www.eife-l.org/publications/eportfolio/proceedings2/ep06/ep2006_papers/homik

Honegger, B. D. (2005). Wikis—a rapidly growing phenomenon in the German-speaking school community. In D. Riehle (Ed.), *Proceedings of the 2005 International Symposium on Wikis* (pp. 113–116). New York: Association for Computing Machinery. Retrieved June 6, 2008, from http://www.wikisym.org/ws2005/proceedings/paper-10.pdf

Hornyak, M., Peach, B., & Fekula, M. (2003). Blogging: A new threat to student research? *Developments in Business Simulation and Experiential Learning, 30*, 131–132. Retrieved April 29, 2010, from http://sbaweb.wayne.edu/~absel/bkl/vol30/30ap.pdf

Hotrum, M. (2008, June 20). Personal learning environment and evolutionary pedagogy [Web log post]. *Choice Learning*. Retrieved March 24, 2009, from http://choicelearning.blogspot.com/2008/06/personal-learning-environment-and.html

Howe, N., & Strauss, W. (2000). *Millennials rising: The next great generation*. New York: Random House.

Hruby, G. G. (2001). Sociological, postmodern, and new realism perspectives in social constructionism: Implications for literacy research. *Reading Research Quarterly, 36*(1), 48–62. doi:10.1598/RRQ.36.1.3

Huang, C.-Y., Shen, Y.-Z., Lin, H.-X., & Chang, S.-S. (2007). Bloggers' motivations and behaviors: A model. *Journal of Advertising Research, 47*(4), 472–484. doi:10.2501/S0021849907070493

Hug, T., Lindner, M., & Bruck, P. A. (Eds.). (2006). *Microlearning: Emerging concepts, practices and technologies after e-Learning. Proceedings of Microlearning 2005: Learning & working in new media*. Innsbruck, Austria: Innsbruck University Press. Retrieved October 15, 2007, from http://www.microlearning.org/micropapers/microlearning2005_proceedings_digitalversion.pdf

Hughes, J., & Lang, K. (2006). Transmutability: Digital decontextualization, manipulation, and recontextualization as a new source of value in the production and consumption of culture products. In *Proceedings of the 39th Annual Hawaii International Conference on System*

Sciences (p. 165a). Los Alamitos, CA: IEEE Computer Society.

Huijser, H. J. (2006). Refocusing multiliteracies for the Net Generation. *International Journal of Pedagogies and Learning*, *2*(1), 21–33.

Huijser, H. J. (2008). Exploring the educational potential of social networking sites: The fine line between exploiting opportunities and unwelcome imposition. *Studies in Learning, Evaluation, Innovation and Development, 5*(3), 45–54. Retrieved June 23, 2009, from http://sleid.cqu.edu.au/include/getdoc.php?id=708&article=199&mode=pdf

Ice, P., Curtis, R., Phillips, P., & Wells, J. (2007). Using asynchronous audio feedback to enhance teaching presence and students' sense of community. *Journal of Asynchronous Learning Networks*, *11*(2), 3–25.

Illich, I. (1973). *Deschooling society*. Harmondsworth, UK: Penguin.

Informal Mobile Podcasting and Learning Adaptation. (2007). *A framework for developing your podcasts*. Retrieved June 29, 2008, from http://www2.le.ac.uk/projects/impala/documents/resources-and-tools-for-creating-podcasts/PodcastChoiceFramework

Ipsos, M. O. R. I. (2007). *Student expectations study: Key findings from online research and discussion evenings held in June 2007 for the Joint Information Systems Committee*. London: JISC. Retrieved November 9, 2009, from http://www.jisc.ac.uk/media/documents/publications/studentexpectations.pdf

Ipsos, M. O. R. I. (2008). *Great expectations of ICT: How higher education institutions are measuring up*. Bristol, UK: Joint Information Systems Committee. Retrieved November 20, 2008, http://www.jisc.ac.uk/media/documents/publications/jiscgreatexpectationsfinalreportjune08.pdf

Irving, C., & Crawford, J. (2007). *A National Information Literacy Framework Scotland.* Retrieved November 1, 2008, from http://www.caledonian.ac.uk/ils/framework.html

Ito, M., Baumer, S., Bittanti, M., Boyd, D., Cody, R., & Herr, B. … Yardi, S. (2009). *Hanging out, messing around, and geeking out: Kids living and learning with new media*. Cambridge, MA: MIT Press.

Jacobs, J., & Polson, D. (2006, September 26). Mobile learning, social learning. Paper presented at the Online Learning and Teaching Conference 2006, Brisbane, Australia. Retrieved November 20, 2008, from https://olt.qut.edu.au/udf/OLT2006/gen/static/papers/Jacobs_OLT2006_paper.pdf

Jaffee, D. (2003). Virtual transformation: Web-based technology and pedagogical change. *Teaching Sociology*, *31*(2), 227–236. doi:10.2307/3211312

James, M. (2008). Assessment and learning. In Swaffield, S. (Ed.), *Unlocking assessment: Understanding for reflection and application* (pp. 20–35). London: Routledge.

Jamieson, P. (2004). The university as workplace: Preparing lecturers to teach in online environments. *Quarterly Review of Distance Education*, *5*(1), 21–27.

Jenkins, H. (2006). *Convergence culture: Where old and new media collide*. New York: New York University Press.

Jenkins, H. (2008, November 21). "Hanging out, messing around, geeking out": A conversation with the Digital Youth Project (Part Two) [Web log post]. *Confessions of an Aca-Fan: The Official Weblog of Henry Jenkins*. Retrieved December 4, 2008, from http://henryjenkins.org/2008/11/hanging_out_messing_around_gee.html

Jenkins, H., Purushotma, R., Clinton, K., Weigel, M., & Robison, A. J. (2006). *Confronting the challenges of participatory culture: Media education for the 21st century*. Chicago: MacArthur Foundation. Retrieved August 7, 2009, from http://digitallearning.macfound.org/atf/cf/%7B7E45C7E0-A3E0-4B89-AC9C-E807E1B0AE4E%7D/JENKINS_WHITE_PAPER.PDF

Johnson, M., & Liber, O. (2008). The personal learning environment and the human condition: From theory to teaching practice. *Interactive Learning Environments*, *16*(1), 3–15. doi:10.1080/10494820701772652

Johnson, M., Hollins, P., Wilson, S., & Liber, O. (2006). Towards a reference model for the personal learning environment. In L. Markauskaite, P. Goodyear, & P. Reimann (Eds.), *Who's learning? Whose technology? Proceedings of the 23rd Australasian Society for Computers in Learning in Tertiary Education (ASCILITE) Conference* (pp. 385–389). Sydney: University of Sydney.

Joint Information Systems Committee. (2005). *Innovative practice with e-learning: A good practice guide to embedding mobile and wireless technologies into everyday practice*. Bristol, UK: JISC. Retrieved December 6, 2008, from http://www.jisc.ac.uk/media/documents/publications/innovativepe.pdf

Joint Information Systems Committee. (2006). *Designing spaces for effective learning: A guide to 21st century learning space design*. Bristol, UK: JISC. Retrieved July 2, 2007, from http://www.jisc.ac.uk/media/documents/publications/learningspaces.pdf

Joint Information Systems Committee. (2007). *Effective practice with e-assessment: An overview of technologies, policies and practice in further and higher education*. Bristol, UK: JISC. Retrieved December 6, 2008, from http://www.jisc.ac.uk/media/documents/themes/elearning/effpraceassess.pdf

Joint Information Systems Committee. (2010a). *Learner experiences of e-learning: Phase 1*. Retrieved June 8, 2010, from http://www.jisc.ac.uk/whatwedo/programmes/elearningpedagogy/learneroutcomes.aspx

Joint Information Systems Committee. (2010b). *Learner experiences of e-learning: Phase 2*. Retrieved June 8, 2010, from http://www.jisc.ac.uk/whatwedo/programmes/elearningpedagogy/learnerexperience.aspx

Jonassen, D. H., Davidson, M., Collins, M., Campbell, J., & Bannan Haag, B. (1995). Constructivism and computer-mediated communication in distance education. *American Journal of Distance Education*, *9*(2), 7–26. doi:10.1080/08923649509526885

Jonassen, D. H. (1991). Evaluating constructivistic learning. *Educational Technology*, *31*(9), 28–33.

Jones, B. L. (Ed.). (2008). *Web 2.0 heroes: Interviews with 20 Web 2.0 influencers*. Indianapolis, IN: Wiley.

Jones, C. R., Ramanau, R., Cross, S., & Healing, G. (2010). Net Generation or digital natives: Is there a distinct new generation entering university? *Computers & Education*, *54*(3), 722–732. doi:10.1016/j.compedu.2009.09.022

Jones, C. R., Dirckinck-Holmfeld, L., & Lindström, B. (2006). A relational, indirect, meso-level approach to CSCL design in the next decade. *International Journal of Computer-Supported Collaborative Learning*, *1*(1), 35–56. doi:10.1007/s11412-006-6841-7

Jones, C. R., Ferreday, D., & Hodgson, V. (2008). Networked learning a relational approach: Weak and strong ties. *Journal of Computer Assisted Learning*, *24*(2), 90–102. doi:10.1111/j.1365-2729.2007.00271.x

Jones, C. R., & Ramanau, R. (2009). Collaboration and the net generation: The changing characteristics of first year university students. In C. O'Malley, D. Suthers, P. Reimann, & A. Dimitracopoulou (Eds.), *Proceedings of the Ninth International Conference on Computer Supported Collaborative Learning* (Vol. 1, pp. 237–241). Atlanta, GA: International Society of the Learning Sciences.

Jones, D. (2008). PLEs: Framing one future for lifelong learning, e-learning and universities. In D. Orr, P. A. Danaher, G. Danaher, & R. E. Harreveld (Eds.), *Lifelong learning: Reflecting on successes and framing futures. Keynote and refereed papers from the Fifth International Lifelong Learning Conference* (pp. 231–236). Rockhampton, Australia: Central Queensland University Press.

Jones, D., & Muldoon, N. (2007). The teleological reason why ICTs limit choice for university learners and learning. In R. Atkinson & C. McBeath (Eds.), *ICT: Providing choices for learners and learning. Proceedings of the 24th Australasian Society for Computers in Learning in Tertiary Education (ASCILITE) Conference* (pp. 450–459). Singapore: Nanyang Technological University. Retrieved June 22, 2008, from http://www.ascilite.org.au/conferences/singapore07/procs/jones-d.pdf

Jones, M., & Alony, I. (2008). Blogs—the new source of data analysis. *Issues in Informing Science and Information Technology*, *5*, 433–446. Retrieved April 28, 2010, from http://proceedings.informingscience.org/InSITE2008/IISITv5p433-446Jones530.pdf

Jones, P. (2007). When a wiki is the way: Exploring the use of a wiki in a constructively aligned learning design. In R. Atkinson & C. McBeath (Eds.), *ICT: Providing choices for learners and learning. Proceedings of the 24th Australasian Society for Computers in Learning in Tertiary Education (ASCILITE) Conference* (pp. 460–467). Singapore: Nanyang Technological University. Retrieved May 3, 2008, from http://www.ascilite.org.au/conferences/singapore07/procs/jones-p.pdf

Journal of Online Learning and Teaching. (2009). *Call for papers—Special issue: Integrity and identity authentication in online education*. Retrieved March 20, 2009, from http://jolt.merlot.org/special09.htm

Joyes, G. (2005/2006). When pedagogy leads technology. *The International Journal of Technology. Knowledge & Society*, *1*(5), 107–113.

Kalyuga, S. (2007). Enhancing instructional efficiency of interactive e-learning environments: A cognitive load perspective. *Educational Psychology Review*, *19*(3), 387–399. doi:10.1007/s10648-007-9051-6

Kamel Boulos, M. N., & Wheeler, S. (2007). The emerging Web 2.0 social software: An enabling suite of sociable technologies in health and healthcare education. *Health Information and Libraries Journal*, *24*(1), 2–23. doi:10.1111/j.1471-1842.2007.00701.x

Kamel Boulos, M. N., Maramba, I., & Wheeler, S. (2006). Wikis, blogs and podcasts: A new generation of web-based tools for virtual collaborative clinical practice and education. *BMC Medical Education*, *6*(41). Retrieved November 4, 2008, from http://www.biomedcentral.com/1472-6920/6/41

Kates, R. (1998). Tape recorders and the commuter student: Bypassing the red pen. *Teaching English in the Two-Year College*, *25*(1), 21–24.

Katz, I. R., & Macklin, A. S. (2007). Information and communication technology (ICT) literacy: Integration and assessment in higher education. *Systemics, Cybernetics and Informatics*, *5*(4), 50–55. Retrieved November 1, 2008, from http://www.iiisci.org/Journal/CV$/sci/pdfs/P890541.pdf

Kay, J., & FitzGerald, S. (2008). *Educational uses of Second Life*. Retrieved December 6, 2008, from http://sleducation.wikispaces.com/educationaluses

Keegan, D. (1996). *Foundations of distance education* (3rd ed.). London: Routledge.

Keegan, V. (2008, February 14). From global village to a local village. *The Guardian*. Retrieved November 20, 2008, from http://www.guardian.co.uk/technology/2008/feb/14/mobilephones.socialnetworking

Keen, A. (2007). *The cult of the amateur: How today's Internet is killing our culture and assaulting our economy*. London: Nicholas Brealey.

Kelton, A. J. (2007). *Second Life: Reaching into the virtual world for real-world learning*. Boulder, CO: EDUCAUSE. Retrieved December 5, 2008, from http://www.educause.edu/ir/library/pdf/ERB0717.pdf

Kennedy, G. E., Judd, T. S., Churchward, A., Gray, K., & Krause, K.-L. (2008). First year students' experiences with technology: Are they really digital natives? *Australasian Journal of Educational Technology, 24*(1), 108–122. Retrieved December 21, 2008, from http://www.ascilite.org.au/ajet/ajet24/kennedy.pdf

Kennedy, G., Dalgarno, B., Gray, K., Judd, T., Waycott, J., & Bennett, S. … Churchward, A. (2007). The Net Generation are not big users of Web 2.0 technologies: Preliminary findings. In R. Atkinson & C. McBeath (Eds.), *ICT: Providing choices for learners and learning. Proceedings of the 24th Australasian Society for Computers in Learning in Tertiary Education (ASCILITE) Conference* (pp. 517–525). Singapore: Nanyang Technological University. Retrieved January 12, 2008, from http://www.ascilite.org.au/conferences/singapore07/procs/kennedy.pdf

Kennedy, G., Krause, K.-L., Gray, K., Bennett, S., Maton, K., Dalgarno, B., & Bishop, A. (2006). Questioning the Net Generation: A collaborative project in Australian higher education. In L. Markauskaite, P. Goodyear, & P. Reimann (Eds.), *Who's learning? Whose technology? Proceedings of the 23rd Australasian Society for Computers in Learning in Tertiary Education (ASCILITE) Conference* (pp. 413–417). Sydney: University of Sydney. Retrieved December 21, 2008, from http://www.ascilite.org.au/conferences/sydney06/proceeding/pdf_papers/p160.pdf

Kenway, J., & Bullen, E. (2005). Globalizing the young in the age of desire: Some educational policy issues. In Apple, M. W., Kenway, J., & Singh, M. (Eds.), *Globalizing education: Policies, pedagogies, & politics* (pp. 31–43). New York: Peter Lang.

Kerawalla, L., Minocha, S., Kirkup, G., & Conole, G. (2008). Characterising the different blogging behaviours of students on an online distance learning course. *Learning, Media and Technology*, *33*(1), 21–33. doi:10.1080/17439880701868838

Kerawalla, L., Minocha, S., Kirkup, G., & Conole, G. (2009a). An empirically grounded framework to guide blogging in higher education. *Journal of Computer Assisted Learning, 25*(1), 31–42. doi:10.1111/j.1365-2729.2008.00286.x

Kerawalla, L., Minocha, S., Kirkup, G., & Conole, G. (2009). Supporting student blogging in higher education. In Hatzipanagos, S., & Warburton, S. (Eds.), *Handbook of research on social software and developing community ontologies* (pp. 231–247). Hershey, PA: Information Science Reference.

Kesim, E., & Agaoglu, E. (2007). A paradigm shift in distance education: Web 2.0 and social software. *Turkish Online Journal of Distance Education, 8*(3), 66–75. Retrieved June 16, 2008, from http://tojde.anadolu.edu.tr/tojde27/pdf/article_4.pdf

Kim, K. J., & Bonk, C. J. (2006). The future of online teaching and learning in higher education: The survey says.... *EDUCAUSE Quarterly, 29*(4), 22–30. Retrieved June 22, 2008, from http://www.educause.edu/ir/library/pdf/EQM0644.pdf

Kirkpatrick, D. L. (2006). *Evaluating training programs: The four levels* (3rd ed.). San Francisco: Berrett-Koehler.

Kirkup, G., & Kirkwood, A. (2005). Information and communications technologies (ICT) in higher education teaching—a tale of gradualism rather than revolution. *Learning, Media and Technology, 30*(2), 185–199. doi:10.1080/17439880500093810

Kirkwood, A., & Price, L. (2005). Learners and learning in the 21st century: What do we know about students' attitudes and experiences of ICT that will help us design courses? *Studies in Higher Education, 30*(3), 257–274. doi:10.1080/03075070500095689

Kirschner, P. A. (2002). Can we support CSCL? Educational, social and technological affordances for learning. In Kirschner, P. A. (Ed.), *Three worlds of CSCL: Can we support CSCL?* (pp. 7–47). Heerlen, The Netherlands: Open University of the Netherlands.

Kleiner, C., & Lord, M. (1999). The cheating game: Cross-national exploration of business students' attitudes, perceptions, and tendencies toward academic dishonesty. *Journal of Education for Business, 74*(4), 38–42.

Kling, R. (1999). What is social informatics and why does it matter? *D-Lib Magazine, 5*(1). Retrieved November 20, 2008, from http://www.dlib.org/dlib/january99/kling/01kling.html

Knight, P. T., & Yorke, M. (2003). *Assessment, learning and employability*. Buckingham, UK: Open University Press.

Knowles, M. S. (1984). *Andragogy in action: Applying modern principles in adult learning*. San Francisco: Jossey-Bass.

Kohut, A., Parker, K., Keeter, S., Doherty, C., & Dimock, M. (2007). *How young people view their lives, futures and politics: A portrait of "Generation Next"*. Washington, DC: The Pew Research Center for the People & the Press. Retrieved March 23, 2009 from http://people-press.org/reports/pdf/300.pdf

Kolas, L., & Staupe, A. (2007). The PLExus Prototype: A PLE realized as topic maps. In J. M. Spector, D. G. Sampson, T. Okamoto, Kinshuk, S. A. Cerri, M. Ueno, & A. Kashihara (Eds.), *Proceedings of the Seventh International Conference on Advanced Learning Technologies* (pp. 750–752). Los Alamitos, CA: IEEE Computer Society.

Kolmos, A., Fink, F. K., & Krogh, L. (Eds.). (2004). *The Aalborg PBL model: Progress, diversity and challenges*. Aalborg, Denmark: Aalborg University Press.

Könings, K. D., Brand-Gruwel, S., van Merriënboer, J. J. G., & Broers, N. (2006). Does a new learning environment come up to students' expectations? A longitudinal study. *Journal of Educational Psychology, 100*(3), 535–548. doi:10.1037/0022-0663.100.3.535

Kop, R. (2007). Blogs and wikis as disruptive technologies: Is it time for a new pedagogy? In Osborne, M., Houston, M., & Toman, N. (Eds.), *The pedagogy of lifelong learning: Understanding effective teaching and learning in diverse contexts* (pp. 192–202). Abingdon, UK: Routledge.

Koper, R. (2004). Use of the Semantic Web to solve some basic problems in education: Increase flexible, distributed lifelong learning, decrease teachers' workload. *Journal of Interactive Media in Education*. Retrieved April 29, 2010, from http://www-jime.open.ac.uk/2004/6/koper-2004-6.pdf

Koschmann, T. (Ed.). (1996). *CSCL: Theory and practice of an emerging paradigm*. Mahwah, NJ: Lawrence Erlbaum.

Koschmann, T. (2001). Revisiting the paradigms of instructional technology. In G. Kennedy, M. Keppell, C. McNaught, & T. Petrovic (Eds.), *Meeting at the crossroads. Proceedings of the 18th Australasian Society for Computers in Learning in Tertiary Education (ASCILITE) Conference* (pp. 15–22). Melbourne, Australia: Biomedical Multimedia Unit, The University of Melbourne. Retrieved July 3, 2009, from www.ascilite.org.au/conferences/melbourne01/pdf/papers/koschmannt.pdf

Kost, C. (2007, May 24–26). *Using wikis for a collaborative writing project*. Paper presented at the Computer Assisted Language Instruction Consortium (CALICO) Conference, San Marcos, TX.

Kozma, R. B. (1994). A reply: Media and methods. *Educational Technology Research and Development, 42*(3), 11–14. doi:10.1007/BF02298091

Krause, K.-L. (2007). Who is the e-generation and how are they faring in higher education? In Lockhard, J., & Pegrum, M. (Eds.), *Brave new classrooms: Educational democracy and the Internet* (pp. 125–139). New York: Peter Lang.

Krause, K.-L. (2005a, September 5–7). The changing student experience: Who's driving it and where is it going? Keynote paper presented at the Student Experience Conference, Wagga Wagga, Australia. Retrieved April 23, 2008, from http://www.csu.edu.au/division/studserv/sec/papers/krause.pdf

Krause, K.-L. (2005b). *Understanding and promoting student engagement in university learning communities*. Melbourne, Australia: Centre for the Study of Higher Education, The University of Melbourne. Retrieved August 11, 2006, from http://www.cshe.unimelb.edu.au/pdfs/Stud_eng.pdf

Kreijns, K., Kirschner, P. A., & Jochems, W. (2002). The sociability of computer-supported collaborative learning environments. *Journal of Educational Technology & Society, 5*(1), 8–22.

Kuh, G. D., Cruce, T., Shoup, R., Kinzie, J., & Gonyea, R. M. (2007, April 9–13). *Unmasking the effects of student engagement on college grades and persistence.* Paper presented at the 2007 Annual Meeting of the American Educational Research Association (AERA), Chicago. Retrieved December 4, 2008, from http://nsse.iub.edu/uploads/AERA_2007_Kuh_et_al.pdf

Kukulska-Hulme, A. (2005, May 11–12). *The mobile language learner—now and in the future*. Paper presented at Fran Vision till Praktik (Language Learning and ICT Symposium), Umeå, Sweden. Retrieved February 3, 2006, from http://www2.humlab.umu.se/video/Praktikvision/agnes.ram

Kukulska-Hulme, A., Traxler, J., & Pettit, J. (2007). Designed and user-generated activity in the mobile age. *Journal of Learning Design, 2*(1), 52–65. Retrieved November 20, 2008, from http://www.jld.qut.edu.au/publications/vol2no1/documents/designed%20and%20usergenerated.pdf

Kvavik, R. B. (2005). Convenience, communications, and control: How students use technology. In Oblinger, D. G., & Oblinger, J. L. (Eds.), *Educating the Net Generation* (pp. 7.1–7.20). Boulder, CO: EDUCAUSE.

Laaser, W. (1986). Some didactic aspects of audio-cassettes in distance education. *Distance Education, 7*(1), 143–152. doi:10.1080/0158791860070110

Laitner, A. (2008, June 10). EU in working week discussions. *Financial Times*.

Lakoff, G., & Johnson, M. (1980). *Metaphors we live by*. Chicago: University of Chicago Press.

Lamb, B. (2004). Wide open spaces: Wikis, ready or not. *EDUCAUSE Review, 39*(5), 36–46. Retrieved November 30, 2007, from http://www.educause.edu/ir/library/pdf/erm0452.pdf

Lamb, B. (2007). Dr Mashup; or, why educators should learn to stop worrying and love the remix. *EDUCAUSE Review, 42*(4), 12–25. Retrieved January 19, 2008, from http://net.educause.edu/ir/library/pdf/erm0740.pdf

Lampe, C., Ellison, N., & Steinfield, C. (2006). A Face(book) in the crowd: Social searching vs. social browsing. In *Proceedings of the 2006 20th Anniversary Conference on Computer Supported Cooperative Work* (pp. 167–170). New York: Association for Computing Machinery.

Lamshed, R., Berry, M., & Armstrong, L. (2002). *Blogs: Personal e-learning spaces*. Melbourne, Australia: TAFE Frontiers. Retrieved April 29, 2010, from http://www.binaryblue.com.au/docs/blogs.pdf

Lankshear, C., Peters, M., & Knobel, M. (2000). Information, knowledge and learning: Some issues facing epistemology and education in a digital age. *Journal of Philosophy of Education*, *34*(1), 17–40. doi:10.1111/1467-9752.00153

Lankshear, C., & Knobel, M. (2007). Researching new literacies: Web 2.0 practices and insider perspectives. *E-learning*, *4*(3), 224–240. doi:10.2304/elea.2007.4.3.224

Lankshear, C. (2003). The challenge of digital epistemologies. *Education Communication and Information*, *3*(2), 167–186. doi:10.1080/1463631032000092000144

Lather, P. (1989, August 25–27). *Deconstructing/deconstructive inquiry: Issues in feminist research methodologies*. Paper presented at the New Zealand Women's Studies Association Conference, Christchurch, New Zealand.

Laurillard, D. (2002). *Rethinking university teaching: A conversational framework for the effective use of learning technologies* (2nd ed.). London: RoutledgeFalmer. doi:10.4324/9780203304846

Lave, J., & Wenger, E. (1991). *Situated learning: Legitimate peripheral participation*. New York: Cambridge University Press.

Leadbeater, C. (2006). *The ten habits of mass innovation*. London: National Endowment for Science, Technology and the Arts. Retrieved November 3, 2007, from http://www.nesta.org.uk/assets/pdf/ten_habits_of_mass_innovation_provocation_NESTA.pdf

LeBlanc, G., & Bearison, D. J. (2004). Teaching and learning as a bi-directional activity: Investigating dyadic interactions between child teachers and child learners. *Cognitive Development*, *19*(4), 499–515. doi:10.1016/j.cogdev.2004.09.004

Lee, M. J. W. (2005). New tools for online collaboration: Blogs, wikis, RSS and podcasting. *Training and Development in Australia*, *32*(5), 17–20.

Lee, M. J. W., & Chan, A. (2007). Pervasive, lifestyle-integrated mobile learning for distance learners: An analysis and unexpected results from a podcasting study. *Open Learning*, *22*(3), 201–218.

Lee, M. J. W. (2005). New tools for online collaboration: Blogs, wikis, RSS and podcasting. *Training and Development in Australia*, *32*(5), 17–20.

Lee, M. J. W. (2005). Mobile learning: Should we get a move on? *Training and Development in Australia*, *32*(4), 8–11.

Lee, M. J. W., & Chan, A. (2007). Pervasive, lifestyle-integrated mobile learning for distance learners: An analysis and unexpected results from a podcasting study. *Open Learning*, *22*(3), 201–218.

Lee, M. J. W. (2007). Podcasting and digital audio in L&D: Time to hand over the microphone! *Training and Development in Australia*, *34*(3), 28–29.

Lee, M. J. W., McLoughlin, C., & Chan, A. (2008). Talk the talk: Learner-generated podcasts as catalysts for knowledge creation. *British Journal of Educational Technology*, *39*(3), 501–521. doi:10.1111/j.1467-8535.2007.00746.x

Lee, M. J. W. (2008). Mobile and pervasive technology in education and training: Potential and possibilities, problems and pitfalls. In Godara, V. (Ed.), *Risk assessment and management in pervasive computing: Operational, legal, ethical and financial perspectives* (pp. 73–105). Hershey, PA: Information Science Reference.

Lee, M. J. W., & Tynan, B. (2008). Podcasts and distance learning. In Salmon, G., & Edirisingha, P. (Eds.), *Podcasting for learning in universities* (pp. 92–102). London: McGraw-Hill.

Lee, M. J. W. (2006, October). Using blogs and podcasting to facilitate delivery and self/peer evaluation of oral presentation assessments. *Learning Technology*, 28–30. Retrieved May 2, 2007, from http://lttf.ieee.org/learn_tech/issues/october2006/lt_october2006.pdf

Lee, M. J. W., & Chan, A. (2007). Reducing the effects of isolation and promoting inclusivity for distance learners through podcasting. *Turkish Online Journal of Distance Education*, *8*(1), 85–104. Retrieved February 22, 2008, from http://tojde.anadolu.edu.tr/tojde25/pdf/article_7.pdf

Lee, M. J. W., & McLoughlin, C. (2007). Teaching and learning in the Web 2.0 era: Empowering students through learner-generated content. *International Journal of In-*

structional Technology and Distance Learning, 4(10), 21–34. Retrieved November 29, 2008, from http://www.itdl.org/Journal/Oct_07/Oct_07.pdf

Lee, M. J. W., Chan, A., & McLoughlin, C. (2006). Students as producers: Second year students' experiences as podcasters of content for first year undergraduates. In *Proceedings of the Seventh Conference on Information Technology Based Higher Education and Training* (pp. 832–841). Broadway, Australia: University of Technology, Sydney.

Lee, M. J. W., Chan, A., & McLoughlin, C. (2006a). Educational podcasting using the Charles Sturt University Flexible Publishing platform. In T. Reeves & S. Yamashita (Eds.), *Proceedings of World Conference on E-Learning in Corporate, Government, Healthcare, and Higher Education 2006* (pp. 2894–2901). Chesapeake, VA: Association for the Advancement of Computers in Education.

Lee, M. J. W., Eustace, K., Hay, L., & Fellows, G. (2005). Learning to collaborate, collaboratively: An online community building and knowledge construction approach to teaching computer supported collaborative work at an Australian university. In M. R. Simonson & M. Crawford (Eds.), *Proceedings of the 2005 Association for Educational Communications and Technology International Convention* (pp. 286–306). North Miami Beach, FL: Nova Southeastern University.

Lenhart, A., & Madden, M. (2007). *Teens, privacy & online social networks: How teens manage their online identities and personal information in the age of MySpace.* Washington, DC: Pew Internet & American Life Project. Retrieved July 30, 2008, from http://www.pewinternet.org/~/media//Files/Reports/2007/PIP_Teens_Privacy_SNS_Report_Final.pdf.pdf

Lenhart, A., Madden, M., Rankin Macgill, A., & Smith, A. (2007). *Teens and social media.* Washington, DC: Pew Internet & American Life Project. Retrieved November 4, 2008, from http://www.pewinternet.org/~/media//Files/Reports/2007/PIP_Teens_Social_Media_Final.pdf.pdf

Leont'ev, A. N. (1981). *Problems of the development of mind.* (M. Kopylova, Trans.). Moscow: Progress. (1947).

Leslie, P. H., & Murphy, E. (2008). Post-secondary students' purposes for blogging. *International Review of Research in Open and Distance Learning, 9*(3). Retrieved October 24, 2008, from http://www.irrodl.org/index.php/irrodl/article/view/560/1140

Leslie, S., & Landon, B. (2007). *Social software for learning: What is it, why use it?* London: The Observatory of Borderless Higher Education. Retrieved April 28, 2008, from http://www.obhe.ac.uk/products/reports/pdf/2008-01-01.pdf

Levin, D., & Arafeh, S. (2002). *The digital disconnect: The widening gap between Internet-savvy students and their schools*. Washington, DC: Pew Internet & American Life Project. Retrieved October 28, 2009, from http://www.pewinternet.org/~/media//Files/Reports/2002/PIP_Schools_Internet_Report.pdf.pdf

Lew, A. (2007, August 19). Twitter tweets for higher education [Web log post]. *Web 2.0 Teaching Tools*. Retrieved November 4, 2008, from http://web20teach.blogspot.com/2007/08/twitter-tweets-for-higher-education.html

Ley, D. (2007). Ubiquitous computing. In *Emerging technologies for learning* (Vol. 2, pp. 64–79). Coventry, UK: Becta. Retrieved November 30, 2008, from http://partners.becta.org.uk/upload-dir/downloads/page_documents/research/emerging_technologies07.pdf

Liber, O., & Johnson, M. (2008). Personal learning environments [Special issue]. *Interactive Learning Environments, 16*(1). doi:10.1080/10494820701772645

Light, R. J. (2001). *Making the most of college: Students speak their minds*. Cambridge, MA: Harvard University Press.

Lim, C. P., & Chai, C. S. (2007). Teachers' pedagogical beliefs and their planning and conduct of computer-mediated classroom lessons. *British Journal of Educational Technology, 39*(5), 807–828. doi:10.1111/j.1467-8535.2007.00774.x

Lindblom-Ylänne, S., & Pihlajamäki, H. (2003). Can a collaborative network environment enhance essay-writing processes? *British Journal of Educational Technology, 34*(1), 17–30. doi:10.1111/1467-8535.00301

Linden, G. (2006, May 14). Tim O'Reilly and defining Web 2.0 [Web log post]. *Geeking with Greg*. Retrieved November 20, 2008, from http://glinden.blogspot.com/2006/05/tim-oreilly-and-defining-web-20.html

Lindner, M. (2006). Use these tools, your mind will follow. Learning in immersive micromedia and microknowledge environments. In D. Whitelock & S. Wheeler (Eds.), *The next generation: Research proceedings of the 13th Association for Learning Technology Conference* (pp. 41–49). Oxford, UK: ALT.

Lindstrom, P. (2007). *Securing "Web 2.0" Technologies*. Boulder, CO: EDUCAUSE Center for Applied Research.

Lippincott, J. K. (2006). Learning, engagement, and technology. In Gibson, C. (Ed.), *Student engagement and information literacy* (pp. 169–183). Chicago: Association of College and Research Libraries.

List of social networking websites. (2009, January 7). In *Wikipedia, the free encyclopedia*. Retrieved January 8, 2009, from http://en.wikipedia.org/wiki/List_of_social_networking_websites

Littleton, K., Miell, D., & Faulkner, D. (Eds.). (2004). *Learning to collaborate, collaborating to learn: Understanding and promoting educationally productive collaborative work*. New York: Nova Science.

Littleton, K., & Häkkinen, P. (1999). Learning together: Understanding the processes of computer-based collaborative learning. In Dillenbourg, P. (Ed.), *Collaborative learning: Cognitive and computational approaches* (pp. 20–30). Oxford, UK: Pergamon.

Livingstone, S. (2002). *Young people and new media: Childhood and the changing media environment*. Thousand Oaks, CA: Sage.

Loddington, S., Pond, K., Wilkinson, N., & Willmot, P. (2009). A case study of the development of WebPA: An online peer-moderated marking tool. *British Journal of Educational Technology*, *40*(2), 329–341. doi:10.1111/j.1467-8535.2008.00922.x

Lohnes, S., & Kinzer, C. (2007). Questioning assumptions about students' expectations for technology in college classrooms. *Innovate: Journal of Online Education*, *3*(5). Retrieved November 1, 2008, from, http://www.innovateonline.info/index.php?view=article&id=431

Lokken, F., & Womer, L. (2007). *Trends in e-learning: Tracking the impact of e-learning in higher education. 2006 distance education survey results*. Washington, DC: Instructional Technology Council. Retrieved December 6, 2008, from http://www.itcnetwork.org/file.php?file=/1/ITCAnnualSurveyFeb2007.pdf

Long, M. H. (1991). *Measuring classroom language change*. Unpublished manuscript, University of Hawai`i, Manoa, HI.

Lorenzo, G., & Dziuban, C. (2006). *Ensuring the Net Generation is net savvy*. Boulder, CO: EDUCAUSE. Retrieved November 1, 2008, from http://www.educause.edu/ir/library/pdf/ELI3006.pdf

Lorenzo, G., & Ittelson, J. C. (2005). *An overview of portfolios*. Boulder, CO: EDUCAUSE. Retrieved December 6, 2008, from http://www.educause.edu/ir/library/pdf/ELI3001.pdf

Lowendahl, J.-M., Zastrocky, M., & Harris, M. (2008). *Gartner Higher Education E-Learning Survey 2007: Clear movements in the market*. Stamford, CT: Gartner.

Lubensky, R. (2006, December). The present and future of Personal Learning Environments (PLE) [Web log post]. *Deliberations*. Retrieved January 8, 2009, from http://www.deliberations.com.au/2006/12/present-and-future-of-personal-learning.html

Luca, J., & Oliver, R. (2002). Developing an instructional design strategy to support generic skills development. In A. Williamson, C. Gunn, A. Young, & T. Clear (Eds.), *Winds of change in the sea of learning: Charting the course of digital education. Proceedings of the 19th Australasian Society for Computers in Learning in Tertiary Education (ASCILITE) Conference* (pp. 401–411). Auckland, New Zealand: UNITEC Institute of Technology. Retrieved August 12, 2008, from http://www.ascilite.org.au/conferences/auckland02/proceedings/papers/073.pdf

Luckin, R. (2008). The learner centric ecology of resources: A framework for using technology to scaffold learning. *Computers & Education*, *50*(2), 449–462. doi:10.1016/j.compedu.2007.09.018

Luckin, R. (2010). *Re-designing learning contexts: Technology-rich, learner-centred ecologies*. Abingdon, UK: Routledge.

Luckin, R., Shurville, S., & Browne, T. (2007). Initiating e-learning by stealth, participation and consultation in a late majority institution. *Organisational Transformation and Social Change*, *4*(1), 317–332. doi:10.1386/jots.3.3.317_1

Luckin, R., du Boulay, B., Smith, H., Underwood, J., Fitzpatrick, G., & Holmberg, J. … Pearce, D. (2005). Using mobile technology to create flexible learning contexts. *Journal of Interactive Media in Education*. Retrieved November 29, 2008, from http://jime.open.ac.uk/2005/22/luckin-2005-22.pdf

Luckin, R., Logan, K., Clark, W., Graber, R., Oliver, M., & Mee, A. (2008). *Learners' use of Web 2.0 technologies in and out of school in Key Stages 3 and 4*. Coventry, UK: Becta. Retrieved November 29, 2008, from http://research.becta.org.uk/upload-dir/downloads/page_documents/research/web2_technologies_ks3_4.pdf

Luppicini, R. (Ed.). (2007). *Online learning communities*. Charlotte, NC: Information Age.

Luzón, M. J. (2009). Scholarly hyperwriting: The function of links in academic blogs. *Journal of the American Society for Information Science and Technology*, *60*(1), 65–89. doi:10.1002/asi.20937

Luzón, M. J. (2006). Research group blogs: Sites for self-presentation and collaboration. In *Proceedings of the Fifth Annual Conference of the European Association of Languages for Specific Purposes (AELFE)* (pp. 629–634). Castelló de la Plana, Spain: AELFE. Retrieved April 29, 2010, from http://www.unizar.es/aelfe2006/ALEFE06/5.newtechnologies/87.pdf

Lyotard, J.-F. (1993). A svelte appendix to the postmodern question. In *Political writings* (pp. 25–29). (Readings, B., & Geiman, K. P., Trans.). Minneapolis, MN: University of Minnesota Press.

Lyotard, J.-F. (1984). *The postmodern condition: A report on knowledge*. (G. Bennington & B. Massumi, Trans.). Minneapolis, MN: University of Minnesota Press. (1979).

Lytras, M., & Naeve, A. (2006). Semantic e-learning: Synthesizing fantasies. *British Journal of Educational Technology*, *37*(3), 479–491. doi:10.1111/j.1467-8535.2006.00617.x

Mabrito, M., & Medley, R. (2008). Why Professor Johnny can't read: Understanding the Net Generation's texts. *Innovate: Journal of Online Education, 4*(6). Retrieved July 20, 2008, from http://www.innovate.info/index.php?view=article&id=510

MacManus, R. (2009, October 21). Emerging Internet trends: An analysis of Mary Meeker's Web 2.0 summit presentation [Web log post]. *ReadWriteWeb*. Retrieved November 20, 2008, from http://www.readwriteweb.com/archives/emerging_internet_trends_meeker_2009.php

MacManus, R., & Porter, J. (2005, May 4). Web 2.0 for designers. *Digital Web Magazine*. Retrieved April 15, 2008, from http://www.digital-web.com/articles/web_2_for_designers

Madden, M., & Fox, S. (2006, October 5). *Riding the waves of "Web 2.0": More than a buzzword, but still not easily defined*. Retrieved January 10, 2008, from http://pewresearch.org/pubs/71/riding-the-waves-of-web-20

Maloney, E. J. (2007, January 5). What Web 2.0 can teach us about learning. *The Chronicle of Higher Education*, B26.

Marcus, E. (1952). The cyclical adjustment pattern of an "open economy": Canada, 1927–1939. *The Economic Journal*, *62*(246), 305–317. doi:10.2307/2227006

Marginson, S. (2007, August 8–10). *Rankings: Marketing mana or menace?* Paper presented at the 16th Annual New Zealand International Education Conference, Christchurch, New Zealand. Retrieved December 4, 2008, from http://www.cshe.unimelb.edu.au/people/staff_pages/Marginson?KeyMar8-10Aug07.pdf

Markwell, D. (2007). *A large and liberal education: Higher education for the 21st century*. Melbourne, Australia: Australian Scholarly Publishing.

Marsh, B. (2007). *Plagiarism: Alchemy and remedy in higher education*. Albany, NY: State University of New York Press.

Marshall, L., & Rowland, F. (1993). *A guide to learning independently*. Buckingham, UK: Open University Press.

Martin, A. (2006). Literacies for the digital age: Preview of Part 1. In Martin, A., & Madigan, D. (Eds.), *Digital literacies for learning* (pp. 3–25). London: Facet.

Martin, A., & Ashworth, S. (2004). Welcome to the Journal of eLiteracy! *Journal of eLiteracy, 1*(1), 2–6. Retrieved November 1, 2008, from http://www.jelit.org/archive/00000011/01/JeLit_Editorial.pdf

Martin, M. (2007). My personal learning environment [Web log post]. *The Bamboo Project Blog*. Retrieved July 17, 2008, from http://michelemartin.typepad.com/thebambooprojectblog/2007/04/my_personal_lea.html

Masie, E. (2006). Nano-learning: Miniaturization of design. *Chief Learning Officer, 5*(1), 17. Retrieved August 29, 2007, from http://www.clomedia.com/content/templates/clo_article.asp?articleid=1221

Mason, R., & Rennie, F. (2008). *E-learning and social networking handbook: Resources for higher education*. New York: Routledge.

Mason, R. (1989). An evaluation of CoSy on an Open University course. In Mason, R., & Kaye, A. (Eds.), *Mindweave: Communication, computers, and distance education* (pp. 221–226). New York: Pergamon.

Massachusetts Institute of Technology. (2009). *About OCW*. Retrieved April 8, 2009, from http://ocw.mit.edu/OcwWeb/web/about/about/index.htm

Mayer, R. E. (1998). Cognitive theory for education: What teachers need to know. In Lambert, N. M., & McCombs, B. L. (Eds.), *How students learn: Reforming schools through learner-centered education* (pp. 353–377). Washington, DC: American Psychological Association. doi:10.1037/10258-013

Mayes, T., & Fowler, C. (2006). Learners, learning literacy and the pedagogy of e-learning. In Martin, A., & Madigan, D. (Eds.), *Digital literacies for learning* (pp. 107–123). London: Facet.

Mayfield, A. (2008). *What is social media?* London: iCrossing. Retrieved August 3, 2009, from http://www.icrossing.co.uk/fileadmin/uploads/eBooks/What_is_Social_Media_iCrossing_ebook.pdf

Mazer, J. P., Murphy, R. E., & Simonds, C. J. (2007). I'll see you on "Facebook": The effects of computer-mediated teacher self-disclosure on student motivation, affective learning, and classroom climate. *Communication Education, 56*(1), 1–17. doi:10.1080/03634520601009710

Mazur, E. (1997). *Peer instruction: A user's manual*. London: Prentice Hall.

McAndrew, P. (2006, October 26–27). *Motivations for OpenLearn: The Open University's open content initiative*. Paper presented at the OECD experts meeting on open educational resources, Barcelona. Retrieved December 21, 2008, from http://kn.open.ac.uk/public/getfile.cfm?documentfileid=10026

McCullagh, K. (2008). Blogging: Self presentation and privacy. *Information & Communications Technology Law, 17*(1), 3–23. doi:10.1080/13600830801886984

McFedries, P. (2007). Social-isms. *IEEE Spectrum, 44*(4), 56.

McFedries, P. (2005, December 22). Web 2.0. *Word Spy*. Retrieved November 1, 2008, from http://www.wordspy.com/words/Web2.0.asp

McGarr, O. (2009). A review of podcasting in higher education: Its influence on the traditional lecture. *Australasian Journal of Educational Technology, 25*(3), 309–321. Retrieved August 10, 2009, from http://www.ascilite.org.au/ajet/ajet25/mcgarr.pdf

McGee, P., & Diaz, V. (2007). Wikis and podcasts and blogs! Oh, my! What is a faculty member supposed to do? *EDUCAUSE Review, 42*(5), 28–41. Retrieved November 30, 2007, from http://www.educause.edu/ir/library/pdf/erm0452.pdf

McGill, L., Nicol, D., Littlejohn, A., Grierson, H., Juster, N., & Ion, W. J. (2005). Creating an information-rich learning environment to enhance design student learning: Challenges and approaches. *British Journal of Educational Technology, 36*(4), 629–642. doi:10.1111/j.1467-8535.2005.00540.x

McKigney, E. (2007, February 15). College forms committee to examine use of Facebook. *The Ithacan Online*. Retrieved July 30, 2008, from http://theithacan.org/am/publish/news/200702_College_forms_committee_to_examine_use_of_Facebook.shtml

McLoughlin, C., Lee, M. J. W., & Chan, A. (2006). Using student-generated podcasts to foster reflection and metacognition. *Australian Educational Computing, 21*(2), 34–40.

McLoughlin, C., & Lee, M. J. W. (2007). Social software and participatory learning: Pedagogical choices with technology affordances in the Web 2.0 era. In *ICT: Providing choices for learners and learning. Proceedings of the 24th Australasian Society for Computers in Learning in Tertiary Education (ASCILITE) Conference* (pp.

664–675). Singapore: Nanyang Technological University. Retrieved June 6, 2008, from http://www.ascilite.org.au/conferences/singapore07/procs/mcloughlin.pdf

McLoughlin, C., & Lee, M. J. W. (2008). Future learning landscapes: Transforming pedagogy through social software. *Innovate: Journal of Online Education, 4*(5). Retrieved November 1, 2008, from http://www.innovateonline.info/index.php?view=article&id=539

McLoughlin, C., & Lee, M. J. W. (2010). Personalised and self-regulated learning in the Web 2.0 era: International exemplars of innovative pedagogy using social software. *Australasian Journal of Educational Technology, 26*(1), 28–43. Retrieved February 23, 2010, from http://www.ascilite.org.au/ajet/ajet26/mcloughlin.pdf

McLoughlin, C., & Visser, T. (2003). Quality e-learning: Are there universal indicators? In C. McLoughlin, P. Le-Cornu, & W. Jackson (Eds.), *Sustaining quality learning environments: Proceedings of the 16th Open and Distance Learning Association of Australia (ODLAA) Biennial Conference*. Canberra, Australia: Canberra Institute of Technology.

McLoughlin, C., Brady, J., Lee, M. J. W., & Russell, R. (2007, November 25–29). *Peer-to-peer: An e-mentoring approach to facilitating reflection on professional experience for novice teachers*. Paper presented at the 2007 Australian Association for Research in Education Conference, Fremantle, Australia. Retrieved January 17, 2009, from http://www.aare.edu.au/07pap/mcl07393.pdf

McLoughlin, C., Lee, M. J. W., & Brady, J. (2008). A learning architecture framework (LAF) for developing community, engagement and professional identity for pre-service teachers. In I. Olney, G. Lefoe, J. Mantei, & J. Herrington (Eds.), *Proceedings of the Emerging Technologies Conference 2008* (pp. 147–157). Wollongong, Australia: University of Wollongong. Retrieved January 17, 2009, from http://ro.uow.edu.au/cgi/viewcontent.cgi?article=1016&context=etc08

McLoughlin, C., Lee, M. J. W., & Chan, A. (2007). Promoting engagement and motivation for distance learners through podcasting. In *New Learning 2.0? Emerging digital territories, developing continuities, new divides: Proceedings of the European Distance Education and E-Learning Network (EDEN) Annual Conference 2007*. Budapest, Hungary: EDEN.

McMurtry, K. (2001). e-cheating: Combating a 21st century challenge. *T.H.E. Journal, 29*(4), 36–41.

McPherson, M. A., & Nunes, J. M. (2004). The failure of a virtual social space (VSS) designed to create a learning community: Lessons learned. *British Journal of Educational Technology, 35*(3), 305–321. doi:10.1111/j.0007-1013.2004.00391.x

McWilliam, E. (2008). Unlearning how to teach. *Innovations in Education and Teaching International, 45*(3), 263–269. doi:10.1080/14703290802176147

Meister, J. C. (2006). Keeping learners engaged: Certifying and supporting online instructors. *Chief Learning Officer, 5*(2), 66.

Mejias, U. (2005). A nomad's guide to learning and social software. *The Knowledge Tree: An e-Journal of Learning Innovation, 7*. Retrieved November 10, 2006, from http://knowledgetree.flexiblelearning.net.au/edition07/download/la_mejias.pdf

Mejias, U. (2006). Teaching social software with social software. *Innovate: Journal of Online Education, 2*(5). Retrieved February 12, 2010, from http://innovateonline.info/pdf/vol2_issue5/Teaching_Social_Software_with_Social_Software.pdf

Menell, B. (2005, November). Atomization of learning (Beyond the learning object) [Web log post]. *Learning 2.0*. Retrieved January 8, 2006, from http://learning20.blogspot.com/2005/11/atomization-of-learning-beyond.html

Mentor, K. (2005, November 15–19). *The Online Encyclopedia of Criminal Justice*. Paper presented at the Annual Meeting of the American Society of Criminology, Toronto, ON.

Mercer, N., & Littleton, K. (2007). *Dialogue and the development of children's thinking: A sociocultural approach*. London: Routledge.

Mercer, N. (1992). Culture, context and the construction of knowledge in the classroom. In Light, P., & Butterworth, G. (Eds.), *Context and cognition: Ways of learning and knowing* (pp. 28–46). London: Harvester Wheatsheaf.

Merrill, M. D. (2002). First principles of instruction. *Educational Technology Research and Development, 50*(3), 43–59. doi:10.1007/BF02505024

Middleton, A. (2008, June 18–19). *Audio feedback: Timely media interventions*. Paper presented at the Third International Blended Learning Conference, Hertfordshire, UK. Retrieved August 12, 2008, from http://www.herts.ac.uk/fms/documents/teaching-and-learning/blu/conference2008/Andrew-Middleton-2008.pdf

Midoro, V. (2007). Quale alfabetizzazione per la società della conoscenza (What literacies are needed for the knowledge society)? *TD: Tecnologie Didattiche, 41*, 47–54. Retrieved November 1, 2008, from http://www.itd.cnr.it/tdmagazine/PDF41/8_Midoro_TD41.pdf

Miell, D., & Littleton, K. (Eds.). (2004). *Creative collaborations*. London: Free Association Books.

Miers, J. (2004). *BELTS or braces?* Retrieved June 5, 2007, from http://www.tsof.edu.au/research/Reports04/miers.asp

Millea, J. Green. I., & Putland, G. (2005). *Emerging technologies: A framework for thinking*. Adelaide, Australia: Education.au. Retrieved October 23, 2009, from http://www.det.act.gov.au/__data/assets/pdf_file/0010/74485/ACT_EmTech_Report_v1_2.pdf

Miller, D. B. (2006, October 18). Podcasting at the University of Connecticut: Enhancing the educational experience. *Campus Technology*. Retrieved April 10, 2007, from http://campustechnology.com/news_article.asp?id=19424&typeid=156

Milne, A. J. (2007). Entering the interaction age: Implementing a future vision for campus learning spaces. *EDUCAUSE Review, 42*(1), 12–31. Retrieved August 30, 2008, from *http://*net.educause.edu/ir/library/pdf/ERM0710.pdf

Mindel, J. L., & Verma, S. (2006). Wikis for teaching and learning. *Communications of the Association for Information Systems, 18*(1), 2–38.

Miniwatts Marketing Group. (2008, July 1). *World Internet usage*. Retrieved July 17, 2008, from http://www.internetworldstats.com/stats.htm

Minocha, S., Petre, M., & Roberts, D. (2008). Using wikis to simulate distributed requirements development in a software engineering course. *International Journal of Engineering Education, 24*(4), 689–704.

Minocha, S. (2009). *A study on the effective use of social software by further and higher education in the UK to support student learning and engagement*. Bristol, UK: Joint Information Systems Committee. Retrieved April 29, 2010, from http://www.jisc.ac.uk/media/documents/projects/effective-use-of-social-software-in-education-finalreport.pdf

Minocha, S., & Tingle, R. (2008). Socialisation and collaborative learning of distance learners in 3-D virtual worlds. In A. Peachey (Ed.), *Proceedings of ReLIVE 08: Researching Learning in Virtual Environments International Conference* (pp. 216–227). Milton Keynes, UK: The Open University. Retrieved April 28, 2010, from http://www.open.ac.uk/relive08/documents/ReLIVE08_conference_proceedings_Lo.pdf

Mintzberg, H. (1989). *Mintzberg on management: Inside our strange world of organizations*. London: Macmillan.

Mobile Data Association. (2009). *The Q4 2009 UK mobile trends report*. London: MDA. Retrieved November 20, 2008, from http://www.themda.org/mda-press-releases/the-q4-2009-uk-mobile-trends-report.php

Mobile phone users reach 3.3bn. (2008, May 27). *The Australian*. Retrieved July 17, 2008, from http://www.theaustralian.com.au/australian-it/mobile-phone-users-reach-33bn/story-e6frgalx-1111116448670

Moll, L. C. (2000). Inspired by Vygotsky: Ethnographic experiments in education. In Lee, C. D., & Smagorinsky, P. (Eds.), *Vygotskian perspectives on literary research: Constructing meaning through collaborative inquiry* (pp. 256–268). New York: Cambridge University Press.

Moody, G. (2006, February 22). Parallel universes: Open access and open source. *LWN.net*. Retrieved May 17, 2008, from http://lwn.net/Articles/172781/

Moore, M. G. (1973). Towards a theory of independent learning and teaching. *The Journal of Higher Education, 44*(9), 661–679. doi:10.2307/1980599

Moore, J. W. (2003). Are textbooks dispensable? *Journal of Chemical Education, 80*(4), 359. doi:10.1021/ed080p359

Moore, M. G., & Thompson, M. (1990). *The effects of distance education: A summary of the literature*. University Park, PA: American Center for Distance Education, Pennsylvania State University. morebrainsmedia.

(2006, March 26). *Hydro Hijinks Version 2* [Video file]. Retrieved December 6, 2008, from http://www.youtube.com/watch?v=JS2JT9IV3CM

Morgan, G. (1986). *Images of organization*. Newbury Park, CA: Sage.

Morrison, G., & Anglin, G. J. (2006). An instructional design approach for effective shovelware: Modifying materials for distance education. *Quarterly Review of Distance Education*, *7*(1), 63–74.

Mortensen, T., & Walker, J. (2002). Blogging thoughts: Personal publication as an online research tool. In Morrison, A. (Ed.), *Researching ICTs in context* (pp. 249–279). Oslo: InterMedia, University of Oslo.

Morville, P. (2005). *Ambient findability: What we find changes who we become*. Cambridge, MA: O'Reilly.

Moses, A. (2007, October 31). Wikipedia project is a class act. *The Sydney Morning Herald*. Retrieved February 12, 2008, from http://www.smh.com.au/news/web/wikipedia-project-is-a-class-act/2007/10/31/1193618940842.html

Muldoon, N. (2008). Self-direction and lifelong learning in the information age: Can PLEs help? In D. Orr, P. A. Danaher, G. Danaher, & R. E. Harreveld (Eds.), *Lifelong learning: Reflecting on successes and framing futures. Keynote and refereed papers from the Fifth International Lifelong Learning Conference* (pp. 277–283). Rockhampton, Australia: Central Queensland University Press.
Norman, D. O. (1988). *The design of everyday things*. New York: Basic.

Multimedia Educational Resource for Learning and Online Teaching. (2009). *About us*. Retrieved April 8, 2009, from http://taste.merlot.org/index.html

Murphy, P. (2000). Gender identifies and the process of negotiation in social interaction. In Joiner, R., Littleton, K., Faulkner, D., & Miell, D. (Eds.), *Rethinking collaborative learning* (pp. 139–160). London: Free Association Books.

Murray, D. E. (1992). Collaborative learning as literary event: Implications for ESL instruction. In Nunan, D. (Ed.), *Collaborative language learning and teaching* (pp. 100–117). Cambridge, UK: Cambridge University Press.

Murray, J. (2008, August 28). Ericsson debuts next generation solar-powered base station. *BusinessGreen*. Retrieved November 20, 2008, from http://www.businessgreen.com/business-green/news/2224857/ericsson-debuts-generation

Naismith, L., Lonsdale, P., Vavoula, G., & Sharples, M. (2006). *Literature review in mobile technologies and learning*. Bristol, UK: Futurelab. Retrieved November 20, 2008, from http://www.futurelab.org.uk/resources/documents/lit_reviews/Mobile_Review.pdf

Naismith, L., Sharples, M., & Ting, J. (2005, October 25–28). *Evaluation of CAERUS: A context-aware mobile guide*. Paper presented at the Fourth World Conference on mLearning (mLearn 2005), Cape Town, South Africa. Retrieved November 20, 2008, from http://www.mlearn.org.za/CD/papers/Naismith.pdf

Nardi, B. A. (1996). *Context and consciousness: Activity theory and human–computer interaction*. Cambridge, MA: MIT Press.

Nardi, B. A., Schiano, D. J., Gumbrecht, M., & Swartz, L. (2004). Why we blog. *Communications of the ACM*, *47*(12), 41–46. doi:10.1145/1035134.1035163

National School Boards Association. (2007). *Creating and connecting: Research and guidelines on online social—and educational—networking*. Alexandria, VA: National School Boards Association. Retrieved June 2, 2008, from http://www.nsba.org/site/docs/41400/41340.pdf

National Science Foundation. (2008). Fostering learning in a networked world: the cyberlearning opportunity and challenge. *A 21st century agenda for the National Science Foundation* (Report of the NSF task force on cyberlearning). Retrieved December 21, 2008, from http://www.nsf.gov/pubs/2008/nsf08204/nsf08204.pdf

National Survey of Student Engagement. (2008). *Our origins and potential*. Retrieved October 23, 2009, from http://nsse.iub.edu/html/origins.cfm

New Media Consortium. (2007). *The Horizon Report: 2007 edition*. Austin, TX: NMC. Retrieved December 4, 2008, from http://www.nmc.org/pdf/2007_Horizon_Report.pdf

New Media Consortium. (2008). *The Horizon Report: 2008 edition*. Austin, TX: NMC. Retrieved June 8, 2010, from http://www.nmc.org/pdf/2008-Horizon-Report.pdf

New Media Consortium. (2009). *The Horizon Report: 2009 edition*. Austin, TX: NMC. Retrieved June 8, 2010, from http://www.nmc.org/pdf/2009-Horizon-Report.pdf

New Media Consortium. (2010). *The Horizon Report: 2010 edition*. Austin, TX: NMC. Retrieved June 8, 2010, from http://www.nmc.org/pdf/2010-Horizon-Report.pdf

Newnham, L., & Miller, C. (2007). Student perceptions of podcasting to enhance learning and teaching in an information systems course. In S. Wheeler & N. Whitton (Eds.), *Beyond control: Learning technology for the social network generation. Research Proceedings of the 14th Association for Learning Technology Conference* (pp. 104–115). Oxford, UK: ALT.

Nicol, D. (2007). Laying a foundation for lifelong learning: Case studies of e-assessment in large 1st-year classes. *British Journal of Educational Technology*, *38*(4), 668–678. doi:10.1111/j.1467-8535.2006.00657.x

Nicol, D. J. (1997). *Research on learning and higher education teaching. UCoSDA Briefing Paper 45*. Sheffield, UK: Universities and Colleges Staff Development Agency.

Nicol, D. J., & Macfarlane-Dick, D. (2006). Formative assessment and self-regulated learning: A model and seven principles of good feedback practice. *Studies in Higher Education*, *32*(2), 199–216. doi:10.1080/03075070600572090

Nicol, D. J. (2007, May 29–31). *Principles of good assessment and feedback: Theory and practice*. Keynote paper presented at the Re-Engineering Assessment Practices (REAP) International Online Conference. Retrieved August 12, 2008, from http://www.reap.ac.uk/public/Papers/Principles_of_good_assessment_and_feedback.pdf

Nie, M., Cashmore, A., & Cane, C. (2008). The educational value of student-generated podcasts. In N. Whitton & M. McPherson (Eds.), *Rethinking the digital divide. Research Proceedings of the 15th Association for Learning Technology Conference* (pp. 116–128). Oxford, UK: ALT.

Nonaka, I., & Takeuchi, H. (1995). *The knowledge-creating company: How Japanese companies create the dynamics of innovation*. New York: Oxford University Press.

Nonaka, I., & Toyama, R. (2003). The knowledge-creating theory revisited: Knowledge creation as a synthesizing process. *Knowledge Management Research and Practice*, *1*(1), 2–10. doi:10.1057/palgrave.kmrp.8500001

Norman, D. A. (1988). *The psychology of everyday things*. New York: Basic.

Norman, D. A. (1999). Affordance, conventions, and design. *Interaction*, *6*(3), 38–43. doi:10.1145/301153.301168

Norman, D. A. (1990). *The design of everyday things*. London: Doubleday.

Norman, D. (2008, March 5). On the PLE [Web log post]. *D'Arcy Norman dot net*. Retrieved July 12, 2008, from http://www.darcynorman.net/2008/03/05/on-the-ple/

O'Brien, C. (2008). How the Google generation thinks differently. *The Times*, Retrieved January 23, 2009, from http://women.timesonline.co.uk/tol/life_and_style/women/families/article4295414.ece

O'Connell, M., Benson, R., & Samarawickrema, G. (2006). Professional development for professional developers: Who's learning about e-learning from whom? In L. Markauskaite, P. Goodyear, & P. Reimann (Eds.), *Who's learning? Whose technology? Proceedings of the 23rd Australasian Society for Computers in Learning in Tertiary Education (ASCILITE) Conference* (pp. 599–602). Sydney: University of Sydney. Retrieved February 12, 2008, from http://www.ascilite.org.au/conferences/sydney06/proceeding/pdf_papers/p169.pdf

O'Reilly, T. (2004). *Open source paradigm shift*. Retrieved February 15, 2008, from http://tim.oreilly.com/articles/paradigmshift_0504.html

O'Reilly, T. (2004). *The architecture of participation*. Retrieved December 21, 2008, from http://www.oreillynet.com/pub/a/oreilly/tim/articles/architecture_of_participation.html

O'Reilly, T. (2005). *What is Web 2.0: Design patterns and business models for the next generation of software*. Retrieved December 21, 2008, from http://www.oreillynet.com/pub/a/oreilly/tim/news/2005/09/30/what-is-web-20.html

O'Reilly, T. (2005, October 10). Web 2.0: Compact definition? [Web log post]. *O'Reilly Radar*. Retrieved July 23, 2006, from http://radar.oreilly.com/archives/2005/10/web_20_compact_definition.html

O'Reilly, T. (2007, July 17). Levels of the game: The hierarchy of Web 2.0 applications [Web log post]. *O'Reilly Radar*. Retrieved January 23, 2008, from http://radar.oreilly.com/archives/2006/07/levels_of_the_game.html

Obasanjo, D. (2004, October 5). Social software is the platform of the future [Web log post]. *Dare Obasanjo aka Carnage4Life*. Retrieved October 10, 2004, from http://www.25hoursaday.com/weblog/PermaLink.aspx?guid=06ff2206-27a3-4d55-81d8-bbee37073d6d

Oblinger, D. G., & Oblinger, J. L. (Eds.). (2005a). *Educating the Net Generation*. Boulder, CO: EDUCAUSE.

Oblinger, D. G., & Oblinger, J. L. (2005b). Is it age or IT: First steps toward understanding the Net Generation. In Oblinger, D. G., & Oblinger, J. L. (Eds.), *Educating the Net Generation* (pp. 2.1–2.20). Boulder, CO: EDUCAUSE.

Oblinger, D. G. (2007). Becoming net savvy. *EDUCAUSE Quarterly, 30*(3), 11–13. Retrieved November 14, 2008, from http://www.educause.edu/ir/library/pdf/eqm0731.pdf

Oblinger, D. G. (2008). Growing up with Google: What it means to education. In *Emerging technologies for learning* (Vol. 3, pp. 11–29). Coventry, UK: Becta. Retrieved November 2, 2009, from http://partners.becta.org.uk/upload-dir/downloads/page_documents/research/emerging_technologies08_chapter1.pdf

OECD. (2005). *E-learning in tertiary education: Where do we stand?* Paris: OECD.

Okada, A., Buckingham Shum, S., & Sherborne, T. (Eds.). (2008). *Knowledge cartography: Software tools and mapping techniques*. London: Springer-Verlag.

Okada, A., & Buckingham Shum, S. (2006, September 3–6). *Knowledge mapping with Compendium in academic research and online education*. Paper presented at the 22nd International Council for Open and Distance Education (ICDE) World Conference, Rio de Janeiro.

Oliver, R. (2005). Quality assurance and e-learning: Blue skies and pragmatism. *ALT-J Research in Learning Technology, 13*(3), 173–187.

Oliver, B., & Goerke, V. (2007). Australian undergraduates' use and ownership of emerging technologies: Implications and opportunities for creating engaging learning experiences for the Net Generation. *Australasian Journal of Educational Technology, 23*(2), 171–186. Retrieved December 4, 2008, from http://www.ascilite.org.au/ajet/ajet23/oliver.html

Oliver, R. (2003). Exploring benchmarks and standards for assuring quality online teaching and learning in higher education. In C. McLoughlin, P. LeCornu, & W. Jackson (Eds.), *Sustaining quality learning environments: Proceedings of the 16th Open and Distance Learning Association of Australia (ODLAA) Biennial Conference*. Canberra, Australia: Canberra Institute of Technology.

Online Encyclopedia of Criminal Justice. (2009). Retrieved November 19, 2009, from http://cjencyclopedia.com

Oravec, J. A. (2003). Blending by blogging: Weblogs in blended learning initiatives. *Journal of Educational Media, 28*(2/3), 225–233.

Owen, M., Grant, L., Sayers, S., & Facer, K. (2006). *Social software and learning*. Bristol, UK: Futurelab. Retrieved April 29, 2010, from http://www.futurelab.org.uk/resources/documents/opening_education/Social_Software_report.pdf

Owyang, J. (2008, January 9). Social network stats: Facebook, MySpace, Reunion (Jan, 2008) [Web log post]. *Web Strategy by Jeremiah Owyang*. Retrieved February 12, 2008, from http://www.web-strategist.com/blog/2008/01/09/social-network-stats-facebook-myspace-reunion-jan-2008/

Oxford University Press. (2005). *All hail "podcasting": More also-rans for the 2005 WOTY*. Retrieved July 3, 2006, from http://blog.oup.com/oupblog/2005/12/podcasting_is_t.html

Paavola, S., & Hakkarainen, K. (2005). The knowledge creation metaphor—An emergent epistemological approach to learning. *Science and Education, 14*(6), 535–557. doi:10.1007/s11191-004-5157-0

Palfrey, J., & Gasser, U. (2008). *Born digital: Understanding the first generation of digital natives*. New York: Basic.

Palloff, R. M., & Pratt, K. (2007). *Building online learning communities Effective strategies for the virtual classroom*. San Francisco: Jossey-Bass.

Pan, B., MacLaurin, T., & Crotts, J. C. (2007). Travel blogs and their implications for destination marketing. *Journal of Travel Research, 46*(1), 35–45. doi:10.1177/0047287507302378

Parashar Panday, P., & Lee, M. J. W. (2007). Graduate education students' perceptions of podcasting as teachers and learners. In T. J. Bastiaens & S. Carliner (Eds.), *Proceedings of World Conference on E-Learning in Corporate, Government, Healthcare, and Higher Education 2007* (pp. 7313–7318). Chesapeake, VA: Association for the Advancement of Computers in Education.

Parker, K. R., & Chao, J. T. (2007). Wiki as a teaching tool. *Interdisciplinary Journal of Knowledge and Learning Objects, 3*, 57–72. Retrieved February 15, 2008, from http://www.ijklo.org/Volume3/IJKLOv3p057-072Parker284.pdf

Parry, D. (2008, January 23). Twitter for academia [Web log post]. *AcademHack*. Retrieved November 4, 2008, from http://academhack.outsidethetext.com/home/2008/twitter-for-academia/

Parsons, C. (2008, July 13). Second Life offers healing, therapeutic options for users. *San Francisco Chronicle*. Retrieved December 6, 2008, from http://www.sfgate.com/cgi-bin/article.cgi?f=/c/a/2008/07/11/LVL211GP5C.DTL

Pata, K., & Väljataga, T. (2007). Collaborating across national and institutional boundaries in higher education—the decentralized iCamp approach. In C. Montgomerie & J. Seale (Eds.), *Proceedings of World Conference on Educational Multimedia, Hypermedia and Telecommunications 2007* (pp. 353–362). Chesapeake, VA: Association for the Advancement of Computers in Education.

Pea, R. (2008, November 6). *Fostering learning in the networked world*. Keynote presentation delivered at Becta's Research Conference 2008: Exploring technology-enabled change in education, Sheffield, UK. Retrieved December 21, 2008, from http://events.becta.org.uk/download.cfm?resID=38800&download_url=http://events.becta.org.uk/content_files/corporate/resources/events/2008/november/pea_fostering_learning.pdf

Pedró, F. (2006). *The new millennium learners: Challenging our views on ICT and learning*. Retrieved December 21, 2008, from http://www.oecd.org/dataoecd/1/1/38358359.pdf

Perkins, D. N. (1992). Technology meets constructivism: Do they make a marriage. In Duffy, T. M., & Jonassen, D. H. (Eds.), *Constructivism and the technology of instruction: A conversation* (pp. 45–55). Hillsdale, NJ: Lawrence Erlbaum.

Pesce, M. (2007). *Challenges and opportunities: Peer-produced knowledge and Australian education*. Adelaide, Australia: Education.au. Retrieved April 23, 2008, from http://api.edna.edu.au/attachment/2150/39455/1/pesce_seminar_report.pdf

Peterson, E. (2006). Beneath the metadata: Some philosophical problems with folksonomy. *D-Lib Magazine, 12*(11). Retrieved March 16, 2007, from http://www.dlib.org/dlib/november06/peterson/11peterson.html

Pettenati, M. C., & Cigognini, M. E. (2007). Social networking theories and tools to support connectivist learning activities. *International Journal of Web-Based Learning and Teaching Technologies, 2*(3), 39–57.

Pettenati, M. C., Cigognini, M. E., Guerin, E. M. C., & Mangione, G. R. (2009). Personal knowledge management skills for Lifelong-Learners 2.0. In Hatzipanagos, S., & Warburton, S. (Eds.), *Handbook of research on social software and developing community ontologies* (pp. 298–315). Hershey, PA: Information Science Reference.

Pettenati, M. C. (2009). Social networking theories and tools to support connectivist learning activities. In Zaphiris, P., & Ang, C. S. (Eds.), *Human computer interaction: Concepts, methodologies, tools, and applications* (pp. 961–978). Hershey, PA: Information Science Reference.

Pettenati, M. C., Cigognini, M. E., & Edirisingha, P. (2007). *Educating today's learners to become net savvy*. Retrieved November 1, 2008, from http://ltc.umanitoba.ca/wiki/Oblinger

Pettenati, M. C., Cigognini, M. E., & Sorrentino, F. (2007, June 13–16). *Methods and tools for developing personal knowledge management skills in the connectivist era*. Paper presented at the European Distance and E-learning Network (EDEN) 2007 Annual Conference, Naples, Italy.

Pettenati, M. C., Cigognini, M. E., Mangione, G. R., & Guerin, E. (2007). Using social software for personal knowledge management in formal online learning. *Turkish Online Journal of Distance Education, 8*(3), 52–65. Retrieved November 1, 2008, from http://tojde.anadolu.edu.tr/tojde27/pdf/article_3.pdf

Pettit, J., & Kukulska-Hulme, A. (2007). Going with the grain: Mobile devices in practice. *Australasian Journal of Educational Technology, 23*(1), 17–33. Retrieved November 20, 2008, from http://www.ascilite.org.au/ajet/ajet23/pettit.html

Piaget, J. (1930). *The child's conception of physical causality*. London: Kogan Paul.

Pilati, M., & Perry, E. (Eds.). (2009). Integrity and identity authentication in online education [Special issue]. *Journal of Online Learning and Teaching, 5*(2). Retrieved November 8, 2009, from http://jolt.merlot.org/Vol5_No2.htm

Pollard, D. (2005, November 23). Personal knowledge management (PKM)—an update [Web log post]. *How to Save the World*. Retrieved November 1, 2008, from http://blogs.salon.com/0002007/2005/11/23.html

Pollock, J. (2006). Suddenly, it's the podcast era. *Des Moines Business Record, 24*(16), 1–12.

Polsani, P. R. (2003). Network learning. In Nyíri, K. (Ed.), *Mobile learning: Essays on philosophy, psychology and education*. Vienna: Pasagen Verlag.

Pond, K., Coates, D., & Palermo, O. (2007). Student experiences of peer review marking of team projects. *International Journal of Management Education, 6*(2), 30–43. Retrieved August 12, 2008, from http://www.heacademy.ac.uk/assets/bmaf/documents/publications/IJME/Vol6No2/IJME62Pond.pdf

Popper, K. (1972). *Objective knowledge: An evolutionary approach*. London: Oxford University Press.

Porter, M. E. (1990). *The competitive advantage of nations*. New York: Free Press.

Porter, J. (1992). *Audience and rhetoric: An archaeological composition of the discourse community*. Upper Saddle River, NJ: Prentice Hall.

Poulis, J., Massen, C., Roberts, E., & Gilbert, M. (1998). Physics lecturing with audience paced feedback. *American Journal of Physics, 66*(5), 439–441. doi:10.1119/1.18883

Power, D. J. (1990). The use of audio in distance education. In Timmers, S. (Ed.), *Training needs in the use of media for distance education* (pp. 43–60). Singapore: Asian Mass Communication Research and Information Centre.

Pratt, J. (2005). The fashionable adoption of online learning technologies in Australian universities. *Journal of the Australian and New Zealand Academy of Management, 11*(1), 57–73.

Prensky, M. (2001). Digital natives, digital immigrants. *Horizon, 9*(5), 1–6. doi:10.1108/10748120110424816

Prensky, M. (2006). *Don't bother me Mom—I'm learning: How computer and video games are preparing your kids for 21st century success and how you can help!* St. Paul, MN: Paragon.

Prensky, M. (2005/2006). Listen to the natives. *Educational Leadership, 63*(4), 8–13.

Prensky, M. (2004). *Digital game-based learning*. New York: McGraw-Hill.

Prensky, M. (2005). "Engage me or enrage me": What today's learners demand. *EDUUCAUSE Review, 40*(5), 60–65. Retrieved April 23, 2008, from http://www.educause.edu/ir/library/pdf/ERM0553.pdf

Prensky, M. (2007). How to teach with technology: Keeping both teachers and students comfortable in an era of exponential change. In *Emerging technologies for learning* (Vol. 2, pp. 40–46). Coventry, UK: Becta. Retrieved April 23, 2008, from http://partners.becta.org.uk/upload-dir/downloads/page_documents/research/emerging_technologies07_chapter1.pdf.

Press, L. (1993). Before the Altair—the history of personal computing. *Communications of the ACM, 36*(9), 27–33. doi:10.1145/162685.162697

Price, M., & O'Donovan, B. (2008, August 27–29). *Feedback: All that effort, but what is the effect?* Paper presented at the Fourth Biennial European Association for Research on Learning and Instruction (EARLI)/Northumbria Assessment Conference, Potsdam/Berlin, Germany.

Protecting Children in the 21st Century Act, S. 49, 110th Cong. (2007).

Pukunui Technology. (2005). *About Moodle*. Retrieved April 24, 2008, from http://moodle.com.au/index.php

Puttnam, D. (2007, May 8). "In class, I have to power down". *The Guardian*. Retrieved July 4, 2009, from http://education.guardian.co.uk/egweekly/story/0,2074182,00.html

Quality Assurance Agency for Higher Education. (2006). *Code of practice for the assurance of academic quality and standards in higher education. Section 6: Assessment of students* (2nd ed.). Gloucester, UK: QAA. Retrieved July 3, 2009, from http://www.qaa.ac.uk/academicinfrastructure/codeOfPractice/section6/COP_AOS.pdf

Ramsden, P. (2003). *Learning to teach in higher education* (2nd ed.). London: Routledge.

Redecker, C. (2009). *Review of Learning 2.0 practices: Learning 2.0, the impact of Web 2.0 innovations on education and training in Europe*. Saville, Spain: Institute for Perspective Technological Studies.

Redecker, C., Ala-Mutka, K., Bacigalupo, M., Ferrari, A., & Punie, Y. (2009). *Learning 2.0: The impact of Web 2.0 innovations on education and training in Europe*. Saville, Spain: Institute for Perspective Technological Studies.

Redecker, C. (2009). *Review of Learning 2.0 Practices: Study on the impact of Web 2.0 innovations on education and training in Europe*. Luxembourg: European Commission. Retrieved April 30, 2009, from http://ftp.jrc.es/EURdoc/JRC49108.pdf

Reid, J., Hull, R., Cater, K., & Fleuriot, C. (2005, June). Magic moments in situated mediascapes. In S.Z.-Y. Zhou & S. P. Lee (Eds.), *Proceedings of the 2005 ACM SIGCHI International Conference on Advances in Computer Entertainment Technology* (pp. 290–293). New York: Association for Computing Machinery.

Reigeluth, C. M. (Ed.). (1999). *Instructional-design theories and models: A new paradigm of instructional theory* (*Vol. 2*). Mahwah, NJ: Lawrence Erlbaum.

Resnick, M. (2006). Computer as paintbrush: Technology, play, and the creative society. In Singer, D. G., Golinkoff, R. M., & Hirsh-Pasek, K. (Eds.), *Play = learning: How play motivates and enhances children's cognitive and socio-emotional growth* (pp. 30–37). Oxford, UK: Oxford University Press.

Resta, P., & Laferriere, T. (2007). Technology in support of collaborative learning. *Educational Psychology Review*, *19*(1), 65–83. doi:10.1007/s10648-007-9042-7

Rettberg, J. W. (2008). *Blogging*. Cambridge, UK: Polity.

Reynard, R. (2008, October 1). Avoiding the 5 most common mistakes in using blogs with students. *Campus Technology*. Retrieved October 16, 2008, from http://www.campustechnology.com/printarticle.aspx?id=68089

Rheingold, H. (1993). *The virtual community*. Reading, MA: Addison-Wesley.

Rheingold, H. (2002). *Smart mobs: The next social revolution*. New York: Perseus.

Rheingold, H. (2003, May 8). *Re: My working definition of social software ...* [Web log comment]. *Plasticbag.org*. Retrieved June 10, 2005, from http://www.plasticbag.org/archives/2003/05/my_working_definition_of_social_software.shtml

Richardson, W. (2006a). *Blogs, wikis, podcasts, and other powerful tools for classrooms*. Thousand Oaks, CA: Sage.

Richardson, W. (2006b). *The Internet breaks school walls down*. Retrieved November 3, 2007, from http://www.edutopia.org/new-face-learning

Rick, J., Guzdial, M., Carroll, K., Holloway-Attaway, L., & Walker, B. (2002). Collaborative learning at low cost: CoWeb use in English composition. In G. Stahl (Ed.), *Proceedings of the Conference on Computer Support for Collaborative Learning: Foundations for a CSCL Community* (pp. 435–442). Atlanta, GA: International Society of the Learning Sciences.

Roberts, G. (2002). *SET for success: The supply of people with science, technology, engineering and mathematics skills. The report of Sir Gareth Roberts' review.* London: HM Treasury. Retrieved April 29, 2010, from http://www.hm-treasury.gov.uk/ent_res_roberts.htm

Rogers, G. (2006, March 8). Google Reference, a Wikipedia partnership? [Web log post]. *Googling Google*. Retrieved December 21, 2008, from http://www.zdnet.com/blog/google/google-reference-a-wikipedia-partnership/124

Rogers, P. C., Liddle, S. W., Chan, P., Doxey, A., & Isom, B. (2007). Web 2.0 learning platform: Harnessing collective intelligence. *Turkish Online Journal of Distance Education, 8*(3), 16–33. Retrieved December 20, 2007, from http://tojde.anadolu.edu.tr/tojde27/pdf/article_1.pdf

Rorty, R. (1979). *Philosophy and the mirror of nature*. Princeton, NJ: Princeton University Press.

Rorty, R. (1989). *Contingency, irony, and solidarity*. Cambridge, UK: Cambridge University Press.

Rosen, J. (2006, June 27). The people formerly known as the audience [Web log post]. *PressThink*. Retrieved October 2, 2007, from http://journalism.nyu.edu/pubzone/weblogs/pressthink/2006/06/27/ppl_frmr.html

Rotheram, B. (2007). Using an MP3 recorder to give feedback on student assignments. *Educational Developments*, *8*(2), 7–11.

Rowntree, D. (1998). *Learn how to study: A guide for students of all ages* (4th rev. ed.). London: Time Warner.

Rowntree, D. (1987). *Assessing students: How shall we know them?* London: Kogan Page.

RSS Advisory Board. (2005). *Really Simple Syndication: RSS 2.0.1 Specification (revision 6)*. Retrieved March 2, 2006, from http://www.rssboard.org/rss-2-0-1-rv-6

Rudd, T., Gifford, C., Morrison, J., & Facer, K. (2006). *What if ...: Re-imagining learning spaces*. Bristol, UK: Futurelab. Retrieved November 20, 2006, from http://www.futurelab.org.uk/resources/documents/opening_education/Learning_Spaces_report.pdf

Rudd, T., Sutch, D., & Facer, K. (2006). *Towards new learning networks*. Bristol, UK: Futurelab. Retrieved July 5, 2007, from http://www.futurelab.org.uk/resources/documents/opening_education/Learning_Networks_report.pdf

Rumsfeld, D. H. (2002, February 12). *DoD news briefing—Secretary Rumsfeld and Gen. Myers* [News transcript]. Retrieved December 6, 2008, from http://www.defense.gov/transcripts/transcript.aspx?transcriptid=2636

Ryan, Y. (1998). Time and tide: Teaching and learning online. *Australian Universities Review, 41*(1), 14–19. Retrieved August 5, 2009, from http://www.aur.org.au/archive/41-01/aur_41-01.pdf

Ryberg, T., & Larsen, M. C. (2008). Networked identities: Understanding relationships between strong and weak ties in networked environments. *Journal of Computer Assisted Learning*, *24*(2), 103–115. doi:10.1111/j.1365-2729.2007.00272.x

Ryder, M. (1995, February 8–12). *USENET: A constructivist learning environment.* Paper presented at the Association for Educational Communications and Technology (AECT) National Convention, Anaheim, CA.

Sadler, D. R. (1989). Formative assessment and the design of instructional systems. *Instructional Science*, *18*(2), 119–144. doi:10.1007/BF00117714

Saettler, P. (1990). Cognitive science and educational technology: 1950–1980. In Saettler, P. (Ed.), *The evolution of American educational technology* (pp. 318–342). Englewood, CO: Libraries Unlimited.

Salaberry, M. R. (2001). The use of technology for second language learning and teaching: A retrospective. *Modern Language Journal*, *85*(1), 39–56. doi:10.1111/0026-7902.00096

Salaway, G., Caruso, J. B., & Nelson, M. R. (2007). *The ECAR study of undergraduate students and information technology, 2007*. Boulder, CO: EDUCAUSE Center for Applied Research. Retrieved December 21, 2008, from http://www.educause.edu/ir/library/pdf/ers0706/rs/ERS0706w.pdf

Salaway, G., Katz, R. N., Caruso, J. B., Kvavik, R. B., & Nelson, M. R. (2006). *The ECAR study of undergraduate students and information technology, 2006.* Boulder, CO: EDUCAUSE Center for Applied Research. Retrieved November 1, 2008, from http://www.educause.edu/ir/library/pdf/ers0607/ERS0607w.pdf

Säljö, R. (1987). The educational construction of learning. In J. T. E. Richardson, M. W. Eysenck, & D. W. Piper (Eds.), *Student learning: Research in education and cognitive psychology* (pp. 101–108). Milton Keynes, UK: Society for Research into Higher Education and Open University Press.

Salmon, G. (2004). *E-moderating: The key to teaching and learning online* (2nd ed.). London: Routledge Falmer.

Salmon, G. (2002). *E-tivities: The key to active online learning*. London: Kogan Page.

Salmon, G. (2005). Flying not flapping: A strategic framework for e-learning and pedagogical innovation in higher education institutions. *ALT-J Research in Learning Technology*, *13*(3), 201–218.

Scardamalia, M., Bereiter, C., McLean, R. S., Swallow, J., & Woodruff, E. (1989). Computer supported intentional learning environments. *Journal of Educational Computing Research, 5*(1), 51–68.

Scardamalia, M., Bereiter, C., & Lamon, M. (1994). The CSILE project: Trying to bring the classroom into world 3. In K. McGilly (Ed.), *Classroom lessons: Integrating cognitive theory and classroom practice*. (pp. 201–228). MA: MIT Press.

Schaffert, S., Gruber, A., & Westenthaler, R. (2006). A semantic wiki for collaborative knowledge formation. In Reich, S., Güntner, G., Pelligrini, T., & Wahler, A. (Eds.), *Semantic Content Engineering: Proceedings of Semantics 2005*. Linz, Austria: Trauner Verlag.

Schaffert, S., & Hilzensauer, W. (2008). On the way towards personal learning environments: Seven crucial aspects. *eLearning Papers, 9*. Retrieved July 22, 2008, from http://www.elearningeuropa.info/files/media/media15971.pdf

Schaffert, S., Bischof, D., Buerger, T., Gruber, A., Hilzensauer, W., & Schaffert, S. (2006). Learning with semantic wikis. In M. Völkel & S. Schaffert (Eds.), *Proceedings of the First Workshop on Semantic Wikis: From wiki to semantics* (pp. 109–123). Aachen, Germany: Informatik V, RWTH Aachen University. Retrieved June 5, 2007, from http://sunsite.informatik.rwth-aachen.de/Publications/CEUR-WS/Vol-206/paper9.pdf

Schiltz, M., Truyen, F., & Coppens, H. (2007). Cutting the trees of knowledge: Social software, information architecture and their epistemic consequences. *Thesis Eleven, 89*(1), 94–114.

Schlosser, C. A., & Burmeister, M. L. (2006, October 10–13). Audio in online courses: Beyond podcasting. Paper presented at the World Conference on E-Learning in Corporate, Government, Healthcare, and Higher Education 2006, Honolulu, HI. Retrieved October 20, 2006, from http://www.nova.edu/~burmeist/audio_online.html

Schmidt, J. (2007). Social software: Facilitating information-, identity- and relationship management. In Burg, T. N., & Schmidt, J. (Eds.), *BlogTalks reloaded: Social software research & cases* (pp. 31–49). Norderstedt, Germany: Books on Demand.

Schneider, M. L. (1990). Collaborative learning: A concept in search of a definition. *Issues in Writing, 3*(1), 26–39.

Sclater, N. (2008). *Large-scale open source e-learning systems at the Open University UK*. Boulder, CO: EDUCAUSE Center for Applied Research. Retrieved December 21, 2008, from http://www.educause.edu/ir/library/pdf/ERB0812.pdf

Sclater, N. (2008). *Web 2.0, personal learning environments, and the future of learning management systems*. Boulder, CO: EDUCAUSE Center for Applied Research. Retrieved October 28, 2009, from http://www.educause.edu/ir/library/pdf/ERB0813.pdf

Scottish Council for Educational Technology. (1994). Audio. In *Technologies in learning*. Glasgow: Scottish Council for Educational Technology.

Segers, M., Dochy, F., & Cascallar, E. (Eds.). (2003). *Optimising new modes of assessment: In search of qualities and standards*. Dordrecht, The Netherlands: Kluwer. doi:10.1007/0-306-48125-1

Selanikio, J. (2008, January 17). The invisible computer revolution. *BBC News*. Retrieved November 20, 2008, from http://news.bbc.co.uk/1/hi/technology/7106998.stm

Seldow, A. (2007, June 5–7). *Social tagging in education and the workplace*. Paper presented at the 3rd Annual Innovations in e-Learning Symposium, Fairfax, VA. Retrieved October 28, 2009, from http://innovationsinelearning.gmu.edu/2007/presentations/Seldow%20-%20Social%20Tagging%20in%20Education%20and%20the%20Workplace.pdf

Selwyn, N. (2007). Curriculum online? Exploring the political and commercial construction of the UK digital learning marketplace. *British Journal of Sociology of Education, 28*(2), 223–240. doi:10.1080/01425690701192729

Selwyn, N. (2008). An investigation of differences in undergraduates' academic use of the Internet. *Active Learning in Higher Education, 9*(1), 11–22. doi:10.1177/1469787407086744

Selwyn, N. (2007, October 16–17). *Web 2.0 applications as alternative environments for informal learning—a critical review*. Paper presented at the CERI-KERIS International Expert Meeting on ICT and Educational Performance, Cheju Island, South Korea. Retrieved March 2, 2008, from http://www.oecd.org/dataoecd/32/3/39458556.pdf

Selwyn, N. (Ed.). (2008). *Education 2.0? Designing the web for teaching and learning*. London: Teaching and Learning Research Programme, Institute of Education, University of London. Retrieved January 12, 2009, from http://www.tlrp.org/tel/files/2008/11/tel_comm_final.pdf

Sener, J. (2007a). In search of student-generated content in online education. *e-mentor, 21*. Retrieved December 20, 2007, from http://www.e-mentor.edu.pl/_xml/wydania/21/467.pdf

Sener, J. (2007b). *University of Connecticut—Beyond lecturecasting: Using podcasts for discussion and student content creation*. Retrieved March 10, 2007, from http://www.sloan-c-wiki.org/wiki/index.php?title=University_of_Connecticut_--_Beyond_Lecturecasting:_Using_Podcasts_for_Discussion_and_Student_Content_Creation

Sener, J. (2007c). *University of North Carolina at Pembroke—cjencyclopedia.com: Online Encyclopedia of Criminal Justice*. Retrieved March 10, 2007, from http://www.sloan-c-wiki.org/wiki/index.php?title=University_of_North_Carolina_at_Pembroke_--_cjencyclopedia.com:_Online_Encyclopedia_of_Criminal_Justice

Senge, P. M. (1990). *The fifth discipline: The art and practice of the learning organization*. New York: Doubleday.

Senges, M., Praus, T., & Bihr, P. (2007). *Virtual worlds: A Second Life beginner's guide*. Barcelona: Open University of Catalonia. Retrieved December 6, 2008, from http://www.thewavingcat.com/wp-content/uploads/2007/07/uoc_virtual_worlds_a_second_life_beginners_guide.pdf

Sessums, C. D. (2006, January 21). Notes on the significance of the emergence of blogs and wikis [Web log post]. *Christopher D. Sessums: Blog*. Retrieved October 12, 2006, from http://elgg.net/csessums/weblog/6172.html

Severance, C., Hardin, J., & Whyte, A. (2008). The coming functionality mash-up in personal learning environments. *Interactive Learning Environments, 16*(1), 47–62. doi:10.1080/10494820701772694

Sfard, A. (1998). On two metaphors for learning and the dangers of choosing just one. *Educational Researcher, 27*(2), 4–13.

Shadbolt, N., Gibbins, N., Glaser, H., Harris, S., & Schraefel, M. C. (2004). CS AKTive Space or how we learned to stop worrying and love the Semantic Web. *IEEE Intelligent Systems, 19*(3), 41–47. doi:10.1109/MIS.2004.8

Sharma, D. (2007). *SOCIAL NETWORKING GOD: 350+ social networking sites*. Retrieved April 11, 2009, from http://mashable.com/2007/10/23/social-networking-god/

Sharpe, R., Benfield, G., Lessner, E., & DeCicco, E. (2005). *Final report: Scoping study for the pedagogy strand of the JISC e-learning programme*. Bristol, UK: Joint Information Systems Committee. Retrieved July 17, 2008, from http://www.jisc.ac.uk/uploaded_documents/scoping%20study%20final%20report%20v4.1.doc

Shavelson, R. J. (2007). Assessing student learning responsibly: From history to an audacious proposal. *Change: The Magazine of Higher Learning, 39*(1), 26–33. doi:10.3200/CHNG.39.1.26-33

Sheehan, M. C. (2008). *Higher education IT and cyberinfrastructure: Integrating technologies for scholarship*. Boulder, CO: EDUCAUSE Center for Applied Research. Retrieved December 21, 2008, from http://www.educause.edu/ir/library/pdf/ers0803/rs/ERS0803w.pdf

Sheely, S. (2006). Persistent technologies: Why can't we stop lecturing online? In L. Markauskaite, P. Goodyear, & P. Reimann (Eds.), *Who's learning? Whose technology? Proceedings of the 23rd Australasian Society for Computers in Learning in Tertiary Education (ASCILITE) Conference* (pp. 769–774). Sydney: University of Sydney. Retrieved January 12, 2008, from http://www.ascilite.org.au/conferences/sydney06/proceeding/pdf_papers/p167.pdf

Shepard, L. A. (2000). The role of assessment in a learning culture. *Educational Researcher, 29*(7), 4–14.

Shepard, L. A. (2001). The role of classroom assessment in teaching and learning. In Richardson, V. (Ed.), *Handbook of research on teaching* (4th ed., pp. 1066–1101). Washington, DC: American Educational Research Association.

Shepherd, C. (2007, April 17). PLE—what are we talking about here? [Web log post]. *Clive on Learning*. Retrieved July 5, 2008, from http://clive-shepherd.blogspot.com/2007/04/ples-what-are-we-talking-about-here.html

Shepherd, J. (2008, October 31). Universities review plagiarism policies to catch Facebook cheats. *The Guardian*. Retrieved November 23, 2008, from http://

www.guardian.co.uk/education/2008/oct/31/facebook-cheating-plagiarism-cambridge-varsity-wikipedia

Shuen, A. (2008). *Web 2.0: A strategy guide*. Sebastapol, CA: O'Reilly.

Siemens, G. (2006). *Knowing knowledge*. Vancouver, BC: Lulu.

Siemens, G. (2003). *Learning ecology, communities, and networks: Extending the classroom*. Retrieved Decemeber 21, 2008, from http://www.elearnspace.org/Articles/learning_communities.htm

Siemens, G. (2005). Connectivism: A learning theory for the digital age. *International Journal of Instructional Technology and Distance Learning, 2*(1), 3–10. Retrieved Decemeber 21, 2008, from http://www.itdl.org/Journal/Jan_05/Jan_05.pdf

Siemens, G. (2007, April 15). PLEs—I acronym, therefore I exist [Web log post]. *elearnspace: learning, networks, knowledge, technology, community*. Retrieved November 1, 2007, from http://www.elearnspace.org/blog/archives/002884.html

Siemens, G. (2007, October 22). Digital natives and immigrants: A concept beyond its best before date [Web log post]. *Connectivism Blog*. Retrieved November 1, 2008, from http://connectivism.ca/blog/2007/10/digital_natives_and_immigrants.html

Siemens, G. (2008, May 21). A seismic shift in epistemology [Web log post]. *elearnspace*. Retrieved January, 9, 2009, from http://www.elearnspace.org/blog/2008/05/21/a-seismic-shift-in-epistemology/

Sifry, D. (2007, April 5). The state of the live web, April 2007 [Web log post]. *Sifry's Alerts*. Retrieved February 12, 2008, from http://www.sifry.com/alerts/archives/000493.html

Silvertown, J. (2008, August 3–8). *Geographically-referenced teaching and learning (GReTL): Making a virtue out of necessity in distance education and citizen science—the example of the Evolution MegaLab*. Paper presented at 93rd Ecological Society of America Annual Meeting, Milwaukee, WI. Retrieved November 20, 2008, from http://esameetings.allenpress.com/2008/P9955.HTM

Simkins, M. (2008, March 15). 3-D printing a goo goo, *TechLearning*. Retrieved July 1, 2008, from http://www.techlearning.com/showArticle.php?articleID=196605073

Simpson, V., & Oliver, M. (2007). Electronic voting systems for lectures then and now: A comparison of research and practice. *Australasian Journal of Educational Technology, 23*(2), 187–208. Retrieved July 3, 2009, from http://www.ascilite.org.au/ajet/ajet23/simpson.html

Sims, R. (Ed.). (2006). Online distance education: New ways of learning; new modes of teaching? [Special issue]. *Distance Education*, *27*(2).

Sipple, S. (2007). Ideas in practice: Developmental writers' attitudes toward audio and written feedback. *Journal of Developmental Education*, *30*(3), 22–31.

Skene, J., Cluett, L., & Hogan, J. (2007, July 3–6). *Engaging Gen Y students at university: What web tools do they have, how do they use them and what do they want?* Paper presented at the First Year in Higher Education Conference, Brisbane, Australia. Retrieved December 6, 2008, from http://www.fyhe.com.au/past_papers/papers07/final_papers/pdfs/2b.pdf

Skiba, D. J. (2006). The 2005 word of the year: Podcast. *Nursing Education Perspectives*, *27*(1), 54–55.

Smagorinsky, P., & Fly, P. K. (1993). The social environment of the classroom: A Vygotskian perspective on small group process. *Communication Education*, *42*(2), 159–171. doi:10.1080/03634529309378922

Smith, K. H. (2007). *Innovation and growth in resource-based economies*. Melbourne, Australia: Committee for Economic Development of Australia.

Snowden, D. J., & Boone, M. E. (2007). A leader's framework for decision making. *Harvard Business Review*, *85*(11), 68–76.

Sørensen, B. H., Jessen, C., & Olesen, B. R. (Eds.). (2002). *Børn på nettet: Kommunikation og læring (Children on the Internet: Communication and learning)*. Copenhagen: Gads.

Sørensen, B. H., Olesen, B. R., & Audon, L. (2001). *Det hele kører parallelt: De nye medier i børns hverdagsliv (Everything runs in parallel: The new media in children's everyday life)*. Copenhagen: Gads.

Sorrel, C. (2009, February 6). Read Google Books on your iPhone. *Wired.com*. Retrieved November 20, 2008, from http://www.wired.com/gadgetlab/2009/02/read-google-boo/

Sorrentino, F., & Paganelli, F. (2006). *L'intelligenza distribuita—Ambient Intelligence: il futuro delle tecnologie invisibili (Ambient intelligence: The future of invisible technologies)*. Trento, Italy: Erickson.

Sproll, L., & Faraj, S. (1993). Atheism, sex, and databases: The net as a social technology. In Kiesler, S. (Ed.), *Culture of the Internet* (pp. 35–51). Mahwah, NJ: Lawrence Erlbaum.

Stahl, G. (2000). Collaborative information environments to support knowledge construction by communities. *AI & Society*, *14*(1), 71–97. doi:10.1007/BF01206129

Stahl, G. (2006). *Group cognition: Computer support for building collaborative knowledge*. Cambridge, MA: MIT Press.

Staton, M. (2008, February 2). *Best practices for educators using Facebook*. Presentation delivered to Classroom 2.0 LIVE. Retrieved February 9, 2009, from http://www.edumorphology.com/wp-content/uploads/2008/02/fb_classroom1.pdf

Steel, J., & Hudson, A. (2001). Educational technology in learning and teaching: The perceptions and experiences of teaching staff. *Innovations in Education and Teaching International*, *38*(2), 103–111. doi:10.1080/13558000010030158

Storch, N. (2005). Collaborative writing: Product, process, and students' reflections. *Journal of Second Language Writing*, *14*(3), 153–173. doi:10.1016/j.jslw.2005.05.002

Stroud, R. (2008). Social networking: An age-neutral commodity—Social networking becomes a mature web application. *Journal of Direct, Data and Digital Marketing Practice, 9*(3), 278–292. Retrieved August 5, 2009, from http://www.palgrave-journals.com/dddmp/journal/v9/n3/pdf/4350099a.pdf

Stutzman, F. (2006). An evaluation of identity-sharing behavior in social network communities. *International Digital Media and Arts Journal*, *3*(1), 10–18.

Stutzman, F. (2007). *The vibrancy of online social space*. Unpublished manuscript. Retrieved April 11, 2009, from http://fredstutzman.com/papers/MG2008_Stutzman.pdf

Sundén, J. (2003). *Material virtualities: Approaching online textual embodiment*. New York: Peter Lang.

Surowiecki, J. (2004). *The wisdom of crowds: Why the many are smarter than the few and how collective wisdom shapes business, economies, societies, and nations*. New York: Doubleday.

Sutherland, S. A. (2007, July 6). A model relating eportfolios to [portfolio] tools? [Electronic mailing list message]. Retrieved July 3, 2009, from https://www.jiscmail.ac.uk/cgi-bin/webadmin?A2=CETIS-PORTFOLIO;%2FPHwFQ;20070706145351%2B0100

Sutton, A. (1980). Backward children in the USSR: An unfamiliar approach to a familiar problem. In Brine, J., Perrie, M., & Sutton, A. (Eds.), *Home, school and leisure in the Soviet Union* (pp. 160–191). London: Allen & Unwin.

Swain, M., & Lapkin, S. (1998). Interaction and second language learning: Two adolescent French immersion students working together. *Modern Language Journal*, *82*(3), 320–337. doi:10.2307/329959

Swan, K. (2002). Immediacy, social presence, and asynchronous discussion. In Bourne, J., & Moore, J. C. (Eds.), *Elements of quality online education* (*Vol. 3*, pp. 157–172). Needham, MA: Sloan Consortium.

Syed-Khuzzan, S. M., Goulding, J. S., & Underwood, J. (2009). Personalised learning environments—Part 1: Core development issues for construction. *Industrial and Commercial Training*, *40*(6), 310–319. doi:10.1108/00197850810900075

Tabuchi, H. (2007, November 21). Making "Second Life" more like real life. *MSNBC*. Retrieved July 1, 2008, from http://www.msnbc.msn.com/id/21917042/

Takahashi, D. (2008, July 1). Cigna deploys a Second Life island for health education. *VentureBeat*. Retrieved December 6, 2008, from http://venturebeat.com/2008/07/01/cigna-deploys-a-second-life-island-for-health-education/

Tapscott, D. (1998). *Growing up digital: The rise of the Net Generation*. New York: McGraw-Hill.

Tapscott, D., & Williams, A. D. (2006). The prosumers. In *Wikinomics: How mass collaboration changes everything* (pp. 124–150). New York: Penguin.

Tapscott, D. (1999). Educating the Net Generation. *Educational Leadership*, *56*(5), 6–11.

Taylor, J. C. (2001, April 1–5). *Fifth generation distance education*. Keynote address delivered at the 20th International Council for Open and Distance Education (ICDE) World Conference, Düsseldorf, Germany. Retrieved April 24, 2008, from http://www.usq.edu.au/users/taylorj/publications_presentations/2001ProfessorialLecture.ppt

The European e-Skills Forum. (2004). *e-Skills for Europe: Towards 2010 and beyond.* Brussels: European Commission. Retrieved November 1, 2008, from http://ec.europa.eu/enterprise/sectors/ict/files/e-skills-forum-2004-09-fsr_en.pdf

The Facebook classroom: 25 Facebook apps that are perfect for online education. (2008). Retrieved March 28, 2009, from http://www.collegedegree.com/library/college-life/15-facebook-apps-perfect-for-online-education

Thompson, J. (2007). Is Education 1.0 ready for Web 2.0 students? *Innovate: Journal of Online Education, 3*(4). Retrieved April 24, 2008, from http://www.innovateonline.info/index.php?view=article&id=393

Thorne, S. L. (2008). Mediating technologies and second language learning. In Coiro, J., Knobel, M., Lankshear, C., & Leu, D. J. (Eds.), *Handbook of research on new literacies* (pp. 417–449). Mahwah, NJ: Lawrence Erlbaum.

Thorne, S. L., & Payne, S. (2005). Evolutionary trajectories, Internet-mediated expression, and language education. *CALICO Journal, 22*(3), 371–397. Retrieved February 10, 2008, from https://calico.org/html/article_137.pdf

Thornton, P., & Houser, C. (2005). Using mobile phones in English education in Japan. *Journal of Computer Assisted Learning*, *21*(3), 217–228. doi:10.1111/j.1365-2729.2005.00129.x

Tornero, J. M. P. (2004). *Promoting digital literacy, Final report, EAC/76/03: Understanding digital literacy*. Brussels: European Commission. Retrieved November 1, 2008, from http://ec.europa.eu/education/archive/elearning/doc/studies/dig_lit_en.pdf

Tosh, D., & Werdmuller, B. (2004). *Creation of a learning landscape: Weblogging and social networking in the context of e-portfolios*. Retrieved October 30, 2009, from http://eduspaces.net/bwerdmuller/files/61/179/Learning_landscape.pdf van Weert, T. J. (2006). Education of the twenty-first century: New professionalism in lifelong learning, knowledge development and knowledge sharing. *Education and Information Technologies, 11*(3/4), 217–237.

Toulmin, S. E. (1990). *Cosmopolis: The hidden agenda of modernity*. New York: Free Press.

Trentin, G. (2009). Using a wiki to evaluate individual contribution to a collaborative learning project. *Journal of Computer Assisted Learning*, *25*(1), 43–55. doi:10.1111/j.1365-2729.2008.00276.x

Tsinakos, A. A. (2006). Collaborative student modeling: A new perspective using wiki. *WSEAS Transactions on Advances in Engineering Education*, *6*(3), 475–481.

Tu, C.-H., & McIsaac, M. (2002). The relationship of social presence and interaction in online classes. *American Journal of Distance Education*, *16*(3), 131–150. doi:10.1207/S15389286AJDE1603_2

Türker, M. A., & Zingel, S. (2008). Formative interfaces for scaffolding self-regulated learning in PLEs. *eLearning Papers, 9*. Retrieved July 22, 2008, from http://www.elearningeuropa.info/files/media/media15975.pdf

Turoff, M. (2002). *Murray Turoff's homepage.* Retrieved December 23, 2007, from http://is.njit.edu/turoff

Turoff, M., & Hiltz, S. R. (1995). *An overview of research activities in computer mediated communications from 1976 to 1991 conducted by the Computerized Conferencing and Communications Center at NJIT.* Retrieved December 23, 2007, from http://web.njit.edu/~turoff/Administrative/ccc.htm

Tutty, J. I., & Martin, F. (2009). User generated design: Teaching and learning with Web 2.0. In Kidd, T. T., & Chen, I. L. (Eds.), *Wired for learning: An educator's guide to Web 2.0* (pp. 43–58). Charlotte, NC: Information Age.

Tynan, B., & Colbran, S. (2006). Podcasting, student learning and expectations. In L. Markauskaite, P. Goodyear, & P. Reimann (Eds.), *Who's learning? Whose technology? Proceedings of the 23rd Australasian Society for Com-*

puters in Learning in Tertiary Education (ASCILITE) Conference (pp. 825–832). Sydney: University of Sydney. Retrieved January 12, 2008, from http://www.ascilite.org.au/conferences/sydney06/proceeding/pdf_papers/p132.pdf

Ugoretz, J. (2006, June 9). Three stars and a chili pepper: Social software, folksonomy, and user reviews in the college context. *Academic Commons*. Retrieved January 12, 2009, from http://www.academiccommons.org/commons/essay/Ugoretz-social-software-folksonomy

UK GRAD Programme. (2001). *Joint statement of the UK research councils' training requirements for research students*. Retrieved April 29, 2010, from http://www.grad.ac.uk/downloads/documents/general/Joint%20Skills%20Statement.pdf

Underwood, J., & Banyard, P. E. (2008). Understanding the learning space. *eLearning Papers, 9*. Retrieved July 22, 2008, from http://www.elearningeuropa.info/files/media/media15970.pdf van Harmelen, M. (2006). Personal learning environments. In Kinshuk, R. Koper, P. Kommers, P. Kirschner, D. Sampson, & W. Didderen (Eds.), *Proceedings of the Sixth International Conference on Advanced Learning Technologies* (pp. 815–816). Los Alamitos, CA: IEEE Computer Society.

United Nations Conference on Trade and Development. (2009). *Information economy report 2009: Trends and outlook in turbulent times*. New York and Geneva: UNCTAD. Retrieved November 20, 2008, from http://www.unctad.org/en/docs/ier2009_en.pdf

United Nations Educational, Scientific and Cultural Organization. (2004). *The plurality of literacy and its implications for policies and programmes*. Paris: UNESCO. Retrieved November 1, 2008, from http://unesdoc.unesco.org/images/0013/001362/136246e.pdf

United Nations Educational, Scientific and Cultural Organization. (2008). *ICT competency standards for teachers: Competency standards modules*. Paris: UNESCO. Retrieved October 23, 2009, from http://cst.unesco-ci.org/sites/projects/cst/The%20Standards/ICT-CST-Competency%20Standards%20Modules.pdf

University of Maryland Baltimore County. (n. d.). *Student use of Voice Direct*. Retrieved June 5, 2008, from http://www.umbc.edu/oit/newmedia/blackboard/help/VoiceDirect_student.pdf

Unsworth, J. (2008). University 2.0. In Katz, R. N. (Ed.), *The tower and the cloud: Higher education in the age of cloud computing* (pp. 227–237). Boulder, CO: EDUCAUSE.

Usenet. (2007, December 17). In *Wikipedia. The free encyclopedia*. Retrieved December 23, 2007, from http://en.wikipedia.org/wiki/Usenet

Valdivia, R., & Nussbaum, M. (2009). Using multiple choice questions as a pedagogic model for face-to-face CSCL. *Computer Applications in Engineering Education, 17*(1), 89–99. doi:10.1002/cae.20196

Väljataga, T., & Fiedler, S. (2008). Competence advancement supported by social media. In M. Kalz, R. Koper, V. Hornung-Prähauser, & M. Luckmann (Eds.), *Proceedings of the First Workshop on Technology Support for Self-Organized Learners (TSSOL08)* (pp. 54–66). Aachen, Germany: Informatik V, RWTH Aachen University. Retrieved July 22, 2008, from http://sunsite.informatik.rwth-aachen.de/Publications/CEUR-WS/Vol-349/vaeljataga.pdf

Väljataga, T., Pata, K., Laanpere, M., & Kaipainen, M. (2007). Theoretical framework of the iCampFolio—new approach to evaluation and comparison of systems and tools for learning purposes. In E. Duval, R. Klamma, & M. Wolpers (Eds.), *Creating new learning experiences on a global scale: Second European Conference on Technology Enhanced Learning, EC-TEL 2007, Crete, Greece, September 2007, Proceedings: Vol. Lecture Notes in Computer Science* (pp. 349–363). Berlin/Heidelberg, Germany: Springer-Verlag.

van den Brink-Budgen, R. (2000). *Critical thinking for students: Learn the skills of critical assessment and effective argument* (3rd ed.). Oxford, UK: How To Books.

van der Veer, R., & Valsiner, J. (Eds.). (1994). *The Vygotsky reader*. Oxford, UK: Blackwell.

van Harmelen, M. (2008). Design trajectories: Four experiments in PLE implementation. *Interactive Learning Environments, 16*(1), 35–46. doi:10.1080/10494820701772686

Vander Wal, T. (2005). Folksonomy definition and Wikipedia [Web log post]. *Off the Top: vanderwal.net.*

Retrieved March 14, 2007, from http://www.vanderwal.net/random/entrysel.php?blog=1750

Varis, T. (2005). *New literacies and e-learning competences*. Retrieved November 1, 2008, from http://www.elearningeuropa.info/directory/index.php?doc_id=595&doclng=6&page=doc

Villamil, O. S., & de Guerrero, M. C. M. (1996). Peer revision in the L2 classroom: Social-cognitive activities, mediating strategies, and aspects of social behavior. *Journal of Second Language Writing*, *5*(1), 51–75. doi:10.1016/S1060-3743(96)90015-6

Villamil, O. S., & de Guerrero, M. C. M. (1998). Assessing the impact of peer revision on L2 writing. *Applied Linguistics*, *19*(4), 491–514. doi:10.1093/applin/19.4.491

Vossen, G., & Hagemann, S. (2007). *Unleashing Web 2.0: From concepts to creativity*. San Francisco: Morgan Kaufmann.

Vygotsky, L. S. (1986). *Thought and language*. Cambridge, MA: MIT Press.

Vygotsky, L. S. (1978). *Mind in society: The development of higher psychological processes* (Cole, M., Trans.). Cambridge, MA: Harvard University Press.

Wager, J. J. (2005). Support services for the Net Generation. In Oblinger, D. G., & Oblinger, J. L. (Eds.), *Educating the Net Generation* (pp. 10.1–10.18). Boulder, CO: EDUCAUSE.

Wallace, R. (1999). *Learners as users, users as learners: What's the difference?* Retrieved November 1, 2008, from https://www.msu.edu/~mccrory/pubs/HCIC_LCD-boaster.htm

Walsh, S. (2004). Appendix: IPod, therefore I learn. In *iPod-learning* (pp. 23–29). Brighton, UK: Epic Group.

Walton, A., Weller, M., & Conole, G. (2009). SocialLearn—widening participation and sustainability of higher education. In Tait, A., Vidal, M., Bernath, U., & Szucs, A. (Eds.), *Distance and e-learning in transition: Learning innovation, technology and social challenges* (pp. 691–699). London and Hoboken, NJ: International Society for Technology in Education and John Wiley & Sons.

Wang, H.-C., Lu, C.-H., Yang, J.-Y., Hu, H.-W., Chiou, G.-F., Chiang, Y.-T., & Hsu, W.-L. (2005). An empirical exploration of using wiki in an English as a second language course. In P. Goodyear, D. Sampson, D. J.-T. Yang, Kinshuk, T. Okamoto, R. Hartley, & N.-S. Chen (Eds.), *Proceedings of the Fifth IEEE International Conference on Advanced Learning Technologies* (pp. 155–157). Los Alamitos, CA: IEEE Computer Society.

Ward, C. B. (2008). Information fluency: A literary review. *Journal for Computing Teachers, 1*(1). Retrieved May 9, 2009, from http://www.iste.org/Content/NavigationMenu/Membership/SIGs/SIGCS_Computer_Science_/JCTJournalforComputingTeachers/PastIssues/2008/Fall/Ward.pdf

Ward, M.-H., & West, S. (2008). Blogging PhD candidature: Revealing the pedagogy. *International Journal of Emerging Technologies and Society, 6*(1), 60–71. Retrieved April 28, 2010, from http://www.swin.edu.au/hosting/ijets/journal/V6N1/pdf/Article4Ward&West.pdf

Warlick, D. F. (2004). *Redefining literacy for the 21st century*. Worthington, OH: Linworth.

Warschauer, M. (2003). *Technology and social inclusion: Rethinking the digital divide*. Cambridge, MA: MIT Press.

Waters, D. (2008, January 8). Intel predicts the personal net. *BBC News*. Retrieved November 20, 2008, from http://news.bbc.co.uk/1/hi/technology/7176177.stm

Watson, K., & Harper, C. (2008). Supporting knowledge creation: Using wikis for group collaboration. EDUCAUSE Center for Applied Research. Retrieved October 28, 2009, from http://www.educause.edu/ir/library/pdf/ERB0803.pdf

Wayner, P. (2007, April 5). Beaming up 3-D objects on a budget. *New York Times*. Retrieved July 1, 2008, from http://www.nytimes.com/2007/04/05/business/05scan.html?ex=1336190400&en=0344a82aae2a277b&ei=5124&partner=permalink&exprod=permalink

Weaver, M. R. (2006). Do students value feedback? Student perceptions of tutors' written responses. *Assessment & Evaluation in Higher Education*, *31*(3), 379–394. doi:10.1080/02602930500353061

Weaver, D., Spratt, C., & Nair, C. S. (2008). Academic and student use of a learning management system: Implications for quality. *Australasian Journal of Educational*

Technology, 24(1), 30–41. Retrieved February 19, 2008, from http://www.ascilite.org.au/ajet/ajet24/weaver.pdf

Web 2.0. (2009, January 7). In *Wikipedia, the free encyclopedia*. Retrieved January 8, 2009, from http://en.wikipedia.org/wiki/Web_2.0

Weinberger, D. (2002). *Small pieces loosely joined: A unified theory of the Web*. New York: Perseus.

Weinberger, D. (2007). *Everything is miscellaneous: The power of the new digital disorder*. New York: Times.

Weinberger, D. (2006). *The new shape of knowledge: From trees to piles of leaves* [Webcast]. Retrieved January 16, 2009, from http://webcast.oii.ox.ac.uk/?view=Webcast&ID=20051130_109

Weiss, S. (2009). Privacy threat model for data portability in social network applications. *International Journal of Information Management, 29*(4), 249–254. doi:10.1016/j.ijinfomgt.2009.03.007

Welch, D. J. (2008) Virtual worlds: Moving beyond today. *EDUCAUSE Review, 43*(5), 12–13. Retrieved January 16, 2009, from http://www.educause.edu/ir/library/pdf/ERM0858.pdf

Wellman, B. (2002). Little boxes, glocalization, and networked individualism. In M. Tanabe, P. van den Besselaar, & T. Ishida (Eds.), *Digital cities II. Computational and sociological approaches. Second Kyoto Workshop on Digital Cities, Kyoto, Japan, October 18–20, 2001. Revised papers: Vol. 2362 Lecture Notes in Computer Science* (pp. 10–25). London: Springer-Verlag.

Wells, G., & Claxton, G. (Eds.). (2002). *Learning for life in the 21st century: Sociocultural perspectives on the future of education*. Oxford, UK: Blackwell.

Wenger, E. (1998). *Communities of practice: Learning, meaning, and identity*. Cambridge, UK: Cambridge University Press.

Wenger, E., McDermott, R., & Snyder, W. M. (2002). *Cultivating communities of practice: A guide to managing knowledge*. Cambridge, MA: Harvard Business School Press.

Wenger, E. (2006). *Learning for a small planet: A research agenda*. Retrieved December 5, 2008, from http://ewenger.com/research/LSPfoundingdoc.doc

Wertsch, J. V., & Sohmer, R. (1995). Vygotsky on learning and development. *Human Development, 38*(6), 332–337. doi:10.1159/000278339

Wertsch, J. V. (1994). The primacy of mediated action in sociocultural studies. *Mind, Culture, and Activity, 1*(4), 202–208.

Wertsch, J. V. (1998). *Mind as action*. New York: Oxford University Press.

Wesch, M. (2007a, October 12). *A vision of students today* [Video file]. Retrieved June 8, 2010, from http://www.youtube.com/watch?v=dGCJ46vyR9o

Wesch, M. (2007b, March 8). *Web 2.0 ... The machine is us/ing us* [Video file]. Retrieved November 4, 2008, from http://www.youtube.com/watch?v=6gmP4nk0EOE

Wesch, M. (2008, June 17). *A portal to media literacy*. Guest lecture delivered at the University of Manitoba, Winnipeg, MB. Retrieved June 8, 2010, from http://umanitoba.ca/ist/production/streaming/podcast_wesch.html

Wheeler, S., Yeomans, P., & Wheeler, D. (2008). The good, the bad and the wiki: Evaluating student-generated content for collaborative learning. *British Journal of Educational Technology, 39*(6), 987–995. doi:10.1111/j.1467-8535.2007.00799.x

Wheeler, S. (2009). Destructive creativity on the social web: Learning through wikis in higher education. In Hatzipanagos, S., & Warburton, S. (Eds.), *Handbook of research on social software and developing community ontologies* (pp. 497–510). Hershey, PA: Information Science Reference.

White, D. (2007). *Results and analysis of the Web 2.0 services survey undertaken by the SPIRE project*. Bristol, UK: Joint Information Systems Committee. Retrieved March 28, 2009, from http://www.jisc.ac.uk/media/documents/programmes/digitalrepositories/spiresurvey.pdf

White, D. (2007). Some real data on Web 2.0 use [Web log post]. *Tall Blog*. Retrieved April 23, 2008, from http://tallblog.conted.ox.ac.uk/index.php/2007/03/16/some-real-data-on-web-20-use/

Whitelock, D. (2006). Electronic assessment: Marking, monitoring and mediating learning. *International Journal of Learning Technology., 2*(2/3), 264–276. doi:10.1504/IJLT.2006.010620

Whitelock, D., Watt, S., Raw, Y., & Moreale, E. (2004). Analysing tutor feedback to students: First steps towards constructing an electronic monitoring system. *ALT-J Research in Learning Technology*, *11*(3), 31–42.

Whitelock, D., & Raw, Y. (2003). Taking an electronic mathematics examination from home: What the students think. In C. P. Constantinou & Z. C. Zacharia (Eds.), *New technologies and their applications in education: Proceedings of the Sixth International Conference on Computer-Based Learning in Science (CBLIS), Volume I* (pp. 701–713). Nicosia, Cyprus: University of Cyprus.

Whitelock, D., & Watt, S. (2007). Supporting tutors with their feedback to students. In F. Khandia (Ed.), *Proceedings of the 11th International Computer-Assisted Assessment Conference* (pp. 421–432). Loughborough, UK: Loughborough University.

Whitelock, D., Ruedel, C., & Mackenzie, D. (2006). *e-Assessment: Case studies of effective and innovative practice*. Bristol, UK: Joint Information Systems Committee. Retrieved May 30, 2009, from http://kn.open.ac.uk/public/getfile.cfm?documentfileid=12880

Whitworth, A. (2009). *Information obesity*. Oxford, UK: Chandos.

Whitworth, A., & Benson, A. D. (2007, January 8–10). *Taming the Lone Ranger: The creative development of e-learning technologies within UK and US higher education institutions.* Paper presented at Creativity or conformity? Building cultures of creativity in higher education, Cardiff, UK.

Wiggins, G. (1998). *Educative assessment*. San Francisco: Jossey-Bass.

Wikipedia. (2007, December 23). In *Wikipedia, the free encyclopedia*. Retrieved December 23, 2007, from http://en.wikipedia.org/wiki/Wikipedia

Wild, F., Mödritscher, F., & Sigurdarson, S. E. (2008). Designing for change: Mash-up personal learning environments. *eLearning Papers, 9*. Retrieved July 22, 2008, from http://www.elearningeuropa.info/files/media/media15972.pdf

Wiley, D., & Edwards, E. K. (2002). *Online self-organizing social systems: The decentralized future of online learning*. Retrieved July 7, 2008, from http://opencontent.org/docs/ososs.pdf

Williams, J. B., & Wong, A. (2009). The efficacy of final examinations: A comparative study of closed-book, invigilated exams and open-book, open-web exams. *British Journal of Educational Technology*, *40*(2), 227–236. doi:10.1111/j.1467-8535.2008.00929.x

Williams, J. B., & Jacobs, J. (2004). Exploring the use of blogs as learning spaces in the higher education sector. *Australasian Journal of Educational Technology, 20*(2), 232–247. Retrieved April 28, 2010, from http://www.ascilite.org.au/ajet/ajet20/williams.html

Wilson, S. (2008). Patterns of personal learning environments. *Interactive Learning Environments*, *16*(1), 17–34. doi:10.1080/10494820701772660

Wilson, S., Liber, O., Johnson, M., Beauvoir, P., Sharples, P., & Milligan, C. (2007). Personal learning environments: Challenging the dominant design of educational systems. *Journal of e-Learning and Knowledge Society, 3*(2), 27–38. Retrieved July 22, 2008, from http://je-lks.maieutiche.economia.unitn.it/en/07_02/04Art_wilson_inglese.pdf

Wirth, K. (2007). Teaching for deeper understanding and lifelong learning. *Elements*, *3*(2), 107–111. doi:10.2113/gselements.3.2.107

Wise, L., & Quealy, J. (2006). At the limits of social constructivism: Moving beyond LMS to re-integrate scholarship. In L. Markauskaite, P. Goodyear, & P. Reimann (Eds.), *Who's learning? Whose technology? Proceedings of the 23rd Australasian Society for Computers in Learning in Tertiary Education (ASCILITE) Conference* (pp. 899–907). Sydney: University of Sydney. Retrieved February 20, 2008, from http://www.ascilite.org.au/conferences/sydney06/proceeding/pdf_papers/p158.pdf

Wojtas, O. (1998, September). Feedback? No, just give us the answers. *Times Higher Education Supplement*, 7.

Wolpert, L. (2003). Causal belief and the origin of technology. *Philosophical Transactions of the Royal Society A: Mathematical, Physical & Engineering Sciences, 361*(1809), 1709–1719.

Wood, D., Underwood, J., & Avis, P. (1999). Integrated learning systems in the classroom. *Computers*

& *Education*, *33*(2/3), 91–108. doi:10.1016/S0360-1315(99)00027-5

Wood, D. J., Bruner, J. S., & Ross, G. (1976). The role of tutoring in problem solving. *Journal of Child Psychology and Psychiatry, and Allied Disciplines*, *17*(2), 89–100. doi:10.1111/j.1469-7610.1976.tb00381.x

Woods, R., & Baker, J. (2004). Interaction and immediacy in online learning. *International Review of Research in Open and Distance Learning, 5*(2). Retrieved July 7, 2008, from http://www.irrodl.org/index.php/irrodl/article/view/186/268

World Bank. (2000). *Technology—Broadcast and computer-based: Radio*. Retrieved May 31, 2005, from http://www1.worldbank.org/disted/Technology/broadcast/broad_radio.html

World Wide Web. (2008, December 3). In *Wikipedia, the free encyclopedia*. Retrieved December 3, 2008, from http://en.wikipedia.org/wiki/World_Wide_Web

Woukeu, A., Millard, D. E., Tao, F., & Davis, H. C. (2005, November 27–December 1). *Challenges for semantic grid based mobile learning*. Paper presented at First International Conference on Signal-Image Technology and Internet-Based Systems, Yaounde, Cameroon. Retrieved November 20, 2008, from http://www.u-bourgogne.fr/SITIS/05/download/Proceedings/Files/f135.pdf

Wozniak, H., Scott, K., & Atkinson, S. (2005). The balancing act: Managing emerging issues of elearning projects at the University of Sydney. In H. Goss (Ed), *Balance, fidelity, mobility: Maintaining the momentum? Proceedings of the 22nd Australasian Society for Computers in Learning in Tertiary Education (ASCILITE) Conference* (pp. 735–745). Brisbane, Australia: Queensland University of Technology. Retrieved February 20, 2008, from http://www.ascilite.org.au/conferences/brisbane05/blogs/proceedings/86_Wozniak.pdf

Wray, R. (2008, February 26). Small and thin—but the phone of the future must bend too. *The Guardian*. Retrieved November 20, 2008, from http://www.guardian.co.uk/business/2008/feb/26/mobilephones

Wray, R. (2009, January 21). Mobile broadband providers promise more clarity over download speeds. *The Guardian*. Retrieved November 20, 2008, from http://www.guardian.co.uk/technology/2009/jan/21/broadband-mobilephones

Wright, K. (2005). Personal knowledge management: Supporting individual knowledge worker performance. *Knowledge Management Research & Practice*, *3*(3), 156–165. doi:10.1057/palgrave.kmrp.8500061

Wright, A. (2003). *Forgotten forefather: Paul Otlet*. Retrieved July 7, 2008, from http://www.boxesandarrows.com/view/forgotten_forefather_paul_otlet

Wuensch, K. L., Shahnaz, A., Ozan, E., Kishore, M., & Tabrizi, M. H. N. (2008). Pedagogical characteristics of online and face-to-face classes. *International Journal on E-Learning*, *7*(3), 523–532.

Xu, Y. (2005). Creating social presence in online environment. In B. Hoffman (Ed.), *Encyclopedia of educational technology*. San Diego, CA: San Diego State University. Retrieved January 11, 2008, from http://coe.sdsu.edu/eet/articles/creatsp/start.htm

Young, R. E. (1990). *A critical theory of education: Habermas and our children's future*. New York: Teachers College Press.

Young, J. (2008, August 18). When professors create social networks for classes, some students see a "creepy treehouse". *The Chronicle of Higher Education*. Retrieved February 9, 2009, from http://chronicle.com/wiredcampus/article/3251/when-professors-create-social-networks-for-classes-some-students-see-a-creepy-treehouse

Yuen, S., & Wang, S. (2004). M-learning: Mobility in learning. In G. Richards (Ed.), *Proceedings of World Conference on E-Learning in Corporate, Government, Healthcare, and Higher Education 2004* (pp. 2248–2252). Chesapeake, VA: Association for the Advancement of Computers in Education.

Zemsky, R., & Massy, W. F. (2004). *Thwarted innovation: What happened to e-learning and why*. Philadelphia, PA: The Learning Alliance at the University of Pennsylvania. Retrieved April 11, 2009, from http://www.irhe.upenn.edu/Docs/Jun2004/ThwartedInnovation.pdf

Zhang, H., & Su, H. (2007). Reforming computing education with new web technologies. *Journal of Computing Sciences in Colleges*, *23*(2), 150–156.

Zimmerman, B. J. (2000). Attaining self-regulation: A social cognitive perspective. In Boekaerts, M., Pintrich, P. R., & Zeidner, M. (Eds.), *Handbook of self-regulation* (pp. 13–39). San Diego: Academic Press. doi:10.1016/B978-012109890-2/50031-7

Zwier, L. J., & Mathes, G. (2005). *Study skills for success*. Ann Arbor, MI: University of Michigan Press.

About the Contributors

Mark J. W. Lee is an Adjunct Senior Lecturer with the School of Education at Charles Sturt University. He concurrently holds Adjunct Senior Lecturer and Honorary Research Fellow appointments with the Distance Education Hub (DE Hub) research institute at the University of New England and the Graduate School of Information Technology and Mathematical Sciences at the University of Ballarat, respectively. Previously, he worked in a variety of teaching, instructional design, and managerial roles within the private vocational education and higher education sectors. Mark has published extensively in the areas of educational technology, e-learning, and innovative pedagogy in tertiary education, with 50 refereed publications to his name. He is the immediate past Chair of the New South Wales Chapter of the Institute of Electrical and Electronics Engineers (IEEE) Education Society, a former director of the International Board of Standards for Training, Performance and Instruction (ibstpi), and a former executive committee member of the Open and Learning Distance Association of Australasia (ODLAA). Presently, he serves as Editor-in-Chief of Impact: Journal of Applied Research in Workplace E-learning, in addition to being on the editorial boards of several other highly reputable international journals. He is a Senior Member of the IEEE, Australian Computer Society (ACS), and Association for Computing Machinery (ACM), and an Associate Fellow of the Australian Institute of Management (AIM).

Catherine McLoughlin, Ph.D., is an Associate Professor with the School of Education at the Australian Catholic University, Canberra, where she formerly served as Head of School. She also is the coordinator of the Australian Capital Territory branch of the Research Centre for Science, Information Technology and Mathematics Education for Rural and Regional Australia (SiMERR). With over 20 years' experience in higher education in Europe, Southeast Asia, the Middle East, and Australia, Catherine has experience and expertise in a variety of educational settings, with diverse students and across a wide range of cultural contexts. She is a member of the Executive Committee of the Australasian Society for Computers in Learning in Tertiary Education (ASCILITE), with oversight for the Society's research strategies and initiatives, and Editor of ASCILITE's official journal, the Australasian Journal of Educational Technology (AJET). Last but not least, Catherine is an editorial board member of a number of leading journals, including the British Journal of Educational Technology (BJET).

* * *

Jon Akass is a founder and director of Media Citizens, a multimedia company that has pioneered participant media projects in South London offering training, production, and online publishing for disadvantaged groups in regeneration zones. Originally a print journalist and television producer, and more recently, a lecturer in online journalism, Jon now focuses on web publishing. Media Citizens involves the Learner-Generated Contexts (LGC) group—fellow members of which he co-authored Chapter 4 with—in current participant media practice; this ranges from contributions to Ofcom (the UK Office of Communications) consultations on media literacy and film projects with young people at risk from knife crime, to the development of content management software for a national digital inclusion network.

Cameron Barnes is eAccess Librarian at the University of New England (UNE). He taught interface design at the New England Institute of TAFE for some years. Cameron was part of the team from the UNE Library that won a Carrick Citation for Outstanding Contributions to Student Learning in 2006. His interest in computer-aided learning (CAL) dates back to the mid-1990s, and he has written a number of refereed conference papers and articles in the area. By training, however, he is an economic historian, having received his Master of Arts (with Honours) in that field in 1993.

Tony Bates is a private consultant specializing in e-learning in higher education. He is a member of the World Economic Forum's Global Advisory Council on Technology and Education. Between 1995 and 2003, he was Director of Distance Education and Technology at the University of British Columbia, and Executive Director, Strategic Planning, at the Open Learning Agency, Vancouver from 2000 to 2005. Before that, Tony was Professor of Educational Media Research at the UK Open University. He has written nine books on distance education and learning technologies, and consulted for the World Bank, OECD, UNESCO, Ministries of Education in several countries, state higher education commissions in the USA, Volkswagen AutoUni, the Open Universities of Catalonia and Portugal, and Southern Alberta Institute of Technology. He holds a Ph.D. in educational administration from the University of London, and honorary degrees from Laurentian and Athabasca Universities, as well as from the Open Universities of Portugal, Hong Kong, and Catalonia.

Maria Elisabetta Cigognini completed her Ph.D. in Telematics and Information Society at the Electronics and Telecommunications Department of the University of Florence in 2008, in which her dissertation was on personal knowledge management (PKM). She formerly (in 2003) graduated with an undergraduate degree in communication sciences from IULM University of Milan and (in 2004) with a Master's degree specializing in e-learning project management and design from the University of Florence. Since then she has been working as an e-learning contractor, instructional designer, and e-tutor both in corporate and in academic settings. Currently, she holds a post-doctoral research position in the University of Trieste's Faculty of Psychology. Elisabetta's broad research areas are instructional design, computer-supported collaborative work, and knowledge management, and in addition to PKM skills she has a particular interest in the design and implementation of personal learning environments (PLEs).

Wilma Clark is a Research Fellow at the London Knowledge Lab, Institute of Education, University of London, where she conducts research in the areas of Web 2.0 technologies and participatory design approaches to technology use in support of learners and learning. Previously, she worked as a teacher of ICT in UK secondary schools. She has a particular interest in the exploration of contexts and cultures, with a focus on boundary spaces and learners' boundary-crossing activity and the implications of these for knowledge acquisition, learner development, and pedagogic design in technology-mediated environments. She is also an editor for the interdisciplinary journal, QWERTY: Journal of Technology and Culture.

Lisa Cluett, Ph.D., is based at The University of Western Australia (UWA), where she is the Project Leader for an Australian federally funded leadership grant that uses the "viral" concept to examine how staff learn about, apply, and spread knowledge of emerging technologies. She is also the Senior Project Officer of UWA's Online Student Journey project, and (with Dr. Judy Skene) conducts the annual NODE (Networking Online to Diversify Engagement) survey of student ICT use. She is responsible for initiatives involving the application and incorporation of Web 2.0 tools within the Student Services Division at UWA, and for staff training and development in emerging technologies. Lisa's research interests focus on the success factors required for staff uptake of new tools, online community development, and integration of applications across platforms for the student-centric delivery of services.

Gráinne Conole, Ph.D., is Professor of E-Learning in the Institute of Educational Technology at The Open University, UK. Previously she was Professor of Educational Innovation in Post-Compulsory Education at the University of Southampton, and before that, Director of the Institute for Learning and Research Technology at the University of Bristol. Her interests include the integration, use, and evaluation of ICTs for learning and the impact of technologies on organizational change. Two of her current specific research areas are: (1) the evaluation of students' experiences and perceptions of technologies, and how learning design can help in creating more engaging learning activities; and (2) open educational resources. She has extensive research, development, and project management experience across the educational and technical domains; funding sources have included the European Union (EU), Higher Education Funding Council for England (HEFCE), Economic and Social Research Council (ESRC), Joint Information Systems Committee (JISC), and commercial sponsors. She serves on and chairs a number of national and international advisory boards, steering groups, committees, and international conference programs. Gráinne has published and presented over 300 papers in refereed conference proceedings, workshops, and articles, including over 100 journal publications on a range of topics. She is co-editor of the recently published RoutledgeFalmer book Contemporary perspectives on e-learning research.

John Cook, Ph.D., is Professor of Technology Enhanced Learning (TEL) at the Learning Technology Research Institute, London Metropolitan University. He also has a cross-university role as E-Learning Project Leader. John has published widely in the area of TEL, having a specific interest in five related and overlapping areas: informal learning, mobile learning, appropriation, user-generated contexts, and TEL leadership and innovation. John is a Chartered Engineer (CEng) and Chartered Information Technology Professional (CITP), in addition to being a Member of the British Computer Society (BCS) and a Fellow of the UK Higher Education Academy (HEA).

Matt Crosslin is an instructional designer at The University of Texas at Arlington's Center for Distance Education. Matt has been online since 1991 and involved in education since 1994. He has been active in web-based education in many different forms for over 10 years now, including writing several articles and presenting at a number of national conferences. In March 2007 Matt started EduGeek Journal, an online community promoting educational technology. He is also currently the Chief Information Officer for the Texas Distance Learning Association and an adjunct online instructor for the Educational Technology program at the University of Texas at Brownsville (UTB). Matt is also an alumni of UTB, having received his Master's degree in Educational Technology in 2006.

Nada Dabbagh, Ph.D., is Associate Professor of Instructional Technology in the College of Education and Human Development at George Mason University (GMU). She teaches courses in learning theory, instructional design, and e-learning design and pedagogy. Her research focuses on the pedagogical ecology of technology-mediated learning systems, with the goal of understanding the cognitive and design characteristics of task structuring as the basis for effective learning designs. Nada has an extensive presentation and publication record, including co-authored books titled Online learning: Concepts, strategies, and application (Prentice Hall, 2005) and Learning to learn with integrative learning technologies (ILT): A practical guide for academic success (Information Age Publishing, 2010).

Peter Day, Ph.D., is a Senior Lecturer in the School of Computing, Mathematical and Information Sciences at the University of Brighton in the UK, and an Honorary Senior Research Fellow at Central Queensland University in Australia. Peter's research interests include online community informatics, ICTs in regional areas, digital cities and community networking, the digital divide, community uses of ICTs, and training provision for community and voluntary sector groups in Brighton and Hove. Peter is also a director of the Sussex Community Internet Project (SCIP), a local, not-for-profit community technology organization that raises awareness of the potential of ICTs to support and underpin the social networks upon which community life is based.

Lone Dirckinck-Holmfeld is Professor in ICT, Learning and Design in the Department of Communication at Aalborg University (AAU), and Dean of the Faculty of Humanities at the same university. She was previously Director of the research center E-Learning Lab: Center for User-Driven Innovation, Learning and Design at AAU. She holds a Ph.D. from Roskilde University in computer-mediated communication and learning. Her main areas of research are computer-supported collaborative learning in distributed environments, participatory design, and implementation of ICT in organizations. She has authored and co-authored several books, in addition to more than 100 papers, articles, and reports on ICT and learning.

Peter Duffy has been involved in the education industry, and in the integration of technology with pedagogy, for the last 19 years. He has been an invited keynote speaker at conferences and a presenter at the Minister's Awards for Excellence in both the IT and Arts fields in Australia. In recent years, he has published and presented many articles dealing with e-learning and Web 2.0. Peter is currently working at The Hong Kong Polytechnic University, where he is based in the Educational Development Centre and is leading a strategic institutional initiative relating to blended learning.

Nigel Ecclesfield is currently a Research Manager at Becta, the UK government agency leading the national drive to ensure the effective and innovative use of technology in education. He is responsible for national surveys of technology use and implementation in post-compulsory education, and research on institutional development in both UK and international contexts. Nigel has worked in further education colleges for 30 years, during which he has been involved in student services, teacher training, research, inspection, and computer education. His past research has included studies on staff development needs of support staff, assessment, accreditation of prior learning, and curriculum development. His current research endeavors, in which he works closely with Fred Garnett, focus on the development of learner and community-centric collaborative organizations and the articulation of models for developing public and community value in education.

Palitha Edirisingha, Ph.D., is a Lecturer in E-Learning in the Beyond Distance Research Alliance (BRDA) at the University of Leicester. He is a published author in the areas of online and distance learning and learning technologies, working as an investigator on the BRDA's IMPALA (podcasting), WoLF (mobile learning), and MOOSE (3-D virtual worlds) projects. He also serves on the University of Leicester's e-learning subcommittee, and coordinates the BDRA's visiting researcher program. Palitha's research interests include the use of emerging technologies such as mobile and social web services and tools for facilitating informal learning within academic contexts and for creating social capital and communities of practice among students to support formal learning, as well as open and distance learning for education in developing countries.

Henk Eijkman, Ph.D., is Director of Learning and Teaching Development at the University of New South Wales, Australian Defence Force Academy (ADFA) campus in Canberra. Henk has a particular interest in the sociology of learning and digital technologies in transcultural higher education. He has a reputation as an innovative and strategically focused specialist in higher education research, development, and innovation, with over 15 years' experience that includes work in South Africa, Malaysia, India, and the Palestinian Territories. His professional interests focus on justice, sustainability, and socially inclusive participation, especially in technology enhanced tertiary learning and teaching. He is the incoming Editor of The Learning Organization, as well as being Chair of the Scientific Committee of the Defence Academies & Colleges e-Learning (DACeL) Conference, a member of the Scientific Committee of the International Conference on ICT in Education (ICICTE), and a reviewer for the British Journal of Educational Technology (BJET). He has published widely in international peer-reviewed journals.

Idoia Elola, Ph.D., is an Assistant Professor of Spanish and Applied Linguistics/Second Language Studies at Texas Tech University. She teaches a range of courses at the undergraduate and graduate levels from Spanish grammar to applied linguistics and second language acquisition/instruction. Her research, quantitative and qualitative in nature, focuses predominantly on second language writing with an emphasis on revision, collaborative writing through the use of social web technologies, and issues of writing fluency and grammar among Spanish heritage speakers. She has published articles on the topics of foreign language writing, collaborative writing, and the use of technology in the language classroom.

Mark Frydenberg is a Senior Lecturer in the Computer Information Systems Department at Bentley University in Waltham, Massachusetts, where he teaches an introductory information technology (IT) course illustrating IT concepts through the lens of Web 2.0. Mark was a pioneer of student-created podcasts as a tool for learning. He has published many journal articles and spoken at many conferences on integrating Web 2.0 technologies in the IT classroom. His book, Web 2.0 concepts and applications, co-authored with Gary Shelly, was recently published by Cengage Learning.

Fred Garnett is a Visiting Research Associate at the London Knowledge Lab and a member of the Learner-Generated Contexts Research Group. He has worked in education for 29 years as a lecturer, trainer, curriculum developer, manager, and researcher in universities, colleges, schools, community centers, and prisons. He has delivered invited talks in Brazil, Germany, and Spain and presented many papers at international conferences worldwide. He played a lead role in the Connected Community projects in the London Borough of Lewisham, setting up both the Creekside Environmental Education Trust and the TaLENT Consortium before becoming Head of Community Programmes at Becta, working on social and digital inclusion nationally across the UK. He is interested in developing participative learning strategies that contribute to the building of a citizen-centric knowledge economy, and blogs about the Open Context Model of Learning at The Heutagogic Archives (http://heutagogicarchive.wordpress.com/).

Tom Hamilton is Director of InQbate, the Higher Education Funding Council for England (HEFCE)-funded Centre of Excellence in Teaching and Learning in Creativity, a joint initiative between the Universities of Sussex and Brighton. He is interested in the interrelationship between creativity and learning, and how both are shaped by the wider context. His research centers on how the context in which learning and creativity occur can be enhanced by the effective combination of technology and spatial design. He is member of the UK Joint Information Systems Committee's TELE (Technology-Enhanced Learning Environments) panel, and provides creative-design consultancy to a range of clients, including galleries, universities, and commercial companies.

Henk Huijser, Ph.D., is a Lecturer in Learning Enhancement (Communication) in the Learning and Teaching Support Unit and a researcher in the Public Memory Research Centre, both at the University of Southern Queensland. His overall research interests and output areas include technology-enhanced learning and teaching, cross-cultural communication, and cultural studies. Of late, he has had a particular interest in mobile learning and social networking technology, and their potential applications in higher education.

Chris Jones, Ph.D., is a Reader in the Institute of Educational Technology at The Open University, where he teaches on the Masters in Online and Distance Education (ODE) and coordinates the ODE strand of the Doctorate in Education. He has authored over 40 journal articles and book chapters, and recently edited the collection Analysing networked learning practices in higher education and continuing professional development, published by Sense Publishers. Chris' research focuses on networked learning and the application of the metaphor of networks to the understanding of learning in tertiary education. He has a longstanding interest in the use of collaborative and cooperative methods in teaching and learning. He was recently the principal investigator for a UK Research Council-funded project entitled "The Net Generation encountering e-learning at university."

Lucinda Kerawalla, Ph.D., is a Research Fellow in the Institute of Educational Technology (IET) at The Open University. She has a keen interest in technology-enhanced learning, and has worked and published in the areas of social software, software-supported collaboration, children's home computer use, technology to enhance home-school links, and augmented reality. Her recent work on the Personal Inquiry project, an initiative funded by the UK Economic and Social Research Council (ESRC) and Engineering and Physical Sciences Research Council (EPSRC), focuses using mobile devices to bridge formal and informal settings and support inquiry learning in the geography classroom. She teaches on the IET's Master's program in Online and Distance Education.

Agnes Kukulska-Hulme, Ph.D., is Professor of Learning Technology and Communication in The Open University's Institute of Educational Technology in the UK. She has been researching mobile learning (m-learning) since 2001, and over the years has led several projects investigating learning technology and educational innovation at The Open University and across the UK. Her publications have centered on issues of learner-driven innovation, web and mobile usability, staff development for m-learning, and the evolution and future of mobile-assisted language learning (MALL). Agnes' recent work includes co-editing two books, Mobile learning: A handbook for educators and trainers (published by Routledge in 2005) and Researching mobile learning: Frameworks, tools and research designs (published by Peter Lang in 2009), as well as guest editing a special issue of ReCALL on MALL and special issues of JIME, ALT-J, and Open Learning on m-learning. She was part of the European project MOTILL (2009–10), which gathered evidence on research and practice relating to mobile technologies in lifelong learning. She is on the Executive Committee of the International Association for Mobile Learning (IAmLearn).

Rosemary Luckin, Ph.D., is Professor of Learner-Centred Design at the London Knowledge Lab, Institute of Education, University of London and an EPSRC (Engineering and Physical Sciences Research Council) Advanced Research Fellow. Her research explores how to most effectively scaffold learning across multiple technologies, locations, subjects, and times. This work is interdisciplinary and encompasses education, psychology, artificial intelligence, and human–computer interaction. It investigates the relationship between people, the concepts they are trying to learn and teach, the contexts within which they operate, and the resources at their disposal. Rose is also a non-executive director of Becta, and she chairs its Research Advisory Group. Her recent book, Re-designing learning contexts: Technology-rich, learner-centred ecologies, was published by Routledge.

Shailey Minocha, Ph.D., is a Reader in Computing in the Centre for Research in Computing at The Open University, UK. The focus of her research is on understanding users' interactions with technology and investigating the socio-technical contexts in which computer systems operate. Shailey's research and consultancy activities have led to insights into factors that affect usability, user experience, and user adoption of technology-enabled systems. Her recent research projects have involved investigating the role of social software and 3-D virtual worlds in training and skills development, with a particular emphasis on the virtual team-working, socialization, collaborative learning, and community-building capabilities of these tools.

Ana Oskoz, Ph.D., is an Associate Professor of Spanish in the Department of Modern Languages and Linguistics at the University of Maryland Baltimore County. Ana's research focuses on the use of technology for second language learning and second language acquisition. She has examined the use of synchronous and asynchronous communication tools such as online chats, discussion boards, blogs, and wikis for second language learning, to promote cultural discussions, enhance second language writing, and foster intercultural competence development. She has published articles on the topics of error correction, classroom-based assessment, and the use of technology in the language classroom.

Kai Pata, Ph.D., is a Senior Researcher in the Center of Educational Technology, Tallinn University. She has a background in science education and ICT in learning. She previously worked as a designer and virtual teacher in the e-learning portal Miksike, and as a researcher in science-related ICT projects at the University of Tartu's Science Didactics Department. She is currently engaged in international projects involving the design of ecological e-learning models for learning with Web 2.0 tools. Kai's main expertise is in management of learning in distributed environments; social systems for self-directed, collaborative, and inquiry learning; scaffolding of decision making processes; and model-based learning in chat.

Maria Chiara Pettenati is a Senior Researcher in the Telematics Laboratory of the Electronics and Telecommunications Department at the University of Florence. She received her Ph.D. in Telematics and Information Society from the University of Florence in 2000 with a dissertation entitled Design and development of a web-based environment for teaching and learning. During her Ph.D. studies, she spent two years at the Computer Science Department (DI-LITH) at the Swiss Federal Institute of Technology in Lausanne (EPFL). Before that, she graduated with honours in telecommunications engineering from the University of Florence in 1996. Her research interests and activities adopt an interdisciplinary perspective and are centered around two main areas: (i) the transformation of the World Wide Web from being a collection of static, "read-only" documents maintained by an elite few to a being a participatory, collaborative "read-and-write" platform for all; and (ii) web technologies, tools, methods, and competencies to support effective and efficient personal learning and knowledge management.

John Pettit is a Lecturer at The Open University's Institute of Educational Technology (IET), where he teaches and researches technology-enhanced learning, and has led projects examining the impact of educational innovation on aspects of Open University teaching. Since 2005 he has been studying learner-led activity in audiographics environments, and user-led mobile learning practice. John's publications explore Mobile 2.0 practices among alumni, user-generated mobile activity, the ways in which staff adopt mobile devices for personal and professional purposes, and power relations in educational innovation. He led the development and presentation of Technology-enhanced learning: practices and debates, a recent addition to IET's postgraduate Online and Distance Education program.

Rick Reo is an instructional designer for the Division of Instructional Technology at George Mason University (GMU), where he collaborates with faculty in the Distance Education program on course design and development. He also leads and supports Web 2.0 initiatives across the university, such as iTunes U, multiuser web log and wiki systems, and projects related to the pedagogy of social software tools. Rick has Master's degrees in both cultural anthropology and education (instructional design). He is an adjunct instructor at GMU, teaching graduate courses on Web 2.0 and undergraduate courses in information technology. Rick was GMU's interim Director for the New Media Consortium and currently serves on the board of the Association of Collegiate Computing Services of Virginia.

Judy Robertson, Ph.D., is a Lecturer in Computer Science in the School of Mathematical and Computer Sciences at Heriot-Watt University. Her research has investigated various aspects of learners' narrative development and approaches to developing their inherent narrative skills. This has included: the creation of a story analysis scheme for evaluating characterization and setting in learners' stories; the analysis of a corpus of learners' stories; the design and implementation of an interactive drama; and the design and running of field studies in local schools. Judy has over 20 peer-reviewed publications and was Guest Editor for a special issue of the International Journal of Artificial Intelligence in Education.

Thomas Ryberg is an Associate Professor in the Department of Communication and Psychology at Aalborg University (AAU), where he is affiliated with the research center E-Learning Lab: Center for User-Driven Innovation, Learning and Design. He holds a Ph.D. from AAU, focusing on youth, technology-enhanced learning, and problem solving. He has participated in and continues to participate in European and international research projects and networks, with his primary interests being in the realms of computer-supported collaborative learning, ICT and learning for development, and how new media and technologies transform ways of thinking about and designing for learning. Thomas has authored and co-authored several articles in these areas.

Michael Sankey, Ed.D., is the Director of the Learning and Teaching Support Unit at the University of Southern Queensland. He specializes in the areas of e-learning pedagogies, multimodal and web design, and visual/multiliteracies. His research focuses on the multiple representation of concepts when using multimedia technologies, and how the use of hybridized electronic environments can enhance learning opportunities for students, particularly those studying at a distance. With a background in art and design Michael is passionate about the ways in which aesthetically enhanced learning environments can better transmit concepts to students of all backgrounds.

Judy Skene, Ph.D., is Manager, Student Support Services at The University of Western Australia. She coordinates a year-long transition support program, UniSkills, for students from groups under-represented in higher education and for international students. Her research interests include equity of access and transition to tertiary study, student teamwork, and the role of ICT in engaging students beyond the classroom and providing seamless delivery of support services. In 2008, the UniSkills program won an Australian Learning and Teaching Council (ALTC) award for programs that support student learning, and in 2007 Judy was awarded an individual ALTC citation.

Kairit Tammets is a Research Assistant in the Center of Educational Technology, Tallinn University. In June 2008 she completed an international Master's degree program in interactive media and knowledge environments with Tallinn University's Institute of Informatics. Kairit's Master's thesis focused on a course design model for self-directed learning in distributed learning environments. She is now pursuing her Ph.D. on the topic of cross-border knowledge building in teachers' lifelong professional development.

Belinda Tynan, Ed.D., has held numerous academic positions in the UK, Japan, and Australia. She is presently a Professor and the Academic Director of the Faculty of The Professions at the University of New England. As Academic Director, she contributes to the development of academic policy within the University, with a particular focus on fostering strategic change. She is also the Director of the University's e-University project, and of the Distance Education Hub (DE Hub), a Commonwealth-funded initiative based at UNE, in addition to leading many grants. Belinda is one of the editors of Higher Education Research and Development, a leading refereed international journal published by Taylor & Francis, and serves as Treasurer of the Open and Distance Learning Association of Australia (ODLAA). Her main research interests lie in the areas of academic development and models of research collaboration. Her research and publications cover areas such as distance education, academic staff development, models of research collaboration, new technologies, and regional issues.

Terje Väljataga is an educational technology researcher at Tallinn University's Center of Educational Technology and a Ph.D. student in the Hypermedia Lab at Tampere University of Technology's Department of Informatics. She has been involved in various educational technology projects since 2004. Her background is in natural sciences and teacher education, and she has experience teaching at both the secondary school and university levels. Her research interests are related to adult education in formal and informal settings, strategies for enhancing the advancement of competencies, as well as self- and group-directed learning in personal and distributed learning environments.

Steve Wheeler is Senior Lecturer in Education at the University of Plymouth, UK. He has spent his entire career working with and witnessing the development of educational media and learning technology in health and medical education, and in teacher training. He originally trained as a teacher in the tertiary sector, and now specializes in training teachers to make effective use of learning technology. His research interests include Web 2.0 and social software, distance education, e-learning, visual collaboration and multimedia, individual differences, creativity, and student support. He has published over 150 scholarly papers, chapters, and articles in these fields and is a regular invited speaker at international conferences. Steve is a co-editor of Interactive Learning Environments, and also serves on the boards of several other international peer-reviewed journals including ALT-J, IRRODL, and Digital Culture and Education. He is Chair of the IFIP Technical Committee 3, Working Group 3.6 on Distance Education, and is a member of a number of other high-profile professional and academic bodies. Steve has served as a consultant on several large-scale distance education projects including RATIO (southwest England), EuroNET (UK nationwide), and the Star Schools Project (South Dakota, USA). He is currently an evaluator for the European-funded CONCEDE project, which is investigating the applications of user-generated content in formal education contexts.

Denise Whitelock, Ph.D., is a Senior Lecturer in Information Technology working in the field of new technologies for learning at The Open University's Institute of Educational Technology. She has expertise in the use of interactive multimedia for teaching, computer-supported collaborative learning, virtual reality systems for conceptual learning, and the development of electronic assessment software. Her research has received international recognition since she currently holds a Visiting Chair position at the Autonoma University, Barcelona, a Visiting Readership at Robert Gordon University in Scotland, and an Honorary Research Fellowship at the Open Polytechnic of New Zealand.

Andrew Whitworth, Ph.D., is a Lecturer in the School of Education, University of Manchester, and the Course Director of the Master of Arts in Digital Technologies, Communication and Education. His research is oriented towards developing a critical theory of the use of technology in education, particularly with reference to staff development and professional practice in technology-rich environments. He is the author of Information obesity (2009), published by Chandos, Oxford.

Index

D

E

F

G

H

I

J

K

L

M

S

T

U

V

W

X

Z

Breinigsville, PA USA
13 October 2010
247145BV00003BJ/1/P

9 781605 662947